The Moder
and Science of Mobility

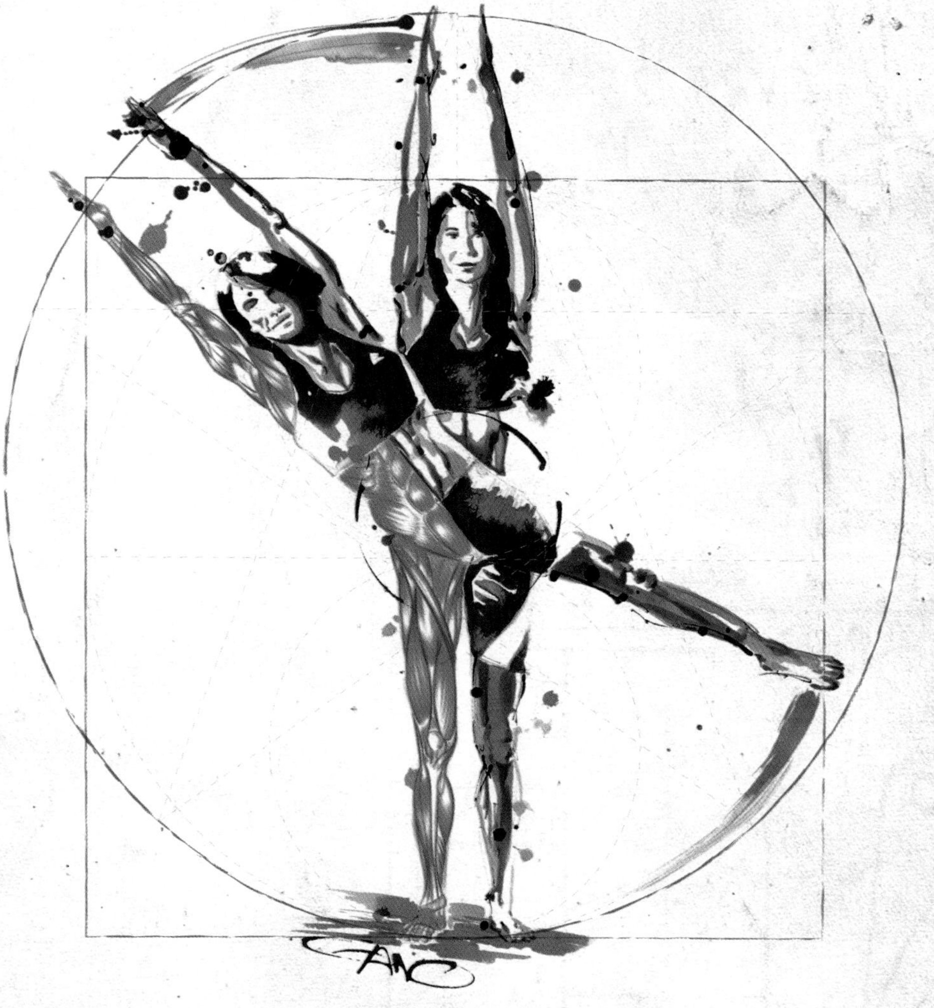

Aurélien Broussal-Derval · Stéphane Ganneau

HUMAN KINETICS

Library of Congress Cataloging-in-Publication Data

Names: Broussal-Derval, Aurélien, author. | Ganneau, Stéphane, author.
Title: The modern art and science of mobility / Aurélien Broussal-Derval, Stéphane Ganneau.
Description: Champaign, IL : Human Kinetics, [2020] | Includes bibliographical references.
Identifiers: LCCN 2018048031 (print) | LCCN 2018060289 (ebook) | ISBN 9781492590507 (epub) | ISBN 9781492571223 (PDF) | ISBN 9781492571216 (print)
Subjects: LCSH: Human mechanics. | Exercise--Physiological aspects. | Myalgia--Treatment. | Breathing exercises. | Stretching exercises. | Massage.
Classification: LCC QP301 (ebook) | LCC QP301 .B8858 2020 (print) | DDC 612.7/6--dc23
LC record available at https://lccn.loc.gov/2018048031

ISBN: 978-1-4925-7121-6 (print)

This book is a revised edition of *L'Art du Mouvement*, published in 2018 by 4Trainers Editions.

Publication/editing: Sen No Sen; **Managing Editor:** Julie Marx Goodreau; **Translator:** Terra Sumstine; **Copyeditor:** Laura Stoffel; **Graphic Designers:** Nicolas Moreau (www.graphiste-pro.com) and Dawn Sills; **Cover Designers:** Nicolas Moreau and Keri Evans; **Cover Design Associate:** Susan Rothermel Allen; **Photographs:** Johann Vayriot; **Models:** Philippe Bas, Arié Elmaleh, Laetitia Fourcade, Dounia Coesens, Aurélien Broussal-Derval, Stéphane Ganneau, Samantha Le Moël; **Illustrations:** Stéphane Ganneau/GANO; **Printer:** Versa Press

Human Kinetics books are available at special discounts for bulk purchase. Special editions or book excerpts can also be created to specification. For details, contact the Special Sales Manager at Human Kinetics.

Printed in the United States of America 10 9 8 7 6 5 4 3 2 1

The paper in this book is certified under a sustainable forestry program.

Human Kinetics
P.O. Box 5076
Champaign, IL 61825-5076
Website: www.HumanKinetics.com

In the United States, email info@hkusa.com or call 800-747-4457.
In Canada, email info@hkcanada.com.
In the United Kingdom/Europe, email hk@hkeurope.com.

For information about Human Kinetics' coverage in other areas of the world, please visit our website: **www.HumanKinetics.com**

E7395

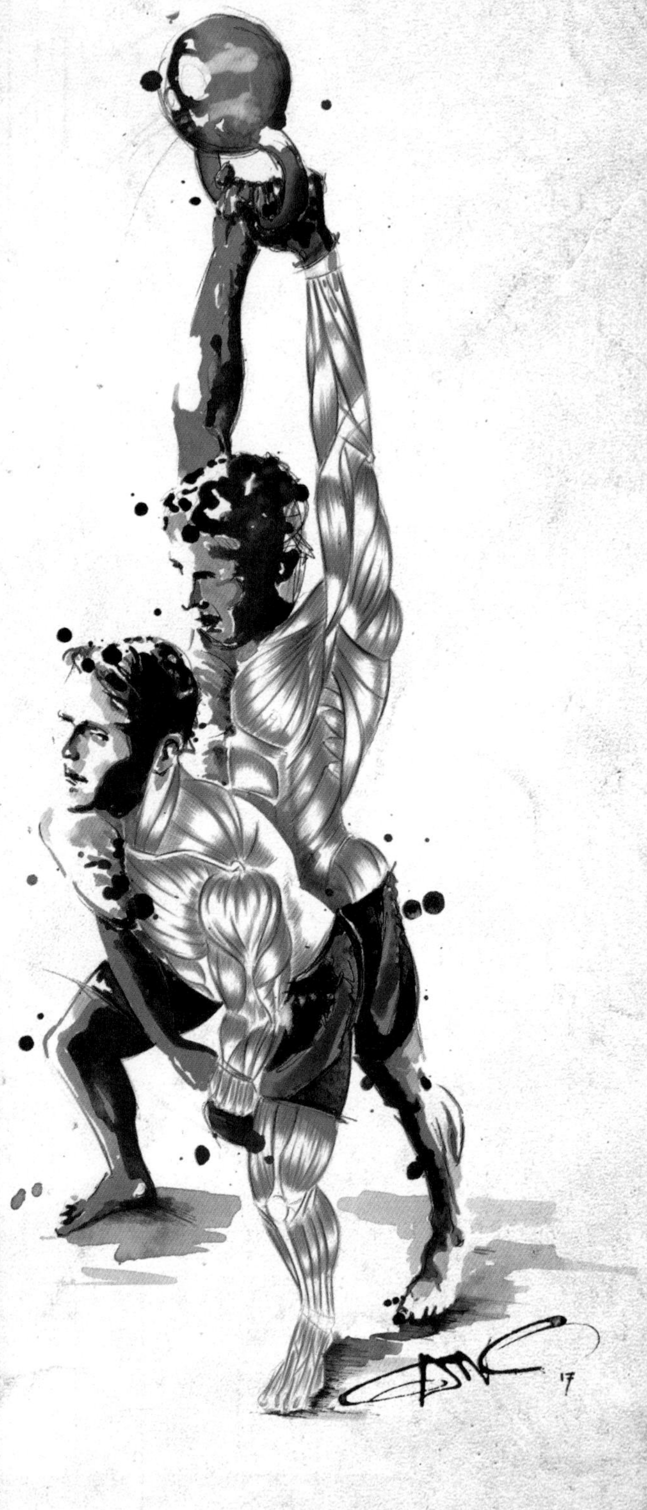

Writing is an adventure . . .

Two months of 20-hour-a-week bibliographical research, note taking, contextual drawings, and other detailed plans are necessary before any writing occurs. A book then requires 6 months of writing—if you are accustomed to writing—or about 30 hours a week. That is only the beginning; then you have to create drawings, take photos, sort and code the photos, design the layout, and reread the book (again and again).

For this book, more so than for any other, I pushed my team to its limits. A single illustration requires about 20 hours of Stéphane Ganneau's time. The book contains 142 illustrations. You can imagine the total time the illustrations required.

Each photo takes about five minutes to edit. The photographer, Johann Vayriot, spent four days and three nights shooting the photos. Of the 6,378 photos that were taken, 1,216 were ultimately used. The models—Arié Elmaleh, Dounia Coesens, Laetitia Fourcade, and Philippe Bas—were especially patient. Simply sorting and coding these images took a complete week of full-time work.

We also wanted to have innovative pedagogical plans, which amounted to about two full days of work for everyone in the group that we formed with Stef Ganneau.

Everything in the book must be harmonious; we created a mock-up with photos and illustrations, all while maintaining the precise instructions that I aimed to provide in this book. The great model artist Nicolas Moreau spent close to 120 hours over many months making this a reality. We spent weeks going back and forth as we decided how to flesh out the anatomy and the technique, as well as on my design ideas.

Finally, you must hunt down all the typos, which could be hiding anywhere: in the text, in the mock-up, or in the images. Olivier Remy and his team at Sen No Sen had a lot of work to do with this gigantic book.

I wish to thank each of these people from the bottom of my heart. It is our book for everyone, and I believe that, together, we have created something exceptional.

Aurélien Broussal-Derval

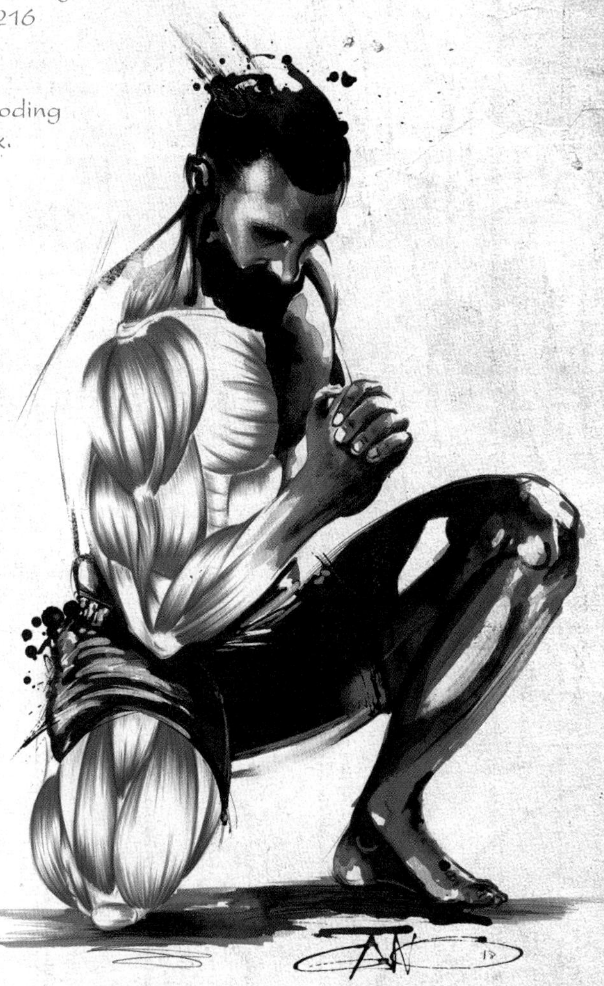

THIS IS NOT A BOOK FOR SELF-DIAGNOSIS

The goal of this book is not to replace doctors, physical therapists, massage therapists, or any other type of health care professional. Instead, it will explain and demonstrate how to detect and resolve fundamental problems that may be caused by a sport you play regularly, a lack of physical activity, or even the effects of your daily life. Pain that persists or that is sharp, consistently failing at certain exercises, or the inability to succeed during a physical test should prompt you to consult this book as fast as possible. Our hope is that, if you take care of your body as we advise you to do in this book, your medical needs will decrease over time. But visiting a general physician or an alternative medicine practitioner at least once a year is, in our opinion, an integral part of the method provided in this book. Taking care of your body also means trusting the professionals.

CONTENTS

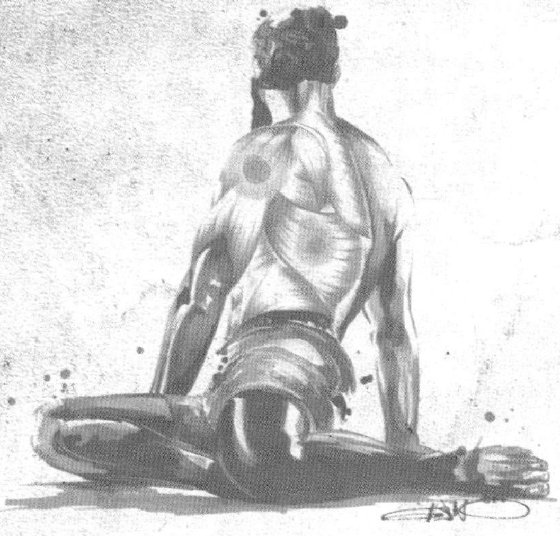

Pain

Pain is not inevitable. In fact, our aim is that after reading this book, your motto might even gradually become this: "The day you no longer hurt anywhere is the day that you're alive."

Part I - page 8

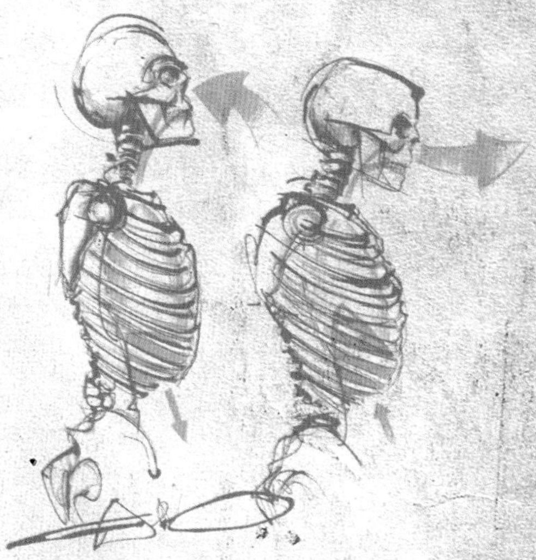

Breathing

On average, we breathe 20,000 times per day. Therefore, this vital element must be taken very seriously; you must train yourself to breathe.

Part II - page 78

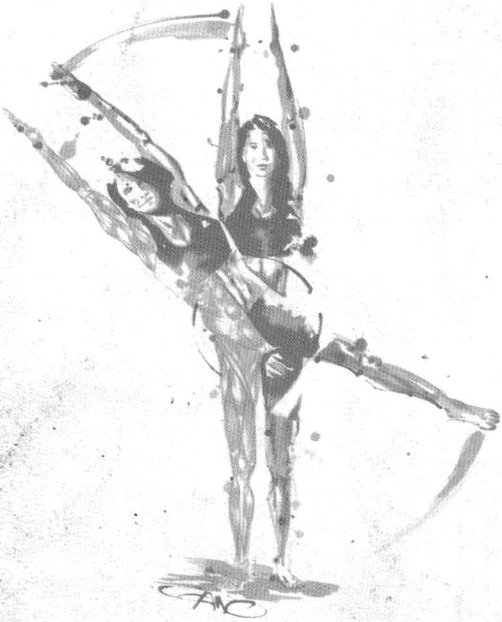

Movement

While many training exercises happen in a single plane, human movement is expressed in three planes and on three axes. To be effective in your training, you must be aware of these planes and axes. But it is only by understanding the global multiplane and multiaxis approach that you can harness the muscle chains to improve mobility to create a functional training approach.

Part III - page 95

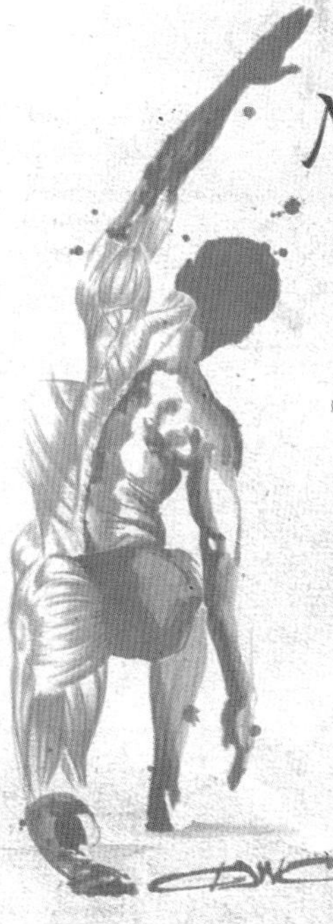

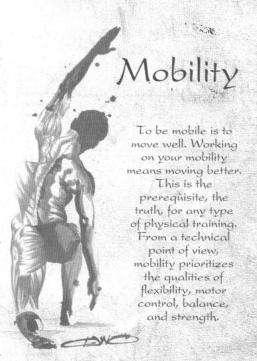

Mobility

To be mobile is to move well. Working on your mobility means moving better. This is the prerequisite, the truth, for any type of physical training. From a technical point of view, mobility prioritizes the qualities of flexibility, motor control, balance, and strength.

Part IV - page 159

MOVEMENT

Human movement has been examined through physiology: The transmission of messages from the central nervous system creates muscle contractions by using the body's energy resources.

Movement has also been examined through anatomy and biomechanics: Here, the body can be thought of as a group of cables and levers that can work together to coordinate movement.

Movement through psychology has also been studied. People must have the will to move as they search for sensations through self-awareness.

Nutrition, sociology, and many other scientific fields can help us to understand human movement and provide a "user's manual" for the powerful machine that is the human body.

Still, it would seem that we have begun to apply this knowledge in a backward fashion.

First, we have forgotten the very human purpose of movement. Why do we really move? What drives us to do more than daily labor and become physically active by choice? What motivates some to become high-level athletes or, on the contrary, pushes others toward complete inactivity?

The problems of a sedentary lifestyle are clear: Our computer-oriented lives are combined with leisure time spent on the sofa. But the concept of the chicken before the egg is still a valid question: Are we only submitting ourselves to this inactive society, or did we actually create it as we would wish it to be? Human nature tends to be lazy and to focus on comfort and idleness. Thus, we have always had a greater tendency to hide in our comfort zone rather than to venture out. *Moving more is not really a natural behavior.*

Beyond that, attempts to play group sports sometimes turn out badly. Even when it is not the intent, a competitive spirit often takes over, shoving aside health and safety concerns.

On the other end of the athletic spectrum—in a more general, collective category that we would call leisure sports—there is an entire fitness industry whose primary economic driver is human narcissism. Using the quest for beauty as a source of motivation, this industry is also missing the main objectives. Even worse, the number of gyms with membership programs and staff is decreasing, the instructors themselves lack training, and the participants lack commitment and seriousness. This means that, quite often, the participants do not reach their aesthetic goals.

The notion of a comfort zone has also suffered a setback: Even though the quest for competition or beauty has driven us for many years—while we told anyone who would listen that the best performance only happens outside of our comfort zone—the "no pain, no gain" approach seems to have come to an end. But constraining your life to a tiny comfort zone with complete safety, the warmth of your sofa, and a refreshing soda in your hand seems, to us, a limited way to live.

What if the solution were to expand your comfort zone? To give yourself the means to be well—if not in every circumstance, at least in all the basic situations you encounter in daily life? What would you say about learning how to expand your comfort zone from a comfortable, reclining position to the most exhilarating effort?

Movement is physiology, biomechanics, psychology, and even sociology. Movement is life.

To do this, you must first become aware.
Movement is physiology, biomechanics, psychology, and even sociology. Movement is life.

At a time when Western social systems are discussing the role of sports in overall health, and some people go so far as to imagine that insurance could one day reimburse sport participation costs in the context of therapeutic or even preventive prescriptions, we think it is time to reimagine the system. *Performance or aesthetic goals are not the most important things.* If our reimagined system is followed, the human body will be optimized beyond today's expectations.

MOVEMENT IS THE KEY

Like any machine, the human body requires maintenance and regular (almost daily) upkeep to function properly.

Like many people, you may not know a lot about mechanics. You drive your car every day; you use it and abuse it without ever opening the hood until the next scheduled maintenance check. Knowledgeable people might add a little oil and remove some grime. But, when it is time for the scheduled maintenance, it is always worse than expected: All the filters and parts must be changed, and the bill is outrageous.

When we look around us, at all performance levels and all ages, the evidence is very instructive: People allow their bodies to wither and get out of shape, and their bodies will not pass the service inspection. Some people may do a little athletic activity or a few stretches; a proper warm-up is clearly only for the minority of people. Worse, almost no one does any kind of maintenance check; they just wait until something breaks or they cannot function any longer before going to see a health care professional, who then has a considerable amount of work to do to get the body back in working order.

ARE YOU WORRIED?

That is normal. Most everyone is worried, from sedentary people to high-performing athletes.

- It is not normal that so many people have back pain.
- It is not normal that so few people can squat, which is an essential function of the hips, knees, and ankles.
- It is not normal when people cannot run or jump comfortably and safely, no matter their age.
- It is not normal to have to choose between movements that people can and cannot do.
- It is not normal for people to have to compensate and modify their posture to perform a simple task.
- It is not normal for people to not be able to move how they want to move.

ALL OF THIS HAS TO CHANGE.

PART I PAIN

"The day when you no longer hurt anywhere is the day that you're dead."

We do not fully agree with the crux of this saying, which creates an attitude in various sports that pain, both acute and chronic, is a way of life.

For many coaches, pain is an integral part of the training process and can even show how difficult and effective the sessions are. Over time, are former athletes who are "ripped to pieces" now more respected because they haven't listened to their bodies throughout their career?

Incidentally, you do not have to be a high-performance athlete or competitor to behave like an idiot. (Do you feel slightly insulted?) Perhaps, like many other people, you have covered up that neck pain for years, buried your head in the sand for months about that chronic backache, or not paid any attention whatsoever to that sore shoulder every morning since you stopped playing sports.

It's not normal, and you know it.
The only real question is this: *Why*?

Why do you allow yourself to suffer like this? When I ask that question of people in a similar situation, they respond by saying they do not have the time to regularly see a health care professional. That, in and of itself, is not an excuse. Almost everyone overlooks the fact that there are daily techniques that can be practiced independently to detect, track, and eradicate common aches and pains.

Pain is not inevitable. In fact, our aim is that after reading this book, your motto might even gradually become this:

"The day you no longer hurt anywhere is the day that you're alive."

WHY ARE WE SO STUBBORN?

The human body is full of protection systems. Whether we're ill, injured, weakened, or dehydrated, backup mechanisms are always working so that, even when it does not make sense, balance is maintained. Because of this, we are free to listen to or ignore a simple piece of information: pain. When pain occurs, the message is not so clear for some people. In that moment when the body says, "Stop or you'll break everything," some people hear, "It hurts, but it will pass." Indeed, when faced with pain, we can be stubborn, even downright narrow-minded. Watch your athletic friends when they complain about a particularly uncomfortable area; how many of them stop, and how many keep going, saying that there's no need to blow things out of proportion? They will even argue that their performance hasn't changed, and, to some extent, they'll be right. This is because pain affects some parts of the body more strongly, disrupting the muscles for posture and stability more than the muscles for movement. In other words, as long as pain is bearable, it only marginally weakens energy levels. It is even commonly acknowledged that 90 percent of world records are beaten by athletes who are suffering from chronic skeletal or muscular pain.

Pain is not inevitable.

"The day when you no longer hurt anywhere is the day that you're dead." We do not fully agree with the crux of this saying, which creates an attitude in various sports that pain, both acute and chronic, is a way of life.

In fact, our aim is that after reading this book, your motto might even gradually become this: "The day you no longer hurt anywhere is the day that you're alive."

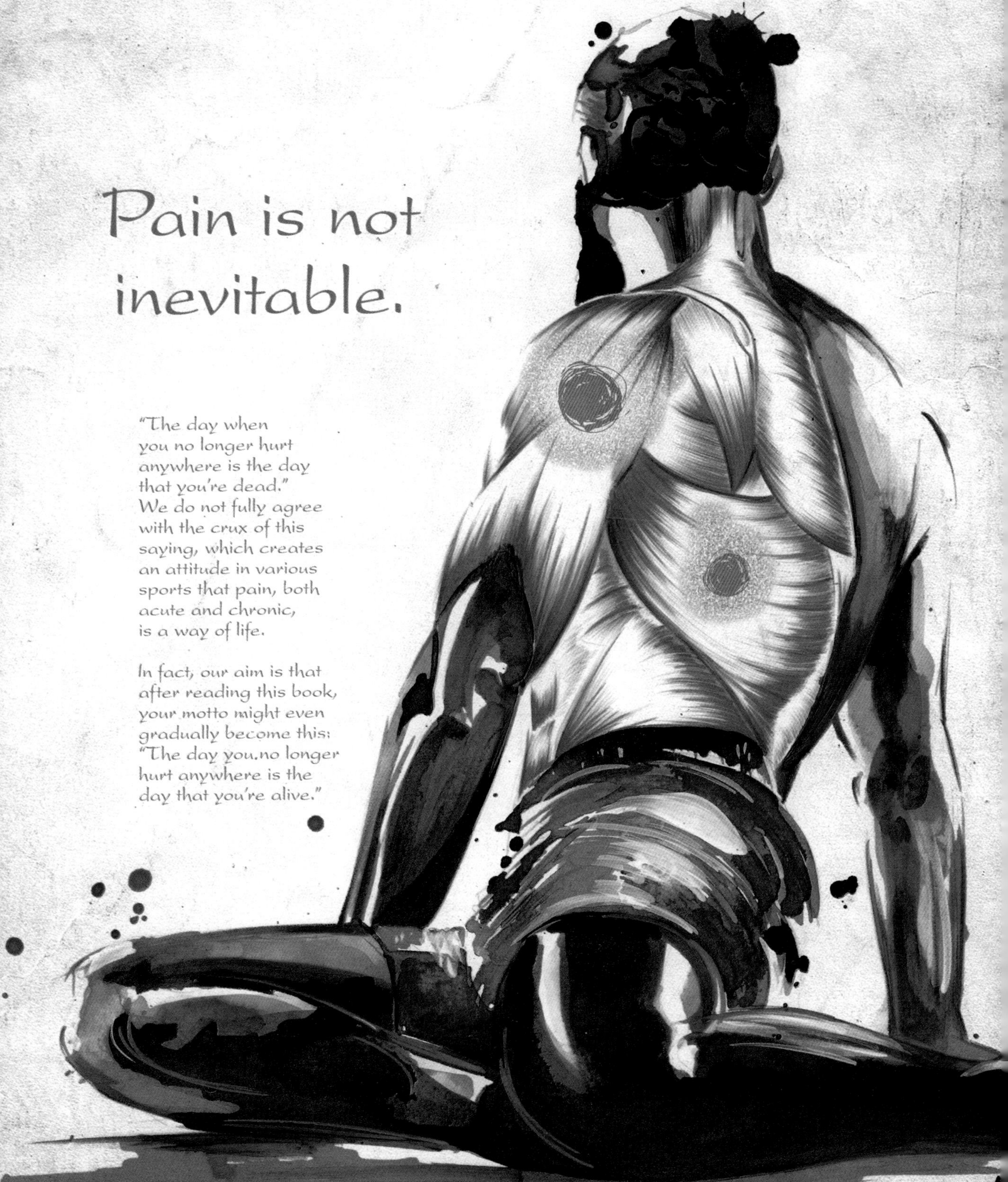

01 PAIN AND MOVEMENT

Pain is not just uncomfortable. It interferes with motor function and limits mobility, creating a vicious cycle of motor inefficiency that causes new postural disorders and chronic pain. We often describe this vicious cycle as a mirror: Pain creates a disorder, which in turn produces more pain.

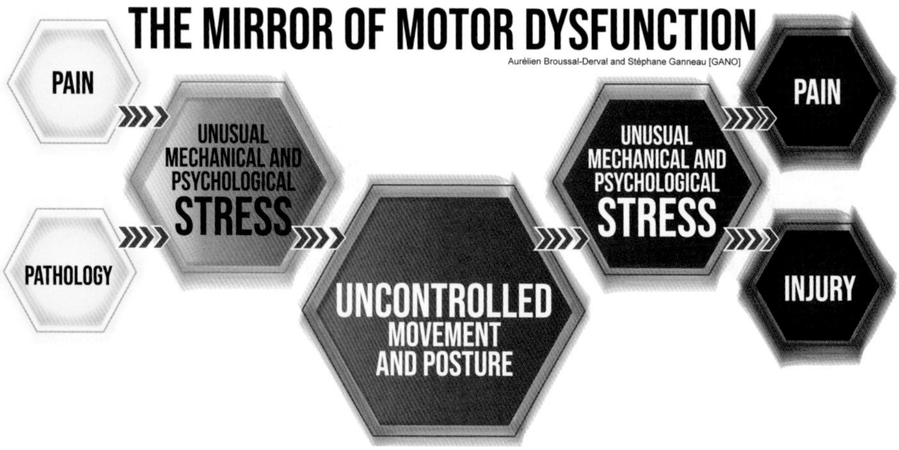

We will now examine two states: pain free and in pain.

- **Pain free:** The brain and central nervous system are capable of learning about or controlling functional movement, balance, and core muscles during both simple and complex tasks. (The authors Hodges and Moseley have spoken passionately about this subject for over 15 years.)
- **In pain:** Pain limits options with regard to adjustment and control of the central nervous system. The deep, postural muscles are overtaken and supplemented by the more powerful motor muscles that are less coordinated and rely on increasingly steady co-contractions, which immobilizes movement, freezes joint freedom, and creates areas of permanent tension within the muscle.

In fact, in the presence of pain, almost all specialists (see the work of Hodges, Lee, Jull, Sahrmann, Richardson, Falla, O'Sullivan, O'Leary, or Dankaerts) agree that they observe large muscles with a high potential for strength or speed instead being used for functional and postural tasks that are much less intense than their usual tasks of jumping, racing, or even resistance training.

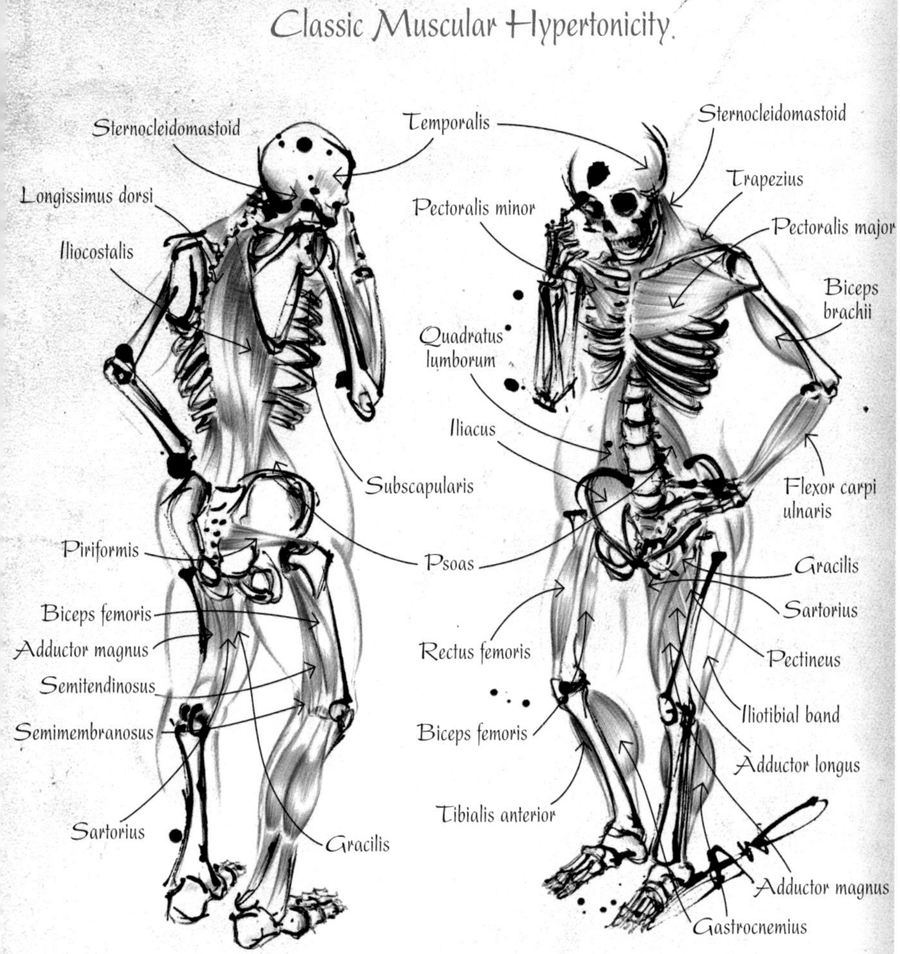

Beyond local treatment for painful or immobile zones, the challenge is to change your movement and posture. It is not just inactivity that creates problems; all activities are responsible. Using the phone, texting, and working at a desk are all motor and postural absurdities that will gradually impact different parts of your joints.

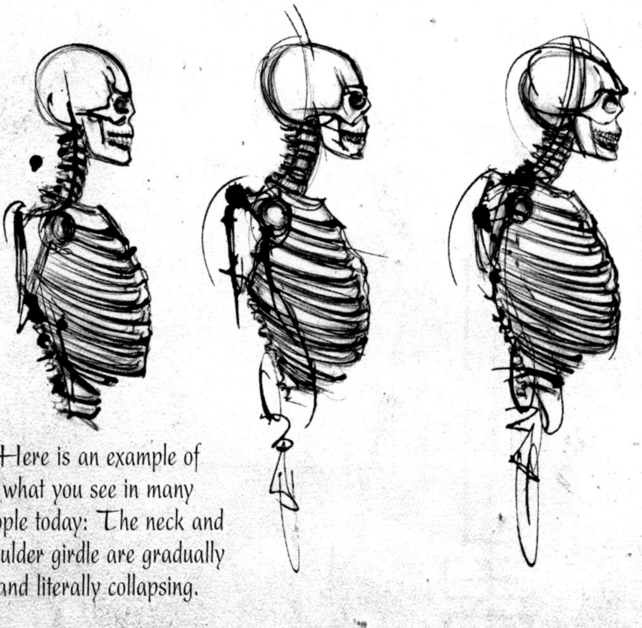

Here is an example of what you see in many people today: The neck and shoulder girdle are gradually and literally collapsing.

The most unfortunate and long-term consequence of pain is decreased activity in the deep and postural muscles, which become less reactive, weaker, and less resistant. The long-term effects on motor and postural efficiency are catastrophic.

Motor muscles are not really affected by pain during their highest performance, as long as the pain is bearable. However, being able to tolerate pain during performance conceals a bigger issue. The imbalances and weaknesses in the postural and deep muscles, which are linked to chronic pain, can only be effectively detected through movements that do not involve bearing weight.

Over time, a painful muscle gradually becomes "disconnected" from the nervous system, and the body's compensating systems allow most movements to be completed with no need for the disconnected link in the chain. Slowly, atrophy ("wasting away" of the muscle) occurs, making the rehabilitation journey longer and more difficult.

Your health care professional or personal trainer may use the following terms to characterize this vicious cycle:

- Replacement strategies
- Compensatory movement
- Muscular imbalances
- Motor deprogramming
- Motor muscle domination
- Uncontrolled co-contraction

In any case, the causes and consequences of the problem are the same.

DID YOU KNOW?

Worrying about injuries or pain (or, perhaps, recurring pain) may be equally destabilizing for posture and movement. In 2003, Moseley and his team also determined that a person's *anxiety* about potential pain affects the nervous system.

We need to radically change our habits by changing how we move, hold ourselves, and live. Of course, it is not likely that you will always be able to check Facebook with your phone perpendicular to the ground, your arms lifted, and your head held high—but when you can do it, you should seize the opportunity. Why not take advantage of the movement opportunities you have? You could, for example, text with your arm raised. Even doing this occasionally can maintain a significant range of diversity in your motor abilities.

Classic Muscular Hypotonicity

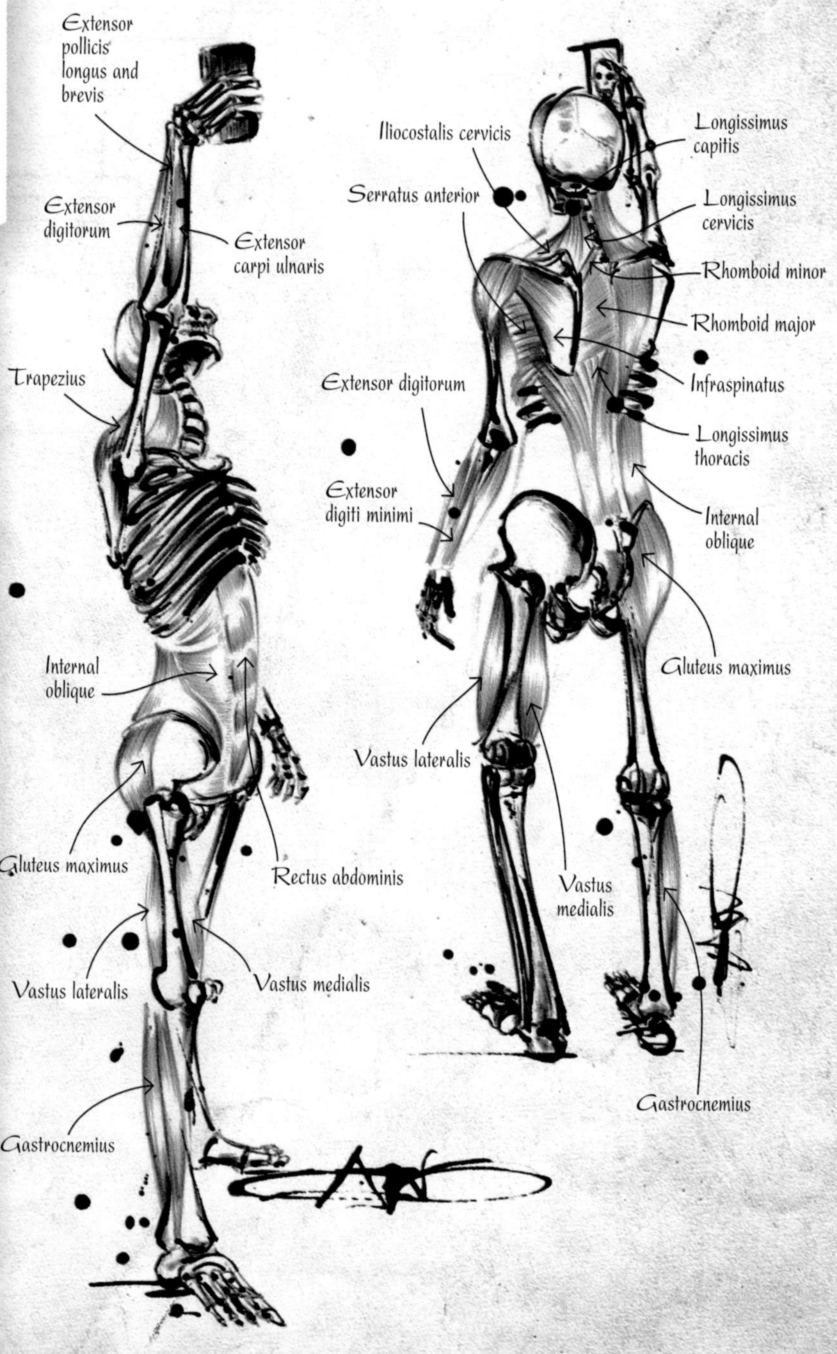

TRIGGER POINTS

02

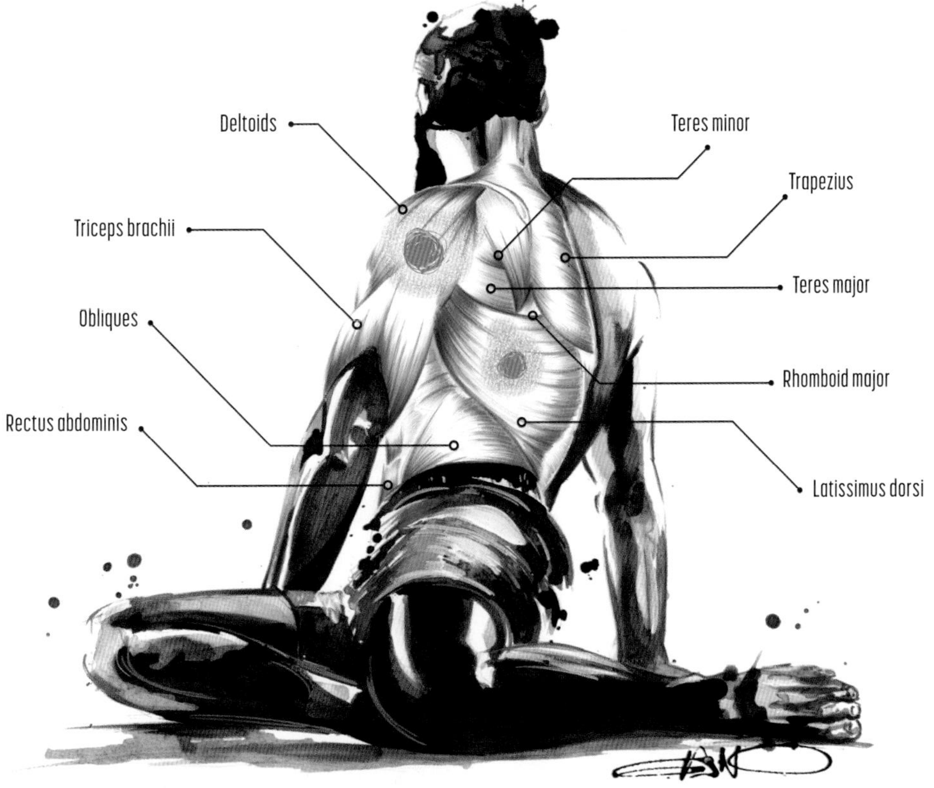

Trigger points are small areas of muscle that are painful to the touch. They can sometimes trigger a larger area of pain, which can be remote, spreading from other muscles. In this way, a trigger point in the buttocks (often called the *gluteals*) could cause back pain for example.

In reality, trigger points take the shape of a pea or a small piece of uncooked spaghetti. They form during unusual or improper movement or positioning of a muscle. The nonuniform tension generated in the muscle leads to areas of stress and adhesion, which often become painful.

For example, if you ride a bike with a seat that is too low, you impair the posture of your back, harm the strength ratios of your quadriceps and hamstrings (the powerful locomotor muscles of the front and back of your thigh, respectively), and overexert the psoas muscle (your hip flexor). The tension in the quadriceps is inconsistent and disordered, and it could create trigger points.

To properly understand the effects of trigger points on human movement, imagine that you are brushing your hair and that the brush is immediately blocked by a knot of hair. You are stopped in your tracks, and you must try another way to untangle the knot.

This is exactly what a trigger point is: a muscular knot that prevents you from moving correctly, pushing you to alter your posture or movement patterns to remain functional without fixing it.

Doctors Travell and Simons (1992 and 1998) identify trigger points according to whether they are *active* or *passive* and *primary or secondary*.

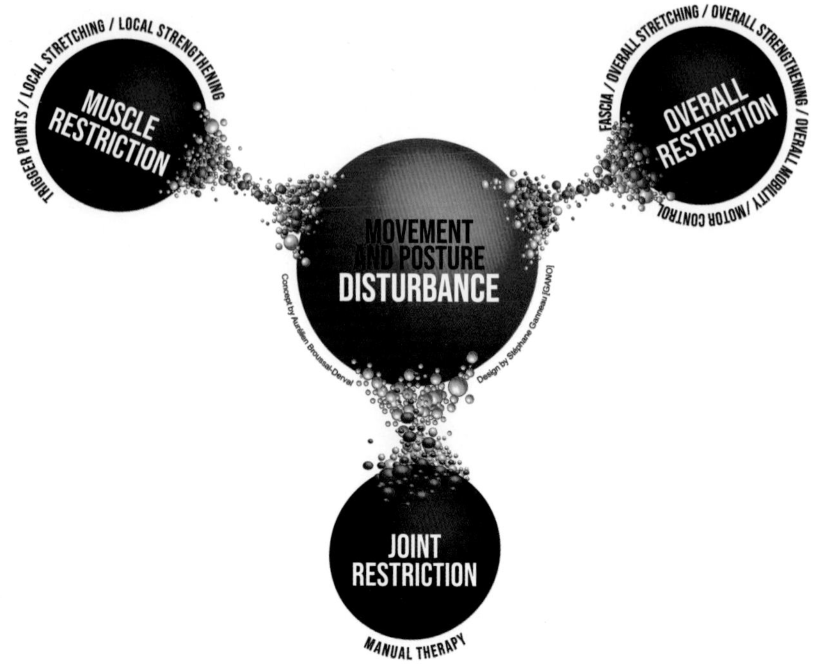

ACTIVE AND PASSIVE TRIGGER POINTS

Passive trigger points are only detectable through spasms or self-massage. They are painful and affect movement and posture, but they go unnoticed in everyday life. On the contrary, *active trigger points* are noticeable even when they are not activated. Because they are more or less constant depending on the time of day and the activity being carried out, their existence should be obvious. Their variable level of irritability affects how much they spread and their intensity, and they appear due to injury, intense (and repeated) stress without an appropriate warm-up, and prolonged improper posture.

> It is necessary to treat both types of trigger points. Rest can force an active trigger point into a passive state at any time, but it does not resolve the problem. Conversely, any passive trigger point can be activated by an unsuitable activity.

MASSAGING TRIGGER POINTS

Take your time: You're not trying to squish a bug but rather to relax a tense muscle fiber. You must therefore be patient and progressive. Pain is part of the game, but it should stay manageable so as not to provoke a further tightening of the trigger point. We aim for a pain intensity of 5 on a scale of 1 to 10 (Davies 2014). If it is really too painful, massage or stretch another nearby area—if possible, one in the same myofascial chain (see the exercises for stretching the functional chain in part III). Remember that frequency is more effective than intensity, so do not hesitate to massage yourself several times a day.

PRIMARY AND SECONDARY TRIGGER POINTS

Primary trigger points can be active or passive and occur along with a motor or postural disorder. When the trigger point radiates, or has previously radiated to other muscles, it causes other disorders at various levels of the *myofascial chain* (a connection of muscle and fascia; *fascia* is a thin sheath of fibrous tissue that encloses a muscle or organ). These lead to *secondary trigger points*. A comprehensive strategy is needed to alleviate all trigger points, not one that is limited to just one area of pain at a given moment. It is possible for a remote primary trigger point to produce secondary trigger points. If these secondary points are treated without addressing the underlying issue, it is likely that new secondary trigger points will appear.

> Several trigger points may be present in the same muscle. We must take time to explore the whole muscle to take care of them.

SELF-MASSAGE 03

Pain is not a weakness in the mind or body to be ignored but a piece of information to examine further. By ignoring pain, your movement will be limited in the short term and long term. Myofascial freedom is required for movement.

In this respect, there will be a lot of discussion in this book about self-massage techniques, or how to free the myofascial chain on your own. With the help of different tools for various parts of the body, you will scan and then detect any stiffness or tension, down to the smallest trigger point.

First, it is necessary to understand that it is not possible to isolate the fascia during self-massage. All of the structures are massaged at the same time: nerve tissue, muscles, and even the skin. Under compression, muscle and skin behave like sponges. Water is pressed out of the tissue when pressure is applied and then drawn in when the pressure eases up or moves to another location.

There are significant effects of self-massage that justify its use both before and after a workout:

- **Effect on recovery time:** In addition to reducing the tension in the muscle that is massaged, self-massage optimizes physical recovery. Further, the loss of muscular performance is limited, and muscle aches are effectively treated (Cheatham et al. 2015).
- **Effect on pain:** By relaxing a tense area, pain retreats. The analgesic effect of self-massage is therefore notable in the short and long term (Pearcey 2015). In 2017, Behm emphasized in his research that there is a decrease in muscle aches (already noted by Macdonald in 2014), a reduction in myofascial pain, and a positive effect on minimizing trigger points.
- **Effect on movement:** In the intermediate term, relaxation of areas of adhesion and decreased pain allow you to move more easily, without compromising muscular performance (Macdonald 2013, Bushell 2015).
- **Effect on warm-ups:** By waking up dormant or even *amnesic sensory-motor areas* (areas that have lost sensation and voluntary control), self-massage is a powerful accelerator during a warm-up by increasing mobility without limiting muscular performance (Halperin et al. 2014, Cheatham et al. 2015).

THE THREE GOLDEN RULES FOR SELF-MASSAGE

1. **Move gently:** Make an effort to feel what you are doing; you should be in the here and now. Self-massage is a time for yourself. The more you work on deeper areas, the more you need to take your time and move gently to relax any painful, tense areas.
2. **Look for unfamiliar areas:** Move toward areas of your body that you never touch or move. These are the ones that need to be stimulated the most.
3. **Alternate between moving your massage tool and moving yourself:** If you use a massage tool, you can also create movement between the layers of soft tissue by keeping the tool in one place and then moving your body. This method is complemented by using a movable massage tool applied to active pressure spots, allowing you to work more effectively on tense or painful areas. For increased fascial movement, the body should move on the tool. For areas of tension, the tool should move on (over) the body.

SHOULD MASSAGE BE PAINFUL?

There are two schools of thought on this. On one hand, there are devoted self-massagers who go far beyond the first level of responsiveness to massage and, as with any addiction, always need more. These people go so far as to use barbells, kettlebells, or weight plates as massage tools and believe that extreme work on active flexibility, which can produce bruising, creates a local adaptation. Often, this method is more painful than the alternative method of remaining within a tolerable pain zone and finishing with a pain-free level of intensity. This more reasonable approach states that, in general, bruises are signs of muscle injury rather than recovery. As is often the case, your instinct and common sense should guide you. Do what you have to do; do what will help you. *Listen to your body.*

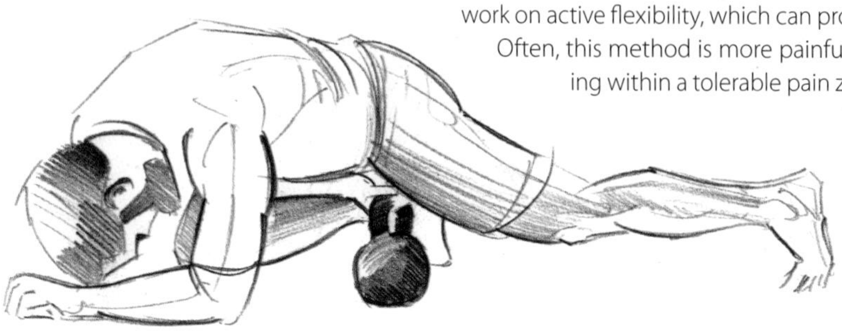

Your body is adaptable. Even in the short term, self-massage eases aches. In the long term, it increases your tolerance to pain (Jay et al. 2014), enabling you to work with tools that allow for more intense and advanced massages.

AVOID OVERLY BONY AREAS!

Remember that self-massage essentially targets soft tissues. There are certain areas that are not very muscular, such as the front of the shin area, that should be treated by self-massage nevertheless. However, other areas should be avoided altogether because they have almost no soft tissue or are often comprised of only ligaments.

A little bit of pain is often necessary to determine the issue, but you should move very slowly; too much pain will lead to a protective reaction in the stimulated muscle when it relaxes. On the other hand, it can sometimes be life changing to work on pain by, for example, working on an old injury under the supervision of your health care professional.

In our opinion, selecting one tool over another, depending on the area being treated, is more important than which paradigm you adhere to. In this respect, Monteiro and his team believe that the range of motion is influenced by the massage tool and the duration of the massage (Monteiro et al. 2017).

TO GUIDE YOU

Here is an anatomy guide for areas to massage with the appropriate tools. In our opinion, you should only switch to more intense tools if you cannot reach the deep areas or stimulate changes.

In this book, we will combine two approaches with some advanced mobility exercises.

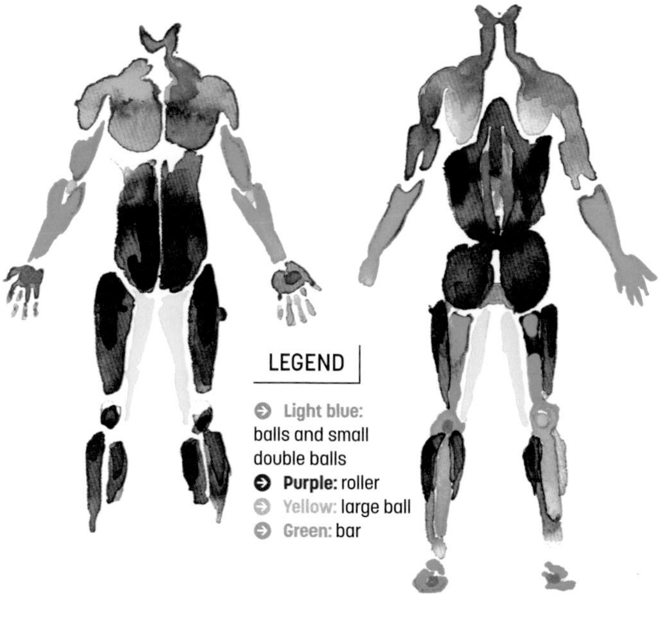

LEGEND

- **Light blue:** balls and small double balls
- **Purple:** roller
- **Yellow:** large ball
- **Green:** bar

THE ILIOTIBIAL BAND

The use of self-massage is starting to appear in research studies and social media. The thigh is one of the most popular areas for self-massage, but massage of the *iliotibial band (IT band)* and the fasciae latae has become especially popular. This area is peculiar because it is not myofascial: Although the deeper layers are comprised of muscle tissue, the IT band itself does not contract. This explains, in part, why the IT band is not an area affected by sensory-motor amnesia; it is stimulated by daily movement. Any effects of a self-massage warm-up of the outer part of the thigh are consequently very limited.

Most of the massage techniques for this area cause pain. In this way, purposely creating friction between the IT band and the deeper tissues is not recommended because it creates more inflammation than pain relief. In fact, it would seem that pressure applied by a massage roller or ball does not isolate the IT band from the underlying vastus lateralis muscle; the pressure actually causes them to crush against one another.

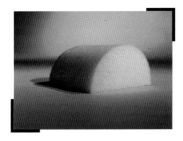

To ensure that these two surfaces "slide" over one another, it may be better to use a stationary tool, such as a roller cut in two pieces and placed on the floor or a roller that is firmly blocked between weights, and then slide your thigh over it. Move your body over the roller, not the roller over your body.

Moreover, the IT band is almost impossible to stretch out through self-massage. The amount of pressure necessary to do this during a massage would be simply unbearable.

It seems more worthwhile to us to concentrate on treating both ends of the IT band as a way to care for the IT band itself. First, treat the area just below the *iliac crest* (the area at the front and outside of the hip bones of your pelvis), at the very top of the gluteals. This area is often missing from both strengthening programs and self-massage programs, and its treatment should produce very quick results. Next, concentrate your self-massage on the opposite end of the IT band on the outside of the knee, between the end of the IT band and the top of the *fibula* (the long bone on the lateral side of the lower leg). This type of massage is particularly useful in sports in which the knee turns repeatedly on a fixed point anchored to the floor, and it will make the top of the fibula more open to rotation.

FROM SELF-MASSAGE TO THE WARM-UP

In this chapter, we have talked a lot about using self-massage as a tool to combat pain. In later chapters, we will discuss developing mobility in the long term through a combination of self-massage and stretching. But what are the short-term effects, for example, of using self-massage in warm-up routines?

The reasons to do self-massage during warm-ups are to increase your range of motion without compromising muscular responsiveness and to maintain (or even improve) the contraction strength of the muscles being used (Halperin et al. 2014).

Muscle Memory Loss

Muscle areas that have "memory loss" can be difficult to find through self-massage. This is for good reason: You may not even be aware they exist. Our advice is very simple: Try to massage everywhere, even the least likely areas. The more you massage the areas that you never touch, the more you increase your chances of finding areas that are experiencing muscle memory. Here is a list of the most common areas:

- → The bottom of the feet (the arch of the foot, the ball of the foot, and the heel)
- → The front of the shins
- → The back of the knees
- → Under the armpits
- → The inner part of the quadriceps
- → The hip rotators
- → The top of the hips
- → The upper neck muscles, just under the head

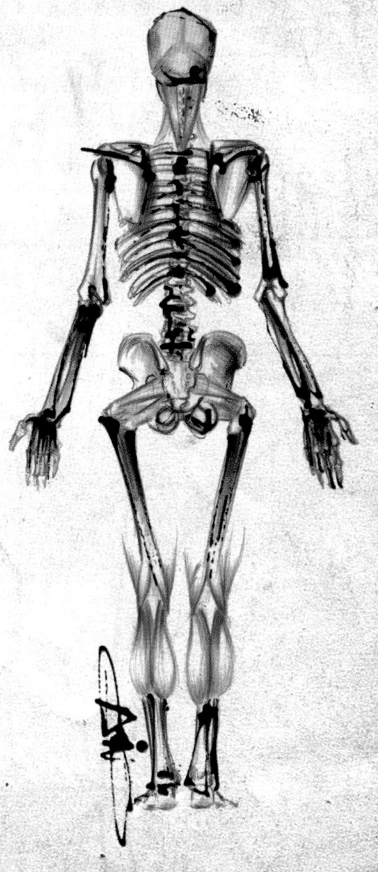

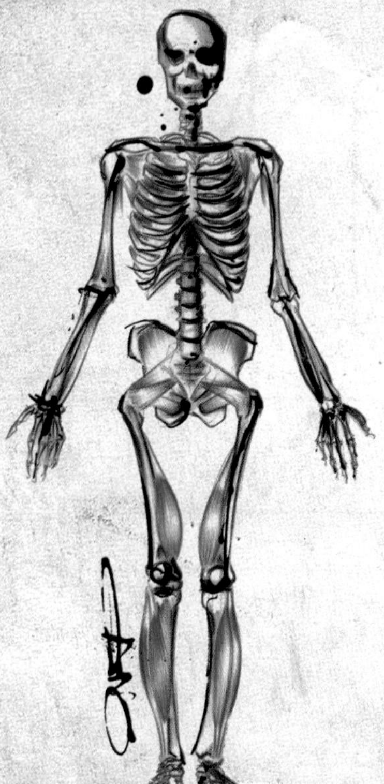

Thus, self-massage has a considerable advantage over passive stretching, which reduces muscular responsiveness.

In 2016, Kelly and Beardsley discovered through their work that sudden increases in mobility happen, on average, in about 9 percent of people and last for about 20 minutes. It should be noted that the effect is also seen in the opposite limb when the arch of the foot is massaged. However, the benefits disappear more quickly (a maximum of 10 minutes on the opposite limb).

We therefore recommend the following during warm-ups:

- Use self-massage just before the target movement, such as a combination of massaging the arch of the foot, the hamstrings, and the gluteal muscles less than 10 minutes before starting squats.
- Use self-massage, when necessary, on the opposite limb when exercising a limb that is stiff for pathological reasons. Even if a foot cannot be massaged, for example, it is possible to increase mobility and help it by massaging the other foot.

Be careful: Not all warm-up activities have been studied yet. In the meantime, use your common sense. At first, self-massage increases the temperature, relaxes the myofascial network, and provides local pain relief in areas of adhesion or trigger points; however, it is still a tool that, when used long term, promotes relaxation. Though we are in favor of implementing it systematically into our warm-ups, self-massage should not be overused at the start of a workout. Here are the methods that we recommend:

SELF-MASSAGE WARM-UP METHOD
Arch of the foot: 1 or 2 times for 60 seconds per foot
All other muscles: 2 or 3 times for 30 seconds per muscle

THINGS TO KEEP IN MIND WHILE WARMING UP

- The more you practice self-massage on a daily basis, the quicker you will see the resulting effects during warm-ups and the more useful self-massage will become during a workout. Do not wait; starting to use self-massage will immediately revolutionize your warm-ups! At first, stiffness and pain will appear, and self-massage during your warm-ups will not last long enough to correct it. On the other hand, if you keep at it too long, you could overrelax your muscles and ligaments. Just as with stretching, it is only by doing it every day that you will see the best results. The clearest study on this subject is by Cavanaugh's team in 2017; they observed a decrease in activation of the hamstring muscles following self-massage of the quadriceps. The authors attributed this effect to the perceived pain in the quadriceps, which led to relaxation of the hamstrings. With regular self-massage, sudden pain disappears, and there are fewer and fewer restrictions to using this technique during warm-ups. However, athletes who are new to self-massage should wait for a few weeks after starting a training program before using self-massage and then only for short durations at first.
- This same study by Cavanaugh advises caution when distinguishing between self-massage for short-term mobility and self-massage for warm-up purposes. When self-massage is used at the beginning of a workout, the intensity should not cause pain. On the other hand, self-massage that aims to improve mobility in the long term, when spaced adequately from other training sessions, can provide relief in terms of pain tolerance.
- Just like warming up the nervous or cardiovascular systems, a progressive approach comes from common sense. For optimal results, gradually increase pressure on soft areas; do not crush them from the outset, or you risk causing physical or even psychological resistance in future sessions.
- Just as with stretching during warm-ups, it is essential to plan a method for neuromuscular reactivation to avoid any risk of overrelaxation. Without fail, your self-massage should be accompanied by energetic and progressive exercise.

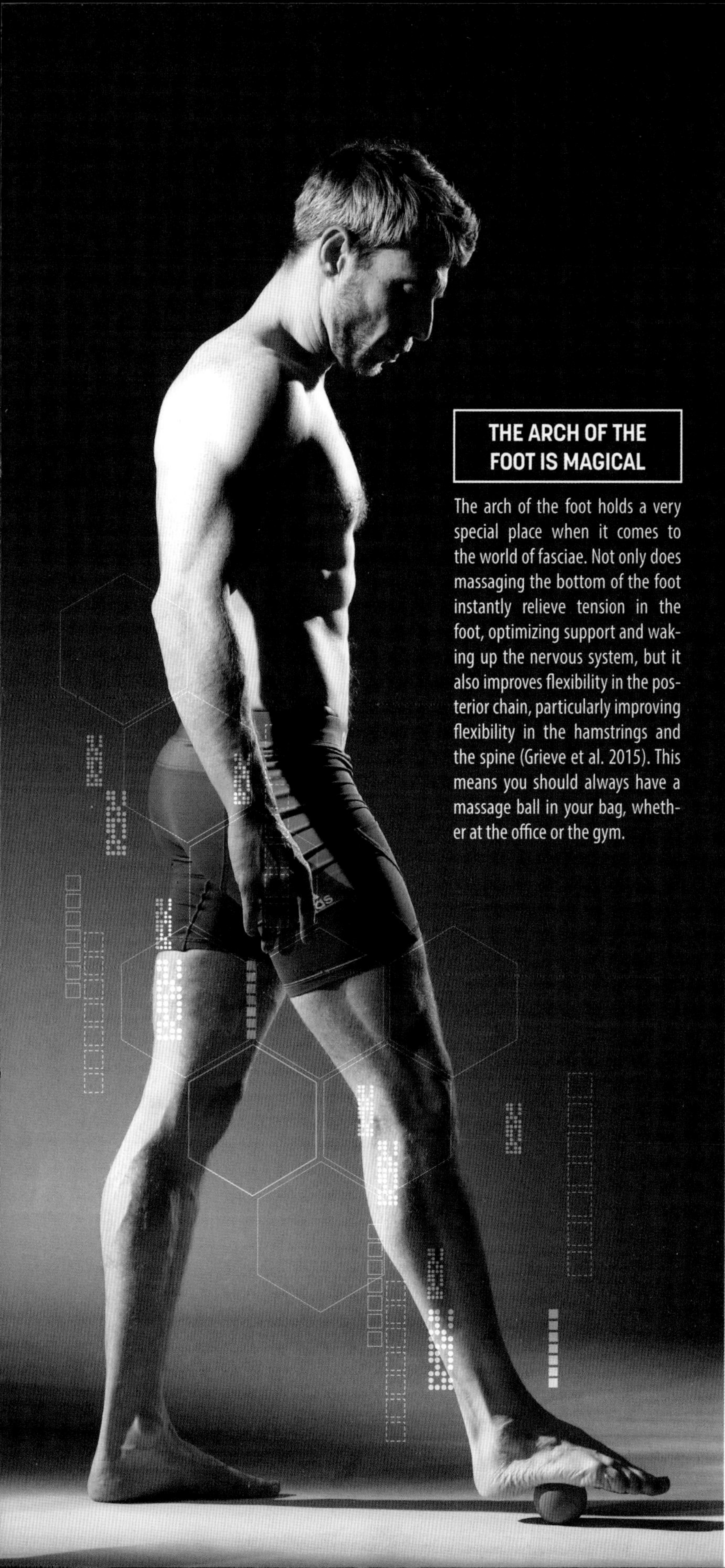

THE ARCH OF THE FOOT IS MAGICAL

The arch of the foot holds a very special place when it comes to the world of fasciae. Not only does massaging the bottom of the foot instantly relieve tension in the foot, optimizing support and waking up the nervous system, but it also improves flexibility in the posterior chain, particularly improving flexibility in the hamstrings and the spine (Grieve et al. 2015). This means you should always have a massage ball in your bag, whether at the office or the gym.

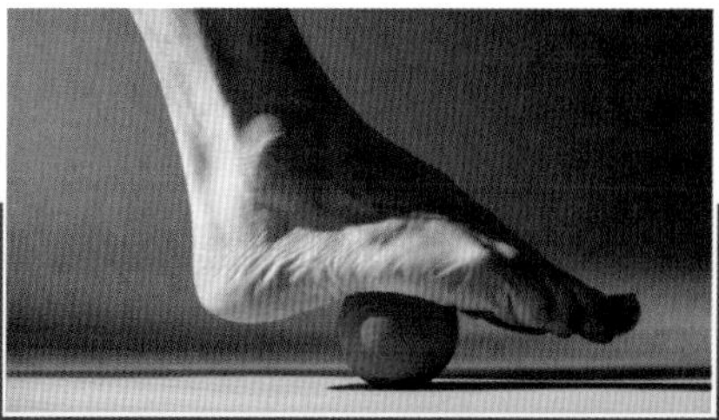

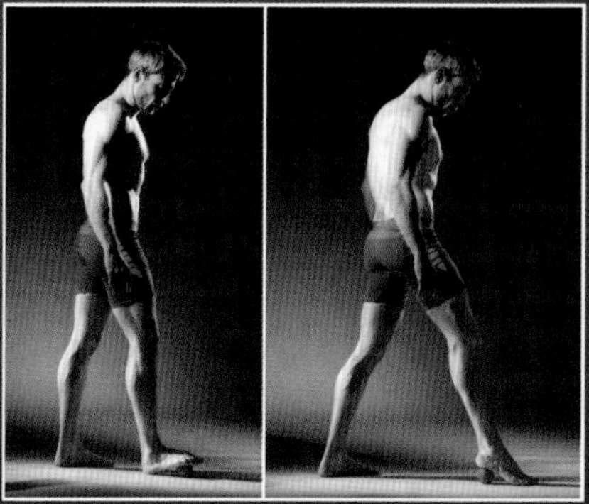

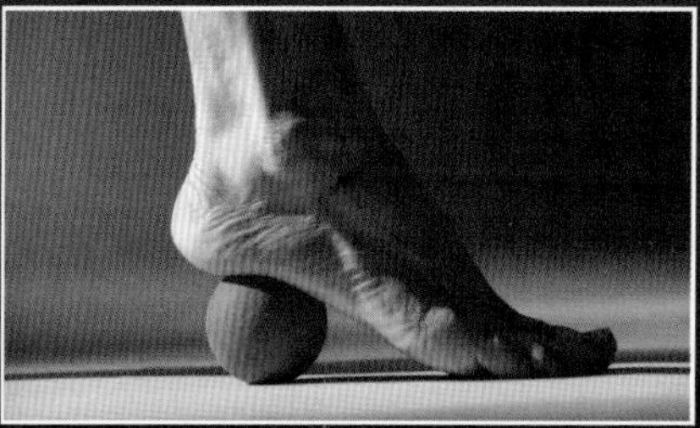

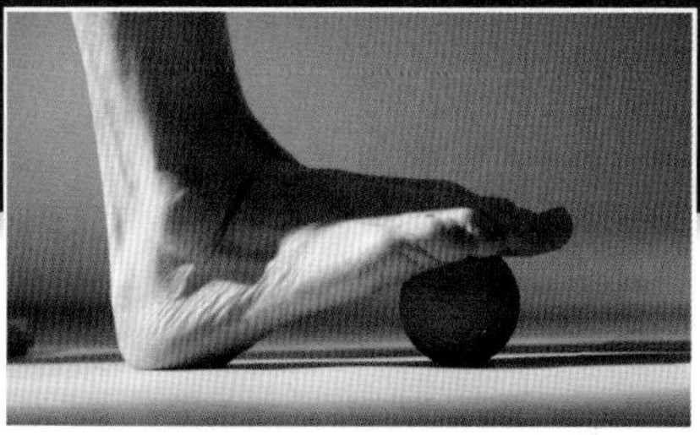

PLEASE NOTE

A roller massage that is brutal, fast, and careless will not produce the "sponge" effect normally created by the combination of pressure and relaxation on the soft tissues. On the contrary, it could create muscular tension and bruising or even damage sensory receptors. You must therefore take your time and be conscientious; your body deserves it.

04 COMBATTING PAIN

Pain is not inevitable.

Local treatment of trigger points, self-massage, stretching, and regular movement, as well as realigning the joints, are all part of the toolkit that you should be making use of every day to maintain your "machine"—your own body.

Using self-massage, "scan" the parts of your body one by one to detect areas that are stiff, painful, or resistant. There are numerous tools available, with varying degrees of precision and appropriateness depending on the areas to be scanned and then treated.

At first, the approach is often healing (we begin these practices in response to persistent pain). At the beginning, healing is often very focused on a certain body part, which takes precedence, but there is no need to wait until these areas are treated to explore the rest of the body and discover other areas to be soothed. Remember that they could be connected.

These first two phases (local and general treatment) should be carried out together every day or every other day as long as tension and pain persist.

Once you have desensitized the areas in question, there is a maintenance period in which daily work is no longer required (although self-massage and stretching can be practiced freely).

EXAMPLE OF A COMPLETE SCANNING METHOD

When should I do these sessions?
All proposed sessions can be carried out completely or in part, depending on the time you have available, at any time of the day. However, doing these exercises when you wake up in the morning will wake up your muscles and tendons. In the evening, they will help with overall relaxation, help to restart the body after a day of stress, and promote restful sleep.

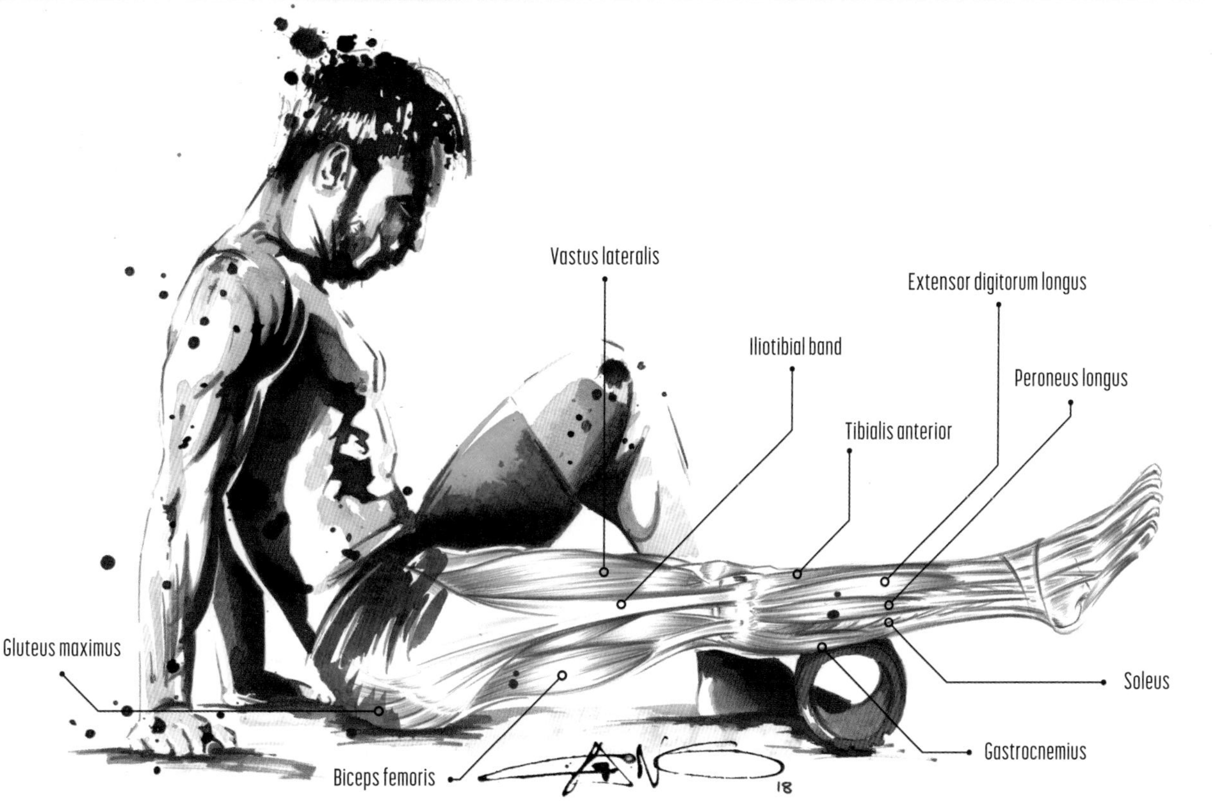

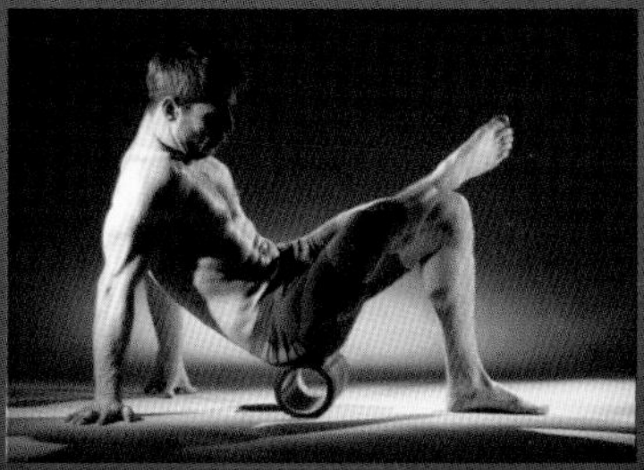

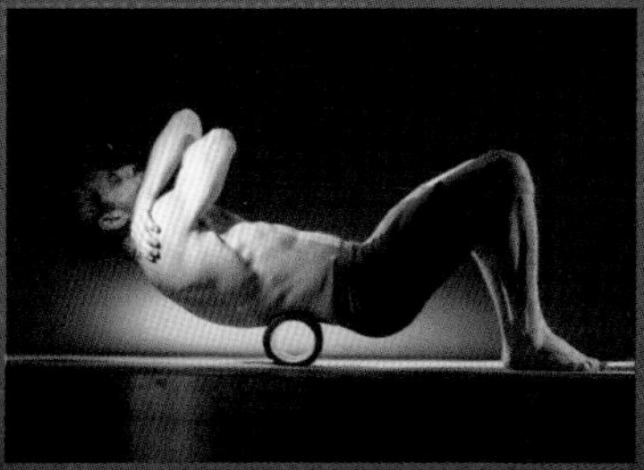

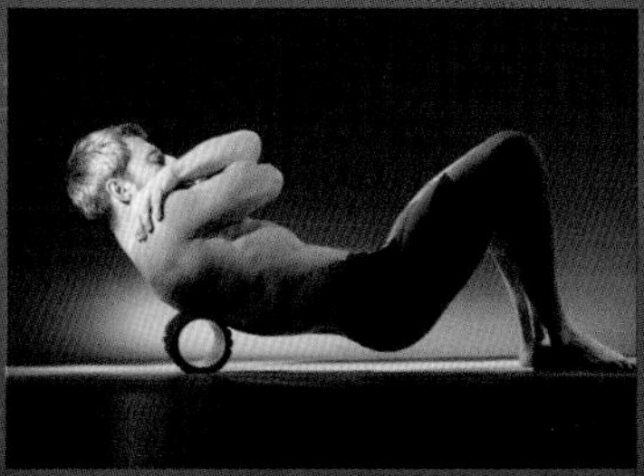

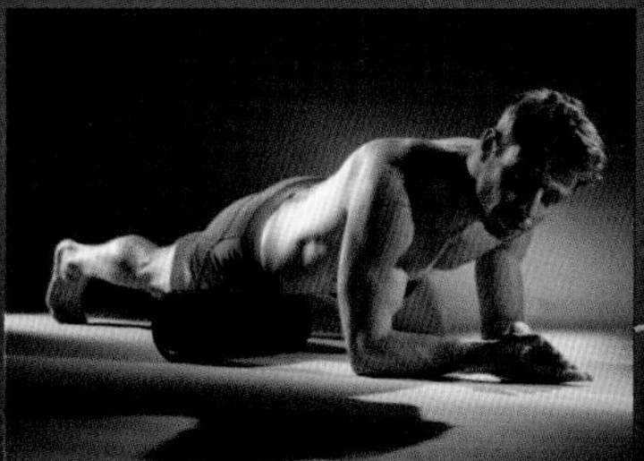

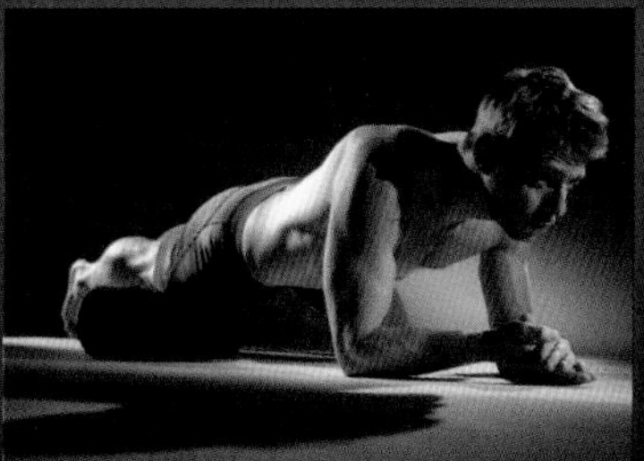

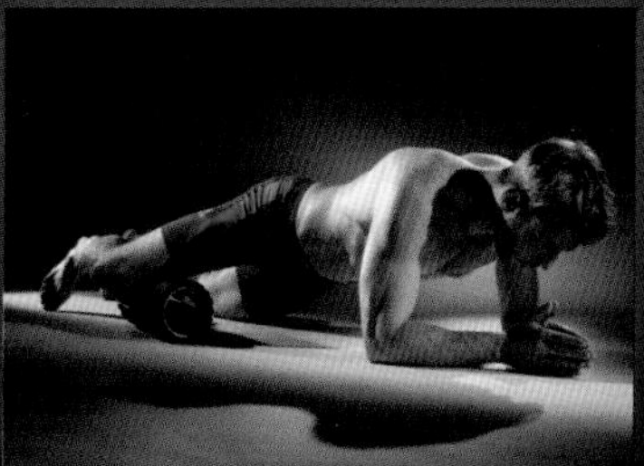

Endless problems are passively linked to sports or movement, to daily activity or inactivity, or to your history of injuries. It is almost impossible to provide an approach that covers everything. We will look at the causes of pain that affect a majority of this book's readers. You will see that there are some exercises that are much more effective than others. You will find a particularly rich selection of exercises, but, naturally, they will not all be of use to you. You can take the exercises you like and spend time on the most urgent areas or consider using the less effective exercises in your next training session.

Above all, this book is for people who suffer from chronic muscular pain linked to psychological or physical stress.

We would like to remind you that this book is written for healthy people who do not suffer from any injuries or trauma that may require surgery, medical treatment, or physical therapy. Above all, this book is for people who suffer from chronic muscular pain linked to psychological or physical stress.

THE BASIC RULES FOR A RESET

Pathological pain can result from a medical cause or be linked to an injury, an accident, a severe postural disorder, or an illness. For all other cases, we believe that pain is unacceptable.

Treating pain is a goal. But as long as postural disorders persist, *pain will return*; as long as bad motor habits exist, *pain will return*. As long as tightness persists, *pain will return*.

It is therefore essential to restore the functional mechanics of movement and posture by following some simple rules. Kelly Starrett, in his book *Deskbound*, suggests four rules.

- **If something is out of place, put it back:** This is the starting point. Take back control of your posture.
- **If something does not move, make it move:** Inactivity locks us into long-term functional limitations. Stiffness becomes more and more common, and pain happens earlier during movement, which can limit mobility.
- **Mobilize areas of localized pain:** Moving a painful area of muscle is essential to alleviate pain. Combined with a pressure point or self-massage, this technique allows you to combat muscular spasms and areas of adhesion effectively.
- **Work above and below the pain to alleviate mechanical restrictions:** Think of the muscles and tendons as a system that goes beyond local pain, which often originates from another blockage point. You should not treat pain only in the painful area or where there is restricted movement. You should also systematically treat above and below this area to treat the zone effectively.

LIMITING THE EXCLUSIVE USE OF SELF-MASSAGE

Because self-massage can be addictive, it is tempting to only use self-massage. But remember that the aim is not just to track down the location of the pain. You must put all that work back into moving and regaining range and motor control. Therefore, do not completely separate self-massage from stretching and motor control exercises.

THE THEORETICAL NEED FOR AN ANALYTICAL APPROACH

If a huge amount of pain is fixed locally, the causes are almost always general (read the chapter dedicated to muscle chains). Keep in mind the rule of "above and below," and do not settle for just treating the place where it hurts and only when it hurts; you must also explore and systematically treat the areas above and below, whether they are painful or not.

You should also regularly maintain each area. For clarity, we have chosen to categorize exercises by painful areas, but do not forget that if your knee is sore, you must also treat the area from the hip to the knee (inclusive) and the area from the ankle to the knee (inclusive). Do not forget to treat the rest of your body a bit too, even if you do not have pain anywhere else!

WHAT DO YOU NEED?

This book, as you will quickly learn, is not enough on its own. Rather, you need a complete toolkit and, depending on the part of the body that you are focusing on, some tools are more appropriate than others.

Power band: At least two elastic bands are required for many stretching, mobility, and joint distraction exercises. We recommend a violet band that provides an average resistance by most manufacturers, as well as a red one, which is more moderate.

Massage roller: The most classic mobility and recovery tool, the massage roller allows you to treat almost all areas of the body. It is particularly appropriate for massaging the posterior muscle chain and lower limbs.

Small-diameter massage ball: Also called a *lacrosse ball*, this ball is generally made of dense rubber and allows you to deeply massage numerous areas of the body.

Double massage ball: This ball allows you to treat two areas side by side at the same time or to work on two parts of a muscle or tendon.

Large-diameter massage ball: This ball allows you to do the work of a massage roller but with more intensity and specificity in certain areas. It also allows you to raise your body and target areas that a small-diameter ball cannot reach, such as the hip flexors and adductors. Rather than having to lie on the floor to use a small ball, it may be better to use a larger ball so you can lift up your body and treat these areas more comfortably.

Exercise ball: Also known as a *stability ball*, this tool is not just for training the core. It is also a powerful mobility tool.

Gym mat: To be effective, self-massage and stretching should be practiced in a comfortable environment. There's no point in staying on your knees on the floor or on your elbows on the tile for several minutes if the goal is to relax. Though it is not a requirement, using a mat is strongly recommended.

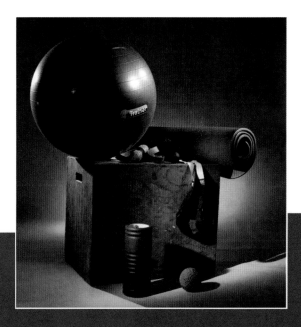

BACK PAIN: THE LUMBAR AREA

One of the most common pains is found in the lower back (also called the *lumbar* area or region), an area that is quite often the origin of many kinds of tension and pain.

Here, many muscles are exposed to significant stress. The lower back is, in effect, a concentration point of force for both posture and movement and a layered collection of many muscles. The quadratus lumborum; the lower insertions of the latissimus dorsi, iliocostalis, and longissimus; and, more deeply, the multifidus and the erector spinae can all become tense, from the *sacrum* (the tail bone) all the way to the 11th or 12th thoracic vertebrae (the base of the ribs) and across the width of the torso.

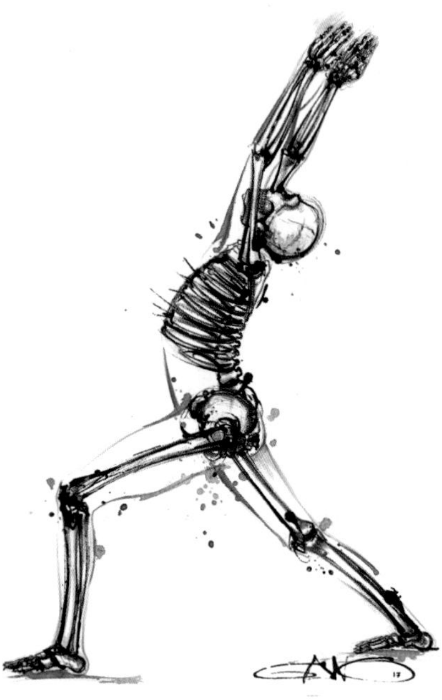

The causes of pain are numerous because this area is complex from a muscular point of view:

→ Because several muscle layers overlap at the curvature of the lumbar region, it is sometimes difficult to pinpoint a sensitive muscle. Often, the whole area must be treated.

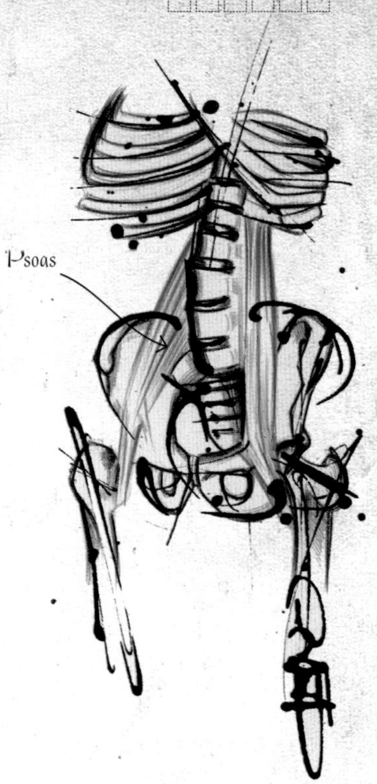

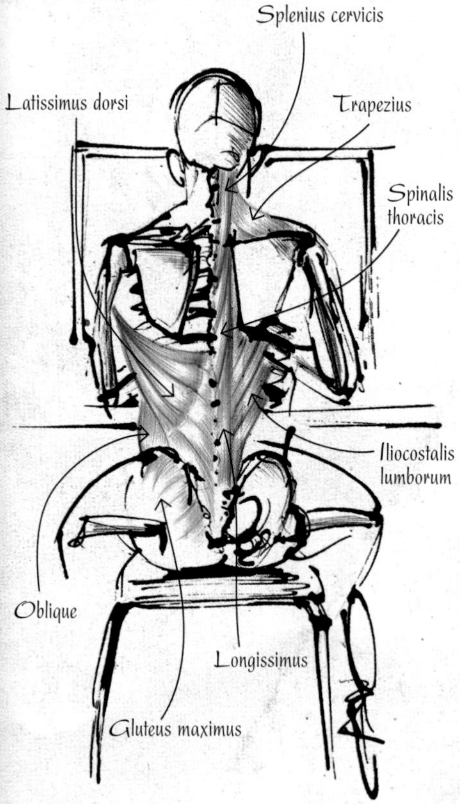

→ The problem is often more general than it seems: The iliopsoas muscles are attached to the lumbar area. If they are too strong, too weak, or too stiff, pain can arise from compensating muscles. Stretching, strengthening, mobilizing, and relaxing the iliopsoas muscles are daily priorities in the struggle against back pain.

→ There is often an imbalance: Abdominal muscles that are overdeveloped compared to the muscles in the lumbar region can also be a source of pain. Therefore, exercises for the abdominals and the lumbar region should always be balanced.

→ Weakness or localized stiffness in the muscles in the lumbar region should not be ignored; it is essential to properly strengthen both the powerful surface muscles as well as the deeper spinal muscles.

THE SCAN

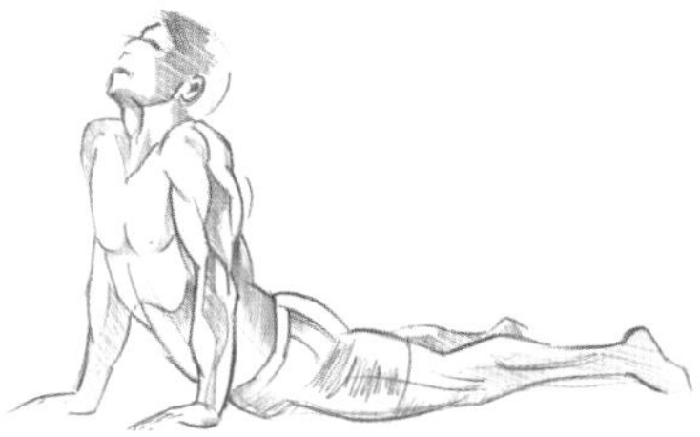

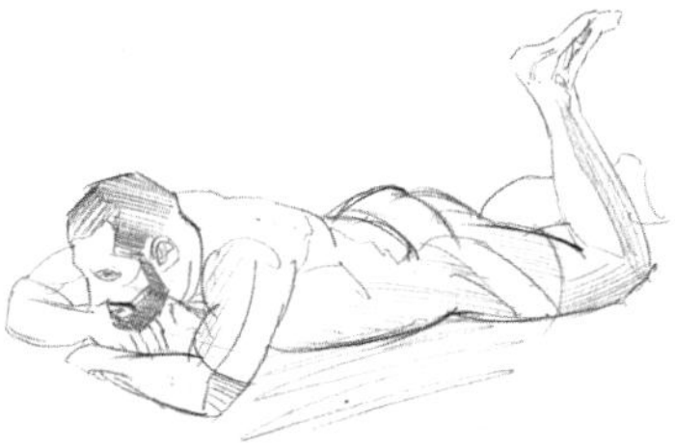

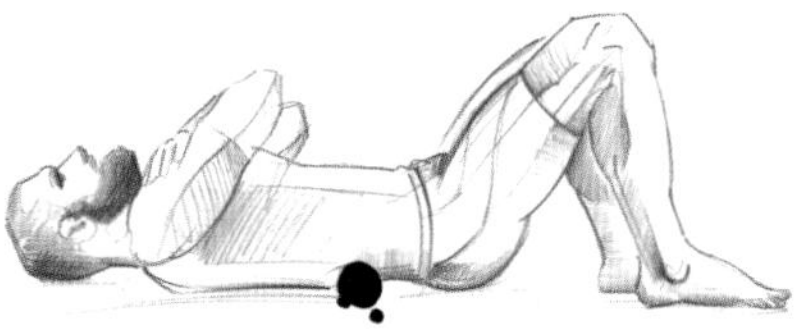

In addition to everyday pain, which often provides sufficient information about the needs in a certain area, a deep scan can reveal areas in the lumbar region that need attention. Here are three exercises to include in the scan:

1

The sphinx position: Lie flat on your stomach with your hands at the sides of your hips. Extend your spine while looking up.

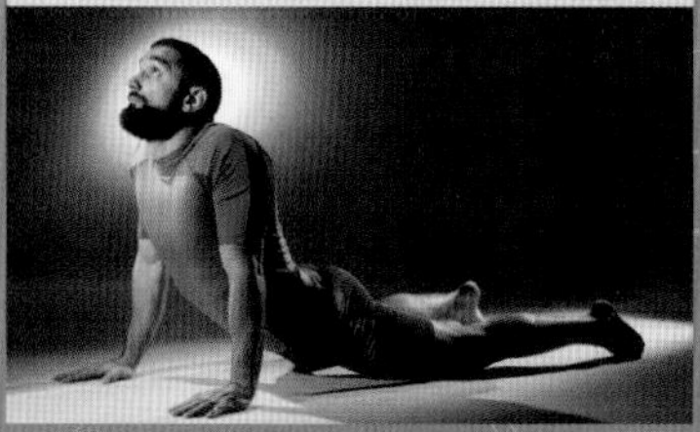

2

The Woolsey test: Stretch out flat on your stomach with your arms crossed under your chin. Try to flex your knee and touch your heel to your buttock. You should be able to flex your knee past 120 degrees without lifting your hip or flexing your pelvis. Do this movement with each leg.

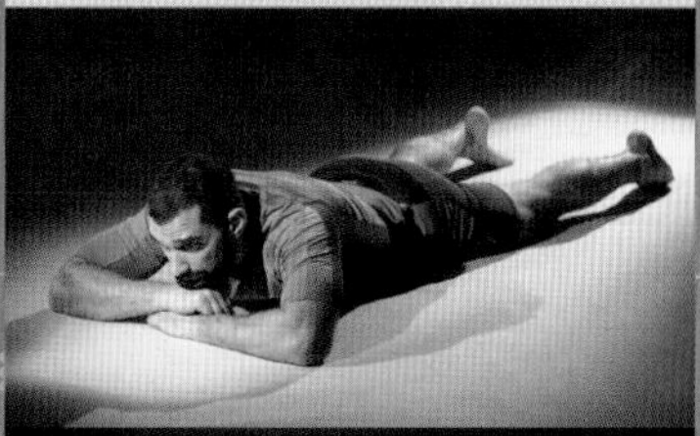

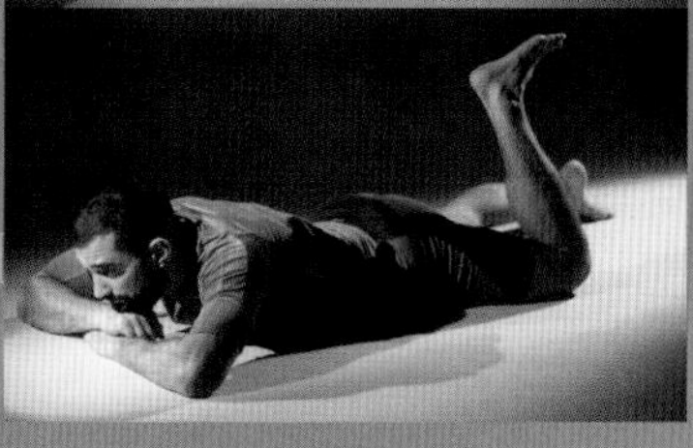

3

Placing the ball between the ribs and the pelvis: Lie on your back, place your feet flat on the floor, and flex your knees to 90 degrees. Slide a ball under the soft lumbar region (avoiding the spine) and move the ball around as you search for painful areas.

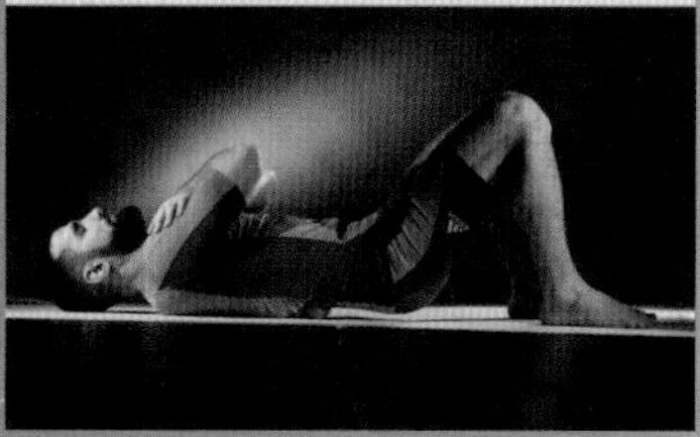

Any acute pain experienced during any of these exercises requires an appointment with your health care professional for a thorough examination. If you experience moderate pain or stiffness during these movements, it means you should perform one or more of the exercises every day.

A1. ROLLER MASSAGE

It is always good to start a muscle exercise session with roller massage, which allows you to gradually relax a large area and to pinpoint more sensitive areas from the outset. To make it more effective, cross your arms over your chest and grab your shoulders. You can roll from the top to the bottom, with your back oriented diagonally to the ground (like in the photo). You can also rotate your torso to the side with your torso parallel to the ground. We encourage you to always work on the links above and below in the muscle chain in equal measures.

Perform 1 to 3 reps of 1 minute.

If you detect a trigger point within the tense area, you can spend more time on it by alternating strong pressure and weak pressure every 5 seconds.

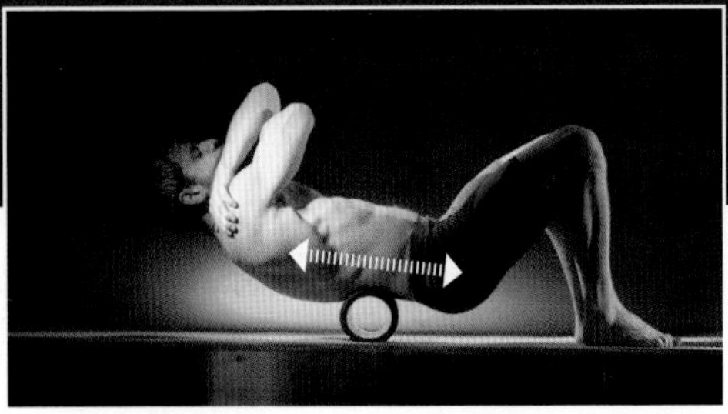

A2. GLUTE MASSAGE USING A ROLLER

Fold your right ankle over your left knee to work on the right gluteal muscles. Look for painful areas by moving bit by bit along the *gluteus maximus* (the thickest part of the buttocks) and the *gluteus medius* (the outer side of the buttocks).

Perform 10 reps front to back and 10 reps left to right before switching legs. Repeat up to 3 times.

If you detect a trigger point within the tense area, you can spend more time on it by alternating strong pressure and weak pressure every 5 seconds.

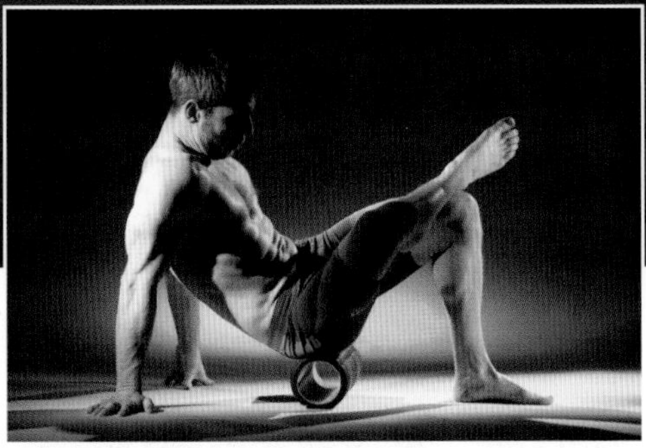

A3. ROLLER STRETCHES

Lie on your back and slide the massage roller under the lumbar area. Relax yourself completely by combining this stretch with breathing exercises (see part II on breathing).

Perform 3 sets of 20 seconds per movement with no rest (2 minutes total).

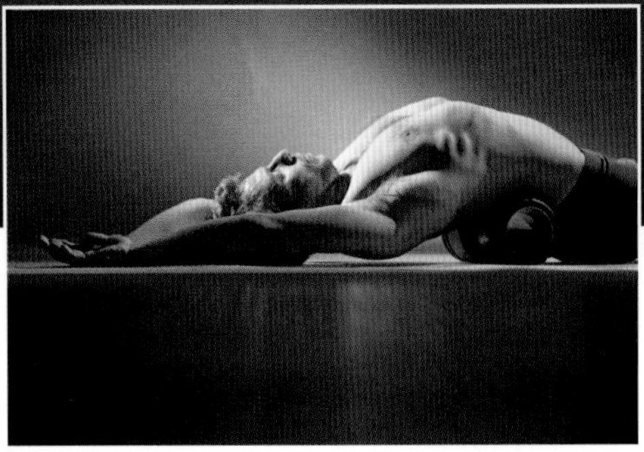

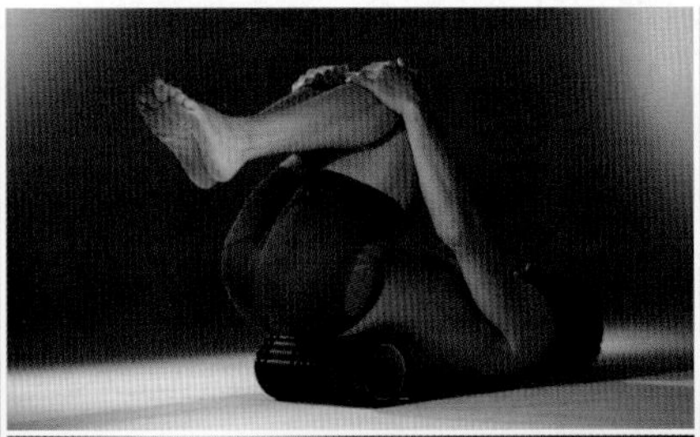

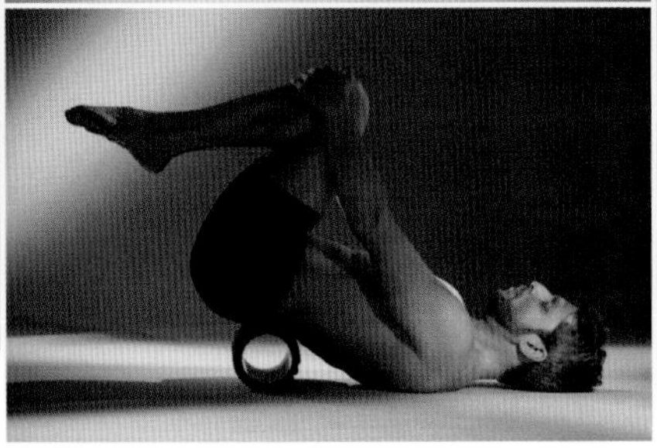

Alternate every 20 seconds between doing this sustained, exaggerated stretch and bringing your knees in toward your chest.

A4. STRETCHING THE FUNCTIONAL CHAIN

Standing with your feet parallel, flex your torso forward and try to relax as you exhale to stretch the lumbar area as much as possible. Inhale again using the diaphragm and move into a forward lunge. Lift your arms overhead and look upward. Repeat this cycle 5 times, or 10 movements, to make 1 set.

Perform 3 sets of 10 movements with 30 seconds of rest between sets.

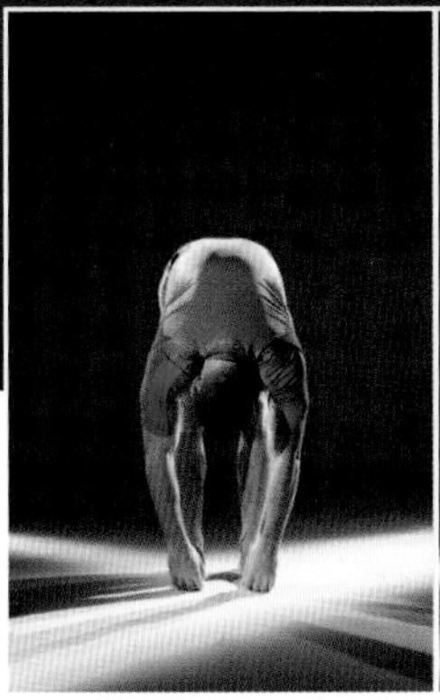

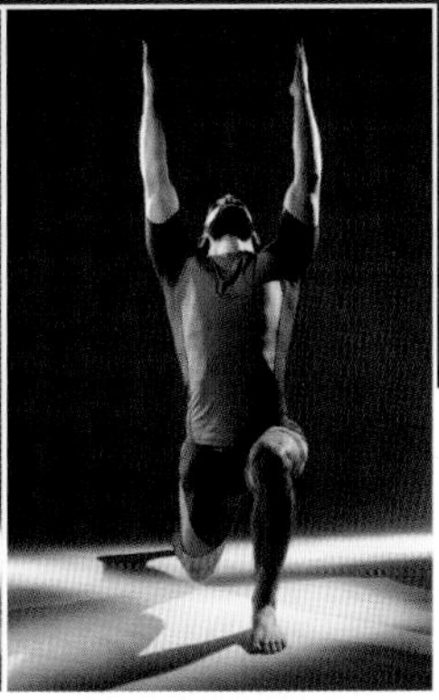

A5. MASSAGE USING A BALL WITH FEET RAISED

Lie on your back, place your feet on a chair or box, and support your head comfortably using a massage roller. Slide a massage ball under the lumbar area and lift your hips to apply pressure on the ball. Move the ball around to explore the area from the top of the gluteals (or the base of the lower back) to the 10th rib; any area could be sensitive depending on your activities and habits. If the whole area is sensitive, start at the bottom and gradually move up until, after several sessions, the pain lessens or disappears.

Perform 3 sets of 1 minute per side. (If painful, 20 seconds is enough.)
If you detect a trigger point within the tense area, you can spend more time on it by alternating strong pressure and weak pressure every 5 seconds.

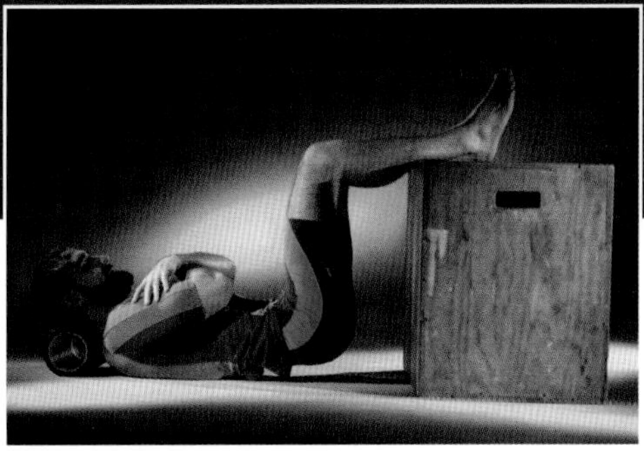

A6. STANDING GLUTE MASSAGE USING A BALL

It is common for lower back pain to radiate from tension in the gluteal muscles. With your back to a wall and knees slightly flexed, place a ball between your glutes and the wall and move the ball around to explore the upper areas of the gluteus maximus.

Perform 3 sets of 1 minute per side. (If painful, 20 seconds is enough.)

If you detect a trigger point within the tense area, you can spend more time on it by alternating strong pressure and weak pressure every 5 seconds.

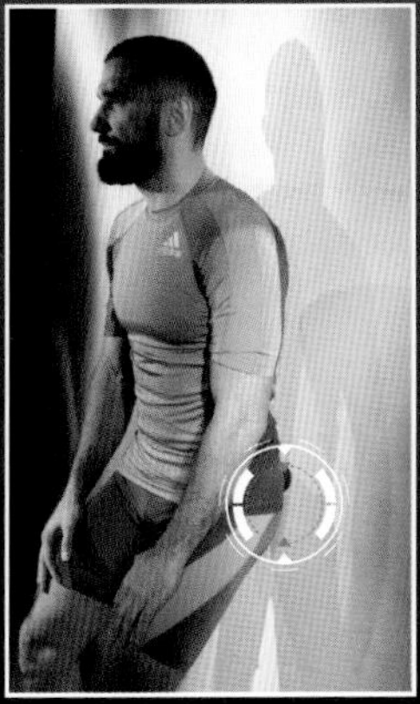

A7. REPOSITIONING JOINTS (WITH OR WITHOUT ANCHORING THE HANDS)

The principle of this exercise is to guide the *femur* (the upper thigh bone) to passively reposition itself within the *ilio-femoral cavity*, commonly called the hip joint. It is also a powerful stretch for the muscles in the lumbar region that are rarely stretched, such as the quadratus lumborum.

Lie on your back and attach a band to a stationary piece of equipment or lock the band in a door. Create a loop around your ankle, as shown in the photo, and move back to place your leg and the band in the extended position, as shown. It is very important to completely relax your leg; do not resist the traction but allow your leg to be pulled straight. A variation is to hold on to a weight plate or kettlebell above your head to allow the traction to pull through the entire muscle chain.

Perform 3 sets of 40 seconds per leg.

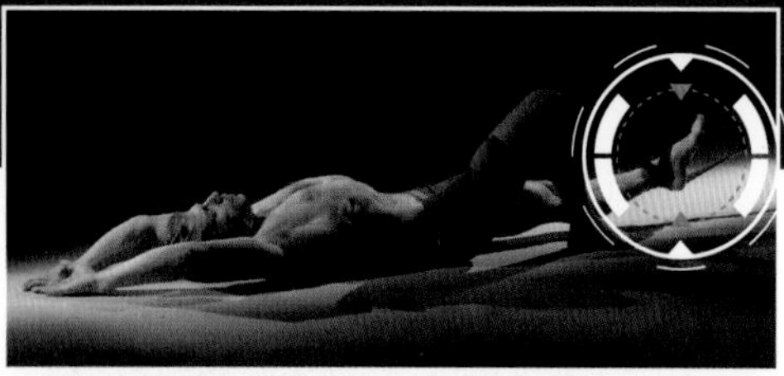

A8. RESETTING THE PELVIS

Back pain often originates from a displacement of the pelvis, which a health care professional must subsequently correct during therapy sessions. This displacement can be limited or even avoided by practicing a simple reset exercise: Lie on your back with your feet and knees raised and apply two opposing pressures on the knees by pushing the right knee downward against the right hand while the left knee pushes upward against the left hand.

Perform 3 sets of 5 seconds per knee.

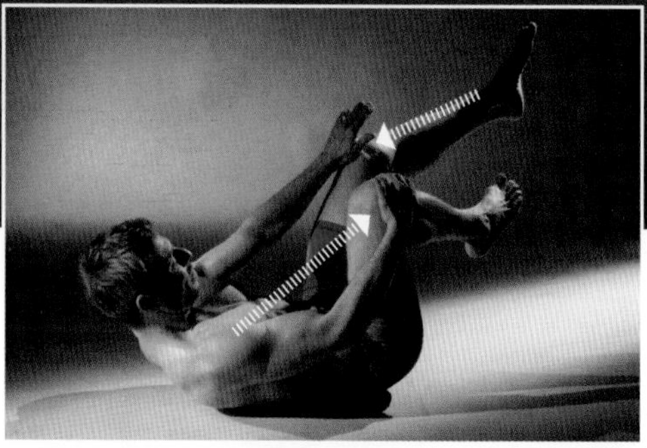

A9. ADVANCED SPHINX

A lack of lumbar mobility is often the cause of pain. It is imperative to return to a normal range of motion of the lumbar area by fixing the hips on or near the floor to prevent other muscles from compensating. A resistance band that anchors your hips and the lumbar area can be used to increase the intensity of this pose.

Perform 3 to 5 sets of 8 reps with a 3- to 5-second hold in full extension.

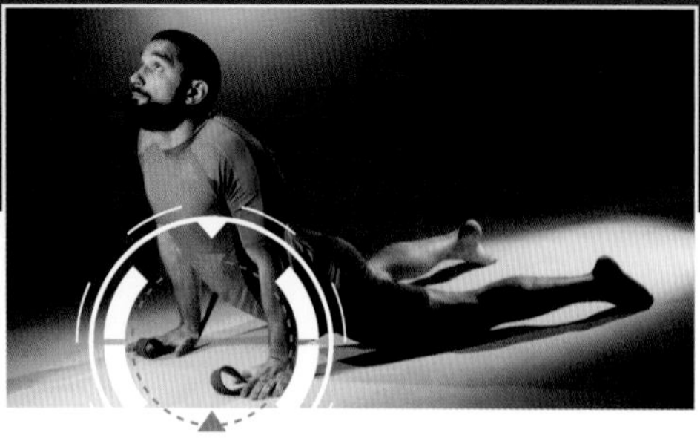

A10. STANDING BACK EXTENSION

To improve movement, sometimes you simply have to move. Often, pain only occurs at the start of an exercise, and you must simply continue to move to alleviate it. Standing with your feet hip-width apart, look at the ceiling to extend the back as much as possible. Avoid compensating with your hips and neck and concentrate on fully extending the lumbar area, which you should aim to increase every time you repeat the exercise. This exercise can be intensified by bracing the thighs against a bar or table before performing the movement.

Perform 3 to 5 sets of 8 reps with a 3- to 5-second hold in full extension.

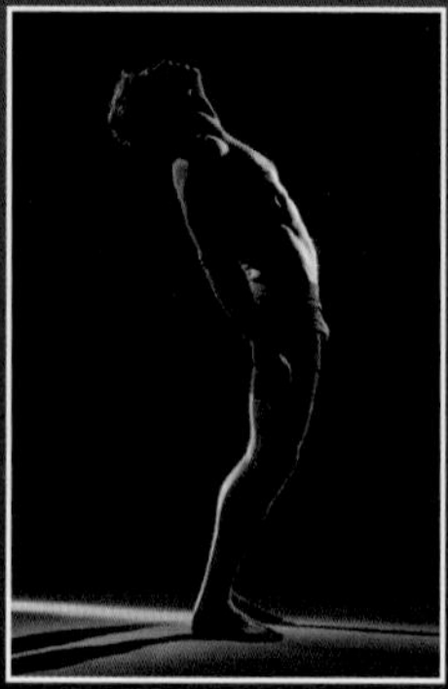

Sample 3-week mobility program targeting the lumbar area (including exercises for neighboring areas)

MONDAY	TUESDAY	WEDNESDAY	THURSDAY	FRIDAY	SATURDAY	SUNDAY
A1*, A2, A10, A3, A4	B10, B2, B5, B4, B6	A1, A8, A7, A6, A9	C7, C12, C13, C9, C10, C17	A1, A5, A10, A5, A9	C12, C2, B2, B4, A5, A10	A7, A1, A2, A5, A4

*These letter/number combinations refer to the exercises and techniques found on pages 26 through 76.

BACK PAIN: THE THORACIC SPINE

The middle or center part of the back is the *thoracic spine*—the part of the spine that serves as the base of the ribs—and it is particularly vulnerable to pain. From a functional point of view, the muscles in this area interact between the shoulders and the back.

There is no doubt that sitting with a curved thoracic spine creates a vicious dynamic between the shoulders and the upper back, pulling the shoulders more and more inward and making the curve in the upper back painful and ineffective. The neck is, to a lesser degree, also linked to this system, particularly by the splenius cervicis muscle, which inserts onto the thoracic vertebrae in this area.

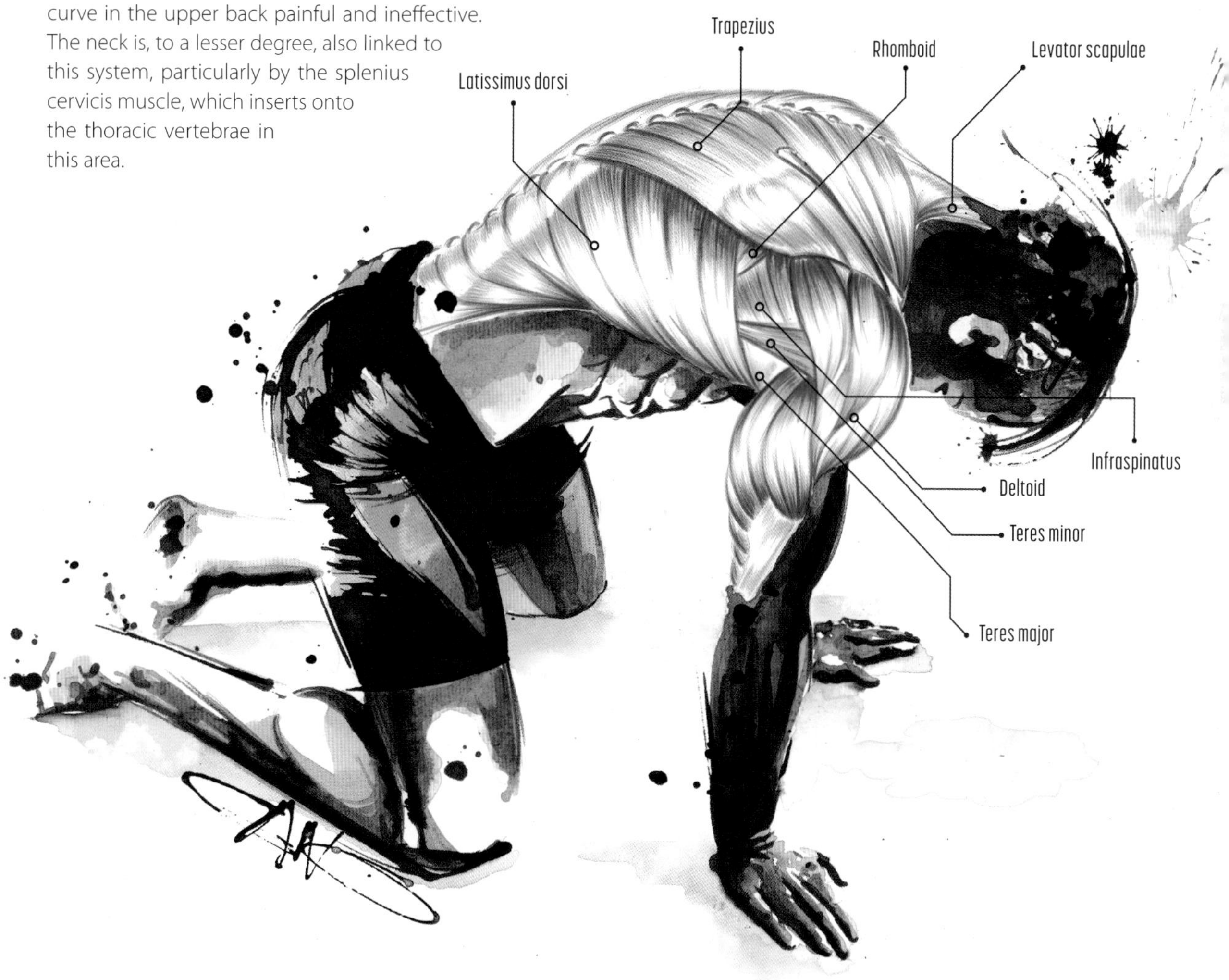

The first layer of the back muscles in the middle region are often strained: The longissimus and the erector spinae are particularly affected. Since the splenius cervicis, rhomboids, and trapezius muscles are also located here, they can be affected too. The rotator cuff muscles and the latissimus dorsi must also be given attention because some of their insertions are in this region and they can radiate negatively into this specific area. Further, psychological stress can also add to an already weakened mechanical system.

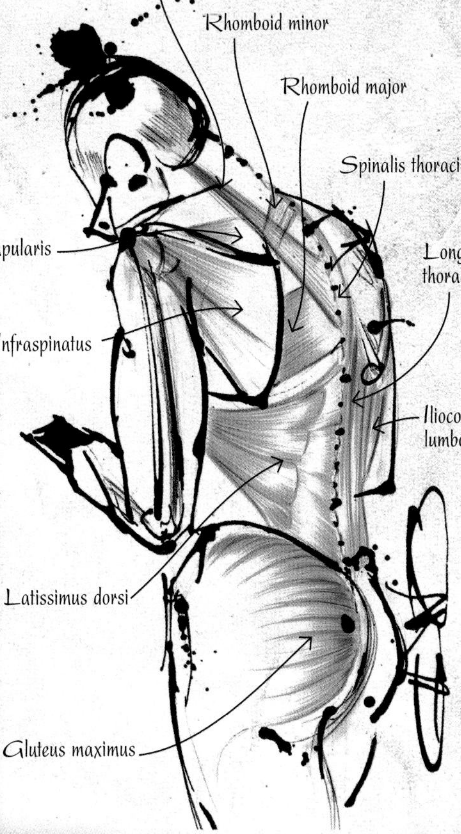

CORRECTING THIS POSTURAL DISORDER RELIEVES BOTH PHYSICAL AND PSYCHOLOGICAL PROBLEMS

- Stop putting up with your default posture: You are in charge, so take back control. Open your chest, pull your shoulders back, and straighten yourself. Ask the people you trust to remind you if necessary. Correcting your posture is a continuous exercise.
- Some people may adopt poor postures due to shyness, lack of confidence, or lack of motivation. Occupy the space; do not hide yourself! Only your posture is changing, not your visibility; do not damage your health by slumping.
- Remember that problems are rarely isolated. Sometimes you must turn around to see the problem more easily. In this case, the issue could simply be caused by stiffness of the pectoralis minor of the chest!
- It is often a flexibility issue rather than a strength issue. Think about testing, stretching, and strengthening the rotator cuff muscles (infraspinatus, supraspinatus, teres minor, teres major, long head of the biceps, and the subscapularis) to strengthen and relax the muscles around the shoulder blades (particularly the rhomboid minor and rhomboid major). Relax the latissimus dorsi, trapezius, and pectoralis minor muscles.

BACK MUSCLES: POTENTIAL TRAPS

A common mistake that some coaches make is to train athletes who have problems in the upper back using pulling exercises. They use exercises that significantly open up the rib cage area such as lat pulldowns, wide-grip low pulley rows, or even bench pulls. This strategy rarely works:

- These exercises essentially target the latissimus dorsi, especially in beginners who struggle to activate their rotator cuff muscles and the muscles around their shoulder blades to lower their shoulders and bring the shoulder blades together. The latissimus dorsi is also rarely the weak link, but it will continue to take over during pulling and balancing movements. This prevents the muscles that are truly responsible for postural problems from getting stronger.
- These exercises create strong tension in the middle area of the back, restricting mobility and control of the area.
- These movements are especially isolated to simple motor movements. If the blockage is coming from another link in the chain, the problem will never be resolved.

We must therefore focus on the muscle and the fascial chains rather than take an analytical approach. If a focus on a link in the chain is required, it is most likely needed in the rotator cuff muscles (strength and/or stiffness), shoulder blade muscles (strength), and the pectoralis minor (stiffness).

THE SCAN

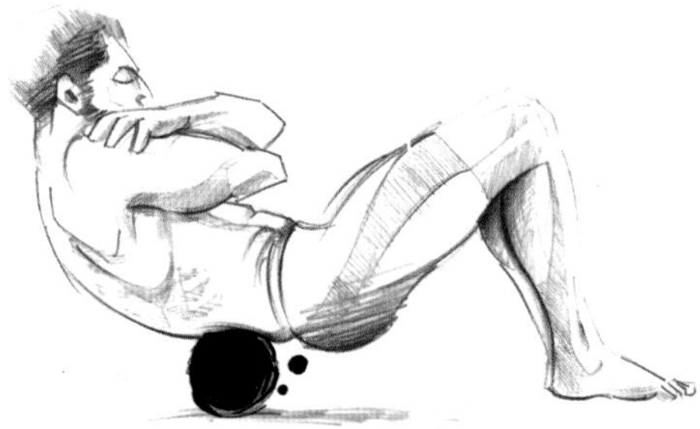

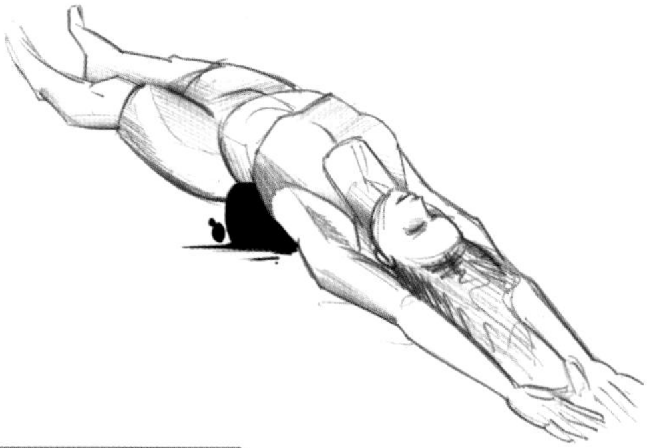

In addition to everyday pain, which often provides sufficient information about the needs in a certain area, a deep scan can reveal areas of the thoracic spine that need attention. Here are two exercises to include in the scan:

1

The rolling pin: Simply roll back and forth on a massage roller, looking for tight or painful areas. Do this as it comes naturally. Do not look for a point to massage; just "listen" to the pain.

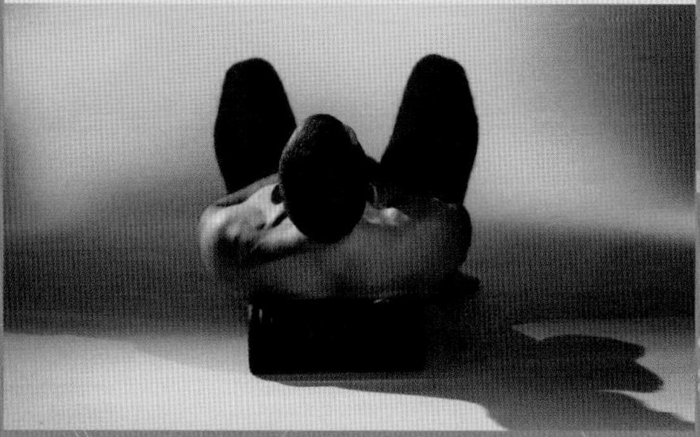

2

Full extension on a roller: Stretch out on your back and slide the roller under your upper back. Try to lengthen yourself as much as possible, using not only your arms and legs but also your head.

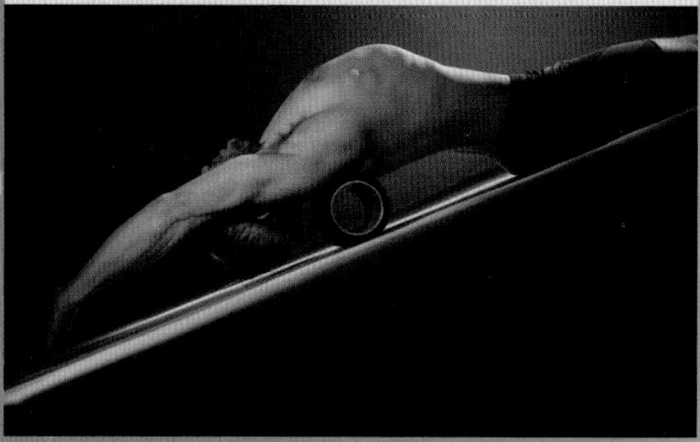

Any acute pain experienced during any of these exercises requires an appointment with your health care professional for a thorough examination. If you experience moderate pain or stiffness during these movements, it means you should perform one or more of the exercises every day.

B1. RELAXATION ON PARALLEL BARS

Supporting yourself with your elbows and forearms, simply suspend yourself on the parallel bars. Lock into the position by contracting your shoulders. The rest of your back should be relaxed.

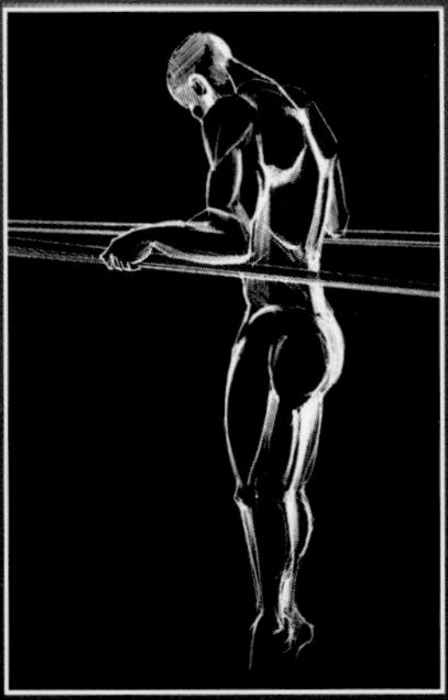

Perform 1 to 3 sets of 15 to 30 seconds, depending on your ability to hold the position.

B2. MASSAGE USING A ROLLER

Lie on your back with your arms crossed over your chest and try to hold onto your shoulders as far back as possible. Roll from the bottom to the top very slowly, rolling over the vertebrae one by one and allowing them to gently fall into place one after the other. Repeat 1 to 3 times if necessary, then work on the stiffest areas by opening up your chest and closing it. Spend at least 5 seconds in the open position and move the roller slightly if necessary to reach the most important areas. For more advanced practitioners, hold the stretch for up to 1 minute.

Perform 1 to 3 slow and controlled sets from bottom to top. Then perform 1 to 3 sets of 6 open/close movements, holding for 5 seconds in the open position.

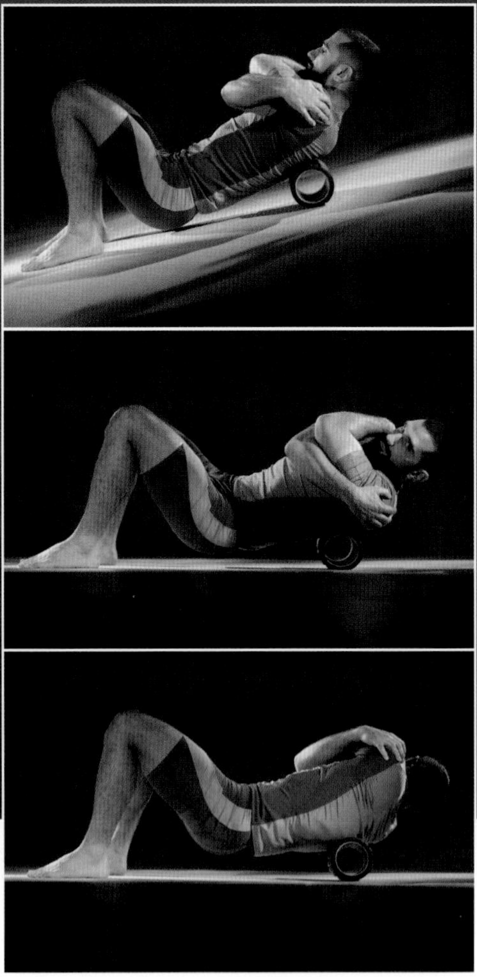

B3. SIDE MASSAGE USING A ROLLER (WITH A LONG ROLLER TO REST THE HEAD)

Lie on your back with the roller along the spine and allow your arms to hang on both sides. Gently roll from left to right 10 times (5 times on each side).

Perform 1 to 3 slow and controlled sets from side to side.

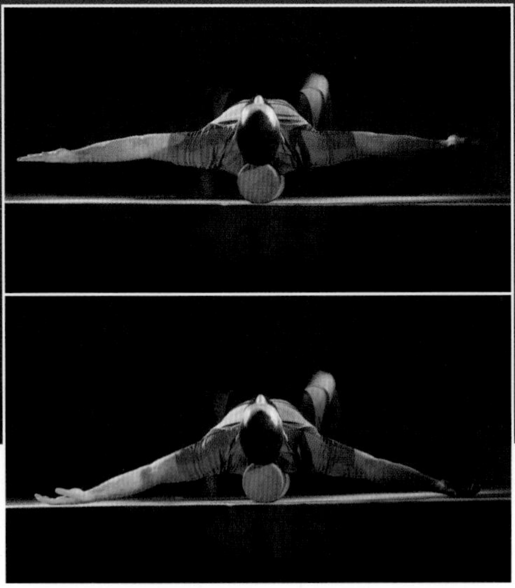

B4. STRETCHING THE THORACIC SPINE

Sit on the floor against a wall, lift your arms, and try to make yourself taller. Bring your feet as close as possible to your gluteals and push backward to flatten your back against the wall as much as you can. Push out your chest and try to make yourself as tall as possible, with your hands reaching over your head.

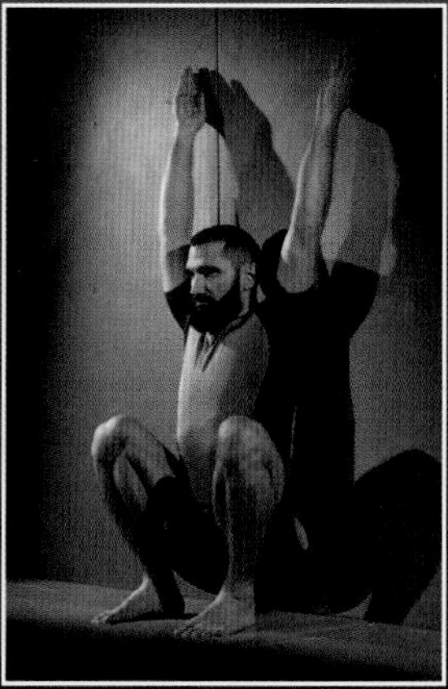

If this exercise is too difficult, simply begin by holding onto the back of a chair. Push out your chest and pull your shoulders back. Straighten your thoracic spine to align your back as much as possible and step back without letting go of the chair. Raise your arms so that your head is between your elbows. Try to push your chest forward.

Perform 2 or 3 stretches of 40 to 60 seconds each.

B5. CAT EXERCISE

On all fours, try to push out the upper back by rounding your back through the shoulder blades, lifting the top of your back as high as possible, and dropping your head. Then do exactly the opposite: Bring your back down as far as you can by slowly raising your head. Try to drive your shoulder blades toward the floor as much as possible.

Perform 3 to 8 reps.

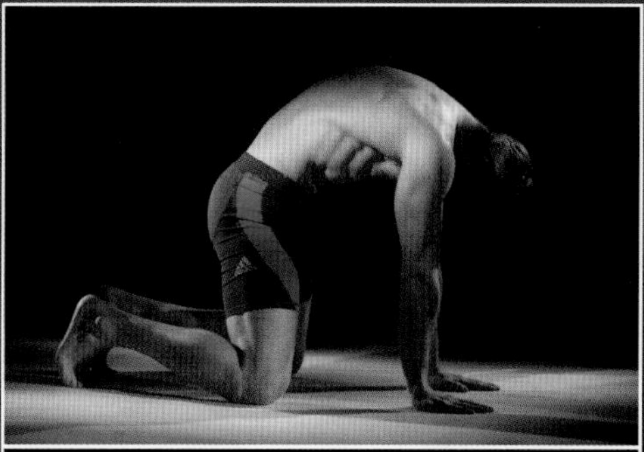

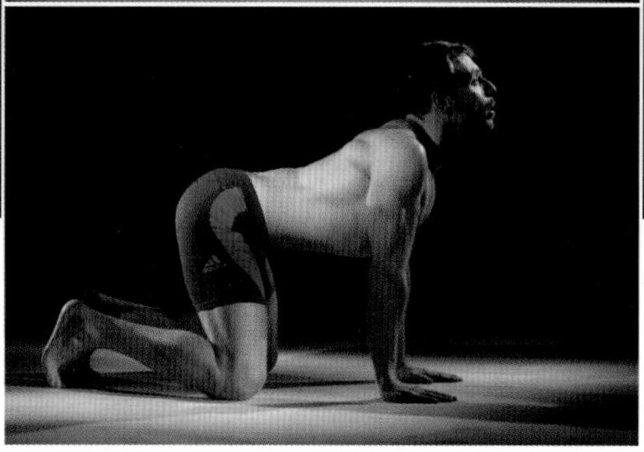

B6. FUNCTIONAL CHAIN STRETCH

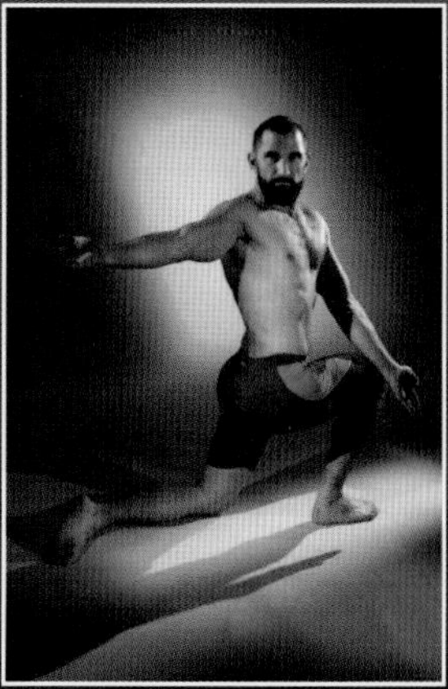

Begin in a lunge position on the floor, with your right knee just in front of your toes, your left knee on the floor, and the instep of your left foot flat on the floor. Put your left hand on the outside of your right knee and lead the rotation of your torso to the right with your right arm (kept parallel to the floor) reaching as far as possible behind you. Hold the position for 15 to 30 seconds then change sides.

Perform 1 to 3 stretches of 15 to 30 seconds per side.

B7. PECTORALIS MINOR MASSAGE AND STRETCH

Alternate between these two exercises. With a massage ball between your chest and the wall, massage the pectoralis minor for 30 seconds using the ball, then sit down with one leg extended. Place the foot of the extended leg in a loop at the end of a band and the hand of the side you massaged in the loop on the other end, as in the photo. Stretch your pectoralis minor by relaxing your shoulder (allow it to move backward). Manage the intensity of the stretch by tightening or loosening the leg and rotating the chest. Stretch for 20 to 30 seconds before starting again on the same muscle using the massage ball. When finished with that side, switch to the other side to alternate the massage and the stretch.

Perform 3 reps of 30 seconds of massage plus 20 to 30 seconds of stretching per side.

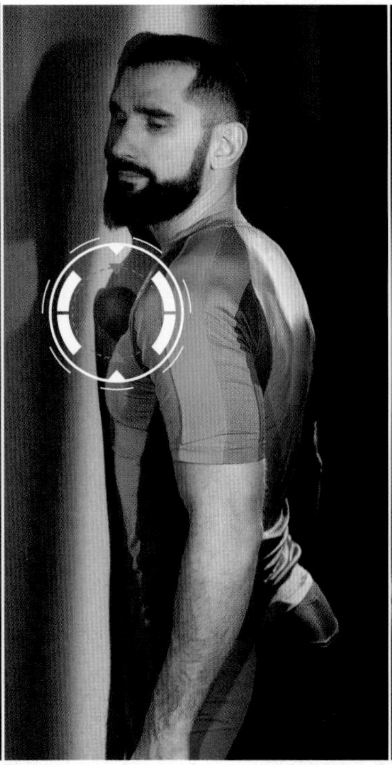

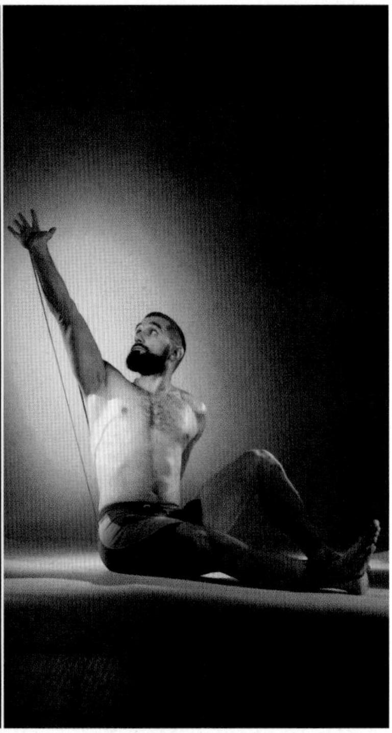

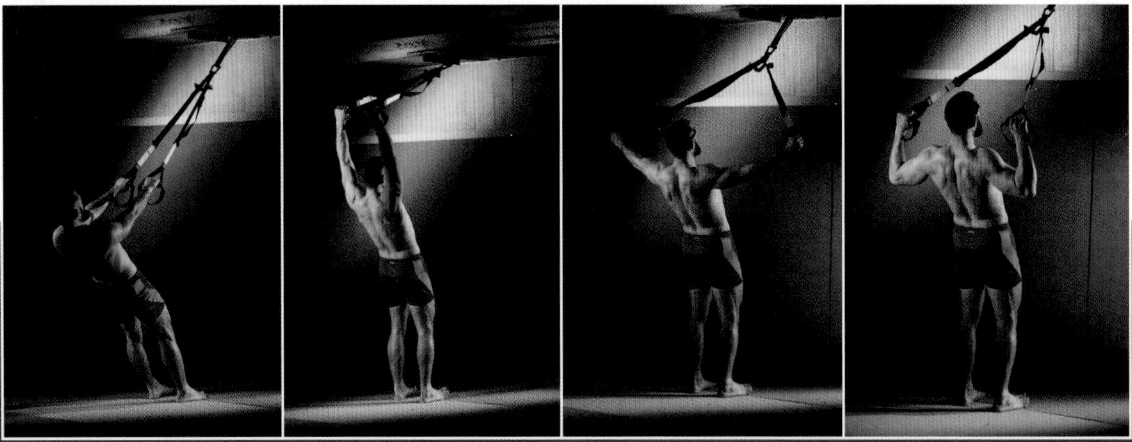

B8. ITW EXERCISES USING A SUSPENSION STRAP

Hang the strap from a fixed bar. Align your body fully and pull your shoulders back by bringing your shoulder blades together. Extend your arms above your head and straighten yourself without disrupting your body's alignment, making the shape of an I. Start again with the arms extended to the sides to form a T-shape, then open your arms and bend them at a 90-degree angle to form a W. The more you recline when starting this exercise, the harder it will be. The more you move your feet back to start the exercise in a raised position, the easier it will be.

Perform 3 to 4 sets of 12 reps (4 of each movement) with 45 seconds of rest between sets.

B9. LATERAL RAISES AND ROTATIONS USING A BAND

Attach a band to a gym ladder or lock it in a door with a strap. Begin the exercise with your arms at your sides and your elbows flexed at a 90-degree angle. Perform a lateral raise to bring your upper arms parallel to the ground. Without changing this position (do not let your elbows drop), rotate your upper arms at the shoulders so that your forearms are perpendicular to the ground. Repeat this sequence in reverse to finish the first set. **Perform 3 to 4 sets of 6 to 12 reps depending on the perceived difficulty.**

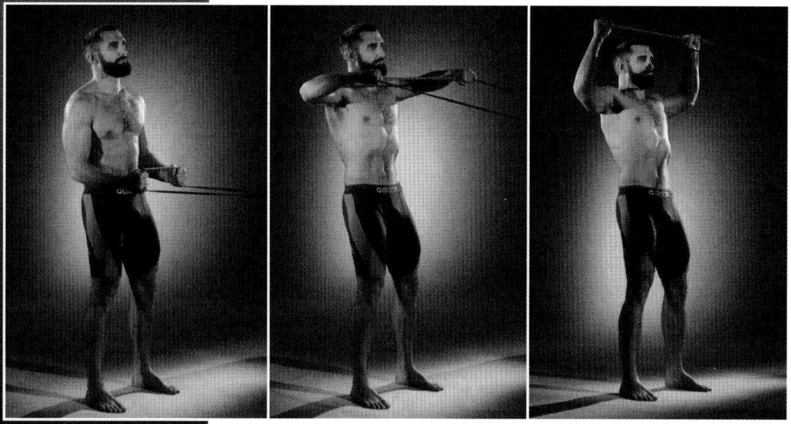

B10. LATISSIMUS DORSI, TERES MINOR, AND TERES MAJOR MASSAGE USING A ROLLER

Lie on your side with the roller under your armpit. Roll gently from top to bottom, then move your body from front to back, and finally rub across the muscle transversely.

Perform 1 to 3 sets of 10 up–down movements, 10 front–back movements, and 10 transverse movements.

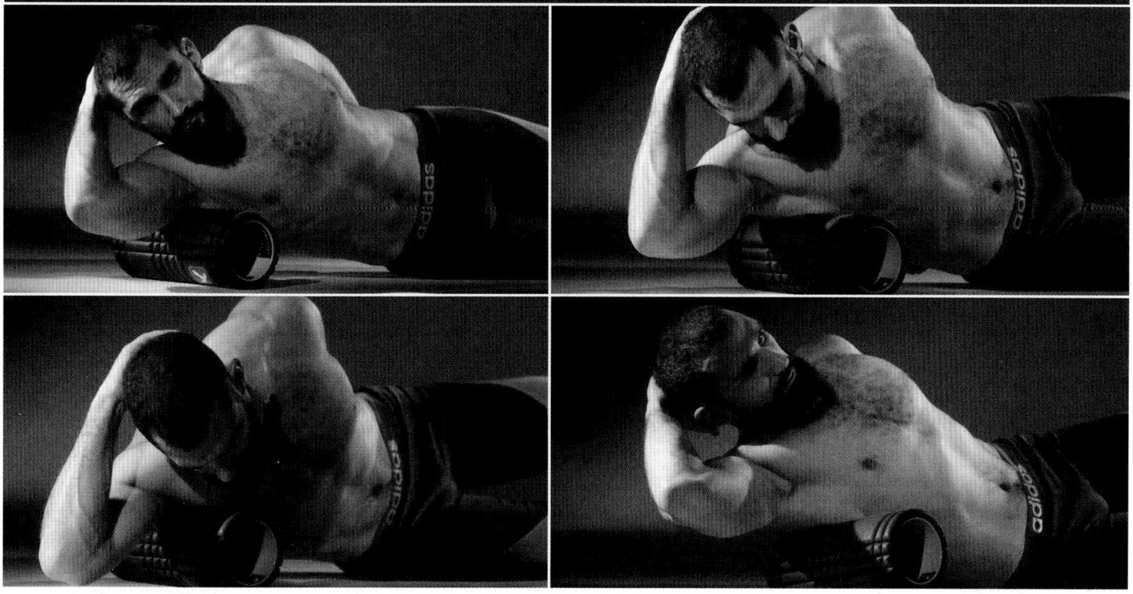

Sample 3-week mobility program targeting the thoracic spine (including exercises for neighboring areas)

MONDAY	TUESDAY	WEDNESDAY	THURSDAY	FRIDAY	SATURDAY	SUNDAY
B2*, B3, B1, B6	A1, A8, A7, A6, A9	B2, B3, B8, B9	C2, C6, C16, C11, C13, C15	B10, B2, B5, B4, B6	C12, C2, B2, B4, A5, A10	B7, B3, B4, B1, B6

*These letter/number combinations refer to the exercises and techniques found on pages 26 through 76.

THE PELVIC AREA

The pelvis is an area of the body that is particularly susceptible to stress.

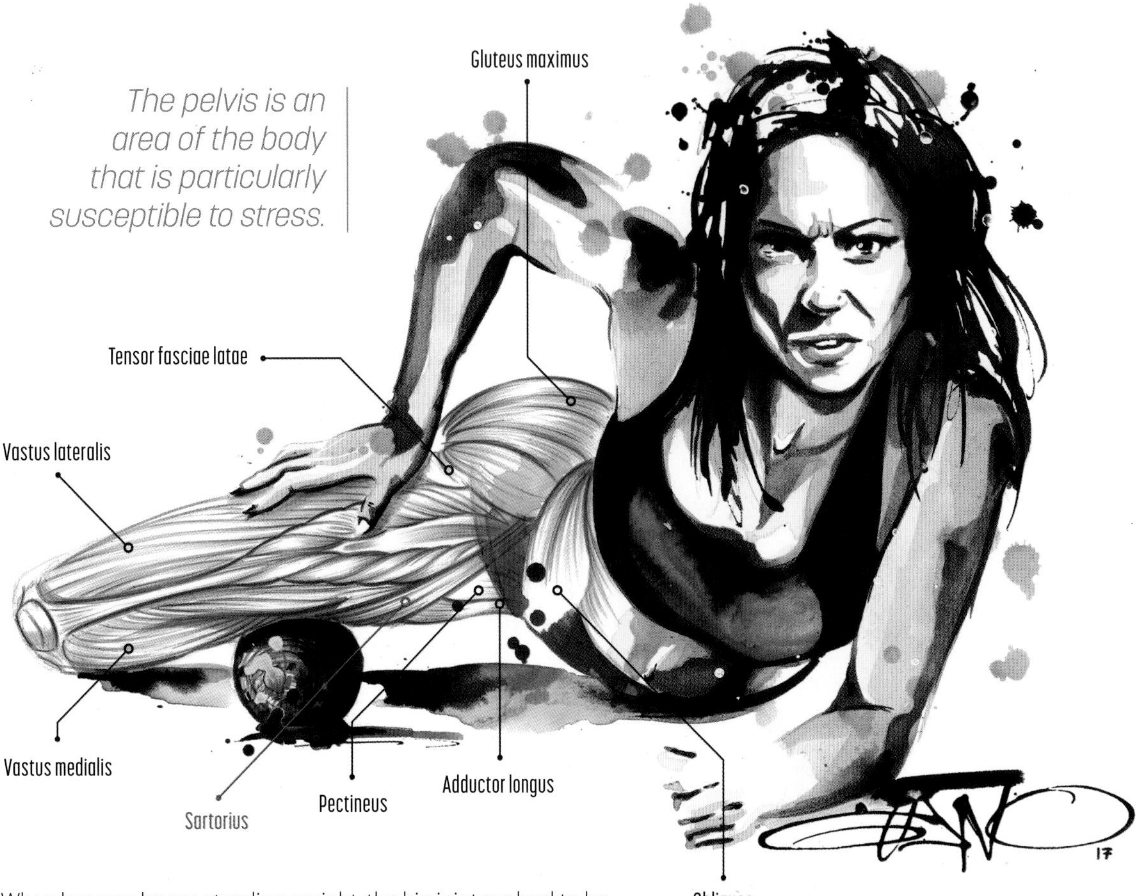
Gluteus maximus
Tensor fasciae latae
Vastus lateralis
Vastus medialis
Sartorius
Pectineus
Adductor longus
Obliques

When humans began standing upright, the hip joint evolved to be significantly more open, allowing for the possibility of many inflammatory mechanisms, numerous imbalances, and a large amount stiffness to appear. Additionally, the hip plays a role in many body positions, helps gather proprioceptive information, and affects movement ability. Its mobility, without pain, is essential for the proper functioning of our human machine.

Normally, the hip joint is especially mobile. Numerous muscle structures surrounding this joint ensure its optimal functioning. Stiffness, an imbalance, or weakness in one of these structures could potentially lead to localized inflammation, which could quickly spread to the whole area and turn into groin strain or hernia because these structures are close to each other and interconnected.

Let's examine the muscles of the pelvic area. First, there are the iliopsoas muscles, which are used almost constantly. From walking to sitting down to climbing stairs: all movements involving lifting the legs or flexing the torso use these muscles. Taking care of the iliopsoas should be a daily priority.

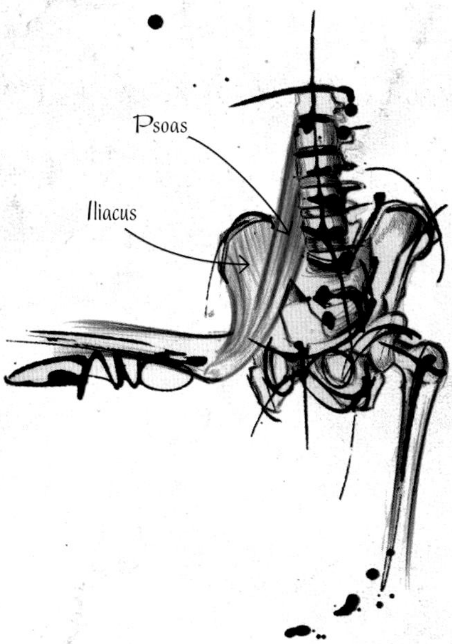

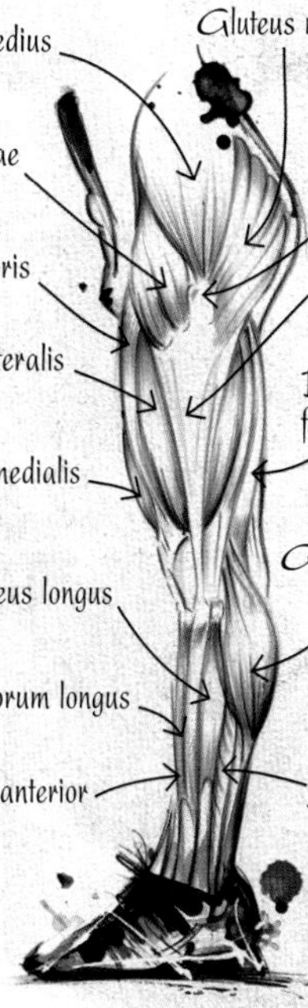

There is a support system on the outer part of the leg: the fasciae latae and its tensor (muscle), the IT band, and the *vastus lateralis* (the outer portion of the front of the thigh). If there is tension here or if an imbalance in strength or use develops between muscle pairs, it can lead to reduced mobility or even pain.

There are also the adductor muscles (gracilis, adductor longus, adductor magnus, sartorius, adductor brevis, and pectineus), which are often too weak and too stiff. The quadriceps and hamstring muscle complex should not be neglected either. These muscles suffer from limitations because they are directly involved in hip mobility, particularly the iliopsoas and gluteal muscles.

You must take the time to massage and stretch them. Then there are the gluteal muscles. Deep squats and lunges are particularly effective tools for developing the glutes in a comprehensive and functional manner.

→ Strengthen, stretch, and massage the iliopsoas muscles daily, even more if you are doing abdominal exercises or leg raises, forward bends, or knee raises. Help them to relax so you can maintain control.
→ Regularly self-massage and stretch the abductor muscles of the hips.
→ Regularly self-massage and stretch the adductor muscles of the hips.
→ Regularly self-massage and stretch the quadriceps and hamstring muscles.

THE SCAN

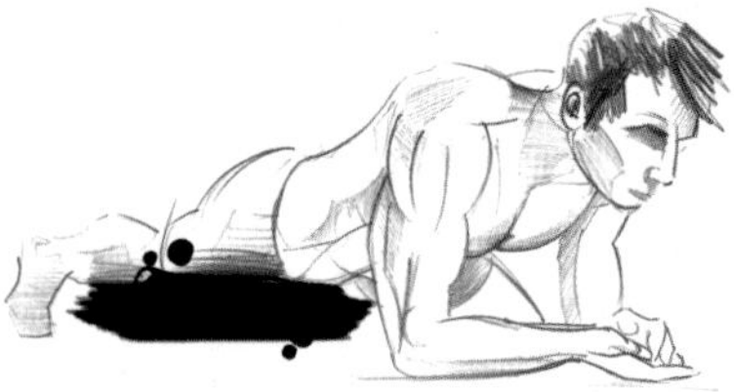

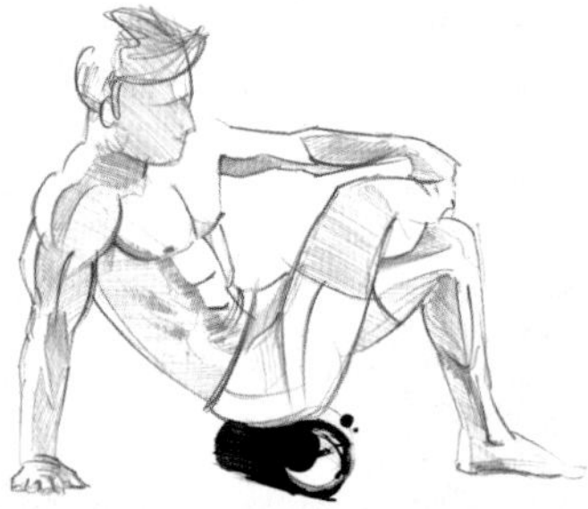

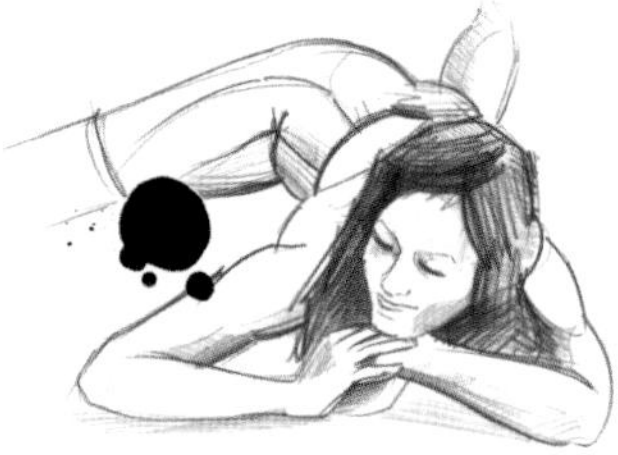

In addition to everyday pain, which often provides sufficient information about the needs in a certain area, a deep scan can reveal parts of the pelvic area that need attention. Here are four exercises to include in the scan:

1

Roller under the hip: Lie face down with the roller under your hip joint and extend the right leg straight back. Support yourself on your elbows and opposite knee, which is flexed, and then roll forward and backward.

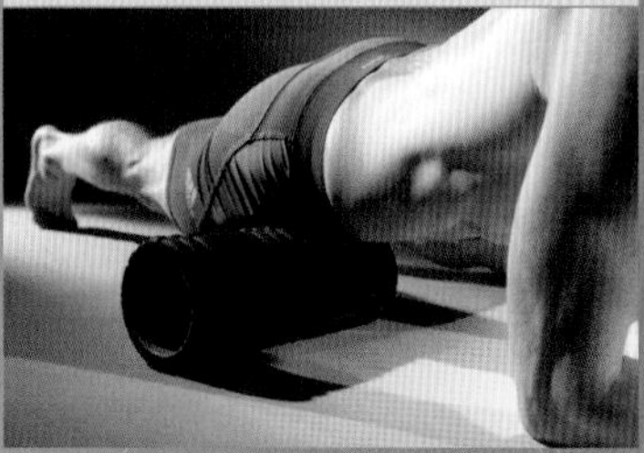

2

Sitting on the roller: Sit on the roller and roll from front to back, passing over one side and then the other. You will immediately feel the painful areas.

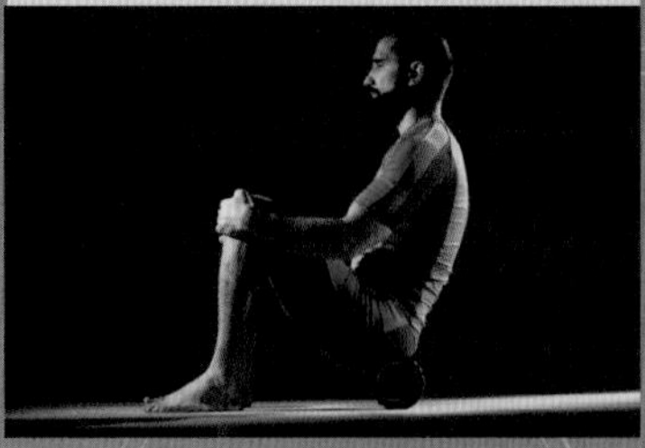

3

Inner thigh on the massage ball: Lie on your side and place a large-diameter massage ball (or a massage roller, but this is less precise) under your inner thigh. Do not try to massage it or place too much weight on it; simply look for any painful areas.

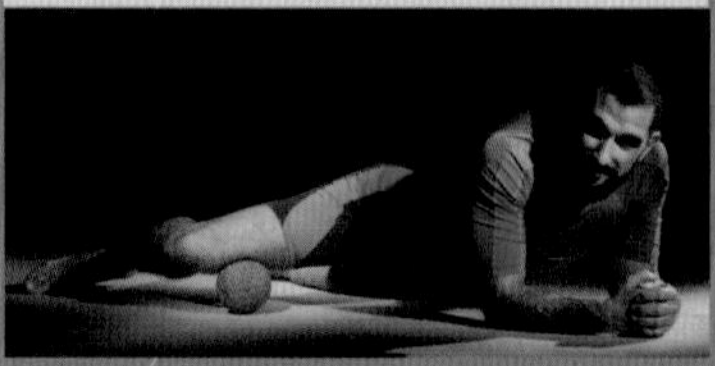

4

The Woolsey test: Stretch out flat on your stomach with your arms crossed under your chin. Try to flex your knee and touch your heel to your buttock. You should be able to flex your knee past 120 degrees without lifting your hip or flexing your pelvis. Do this movement with each leg.

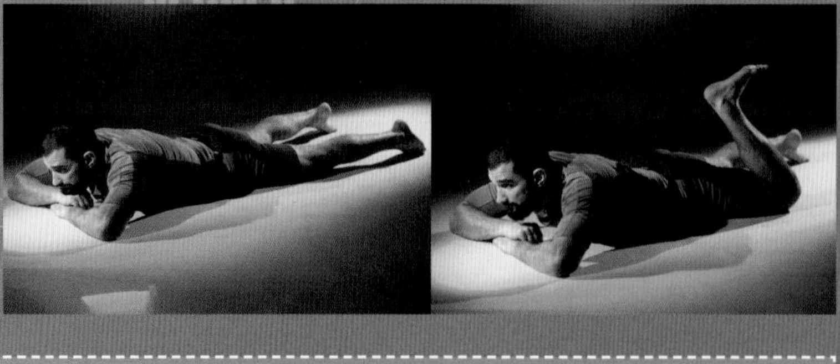

Any acute pain experienced during any of these exercises requires an appointment with your health care professional for a thorough examination. If you experience moderate pain or stiffness during these movements, it means you should perform one or more of the exercises every day.

C1. QUADRICEPS MASSAGE USING A BALL

The larger the diameter of the ball, the better; you can even use a medicine ball. Lie on your stomach, extend one leg, and place the ball under the middle of your thigh. Support yourself on your elbows and opposite knee, which is flexed. As you progress, you can add more weight until you can straighten your other leg and do the exercise with both legs parallel. Move the ball over the whole thigh, looking for painful areas. Each time you experience pain, focus on that spot by using short movements from top to bottom and from front to back.

Perform 1 to 3 movements over each stiff or painful area. Gradually move back up to the psoas area.

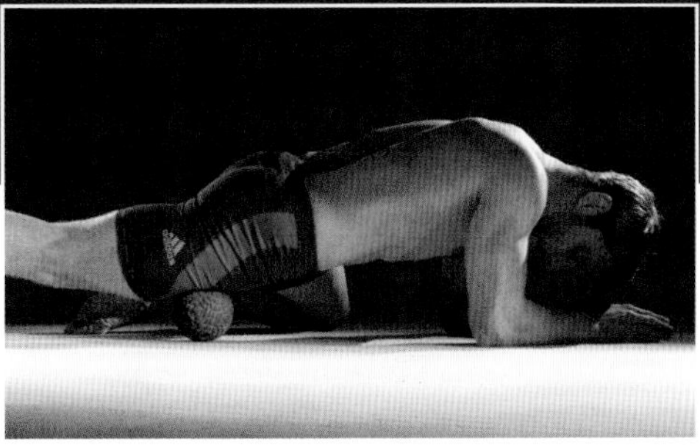

C2. HIP FLEXOR MASSAGE USING A BALL (WITH A HIP FLEXOR STRETCH)

Lie on the massage ball and move the ball over the hip flexor, looking for tense areas. Regulate the amount of weight you place on the ball by supporting yourself with your hands, feet, elbows, or knees. **Roll 10 times front-to-back and 10 times left-to-right. Repeat 1 to 3 times before changing to a different area.** Then do a lunge stretch and laterally flex (tilt) your torso away from the hip flexor that is being stretched. For a greater stretch, reach your arm overhead and away from the side that is being stretched.

Perform the exercise 1 to 3 times, holding the position for 30 seconds per leg.

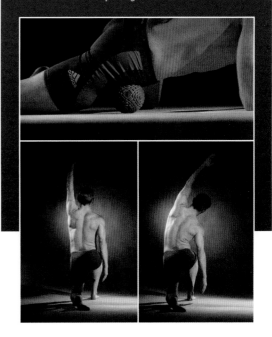

C3. STRETCHING THE QUADRICEPS

Lie face down with your knee comfortably positioned on a foam mat and raise your foot until your shin is perpendicular to the floor. Move back until your knee touches the wall and then gradually lift yourself up as high as possible.

Perform the exercise 1 to 3 times, holding the position for 15 seconds per leg.

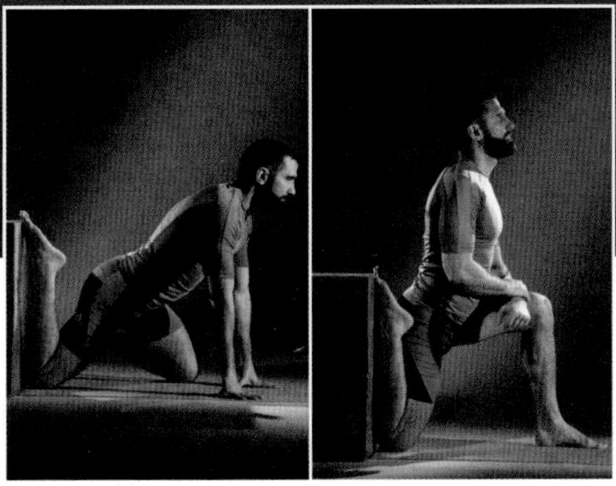

C4. TENSOR FASCIAE LATAE (TFL) MASSAGE USING A ROLLER

Lie on your side and place the roller at hip level on the outer thigh. Cross the top leg over and place that foot flat on the floor. Move the roller over the whole zone to find painful areas. Each time you experience pain, focus on that spot with short movements from top to bottom and front to back.

Perform 1 to 3 times for each stiff or painful area.

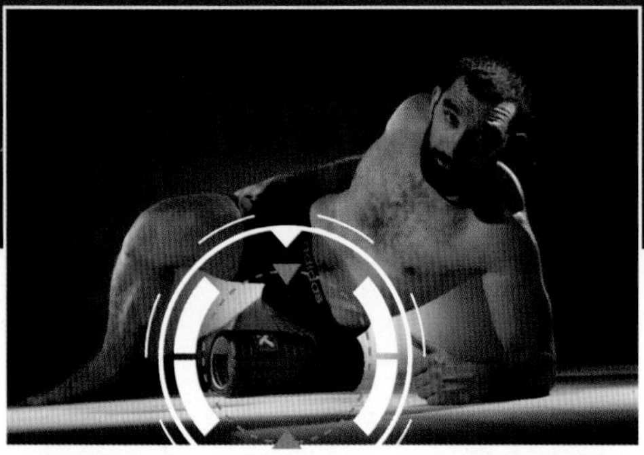

C5. STRETCHING THE ABDUCTORS

Sit with one leg extended in front of you. Cross the other leg over and place that foot flat on the floor. Rotate your torso by folding or crossing your arm over the opposite leg.

Perform 1 to 3 times per leg, holding this pose for 20 to 30 seconds.

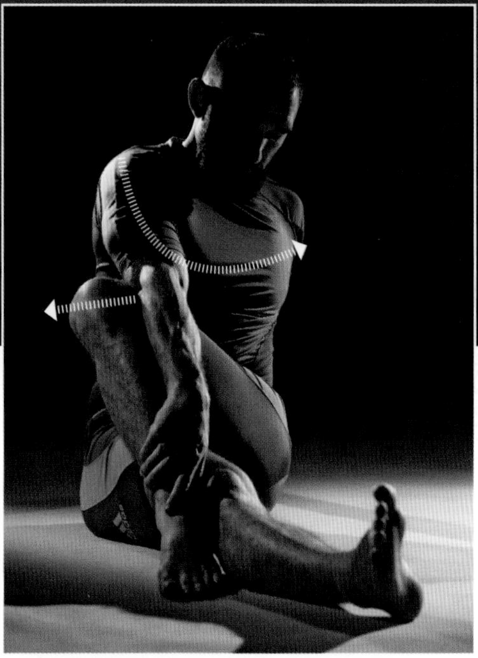

C6. ADDUCTOR MASSAGE USING A ROLLER

Lie on your stomach, flex your knee, and position the roller under your inner thigh, perpendicular to your thigh. Extend your other leg and rest it on the floor. Move the roller over the whole thigh to find painful areas. Each time you experience pain, focus on that spot using short movements from top to bottom and front to back.

Perform 1 to 3 times for each stiff or painful area, then move back to the highest adductor insertion point (which is often more sensitive and stiffer) and repeat the exercise.

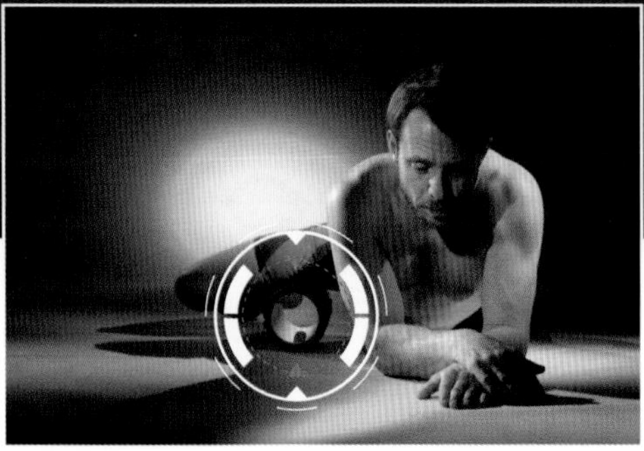

C7. PRESSURE POINT USING A MASSAGE BALL

The region close to the anus plays an essential role in relieving pain in the entire pelvic area. An excellent (although uncomfortable) way to relax the area is to sit on a very dense massage ball, which must be positioned as close as possible to the outer edge of the anus.

Perform 1 to 2 times, holding the position for at least 30 seconds.

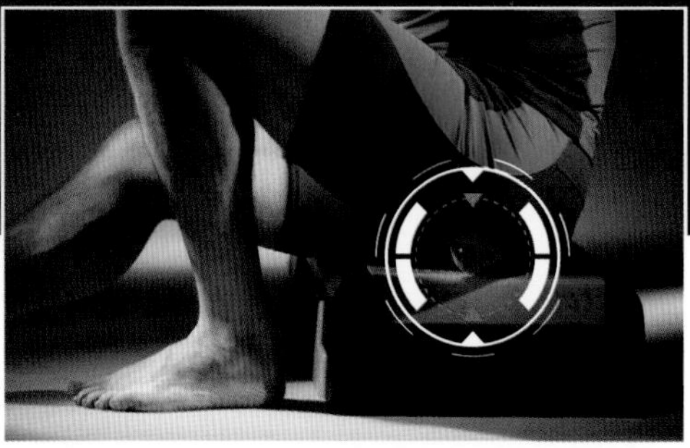

C8. STRETCHING THE ADDUCTORS

Place one knee on the floor and stretch your other leg to the side. Place your extended foot flat on the floor without rolling your ankle to the inside. Consult the photo for the correct position for your foot.

Perform 1 to 3 times per leg, holding this pose for 20 to 30 seconds.

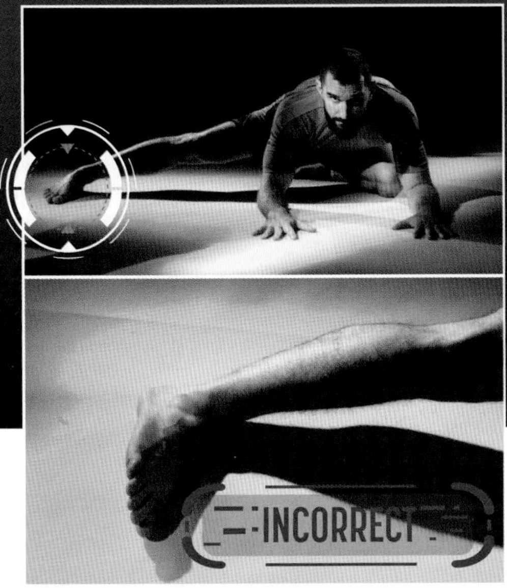

C9. HAMSTRING MASSAGE USING A WEIGHT BAR

This exercise can also be done with a massage roller, but it is much more effective with a weight bar. Place the bar at the height of your pelvis. Extend one leg over the bar so it is at the middle of—and perpendicular to—your thigh. The other leg remains behind the bar. Roll the whole thigh over the bar to find any painful areas. Each time you experience pain, focus on that spot with short movements from top to bottom.

Perform 1 to 3 times for each stiff or painful area then move back up to the glutes.

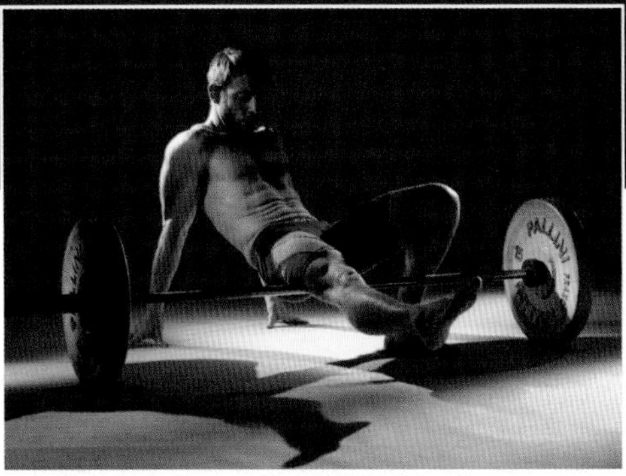

C10. STRETCHING THE HAMSTRINGS

Sit on the floor, extend one leg, and flex the other. Keeping your back flat and the leg extended, lean forward.

Perform 1 to 3 reps, holding for 20 to 30 seconds per leg.

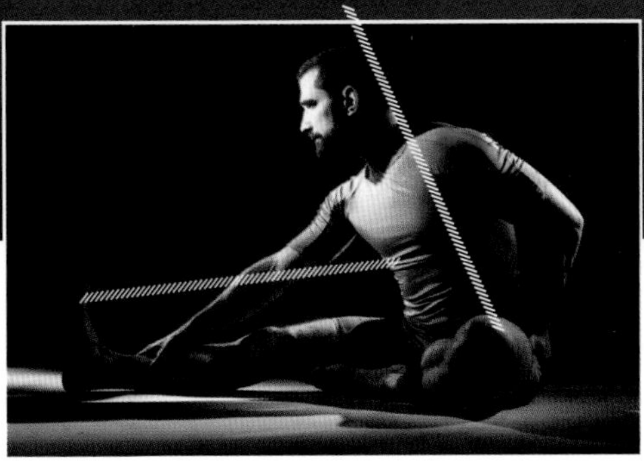

C11. GLUTE MASSAGE USING A ROLLER

Sit on the roller and cross one of your legs by placing your ankle on top of the knee of the opposite leg. The massage is done on the raised leg by moving the roller from front to back and left to right.

Perform 10 times over each stiff or painful area.

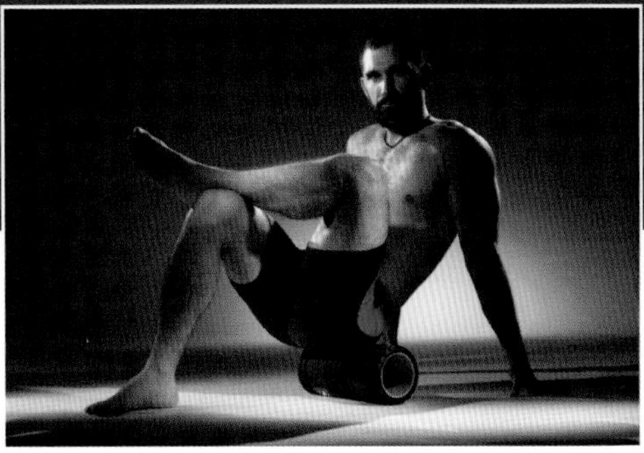

C12. GLUTE MASSAGE USING A BALL

Lie on your back, flex one knee, and place a large-diameter ball on the upper part of the gluteals, just below the pelvis. Grab your flexed knee, keep the other leg extended, relax your whole body, and rock the leg from right to left as you roll over the ball forward and backward.

Perform 10 times for each leg.

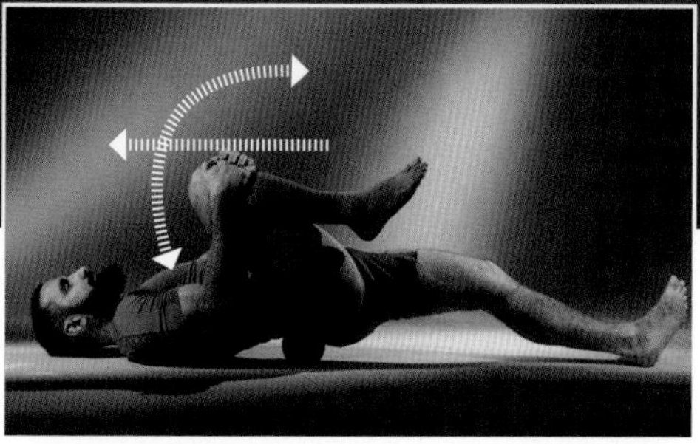

C13. STRETCHING THE GLUTES

Sit on the floor and place one foot on the knee of the other leg to form a triangle. Hold the back of your bottom thigh and bring your foot toward you while keeping your knee and hip open. Do not let your legs cross over one another; hold the triangle shape as much as possible.

Perform 1 to 3 reps, holding for 20 to 30 seconds per leg.

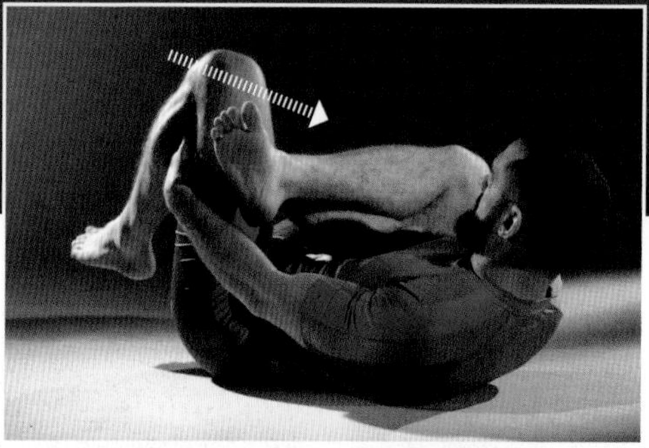

C14. BALLISTIC STRETCHING

Face a wall and place your hands against the wall. Allow your hip to move freely by making a pendular movement with the leg from left to right. Do this exercise very gradually, taking time to slowly increase your range of motion. **Perform 1 to 3 sets of 10 per leg.** Repeat this exercise standing perpendicular to the wall and swing your leg to the front and back.

Perform 1 to 3 sets of 10 per leg.

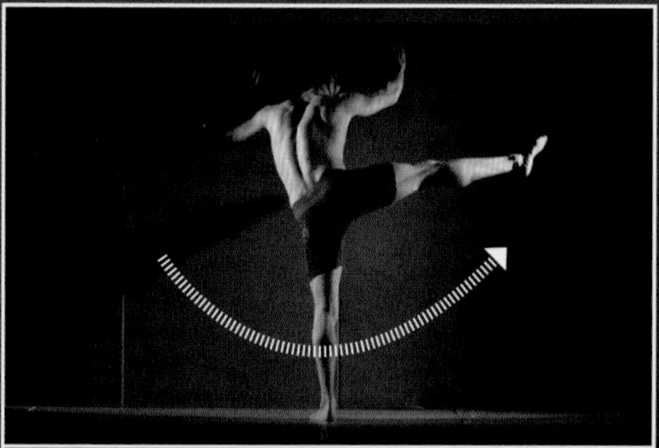

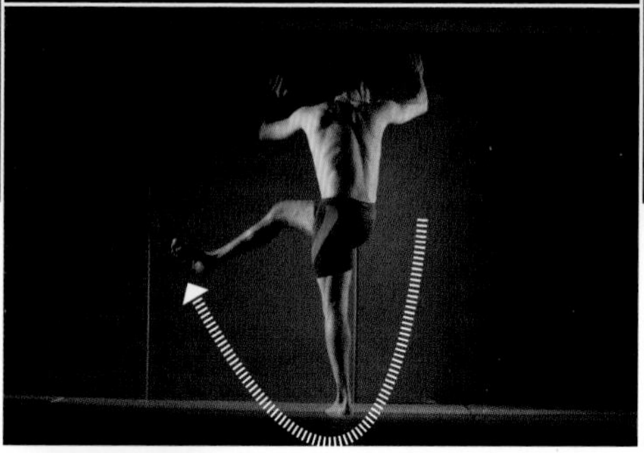

C15. STRETCHING THE HIP ROTATORS

Lie on your stomach, flex your front leg, and extend your back leg as you tilt yourself forward over (or even lie on) the flexed leg on the floor.

Perform 1 to 3 reps, holding for 20 to 30 seconds per leg.

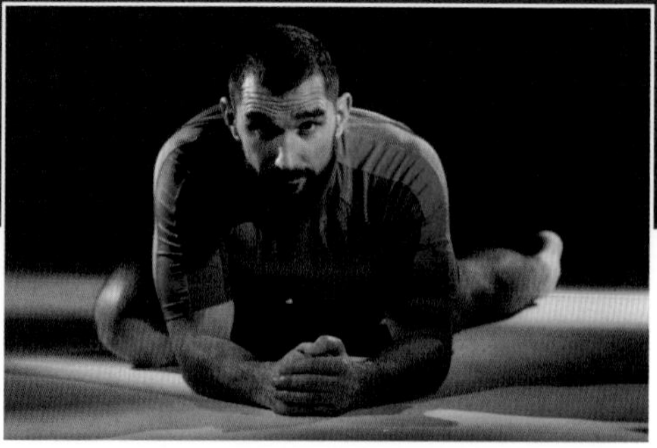

C16. STRETCHING THE QUADRATUS LUMBORUM MUSCLE USING A BAND

Lie on your back, wrap a resistance band around your ankle, and move backward until the band becomes taut. Relax yourself completely and stretch your arms above your head. Make a conscious effort to breathe using your diaphragm. You can work the entire muscle chain by holding a kettlebell.

Perform 1 to 2 reps, holding for 30 seconds to 1 minute per side.

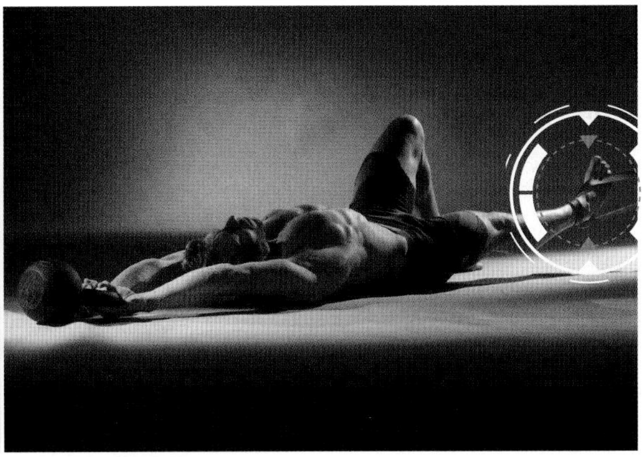

RELAX WITH A SMILE

Self-massages and stretching can be particularly uncomfortable. It is essential to find ways to relax and maximize these mobility techniques. Grimacing during a massage or stretch creates more tension, so try to smile throughout these exercises to encourage relaxation.

C17. HIP PROPRIOCEPTION

Balance yourself on one knee on a proprioception cushion or any soft surface and close your eyes. You can also hold a baton or stick above your head to make the exercise more difficult.

Perform 1 to 3 attempts for as long as possible per side.

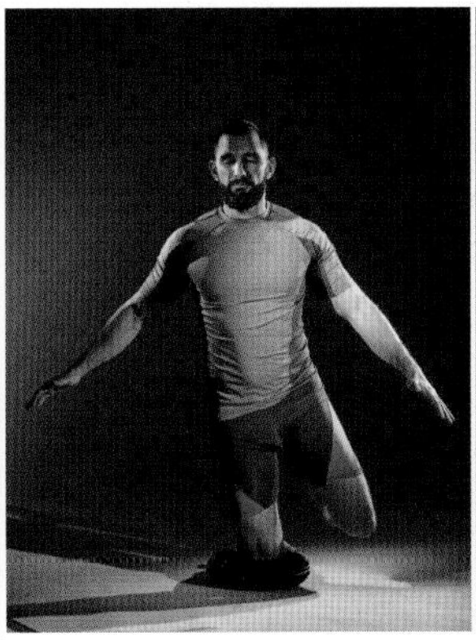

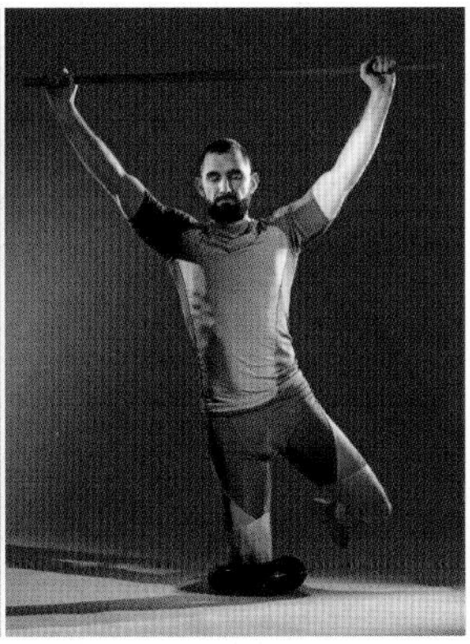

Sample 3-week mobility program targeting the pelvic area (including exercises for neighboring areas)

MONDAY	TUESDAY	WEDNESDAY	THURSDAY	FRIDAY	SATURDAY	SUNDAY
C7*, C12, C13, C9, C10, C17	B10, B2, B5, B4, B6	C1, C3, C4, C5, C11, C2	A1, A5, A10, A5, A9	C6, C8, C13, C15, C14	C12, C2, B2, B4, A5, A10	C2, C6, C16, C11, C13, C15

*These letter/number combinations refer to the exercises and techniques found on pages 26 through 76.

HAMSTRING PAIN

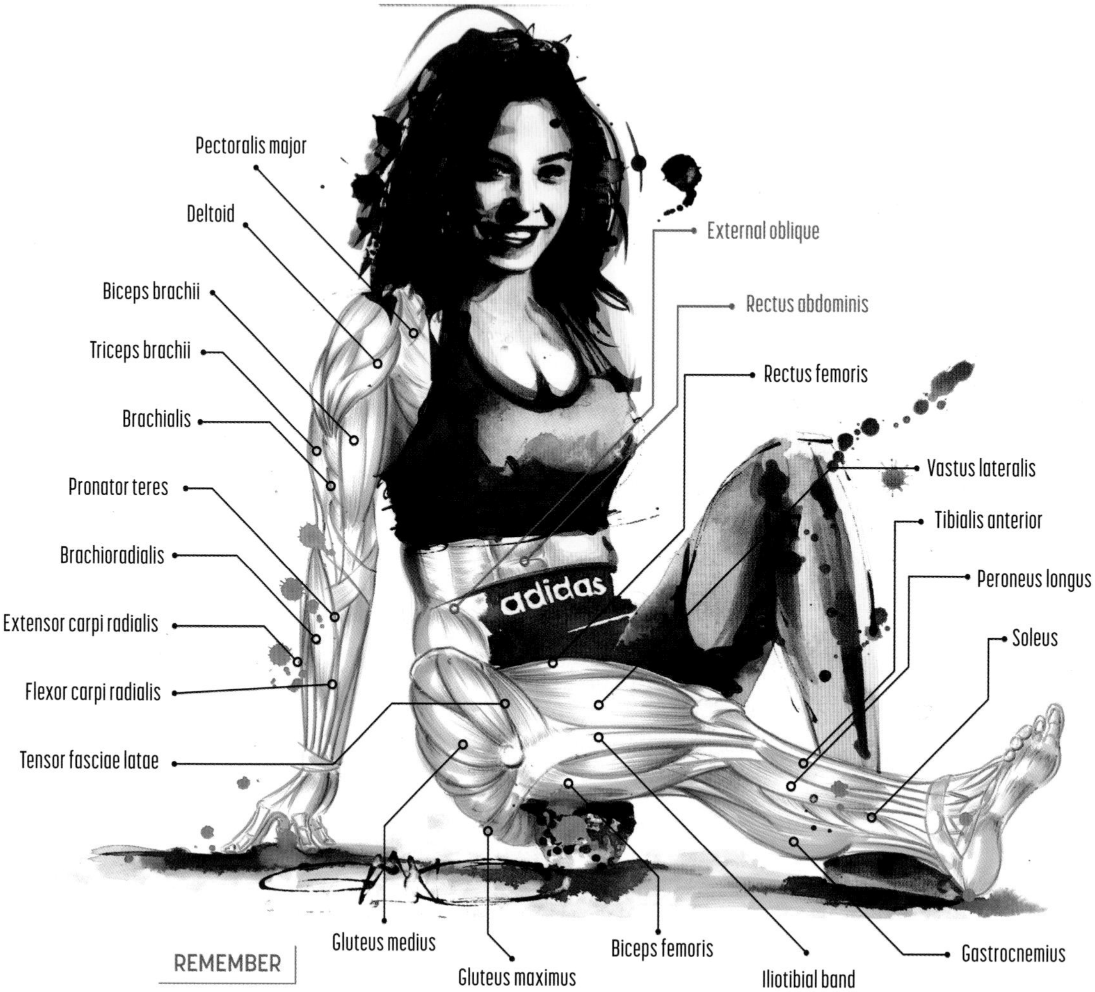

REMEMBER

You cannot always think analytically or in an isolated manner when dealing with pain. Pain often radiates from other areas or can be caused by problems elsewhere in the chain. The hamstring muscles are also vulnerable to radiating pain, in part because of their composition and in part because of their function. These powerful running brakes are also delicate postural supports for various muscle positions. For example, a hypothesis about posture that is gaining more acceptance and that is supported by scientific proof (see, for example, Gabbe et al. 2006) is that an involuntary tilt in the pelvis due to overly tight iliopsoas muscles can in turn cause the hamstrings to become tight, creating stiffness, pain, or both. Therefore, sometimes you need to work on the iliopsoas to resolve hamstring problems.

The powerful brakes of the human body are also especially fragile. Smaller than their large antagonist muscles—the quadriceps—the hamstrings are worked hard during many types of movement. The complex muscles of the hamstrings are of varying lengths, and this makes them very versatile but also prone to injury.

This is the opposite of the triceps brachii muscle, for example, which is made up of three muscles (even more if we include the posterior chain of the arms) that work together in almost all directions. In the hamstrings, however, the semitendinosus, semimembranosus, and the biceps femoris muscles are not recruited equally.

This means it is especially important to properly warm up the hamstrings before any exercise and to care for them when not in training.

THE SCAN

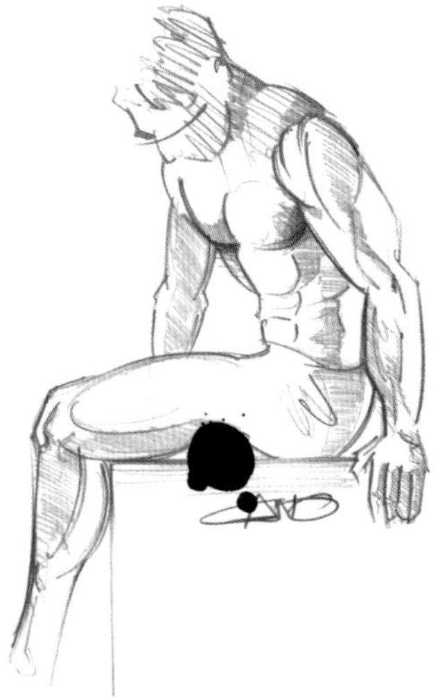

In addition to everyday pain, which often provides sufficient information about the needs in a certain area, a deep scan can reveal areas of the hamstrings that need attention. Here is an exercise to include in the scan:

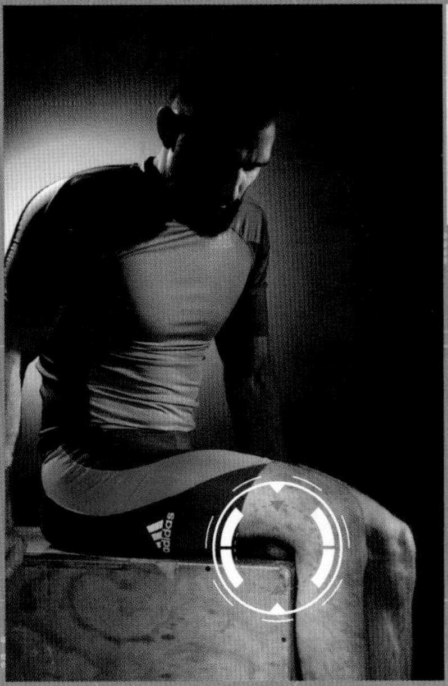

1

Sit on a table or box, place a massage ball under your thigh, and gently roll the ball on your thigh to find any tense areas. Focus on these painful areas.

Any acute pain experienced during this exercise requires an appointment with your health care professional for a thorough examination.
If you experience moderate pain or stiffness during this movement, it means you should perform one or more of the exercises every day.

D1. QUADRICEPS MASSAGE USING A BALL

Using the largest ball you can tolerate, lie on your stomach, extend one leg, and place the ball at the center of that thigh. Bend your other leg and place that knee on the floor. As you progress, you will be able to apply more weight, eventually lifting that knee and keeping both legs parallel. Move the ball over the whole thigh to find painful areas. Each time you experience pain, focus on that spot with short movements from top to bottom and from front to back.

Perform 1 to 3 times for each stiff or painful area. Gradually move up to the psoas area.

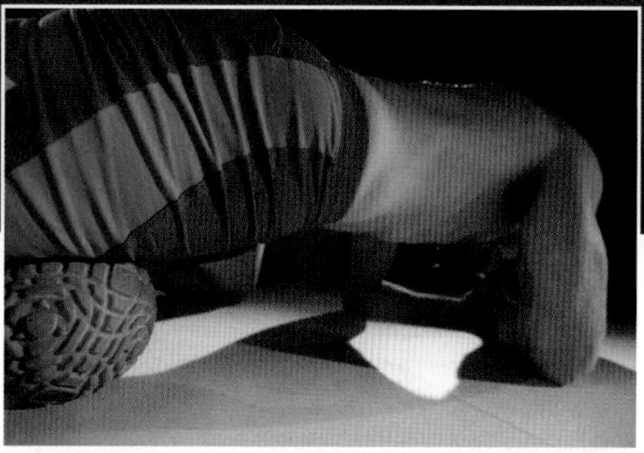

D2. HIP FLEXOR MASSAGE USING A KETTLEBELL (WITH A HIP FLEXOR STRETCH)

Place the kettlebell on the floor at a slight angle to your body. Place your hip on the handle and apply as much weight as you can without causing too much pain. **Massage 10 times from front to back and 10 times from left to right. Repeat 1 to 3 times before changing to a different area.** Then do a lunge stretch and laterally flex (tilt) your torso away from the hip flexor that is being stretched. For a greater stretch, reach your arm overhead and away from the side that is being stretched.

Perform the exercise 1 to 3 times, holding the position for 30 seconds per leg.

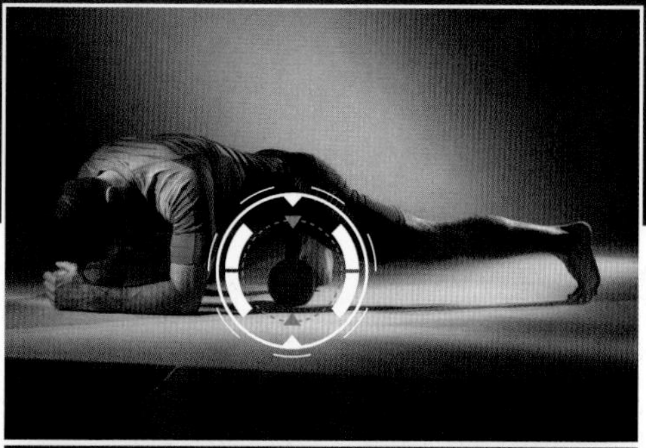

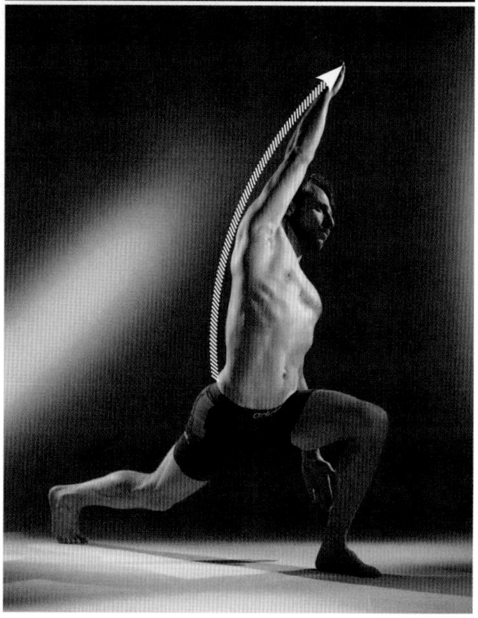

D3. STRETCHING THE QUADRICEPS

In a forward lunge position, grab your back foot and bring your heel to your buttock. Keep your body straight throughout the exercise; do not arch your back.

Perform the exercise 1 to 3 times, holding the position for 15 seconds per leg.

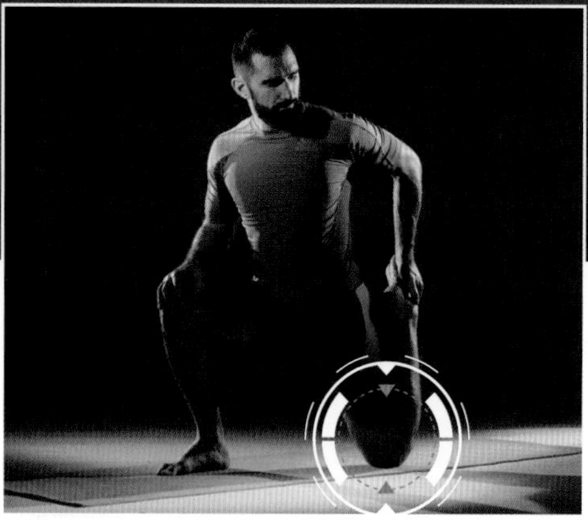

D4. OUTER HAMSTRING MASSAGE USING A ROLLER

Lie on your side and place the roller at the level of your knee, on the outer, back area of the thigh. Move the roller over the whole thigh to find painful areas. Each time you experience pain, focus on that spot using short movements from top to bottom and from front to back.

Perform 1 to 3 times for each stiff or painful area.
Be careful: Self-massage of the IT band area has become popular, but an intense, prolonged massage of this area must be limited (see details on page 17).

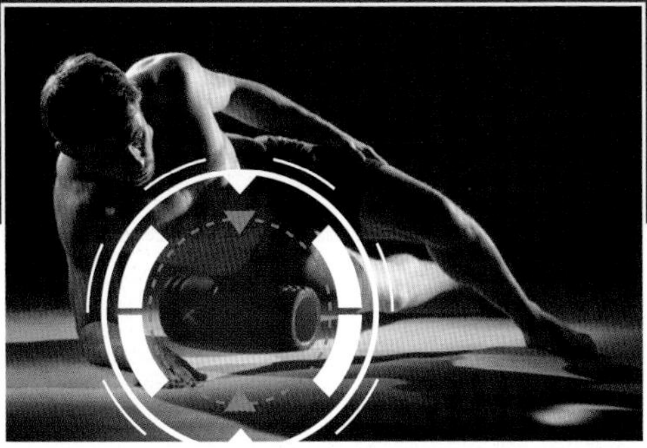

D5. TFL MASSAGE USING A BALL

Massaging the IT band itself may be questionable, but the TFL is, in contrast, an accumulation of tension and trigger points. Tension sometimes leads to compensation by the hamstrings and adductors. It is crucial to take good care of your TFL so that it remains supple and pain free.

Lie your side on a large ball. Extend your bottom leg and cross your upper leg over, placing that foot flat on the floor. Roll from top to bottom and front to back over the most tense or painful areas. Finish with circular movements.

Perform 1 to 3 sets of 10 top-to-bottom, 10 front-to-back, and 10 circular rolls on each stiff or painful area.

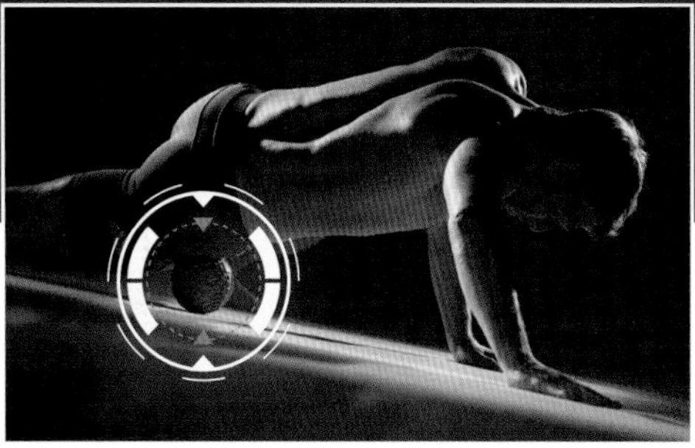

D6. STRETCHING THE TFL

Lie on your side and hold the foot of your bottom leg so that your quadriceps muscles are stretched. Squeeze your glutes to keep your hip forward and your pelvis tilted slightly forward. Cross the ankle of your free leg over your knee, keeping the quadriceps muscles stretched.

Perform 1 to 3 times, holding the stretch for at least 30 seconds.

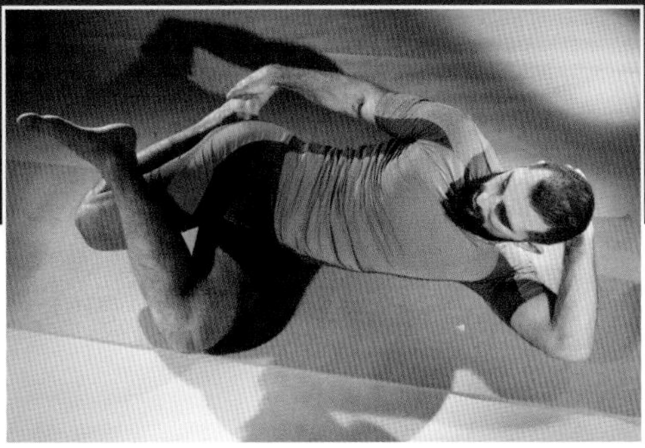

D7. ADDUCTOR MASSAGE USING A BALL

Lie on your stomach, flex your knee, and place the massage ball at your inner thigh. Keep your other leg extended on the floor. Move your whole thigh over the ball to find painful areas. Each time you experience pain, focus on that area with short movements from top to bottom and from front to back.

Perform 1 to 3 times for each stiff or painful area. Move up to the highest adductor insertion (which is often more sensitive and stiffer) and repeat the exercise.

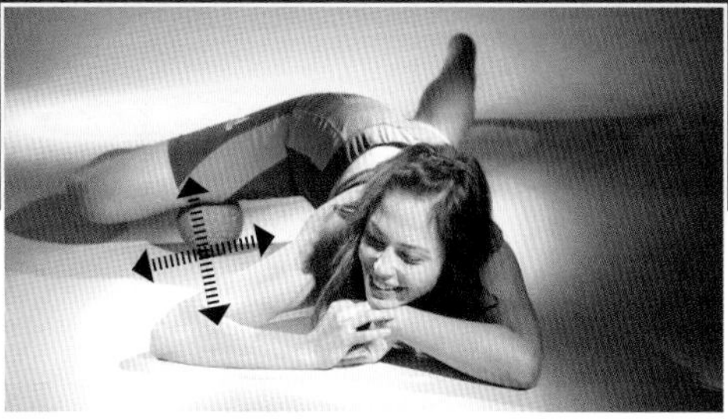

D8. PRESSURE POINT USING A MASSAGE BALL

The region close to the anus plays an essential role in relieving pain in the entire pelvic area. An excellent (although uncomfortable) way to relax the area is to sit on a very dense massage ball, which must be positioned as close as possible to the outer edge of the anus. **Perform 1 to 2 times, holding the position for at least 30 seconds.**

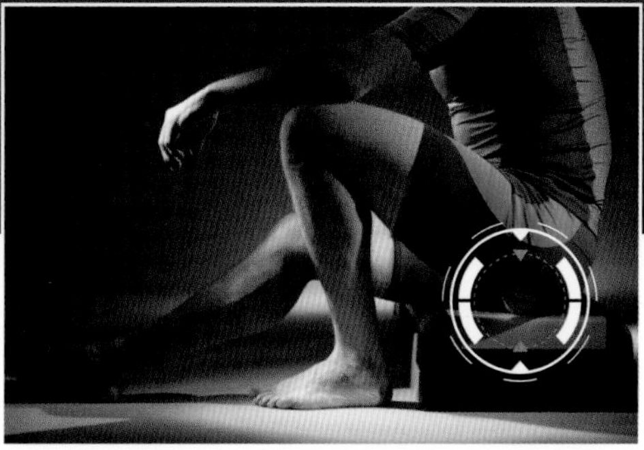

D9. STRETCHING THE ADDUCTORS

Place your knees and elbows on the floor, keep your back straight, and place your femurs at a 90-degree angle to the line of the torso. Spread your knees as far apart as possible. **Perform 1 to 3 times per leg, holding the stretch for 20 to 30 seconds.**

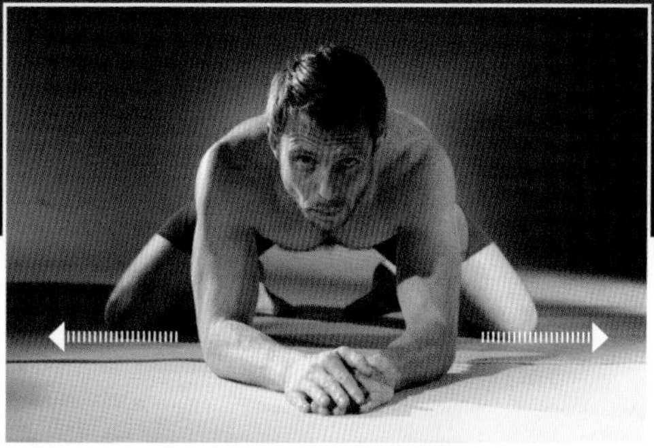

D10. HAMSTRING MASSAGE USING A WEIGHT BAR

Load the bar with weight in the Olympic style and place the bar on the floor. Extend one leg over the bar so it is just above the end of your hamstring above your knee. The other leg remains behind the bar. Move to find any painful and stiff areas. Each time you experience pain, focus on that spot with short movements from front to back. **Perform 1 to 3 times for each stiff or painful area,** then move up to the glutes.

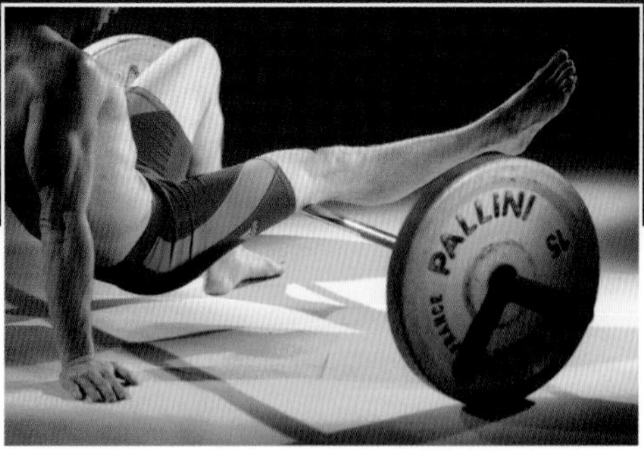

D11. STRETCHING THE HAMSTRINGS

Stand up, keep your legs straight, and place one heel on a raised surface (bench, box, etc.). Flex forward, keeping your back straight. **Perform 1 to 3 reps, holding for 20 to 30 seconds per leg.**

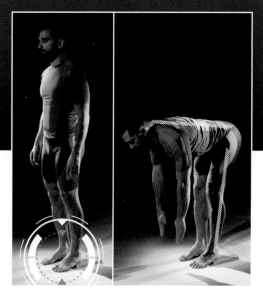

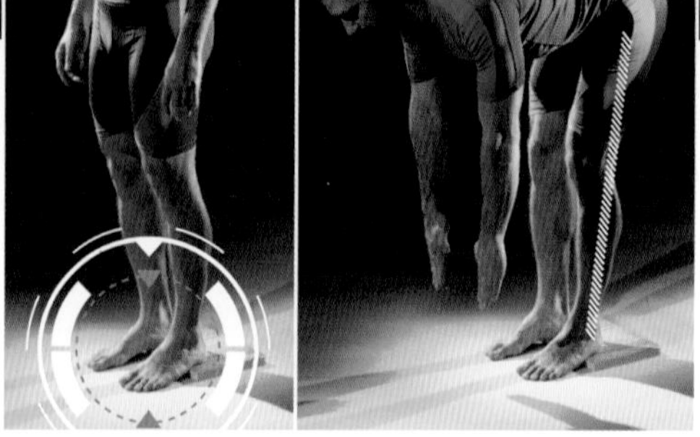

D12. GLUTE MASSAGE USING A BALL

Place the ball on the upper part of your gluteals, just under the pelvis. Lie on your back and move the ball around to explore the area. **Perform 3 sets of 1 minute.**

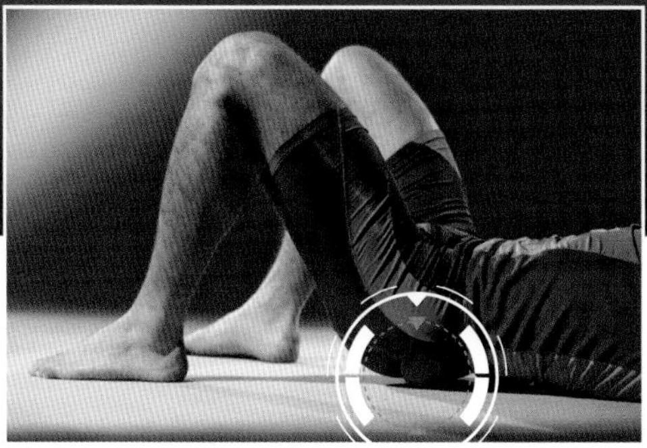

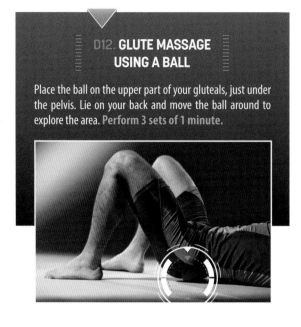

D13. STRETCHING THE GLUTES

Sit cross-legged and lean forward, keeping your back straight. Alternate the top leg. **Perform 1 to 3 reps, holding for 30 seconds per top leg.**

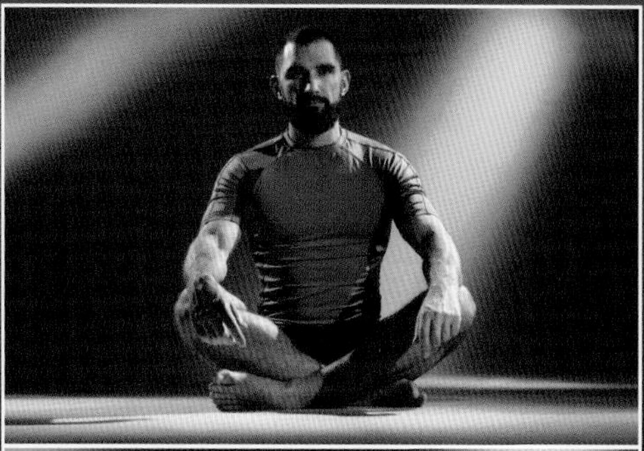

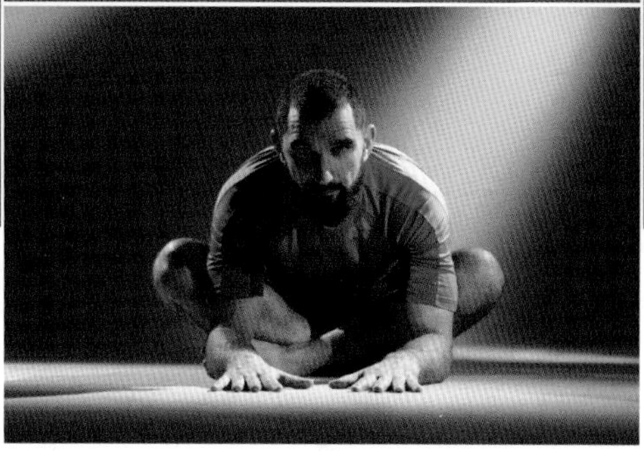

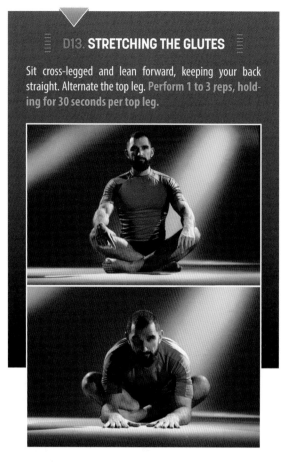

D14. BALLISTIC STRETCHES USING A BAND

Lie on your back with both legs straight. Place one foot in the loop of a band and pull the band taut to quickly raise (and lower) your leg, keeping the speed and incline gradual. **Perform 1 to 3 sets of 10 reps per leg.**

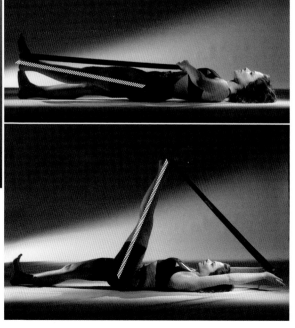

D15. HIP FLEXOR MASSAGE USING A ROLLER (WITH A HIP FLEXOR STRETCH)

Lie on the massage roller and place it at the fold of your hip, slightly off-center so as not to put pressure on the genital area. Move the roller to find tense areas. Regulate your weight by holding yourself up with different supports (hands, feet, elbows, or knees) and concentrate on any tense areas. **Perform 1 to 3 sets of 10 front-to back and 10 left-to-right rolls on each stiff or painful area.** Then do a lunge stretch (see page 46) and laterally flex (tilt) your torso away from the hip flexor that is being stretched. For a greater stretch, reach your arm overhead and away from the side that is being stretched. **Perform the exercise 1 to 3 times, holding the position for 30 seconds per leg.**

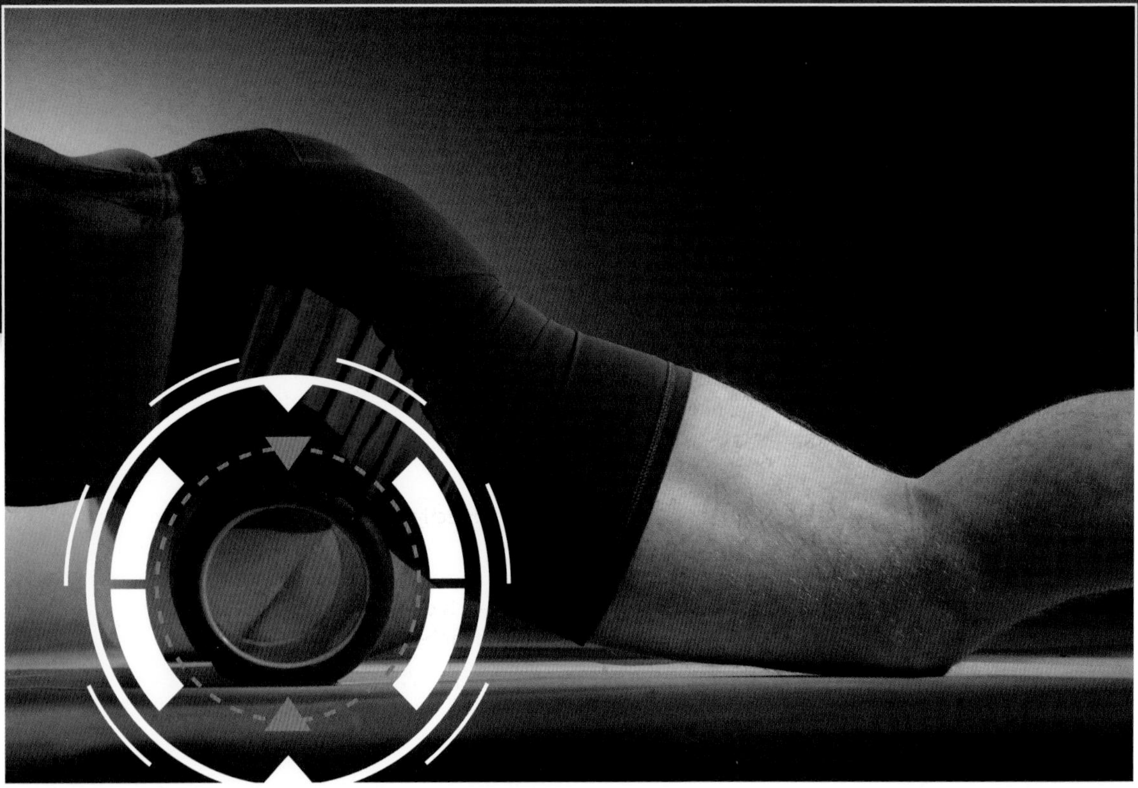

Sample 3-week mobility program targeting the hamstrings (including exercises for neighboring areas)

MONDAY	TUESDAY	WEDNESDAY	THURSDAY	FRIDAY	SATURDAY	SUNDAY
D5*, D6, D1, D3, D14	D2, D8, D12, D13, D15	C1, C3, C4, C5, C11, C2	D7, D9, D10, D11, D14	C6, C8, C13, C15, C14	C12, C2, B2, A5, D15	F3, D6, F5, D4, F7, D11

*These letter/number combinations refer to the exercises and techniques found on pages 26 through 76.

SHOULDER PAIN

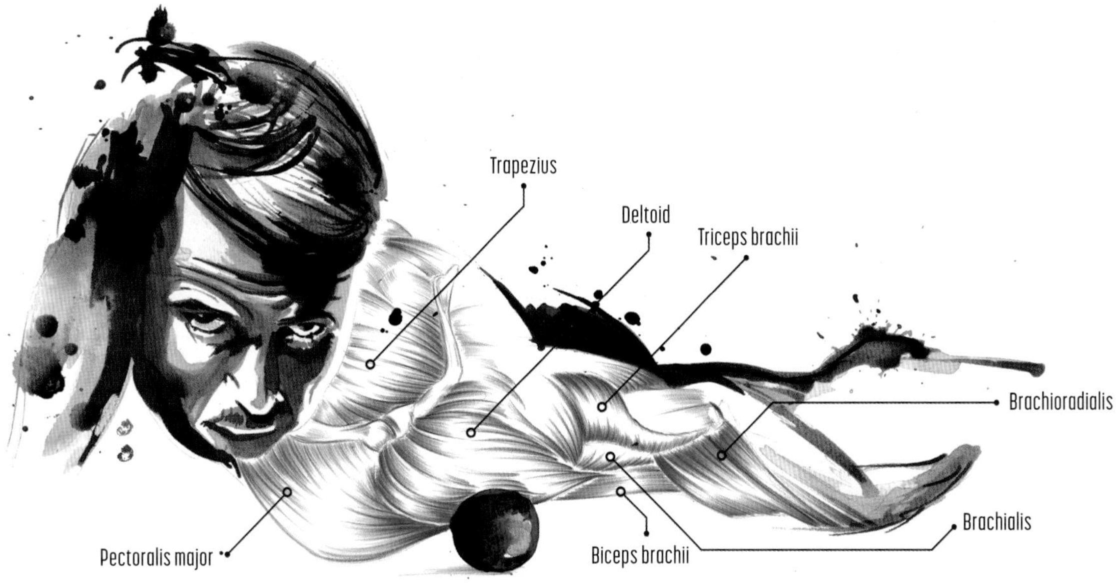

The shoulder is not limited to the deltoids alone. There are many more structures that make up the shoulder than what we see when we look in a mirror. The shoulder joint is the most mobile in the human body, but it can also quickly become unstable. If the shoulder is in a bad position or is consistently moved incorrectly, it will become painful.

The shoulder joint "complex" is comprised of four bones: the collar bone (*clavicle*), the shoulder blade (*scapula*), the head of the upper arm bone (*humerus*), and the upper part of the breast bone (*sternum*). It is stabilized and moved by 12 muscles: deltoids, trapezius, latissimus dorsi, sternocleidomastoid, pectoralis major, and serratus anterior as well as the rotator cuff muscles (subscapularis, supraspinatus, infraspinatus, teres minor, teres major, and rhomboids).

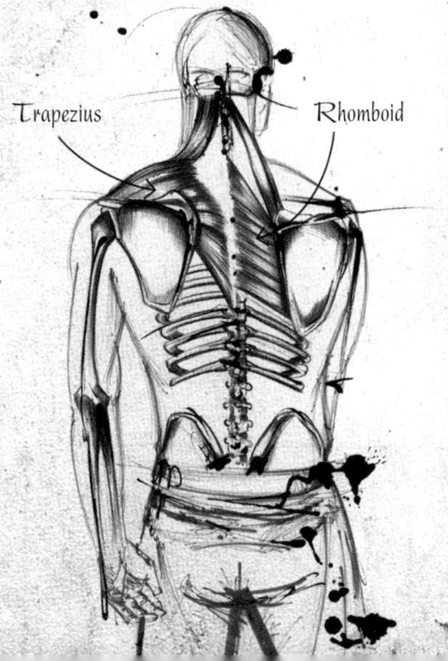

You should explore all of the shoulder muscles and their full range of motion so you can locate the source of any pain:

→ The cause of pain often varies, and the superficial muscles are normally full of trigger points, so often the whole area will need attention.
→ It is important to perform flexibility, stability, and mobility exercises for the shoulder for long-lasting results.
→ The shoulder is one of the most susceptible joints for referred pain. Shoulder pain is often a consequence of numerous other points of tension.

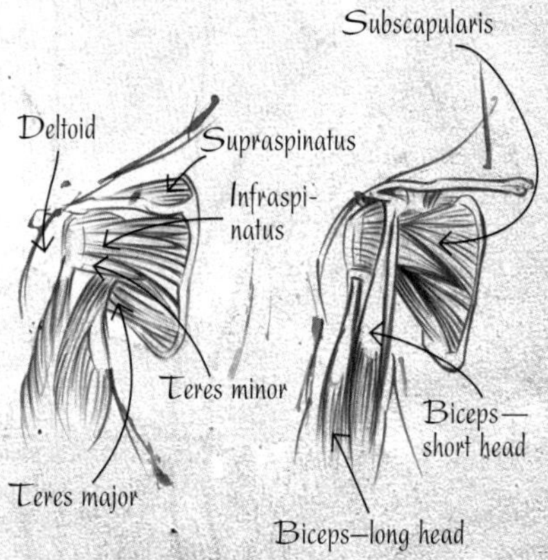

THE SCAN

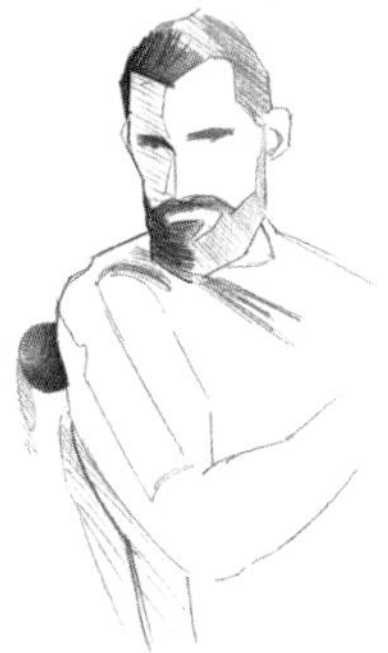

In addition to everyday pain, which often provides sufficient information about the needs in a certain area, a deep scan can reveal areas of the shoulder that need attention. Here are four exercises to include in the scan:

1

Massage ball on the deltoids: Lightly lean against a wall with the ball between the wall and your shoulder. Deeply explore the front, side, and back of the shoulder.

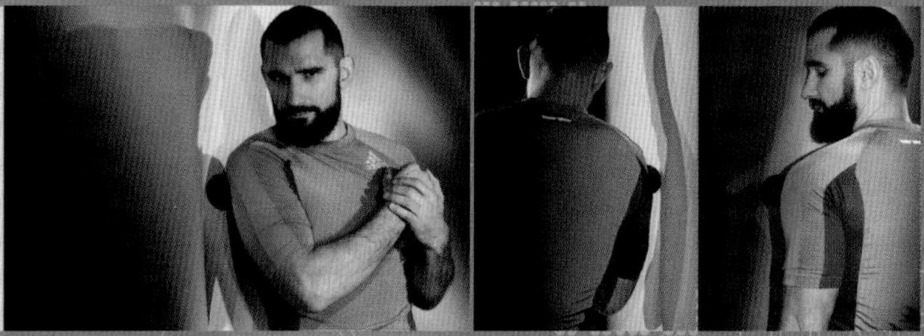

2

Explore the shoulder blades: With a large massage ball (or a small ball, which is more precise but often more uncomfortable), roll over the shoulder blade as you lean against the wall.

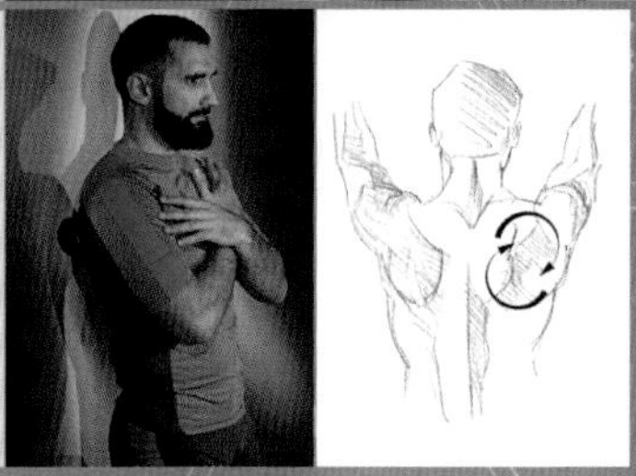

Any acute pain experienced during any of these exercises requires an appointment with your health care professional for a thorough examination. If you experience moderate pain or stiffness during these movements, it means you should perform one or more of the exercises every day.

3

Roll the ball over the trapezius: Roll the ball along your neck from your head down to the edge of your shoulder.

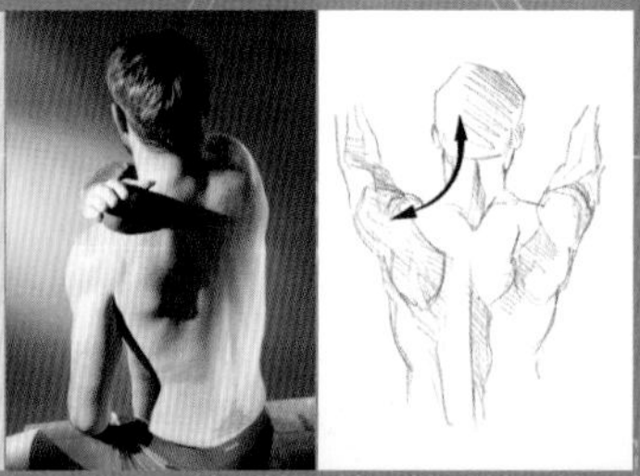

4

Front elbow lift: While resting your hand on the opposite shoulder, raise your elbow in front of you.

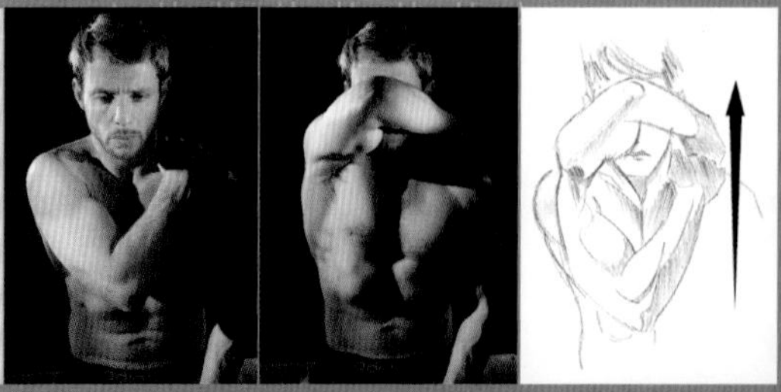

E1. MEDIAL AND POSTERIOR DELTOID MASSAGE USING A BALL

With the massage ball positioned between the wall and your shoulder, look for areas of pain in the deltoids. Massage each painful area using the ball.
Perform 3 sets of 10 back-and-forth massages, 10 top-to-bottom massages, and 10 circular massages.

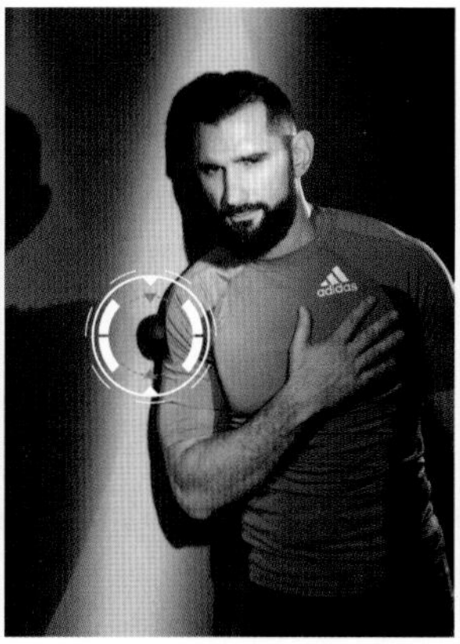

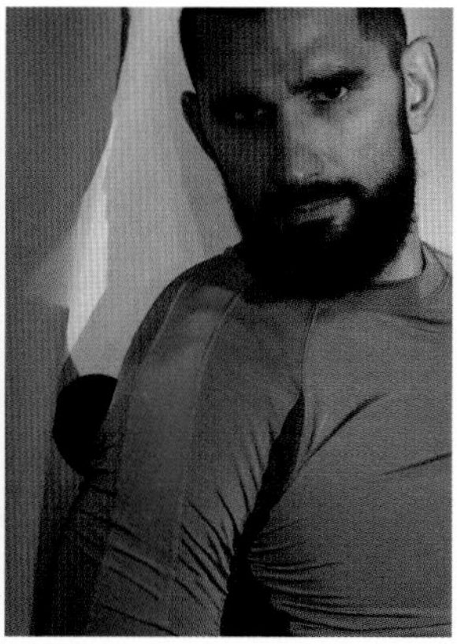

E2. SUPINE DELTOID STRETCH AND MASSAGE

Lie on your side and extend your top arm above your head. Hold your bottom arm perpendicular to your body and roll up and down on this arm. **Perform 1 to 3 times, staying in this stretched position for 20 to 30 seconds. Then roll from left to right 10 times.** Repeat the exercise, varying the angle of the arm (within a range of 20 degrees).

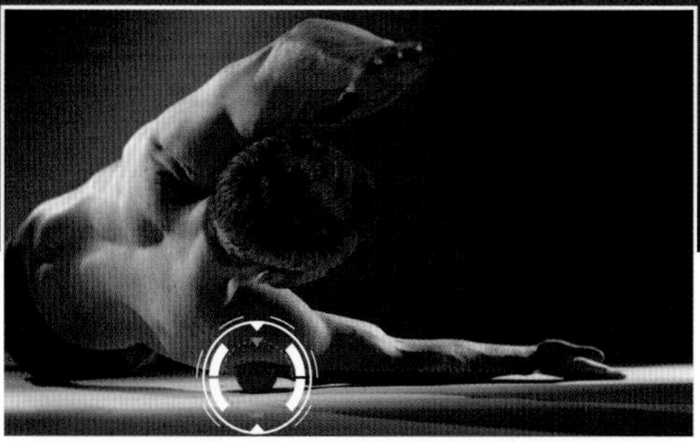

E3. ANTERIOR DELTOID MASSAGE USING A BALL

With the massage ball positioned between the wall and the front of your shoulder, look for areas of pain in the deltoids. With the ball, massage each painful area using small movements.
Perform 3 sets of 10 back-and-forth massages, 10 top-to-bottom massages, and 10 circular massages.

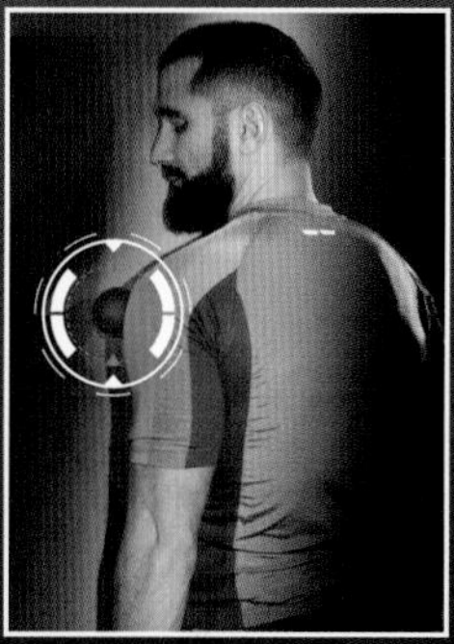

E4. DELTOID STRETCH ON ALL FOURS

On your hands and knees, move your gluteals toward your feet without moving your hands, keeping your arms straight. **Perform 1 to 3 times, holding the stretch for 20 to 30 seconds.**

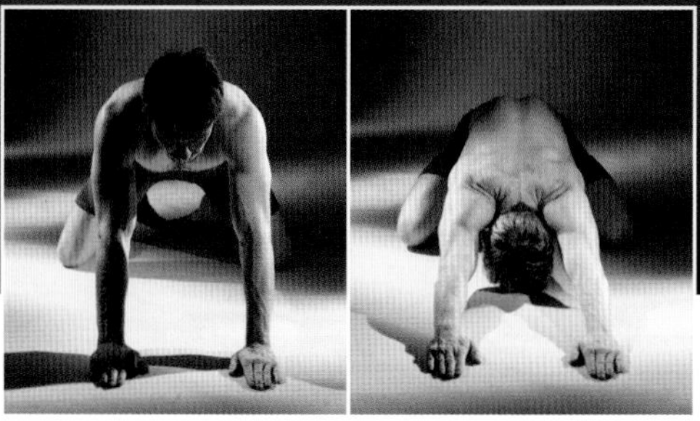

E5. SHOULDER JOINT DISTRACTION

Fold one arm behind your back with your shoulder in the loop of a power band that is perpendicular to the floor. Flex your chest forward so it is parallel to the ground and allow your shoulder to relax as much as possible. Be careful not to rotate your torso in any direction. **Perform 1 to 3 times, holding the stretch for 30 seconds.**

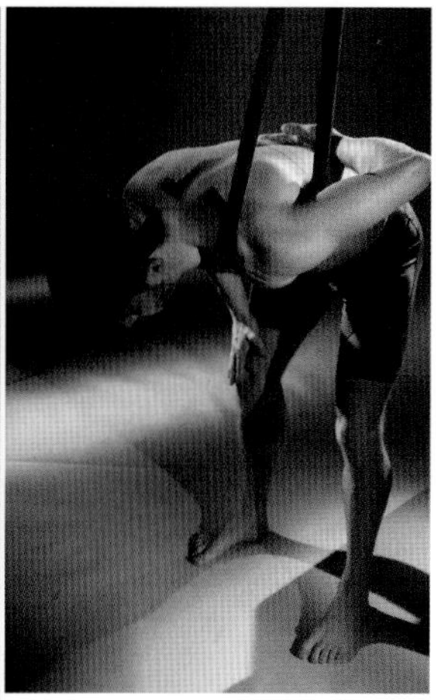

E6. ARM LOCK SHOULDER STRETCH USING A BAND

Put your arm behind your back and grab the loop of a resistance band attached behind you. Do not move your shoulder up or forward. Completely relax and allow your wrist to be pulled up as much as possible. Adjust the intensity of the exercise by varying the position of your leg in a lunge.

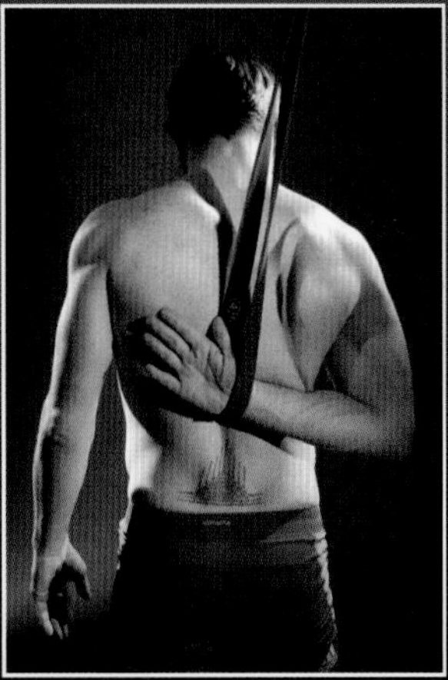

Perform 1 to 3 times, holding the stretch for 30 seconds.

E7. ONE-ARM SHOULDER STRETCH USING AN EXERCISE BALL

On your knees, extend one arm and place your forearm on the top of the ball with your thumb pointing up. Gradually lean your chest toward the floor.

Perform 1 to 3 times, holding the stretch for 30 seconds.

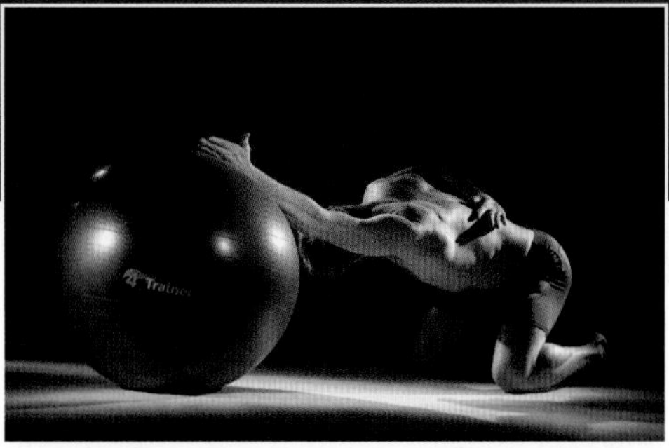

E8. SHOULDER STRETCH USING BOTH ARMS ON AN EXERCISE BALL

On your knees, extend your arms and place your hands palms down or palms up on the ball. Gradually lean your chest toward the floor.

Perform 1 to 3 times, holding the stretch for 30 seconds.

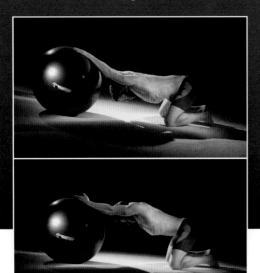

E9. PECTORALIS MINOR MASSAGE USING A BALL

Place a massage ball between the wall and your chest, just below your collarbone, and look for areas of pain in the pectoralis minor. Massage each painful area with the ball.

Perform 3 sets of 10 left-and-right massages, 10 top-to-bottom massages, and 10 circular massages.

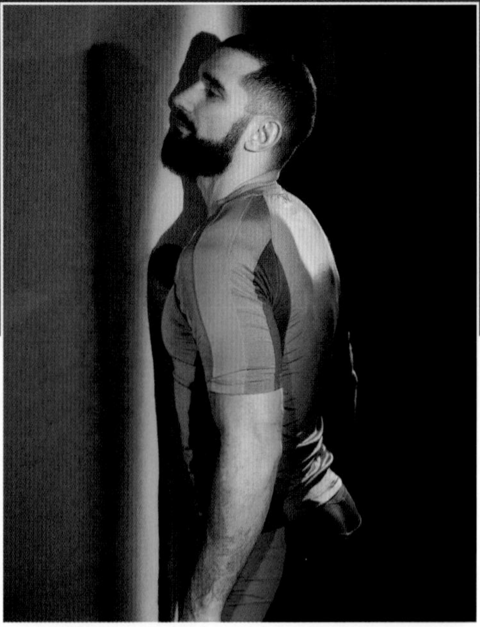

E10. PECTORALIS MAJOR MASSAGE USING A ROLLER

Lie on the floor and place your chest on a massage roller in line with your body. Roll from left to right over the stiffest areas. Gradually vary the orientation of the roller to cover all areas of the chest.

Perform 3 sets of 10 left-to-right massages for each stiff area.

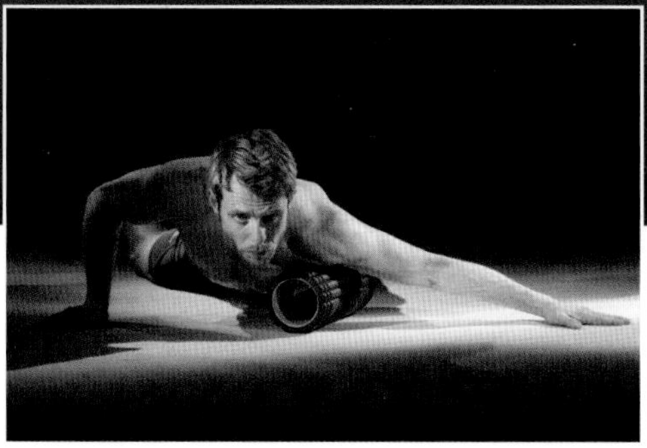

E11. STRETCHING THE CHEST MUSCLES USING A RESISTANCE BAND

Hang a band from a fixed bar overhead. Extend one arm with your thumb pointing toward the ceiling. Move into a lunge position, varying the angle of your arm to stretch different areas of the chest muscles. If you are experience pain, change the orientation of your arms.

Perform 1 to 3 sets of 20- to 30-second stretches.

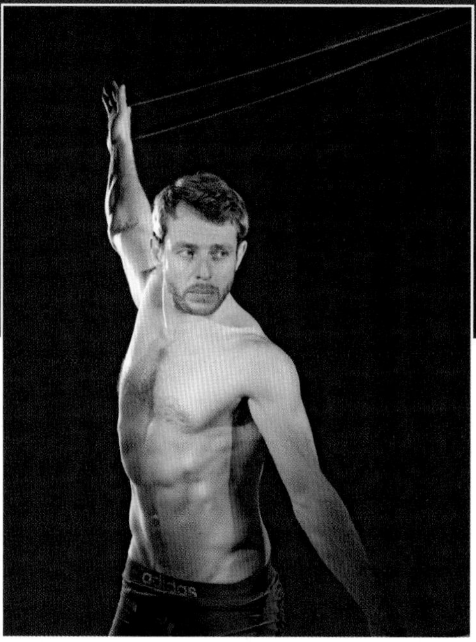

E12. UPPER AND MIDDLE BACK MUSCLE MASSAGE USING A BALL

Place a massage ball between the wall and your back and look for areas of pain in the rotator cuff, trapezius, and latissimus dorsi muscles. Use small movements to apply pressure to each painful spot using the ball. Vary the position of your arm during the massages; stretch your arm overhead, extend it in front or to the side, and lock it behind your back.

Perform 3 sets of 10 right-and-left massages, 10 top-to-bottom massages, and 10 circular massages.

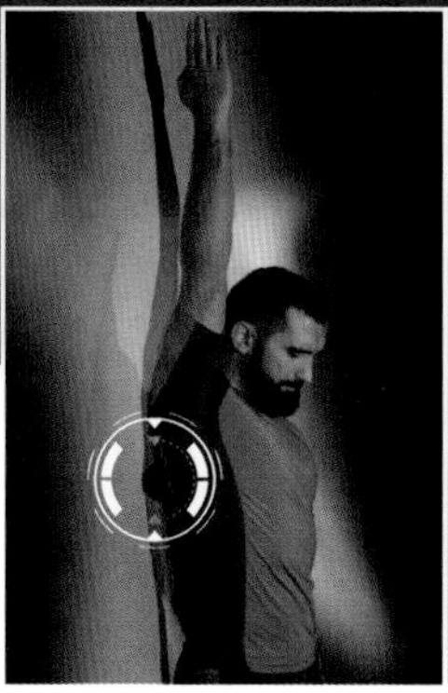

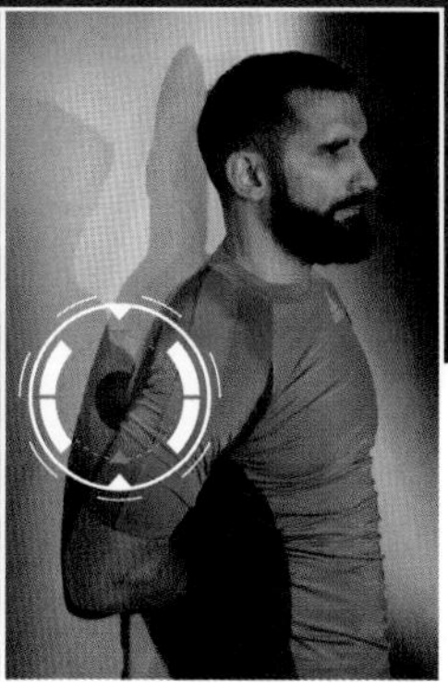

E13. TRICEPS MASSAGE AND STRETCH

Lie on your side with your triceps on a roller. Combine rolling movements from top to bottom on the roller with flexing and bending the elbow, followed by internal and external shoulder rotations. This will vary the length of the triceps muscles and allow you to explore the different orientations of the muscle fibers. Vary the angles as much as possible to reach the largest possible area.

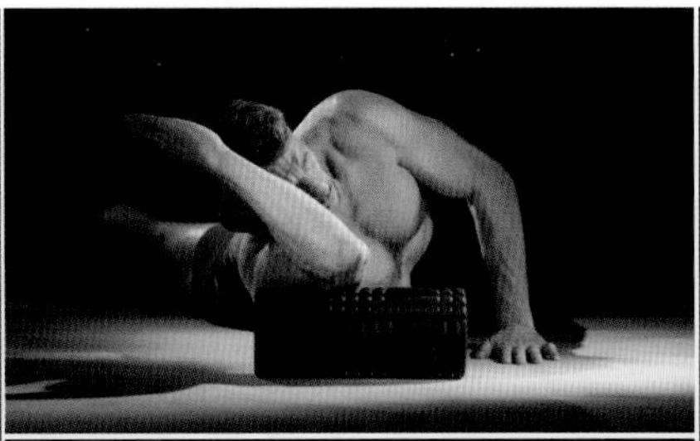

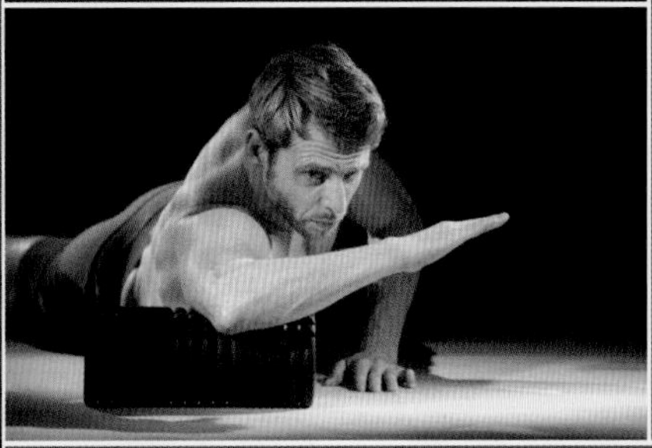

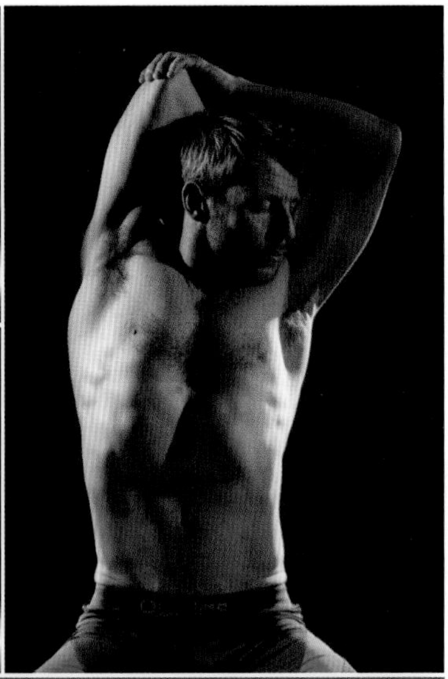

Perform 1 to 3 sets of 10 bending and flexing moves and 10 internal and external rotations. Then stretch your triceps for 20 seconds: Extend the arm over your head and grab the elbow using your other hand. Keep your spine straight and gently turn your head to the side.

E14. TRAPEZIUS MASSAGE USING A BALL

Position the ball above one of your shoulder blades between your neck and shoulder. The arm on the side you are not massaging remains stretched down at your side parallel to the floor. Raise your hips to increase the pressure. There are four possible positions for the moving arm:

- Arm flexed in an arm lock behind the back
- Arm stretched diagonally upward
- Arm stretched upward
- Arm stretched diagonally downward

You can also do this exercise with the ball just below the shoulder blade.
Perform 1 to 3 sets of 10 of each arm movement.

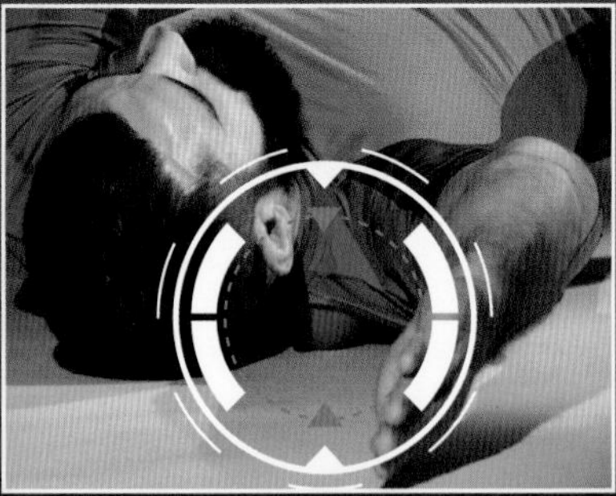

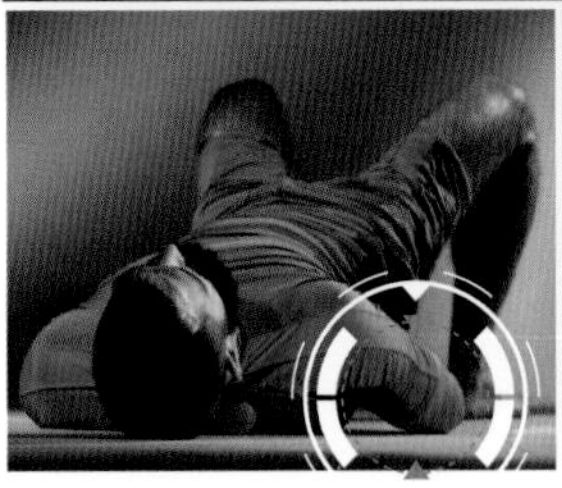

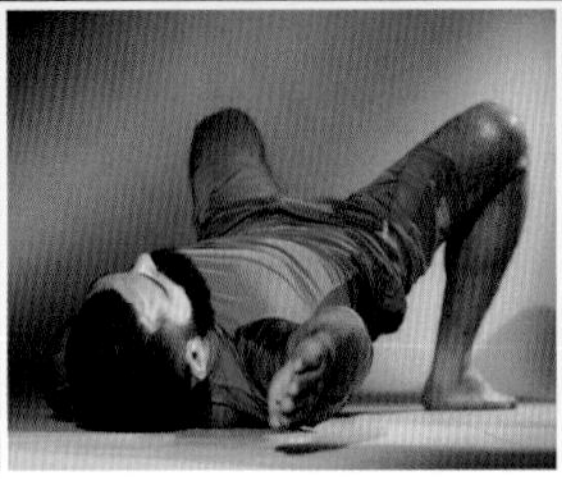

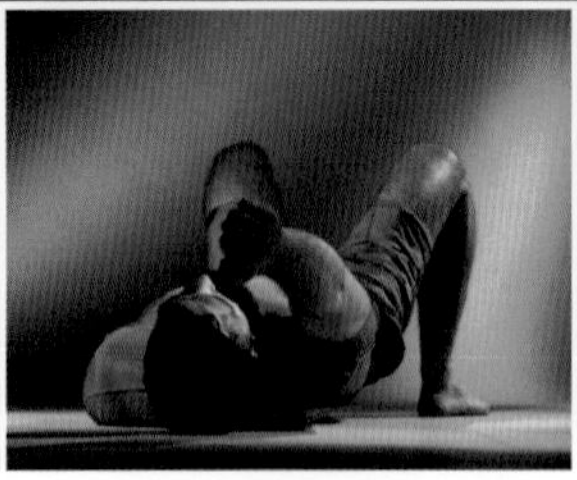

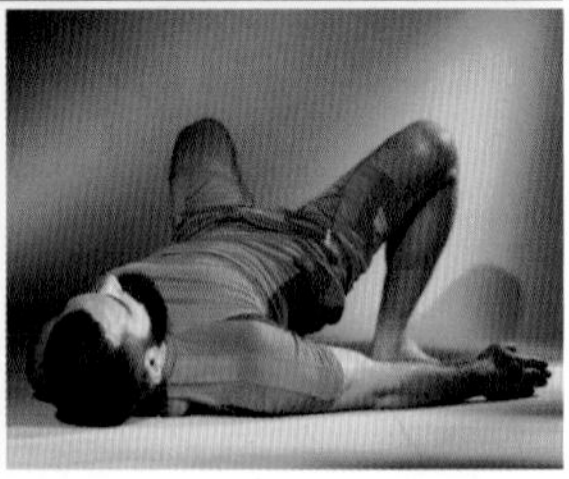

Sample 3-week mobility program targeting the shoulder (including exercises for neighboring areas)

MONDAY	TUESDAY	WEDNESDAY	THURSDAY	FRIDAY	SATURDAY	SUNDAY
E1*, E2, E3, E4, E7	B2, B3, B4, B6	E14, E13, E3, E6, E5	H1, H5, H7, H9, H10	E9, E11, E10, E14	H3, H5, H8, B1, B3	E3, E6, E12, E8, E4

*These letter/number combinations refer to the exercises and techniques found on pages 26 through 76.

KNEE PAIN

The knee is a very complex joint, and everyday mechanical stresses and past injuries often lead to pain that originates in the joint structure itself. Especially susceptible to degenerative joint disease and injuries of its smallest parts (meniscus, kneecap, cartilage, etc.), the knee joint quite often suffers from structural pain.

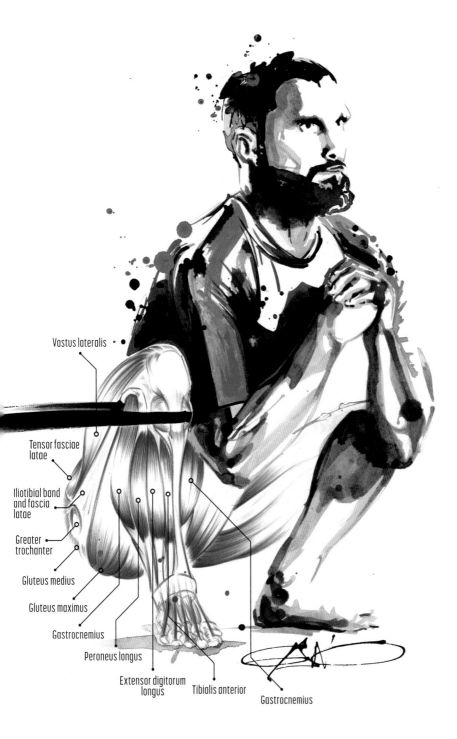

The soft tissues surrounding the knee also work very hard and will benefit from relaxation:

→ Remember the down-up treatment rule for pain. Knee pain can also radiate from other areas such as the hamstrings (biceps femoris, semitendinosus, or even semimembranosus) and the calves (gastrocnemius or even soleus muscles).

→ The posterior chain is not the only one responsible for knee pain. To be comprehensive, you must also pay attention to the front of the leg. The quadriceps and the tibialis anterior muscles are often indirectly responsible for knee pain.

→ The pelvis is also often involved. You should consider performing all the exercises suggested in the section dedicated to caring for the pelvic area.

Vastus lateralis
Tensor fasciae latae
Iliotibial band and fascia latae
Greater trochanter
Gluteus medius
Gluteus maximus
Gastrocnemius
Peroneus longus
Extensor digitorum longus
Tibialis anterior
Gastrocnemius

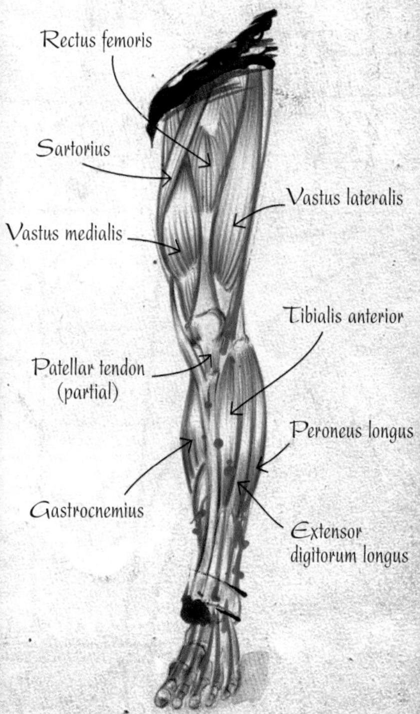
Rectus femoris
Sartorius
Vastus lateralis
Vastus medialis
Tibialis anterior
Patellar tendon (partial)
Peroneus longus
Gastrocnemius
Extensor digitorum longus

THE SCAN

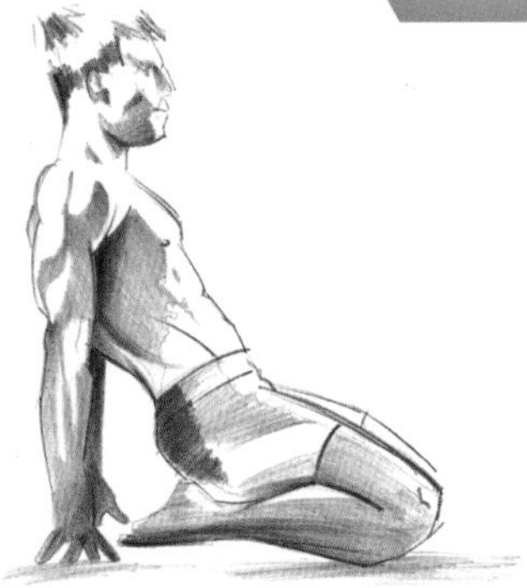

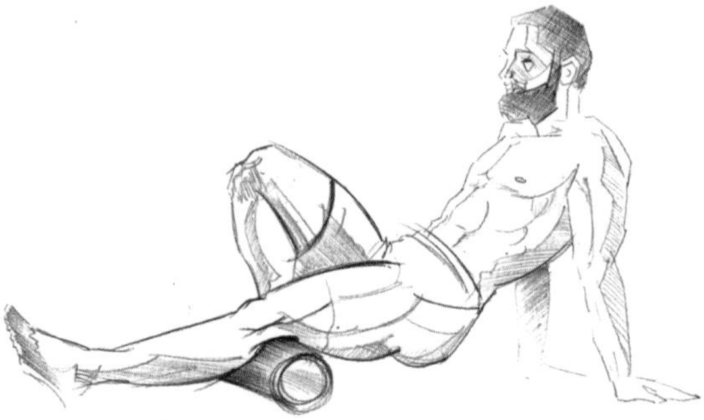

In addition to everyday pain, which often provides sufficient information about the needs in a certain area, a deep scan can reveal areas of the knee that need attention. Here are two exercises to include in the scan:

1

The resting pose: Gently lower yourself onto your knees with the insteps of your feet flat on the floor behind you if possible. You may feel pain when you sit down (compression) or when you bend; be careful.

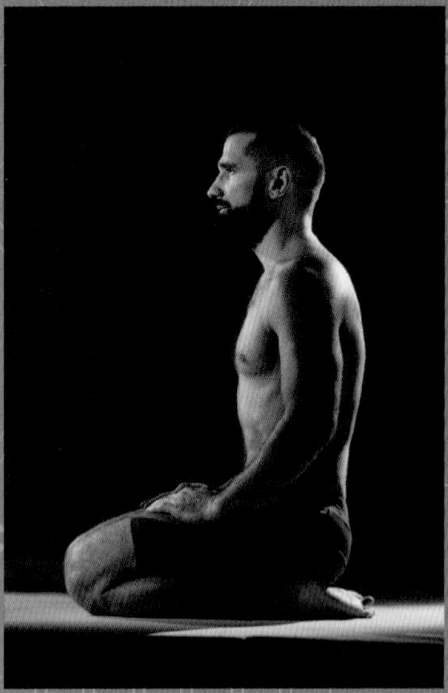

2

Flatten the *popliteal fossa* (the space behind your knee) with a massage roller: Lean back on your hands, place the roller behind your knee, and squeeze your knee against the roller.

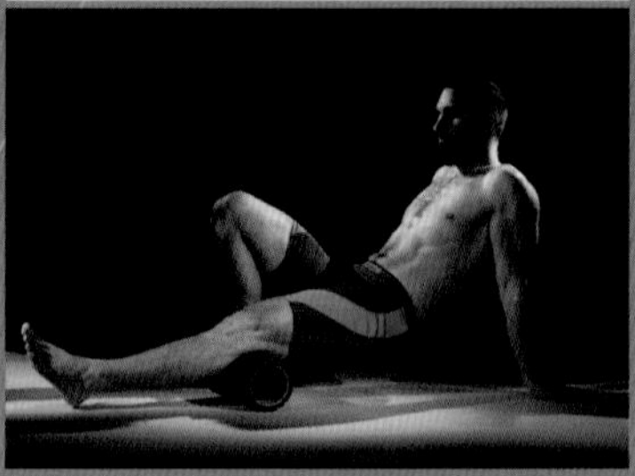

Any acute pain experienced during any of these exercises requires an appointment with your health care professional for a thorough examination. If you experience moderate pain or stiffness during these movements, it means you should perform one or more of the exercises every day.

F1. FLATTENING THE POPLITEAL FOSSA USING A MASSAGE BALL

Sit down and slide a ball into the space behind your knee. Grab your shin to gradually apply pressure. This exercise is especially painful for some people. Do not apply more pressure than you can tolerate.

Perform 1 to 3 sets of 3 seconds to 1 minute.

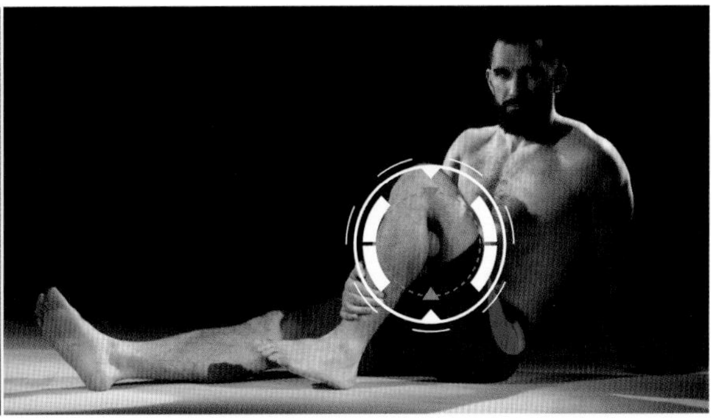

F2. TIBIALIS ANTERIOR MASSAGE USING A DOUBLE BALL

On a box or chair, place a double ball on either side of your shin. Adjust the amount of pressure by regulating how much weight you put on your heel when sitting back. Alternate between flexing, extending, and circling your foot throughout the massage to move the soft tissue in every direction.

Perform 1 to 3 sets of 10 front-to-back rolls, 10 flexions and extensions, and 10 circular movements.

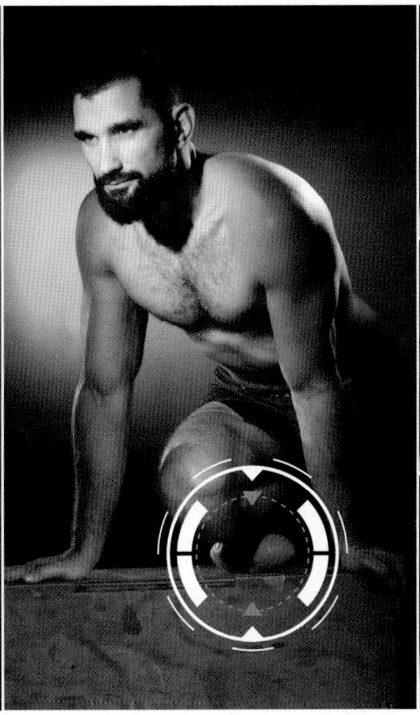

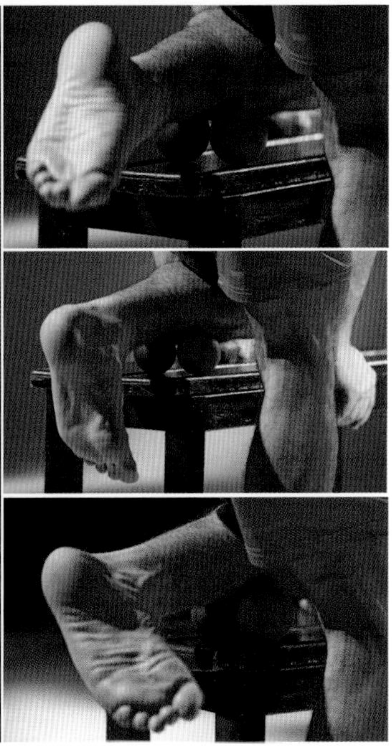

F3. IT BAND MASSAGE

Create a stationary massage tool by blocking a double massage ball or roller; you can also cut a foam roller in two pieces to make a half roller. Slide the layers of soft tissue over one another, especially the IT band over the fasciae latae and the vastus lateralis. During the massage, anchor your massage tool to the floor and move firmly over the tool using short movements. This is undoubtedly the most uncomfortable of all the self-massage exercises. You can vary the internal rotation of the hip to explore different knee positions. Among the exercises done near the knee, this one is generally the most effective for knee pain.

Perform 1 to 3 sets of 10 short massages from top to bottom.

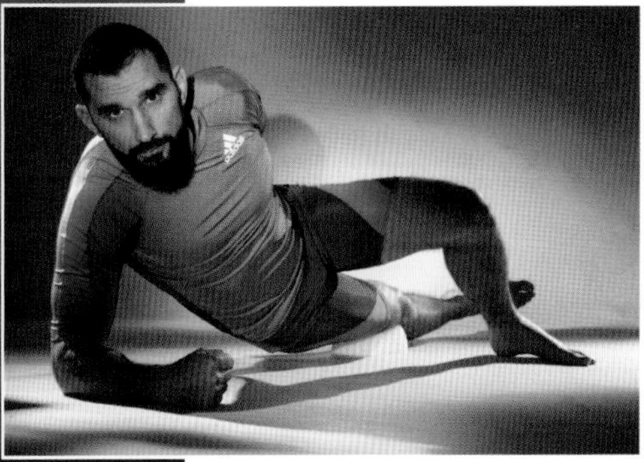

F4. COMPRESSION OF THE KNEECAP AREA USING A ROLLER

Raise one knee and place the other knee on the roller, applying just enough pressure that the exercise is tolerable. Roll from front to back, possibly varying the bend in your hip and knee by a few degrees.

Perform 1 to 3 sets of 10 short massages from front to back.

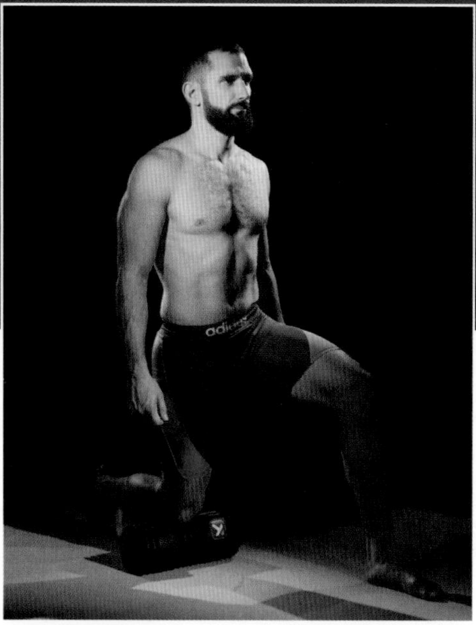

F5. VASTUS MEDIALIS MASSAGE USING A BALL

Lie down and place the vastus medialis of your quadriceps muscle on a ball. Perform this exercise lying flat on your stomach with a flexed leg, flat on your stomach with a straight leg, and on your side. **Perform 1 to 3 sets of 10 top-to-bottom rolls, 10 left-to-right rolls, and 10 circular rolls.** Then change positions.

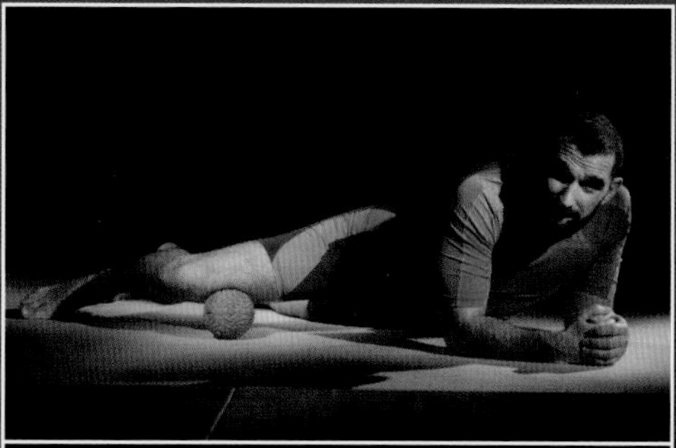

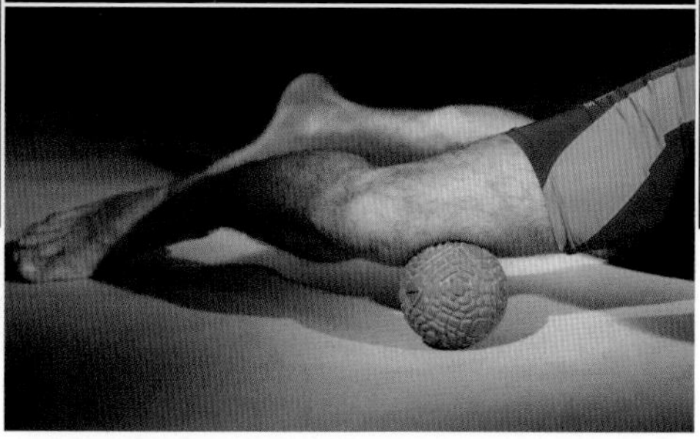

F6. MASSAGE FOR THE UPPER, OUTER PART OF THE CALVES USING A DOUBLE BALL

Sit with your leg flexed in front of you and slide a double massage ball under the upper, outer side of your calf.
Perform 1 to 3 sets of 10 right-to-left massages, then massage the area by tilting yourself forward and backward 10 times.

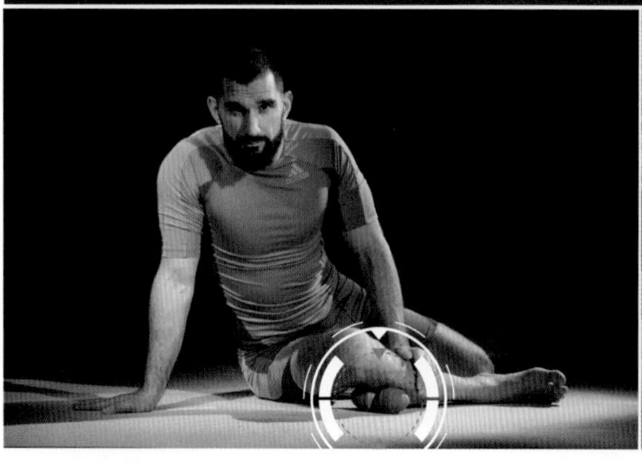

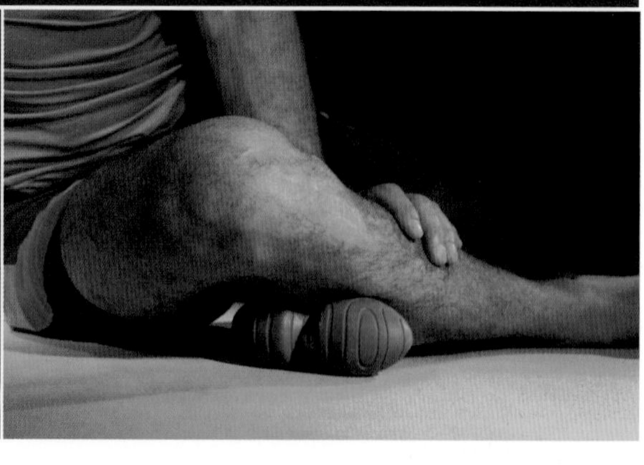

F7. MASSAGE FOR THE LOWER HAMSTRING INSERTIONS USING A BALL

Sit on a box or table and place a ball at the bottom of your hamstrings in the lowest part of the thigh.

Perform 1 to 3 sets of 10 front-to-back rolls, 10 left-to-right rolls, and 10 circular rolls.

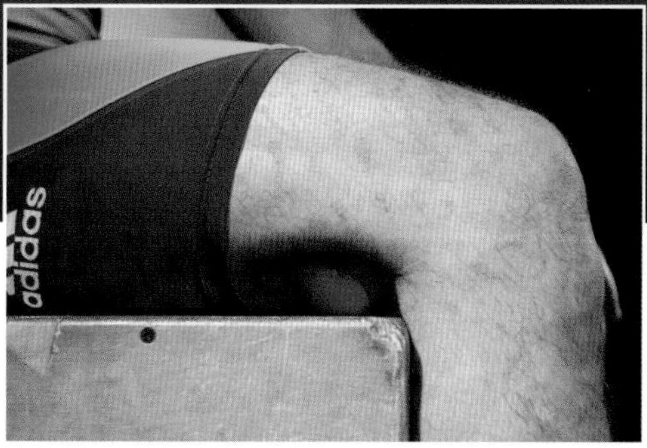

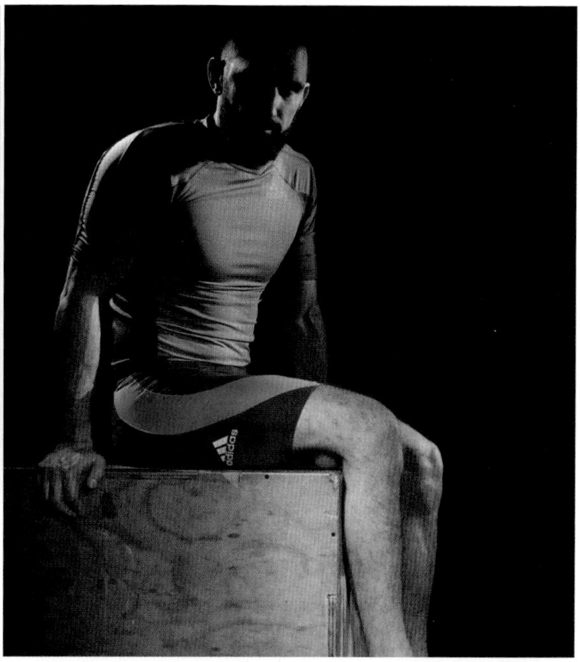

F8. SEATED CALF AND HAMSTRING STRETCH USING A BAND

Sit with one leg completely extended and wrap a band around your foot. Gradually pull your foot toward you without flexing your knee. To activate the hamstrings even more, lean forward while keeping your back as straight as possible.

Perform 1 to 3 times per calf, holding this position for 30 seconds.

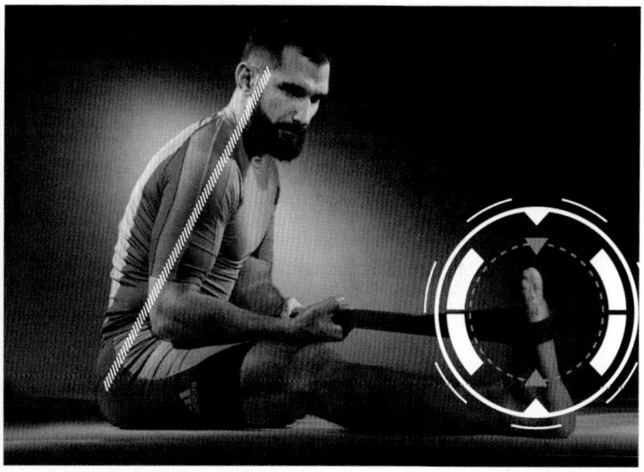

F9. QUADRICEPS STRETCH WHILE LYING ON YOUR SIDE

Lie on your side with one arm extended above your head. Grab your foot with the other hand, flex your knee, and try to bring your heel to your buttock. Do not arch your back or move your knee backward too much.

Perform 1 to 3 times per leg, holding this stretch for 30 seconds.

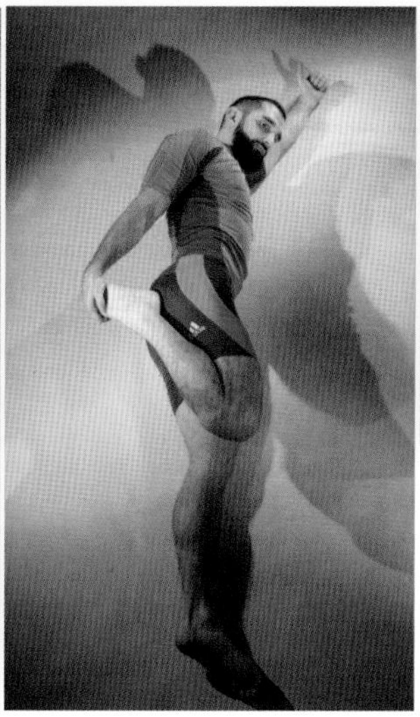

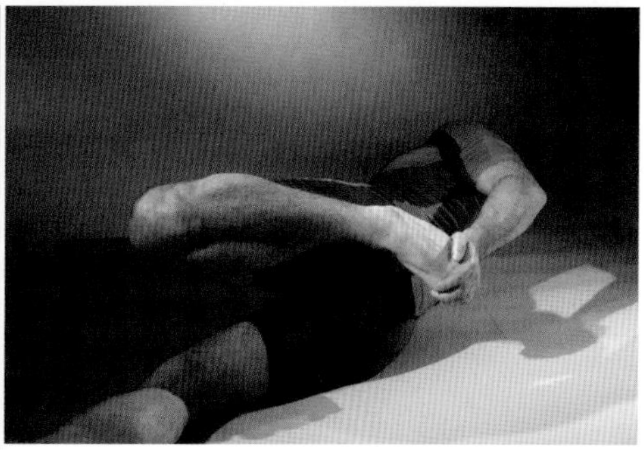

F10. KNEE PROPRIOCEPTION USING A BAND

Stand on one leg with your knee slightly flexed and wrap a taut resistance band around the knee. Slowly flex your knee with your eyes closed. **Perform this move 3 times, keeping your kneecap in line with your toes.** Then move the band to reach different angles.

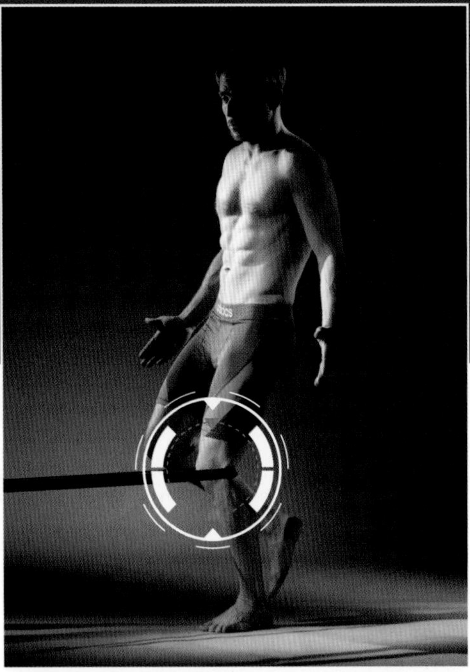

F11. KNEE PROPRIOCEPTION USING A BALANCE DISC

With your eyes closed, stand on a balance disc, soft mat, or pillow and slowly flex your knee to work on stability; try to keep your balance.

Perform 1 to 3 reps, balancing for 30 seconds per knee.

F12. WEIGHT-FREE FLEXION USING SUSPENSION STRAPS

With your body supported from suspension straps in a low position, allow yourself to gradually and slowly descend into a deep squat.

Perform 2 or 3 sets of 5 reps.

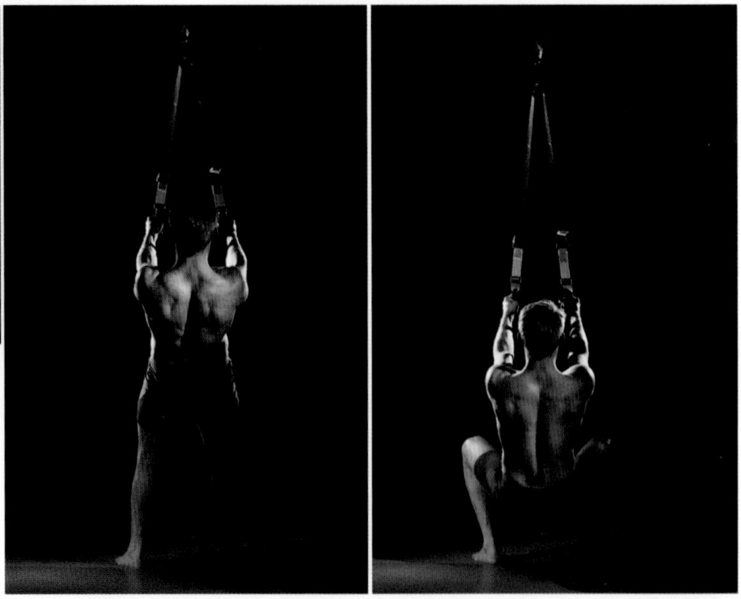

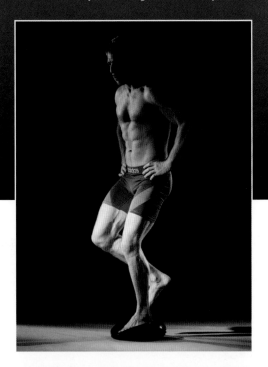

F13. INTERNAL KNEE STRIKE

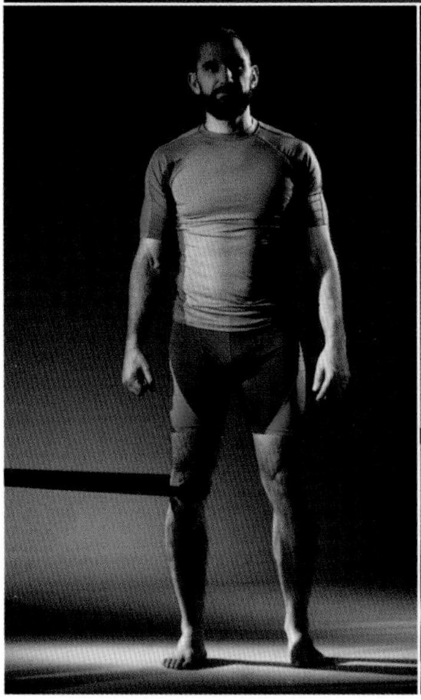

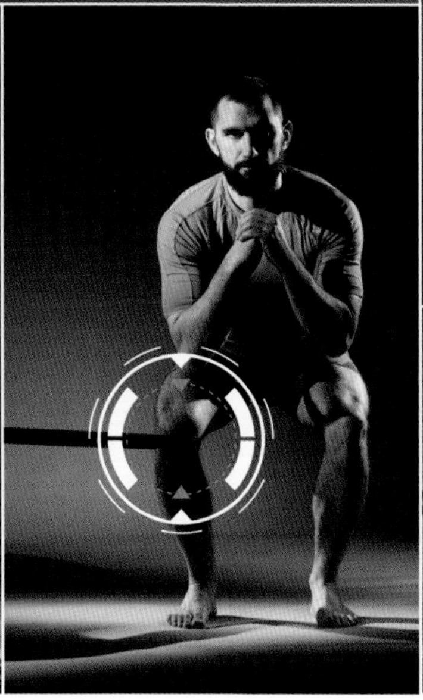

Warning: You should only do this exercise if it does not cause more knee pain than you would experience during normal activity. Using a resistance band that is anchored at a point level with your knee and directly to the side, wrap a taut resistance band around the knee to draw it outward. Squat down and up under full control, aiming for maximum range of motion with minimal lateral movement. **Perform 1 to 3 sets of 10 reps.**

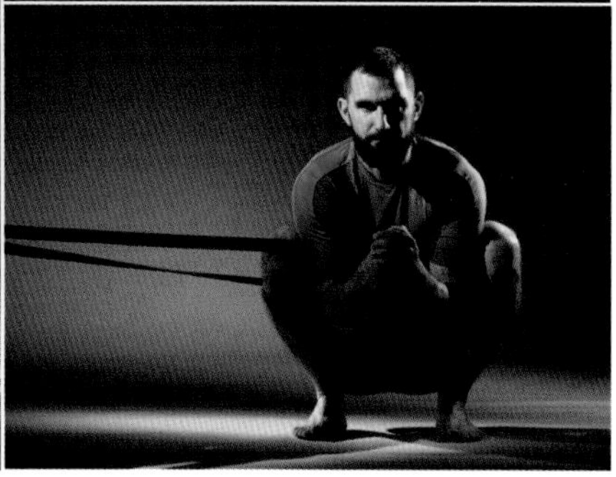

DID YOU KNOW?

Placing the mini band around your knees in the squat position significantly increases the activation of the glutes (gluteus medius and gluteus maximus). A monster squat is both a functional and an aesthetic exercise (Spracklin et al. 2017).

F14. MONSTER SQUAT

Place your knees inside a mini resistance band; this will make it challenging to keep your knees in line with your toes or, even better, pointed outward. Move into a deep squat position, keeping the band where it is. **Perform 2 to 4 sets, holding the position for at least 20 seconds and up to 1 minute** (beyond that, you will not need the band).

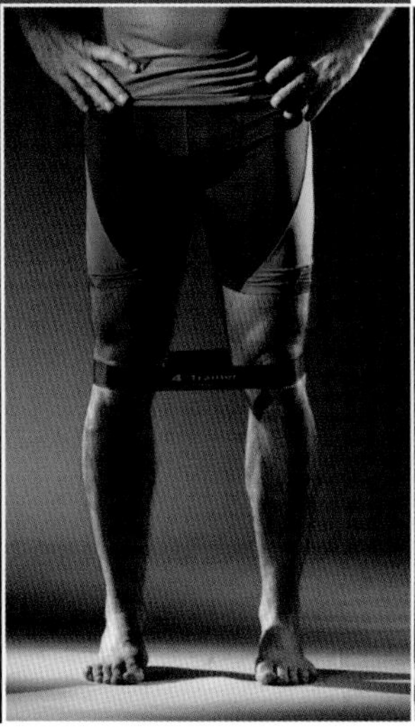

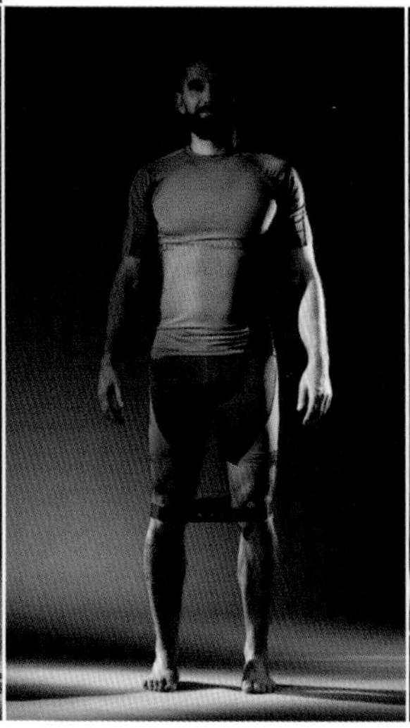

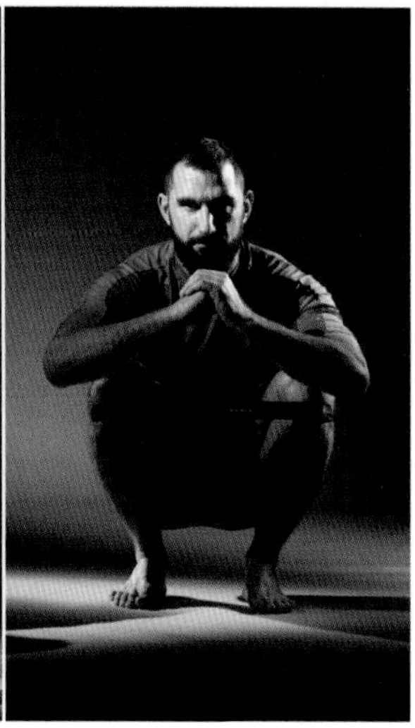

Sample 3-week mobility program targeting the knee (including exercises for neighboring areas)

MONDAY	TUESDAY	WEDNESDAY	THURSDAY	FRIDAY	SATURDAY	SUNDAY
F1, F2, F4, F8, F14	F3, F5, F11, F13, F12	C1, C3, C4, C5, C11, C2	F6, F2, F8, F9, F10	C6, C8, C13, C15, C14	D5, D6, D1, D3, D14	F3, D6, F5, D3, F7, D11

*These letter/number combinations refer to the exercises and techniques found on pages 26 through 76.

ANKLE PAIN

Very susceptible to damage, the ankle often experiences residual pain from past injuries.

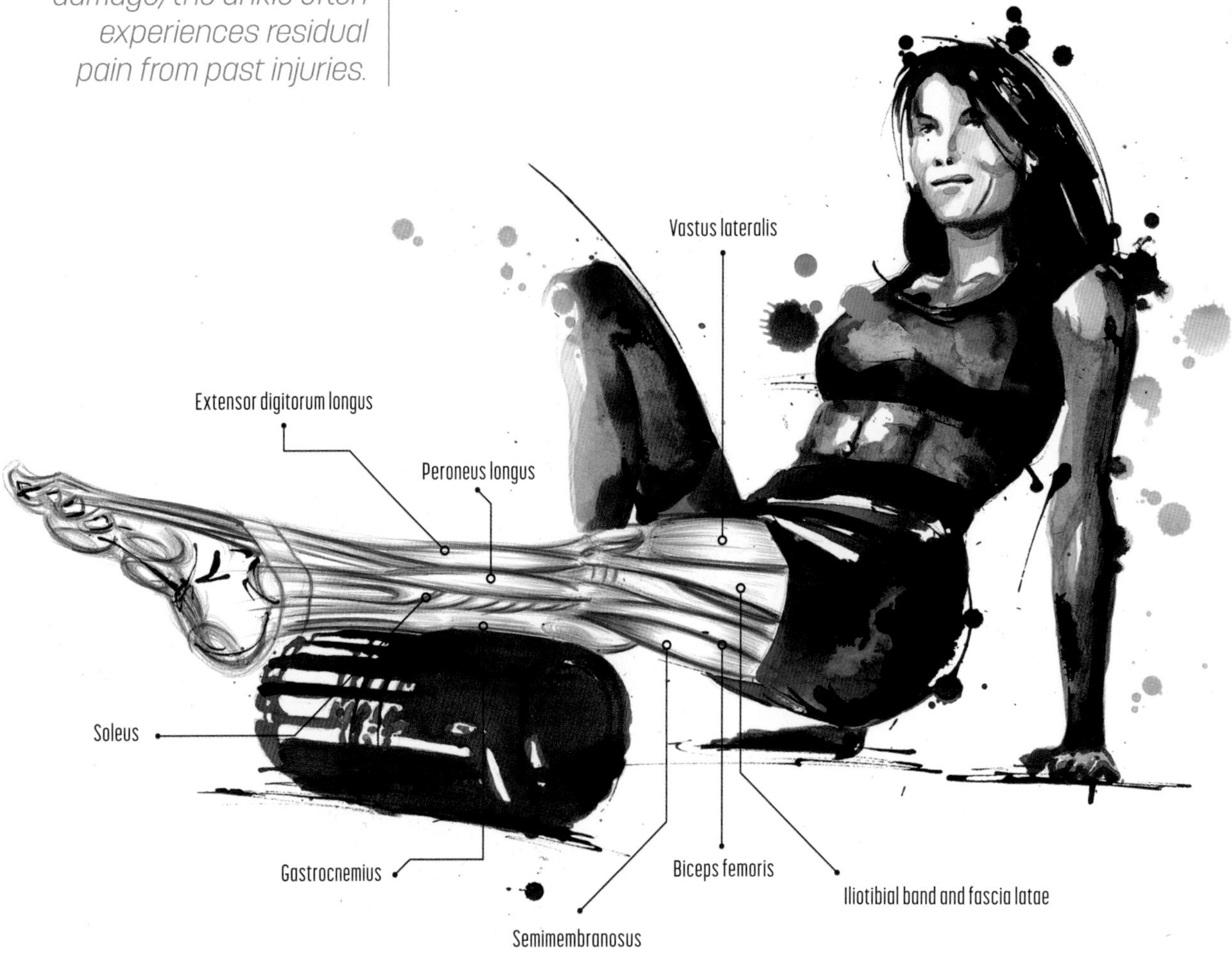

Ankle pain may develop because of imbalances or conflicts from long-standing postural problems or improper walking mechanics. Any chronic ankle pain should prompt you to visit your doctor, podiatrist, or other health care professional. However, in-depth mobility work on this joint is very simple to implement and may fix the root of your problems.

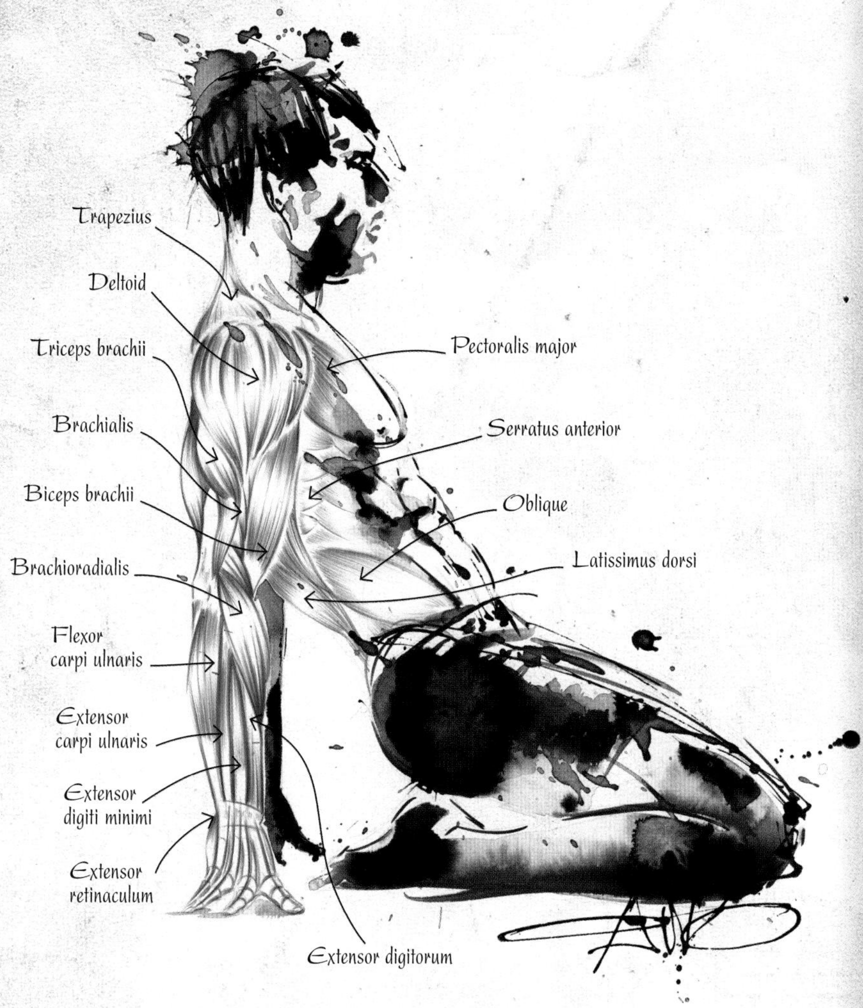

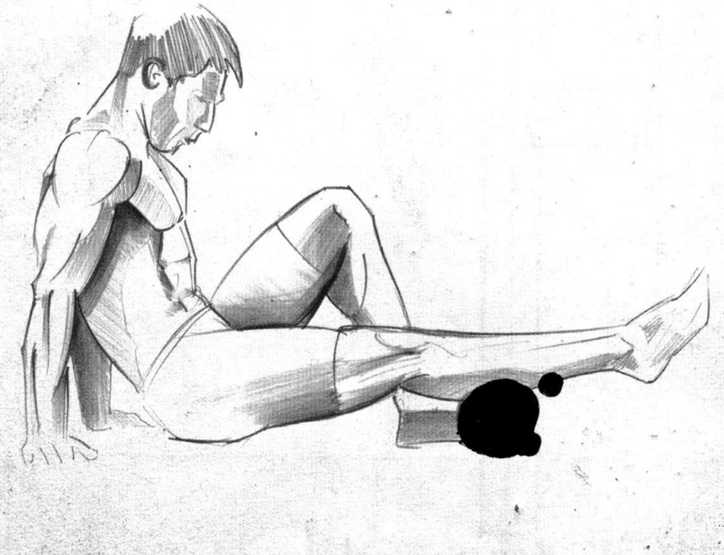

Start by using our rule of "framing" the pain.

Working on the shins and calves is essential for resolving ankle problems, but there is another area that also needs attention: the arch of the foot. This area is almost always forgotten in treatment programs, even though it is directly linked to its mobile upstairs neighbor, the ankle.

Implement the rule of mobility.

Walking on concrete every day, wearing stiff shoes, and a lack of stimulation gradually decrease the ankle's range of motion and limit the flow of information with regard to adjustments in the foot and ankle.

Finish with the rule of stabilization.

Shoes that do not allow control over the foot (untied laces) or that are heavy (leather boots), a loss of sensitivity in the arch sensors, and poor movement habits can all freeze the joint, making it stiff, ineffective, and painful.

THE SCAN

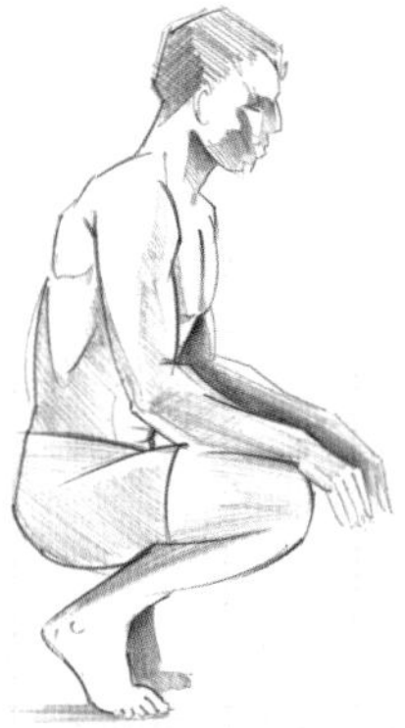

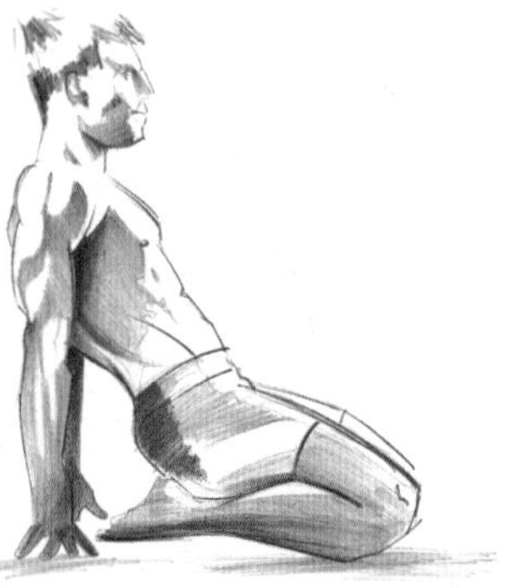

In addition to everyday pain, which often provides sufficient information about the needs in a certain area, a deep scan can reveal whether the ankle needs attention. Here are two exercises to include in the scan:

1

Stand on your tiptoes and move into a crouched position. Any pain and any loss of balance should alert you to an issue. Not being able to lower yourself down or stay in this position for a few seconds is also concerning.

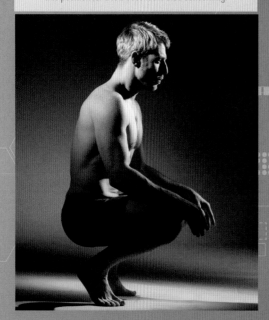

2

Next, sit back on your legs and heels. If you cannot reach this position or even hold it comfortably for several seconds, this is a clear sign that your ankles need attention.

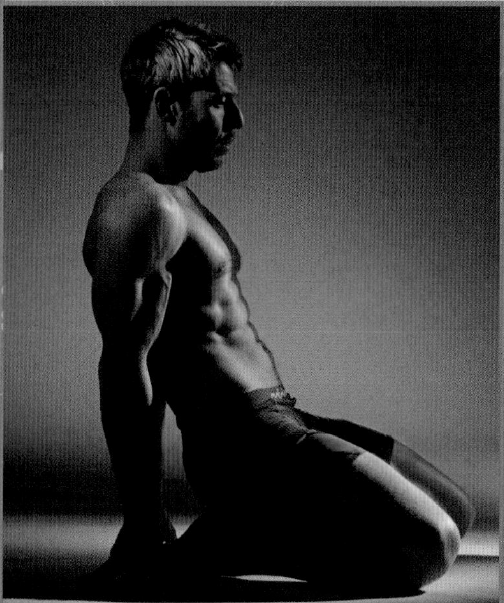

Any acute pain experienced during any of these exercises requires an appointment with your health care professional for a thorough examination. If you experience moderate pain or stiffness during these movements, it means you should perform one or more of the exercises every day.

G1. CALF MASSAGE USING A ROLLER

Support yourself using your hands and sit on your gluteals. Place your calf on the roller, but do not put your full weight on your leg. In this position, roll from front to back, looking for sensitive areas. Increase the pressure by lifting your hips and crossing your free leg over the treated leg.

Perform up to 3 sets of 10 front-to-back massages and 10 left-to-right massages. Add circular foot motions as well.

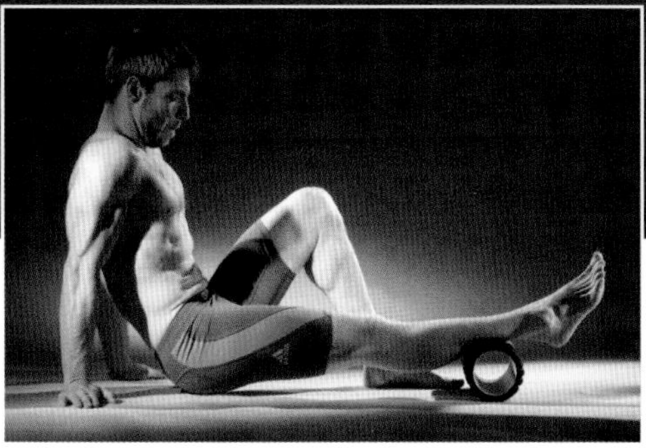

G2. MASSAGE FOR THE SIDE OF THE CALF USING TWO BALLS

Sit on your side with your leg flexed in front of you and place your calf between two massage balls. Look for painful or sensitive areas using the massage balls. Complete this exercise by flexing and extending the foot and then making circles.

Perform 1 to 3 sets of 10 top-to-bottom massages and 10 right-to-left massages on the balls.

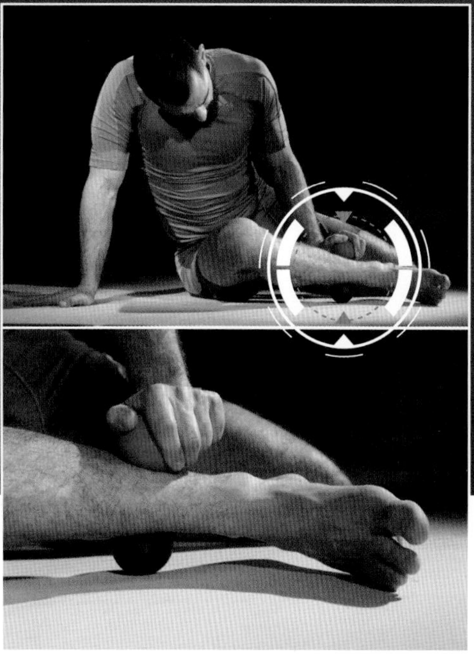

G3. MASSAGE FOR THE BACK OF THE CALF USING A DOUBLE BALL

Start from the lowest part of the calf and gradually move up. Using the double massage ball, look for sensitive areas. Cross your legs to increase pressure on the double ball.

Perform 1 to 3 sets of 10 front-to-back massages, 10 left-to-right massages, and 10 circular massages, holding each for a few seconds.

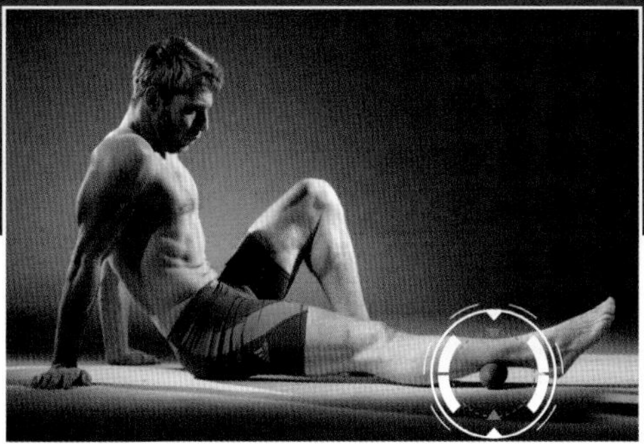

G4. TIBIALIS ANTERIOR MASSAGE USING A DOUBLE BALL

On a box or chair, place the double massage ball on either side of your shin. Adjust the amount of pressure applied by sitting back on your heel. Alternate between flexing, extending, and circling your foot throughout the massage to allow the soft tissue to move in all directions.

Perform 1 to 3 sets of 10 focused front-to-back rolls, 10 flexions and extensions, and 10 circular movements.

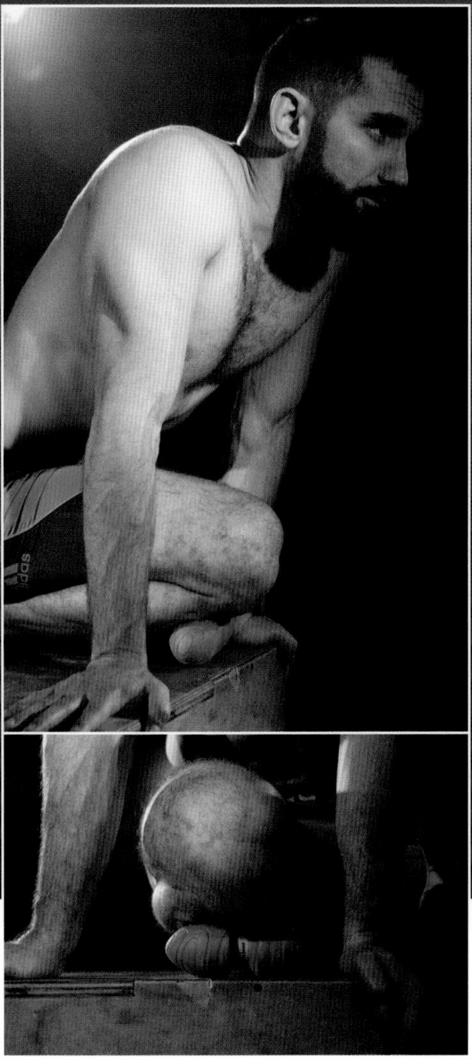

G5. MASSAGE FOR THE ARCH OF THE FOOT USING A BALL

Stand up and place the massage ball under the sole of your foot. Look for stiff areas along the side, then explore the inner part of the foot. Massage from front to back, left to right, and in a circular motion. Take the time to focus on the ball of your foot by putting your heel on the floor with the massage ball underneath the front of the foot. Then massage from left to right. Do not neglect your heel; with your toes on the floor, roll the ball under your heel from right to left.

Perform the massage for 1 to 2 minutes on each foot.

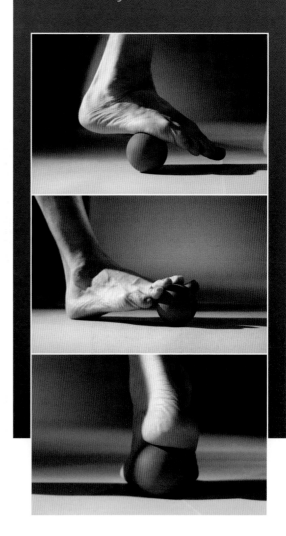

G6. EAGLE CLAW STRETCH

In a seated position, curl your toes. Move as much of your weight as you can to the front of the foot to stretch your toes.

Perform 2 or 3 sets, holding for 30 seconds.

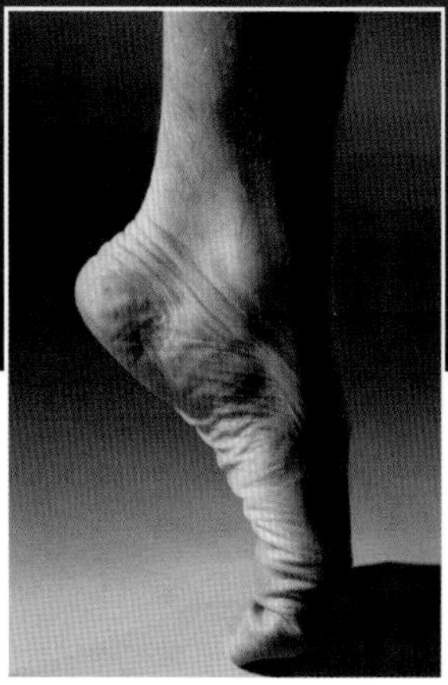

G7. RESTING POSE STRETCH 1

On your knees, extend your toes and sit back onto your heels with your feet in the position shown in the photo.

Perform 2 or 3 sets, holding for 30 seconds.

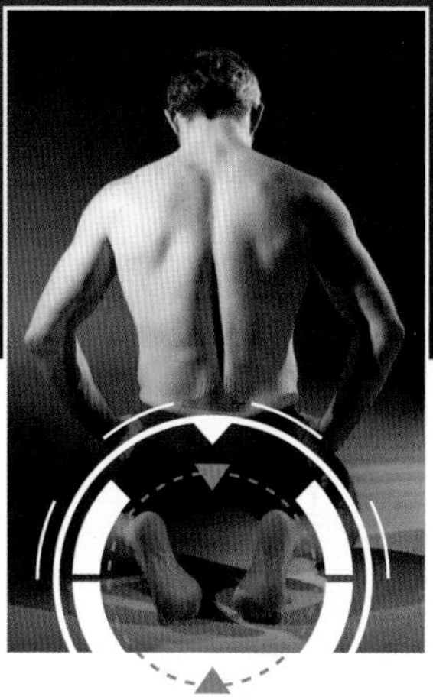

G8. RESTING POSE STRETCH 2

On your knees, extend your feet and sit back onto your heels with your feet in the position shown in the photo.

Perform 2 or 3 sets, holding for 30 seconds.

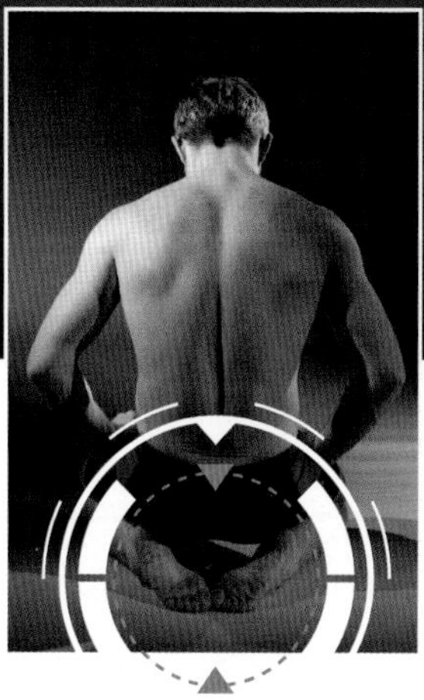

G9. JOINT DECOMPRESSION STRETCH

Place the base of your lower leg in a taut resistance band anchored near the floor behind you, step forward with your other leg, and stretch your rear calf by flexing that knee forward. Be sure to keep the heel of your rear foot flat on the floor.

Perform 1 to 3 times per leg, flexing the leg for 20 seconds then straightening the leg for 20 seconds.

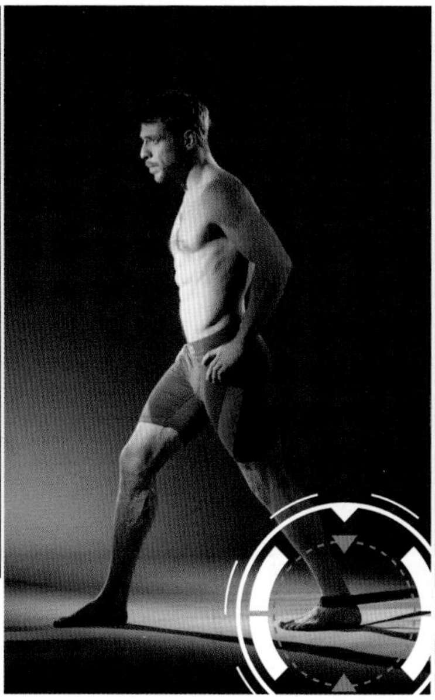

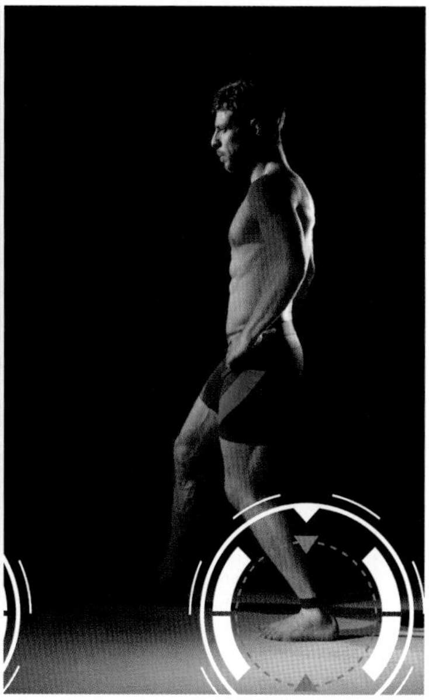

G10. KNIGHTHOOD

Place one knee on the floor and the other knee up with your front shin perpendicular to the ground. Move back to extend the front leg (photo one) and then replant the front foot on the floor and lunge forward so the knee goes past the toes of the front foot (photo two). Gradually increase the time spent in these two extreme positions until you can hold 10 sets of 3 seconds on each side.

Perform this cycle up to 3 times.

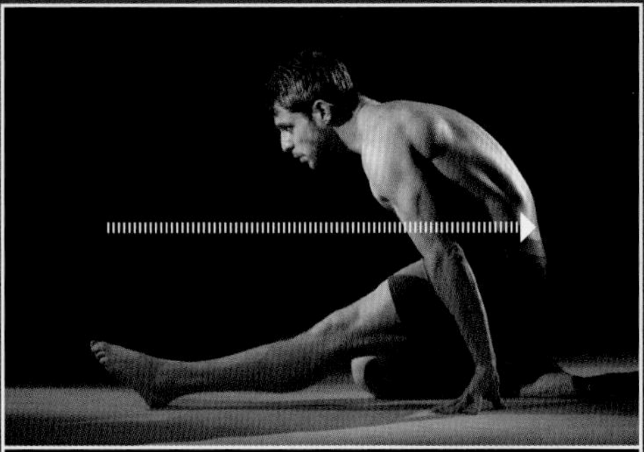

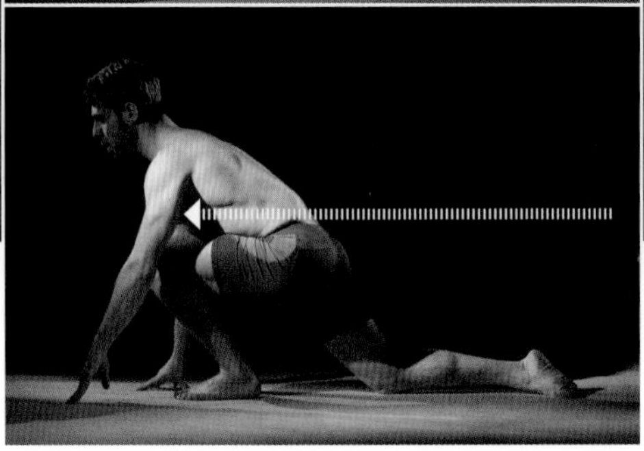

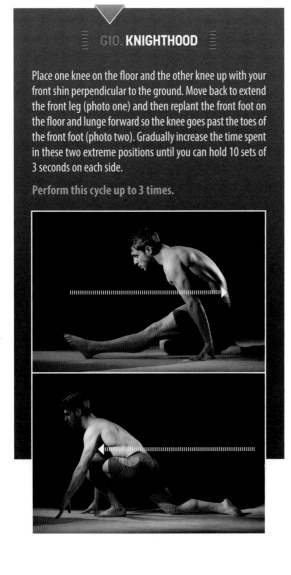

G11. ANKLE PROPRIOCEPTION

On one straight leg, stand on a soft mat, pillow, or balance disc with your eyes closed. Transfer your body weight to the front of the foot, the outside of the foot, the heel, and then the inside of the foot.

Perform this exercise 1 to 3 times in each direction as 1 set. Perform up to 3 sets per leg.

Sample 3-week mobility program targeting the ankle (including exercises for neighboring areas)

MONDAY	TUESDAY	WEDNESDAY	THURSDAY	FRIDAY	SATURDAY	SUNDAY
G1*, G2, G6, G10	G5, G4, G2, G8, G11	F1, G2, F4, G10	G1, G9, G3, G7, G10	F1, F4, F6, F7, F8	G2, G9, G10, G11	F6, F7, G1, F8, F10

*These letter/number combinations refer to the exercises and techniques found on pages 26 through 76.

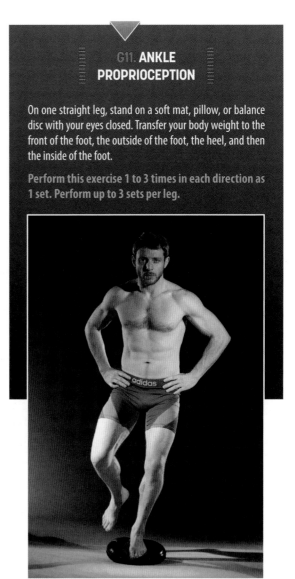

NECK PAIN

There are a host of neck issues, such as pain, stiffness, and immobility, that can cause torticollis *(a twisted neck) and nerve pain. Laptop use can exacerbate neck pain; our posture when using laptops forces our head firmly into a slanted position.*

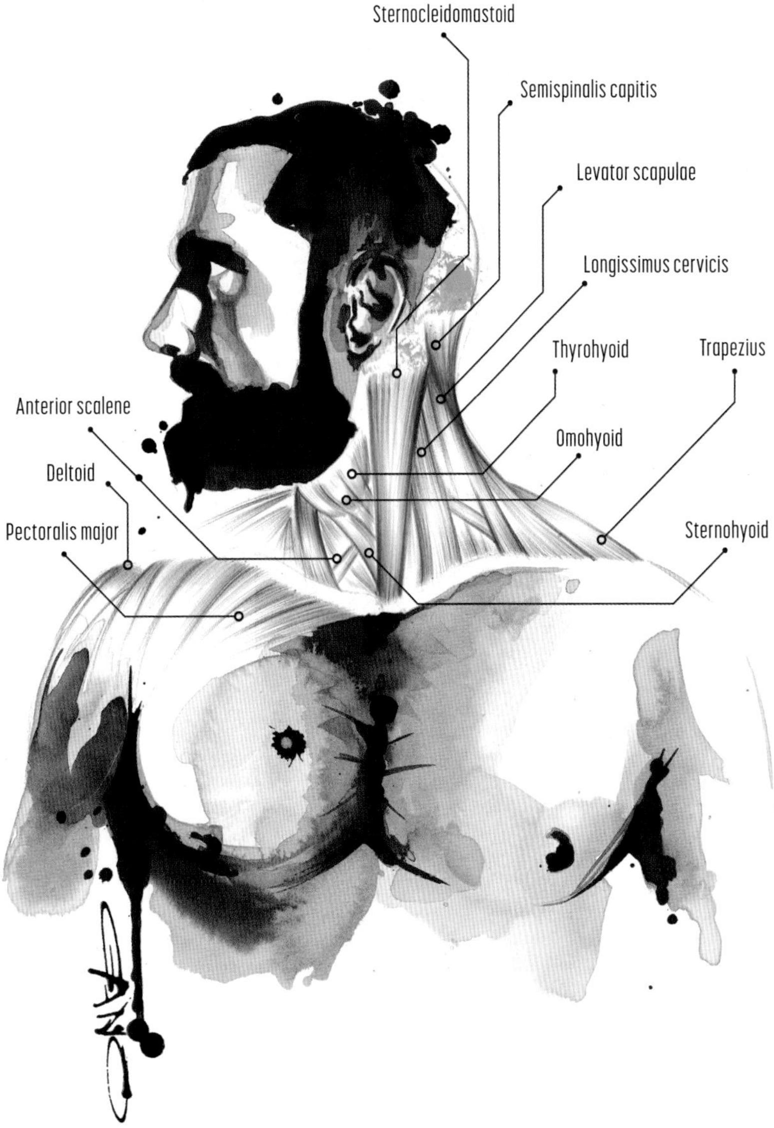

The neck muscles are situated at the end of a muscle chain. When not actually causing problems in movement or posture, they often suffer the consequences. The neck muscles are ideally placed within your body—between your head and respiratory system—to feel the effects of your emotional state.

Therefore, you must spend time relaxing each area, keeping the following points in mind:

- Remind yourself of one of the first rules for beating pain and taking back your mobility: If something no longer moves, or does not move at all, mobilize it.
- Remember the above-below treatment rule for pain. The cause of your problems is just as likely to be found in the lower parts of the trapezius muscles as in the pectoral muscles. The section dedicated to muscle chains will demonstrate how different muscles can be associated with the anterior, posterior, and lateral chains in their final links. Problems radiating to the neck can sometimes be caused by something far below.
- Conversely, the problem could come from higher up, sometimes from the head and often from the eyes. Look at your whole body when considering the source of neck pain.

THE SCAN

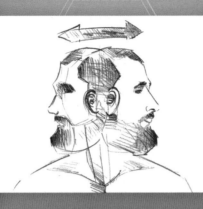

In addition to everyday pain, which often provides sufficient information about the needs in a certain area, a deep scan can reveal areas of the neck that need attention. Here are two exercises to include in the scan:

1

Move: Slowly move your head from left to right and top to bottom. Slowly bring your right ear to your right shoulder, then bring your left ear to your left shoulder, and finish by making circles with your head.

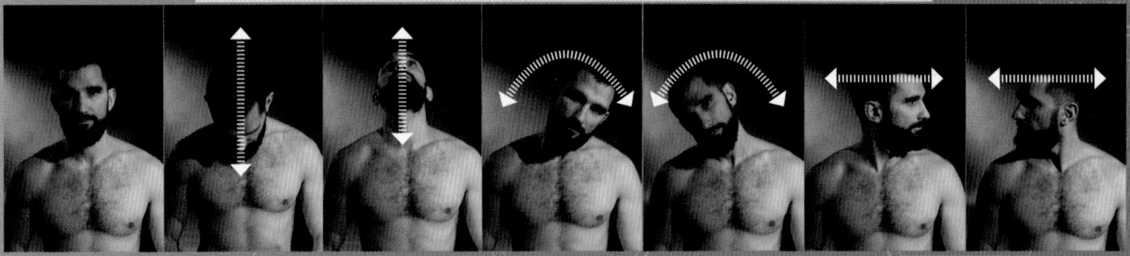

2

Feel: Move your hand gently over all areas of the neck and apply different amounts of pressure. This manual approach will allow you to find any painful or tense areas.

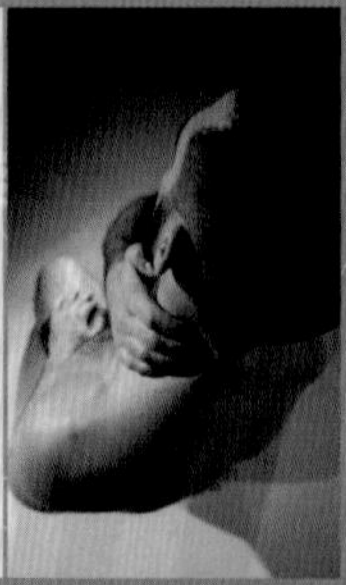

Finish by combining the two exercises: Manually search the neck at different angles by using various head positions. More than ever, the stretches and massages described next should be complemented by breathing exercises (see part II dedicated to breathing). Focus on breathing using your diaphragm and stay relaxed at all times.

H1. NECK ROLLER MASSAGE COMBINED WITH A DOUBLE BALL

Using a massage roller helps reduce tension; inserting a double massage ball between the roller and the nape of your neck will give you more precision and intensity. Lie on your back and let your shoulders fall backward. Let your head hang until you reach the desired pressure on the massage ball then roll up and down, perhaps moving your head gently from left to right.

Perform 1 to 3 sets of 10 to 20 rolls.

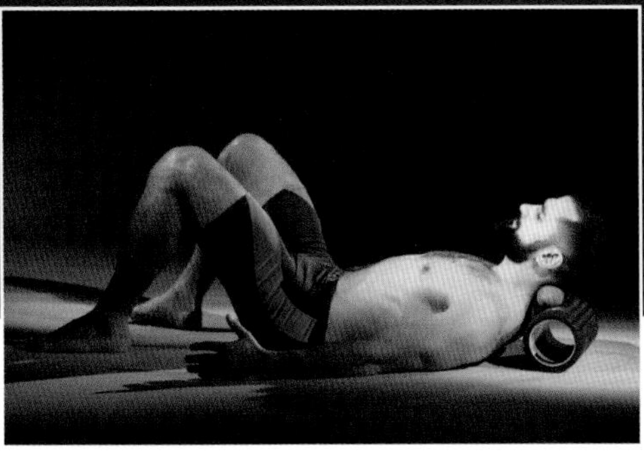

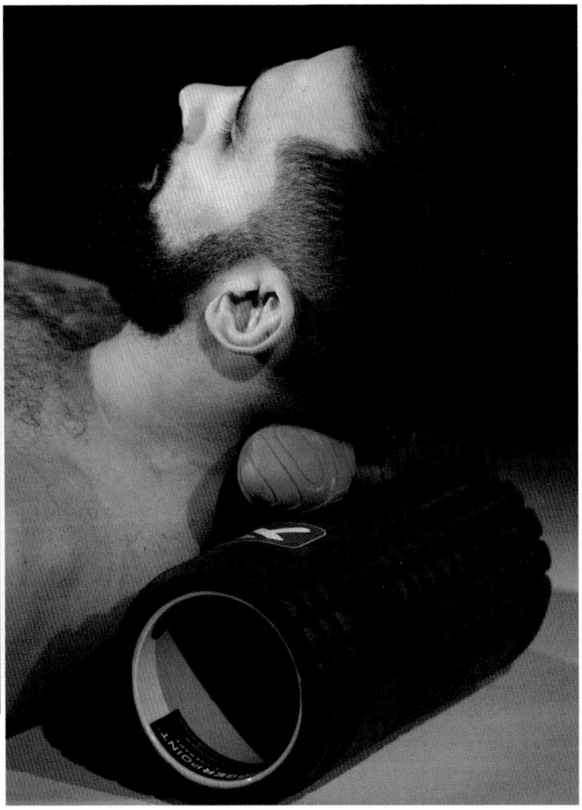

H2. NECK MASSAGE USING A DOUBLE BALL

Lie on your back and place your hands on your thighs or position your arms at your side for balance. Relax your shoulders, allowing them to move down and backward as much as possible (in this case, toward the floor). Slide a double massage ball under your neck and lift your hips to place sufficient pressure on the ball. Roll from front to back and perhaps gently from left to right.

Perform 1 to 3 sets of 10 to 20 rolls.

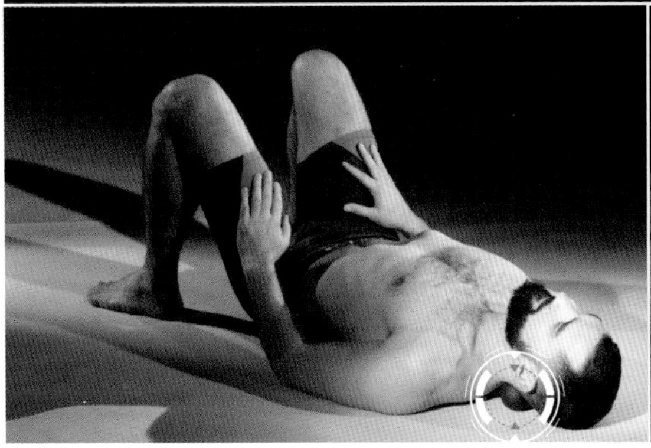

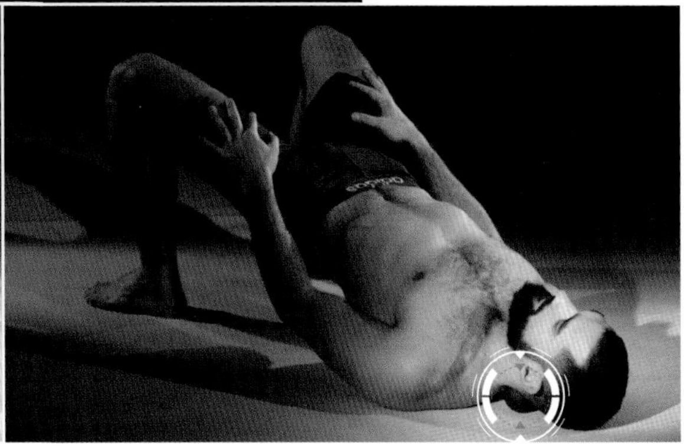

H3. NECK MASSAGE USING A LARGE BALL

Lie on your back and position your arms at your side. Relax your shoulders, allowing them to move down and back as much as possible (in this case, toward the floor). Place the ball in one of the curves on the side of your neck and turn your head from right to left, maintaining pressure on the ball. Increase the intensity by placing the back of your hand on your forehead and your other hand on top of it.

Perform 1 to 3 sets of 10 to 20 rolls.

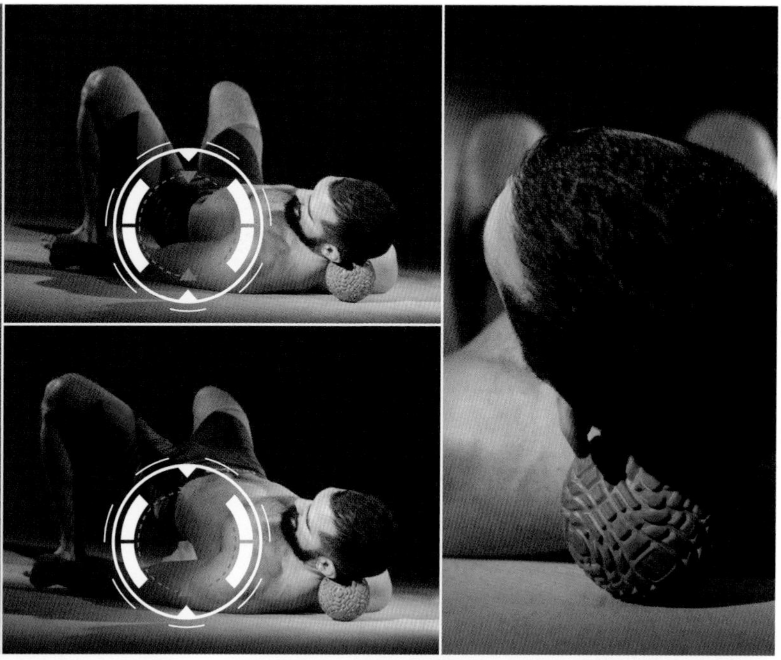

H4. STRETCHING THE ROTATOR MUSCLES

On your knees or standing, straighten your back as much as possible before starting this exercise. Slowly turn your head as far to the left as possible then as far to the right as possible.

Perform 1 to 3 sets, holding for 30 seconds.

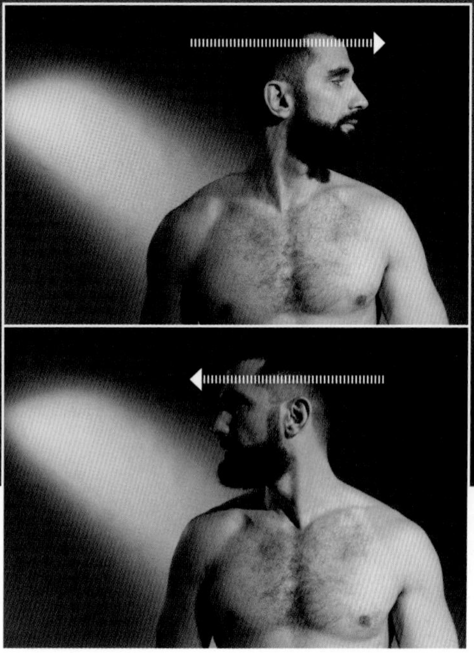

H5. STRETCHING THE EXTENSOR MUSCLES

On your knees or standing, straighten your back as much as possible before starting this exercise. Slowly allow your head to fall forward without changing the posture of your back. If your flexibility allows, grab the top of your head to add additional pressure. Do not try to pull more than is tolerable.

Perform 1 to 3 sets, holding for 30 seconds.

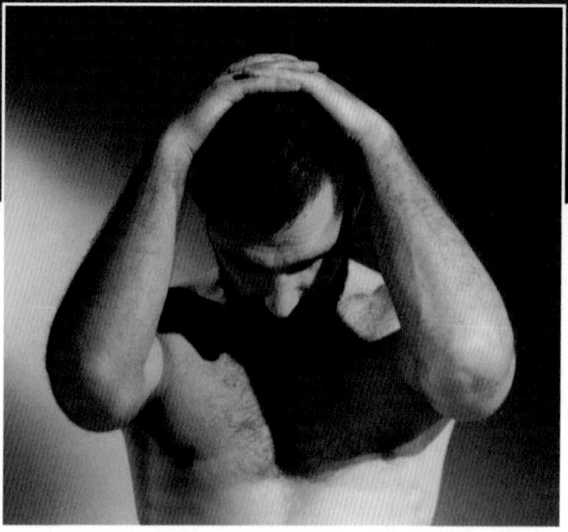

H6. STRETCHING THE FLEXOR MUSCLES

On your knees or standing, straighten your back as much as possible before starting this exercise. Tilt your head backward. Lean slightly backward by opening your hips to increase the stretch in your neck, but be careful not to lean too far back, which could hyperextend your neck and back.

Perform 1 to 3 sets, holding for 30 seconds.

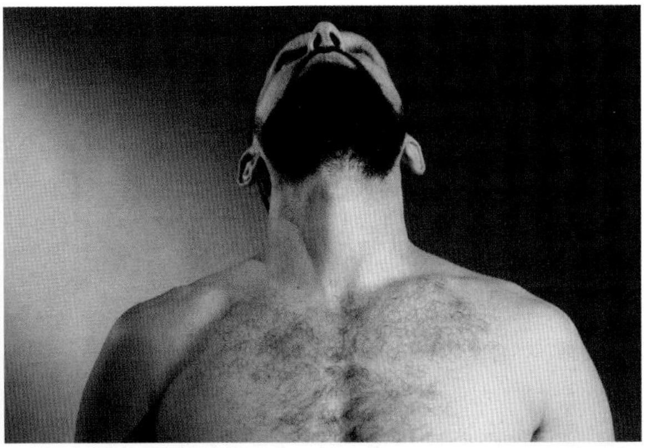

H7. TRAPEZIUS MASSAGE USING A POLE

Lie on your back and place a round-ended pole against a wall and under your trapezius muscle. Do not hesitate to change the contact point as you look for different painful or stiff areas. Although this exercise can be uncomfortable, try to keep your shoulder relaxed and in a neutral position. **Perform 1 to 3 times per shoulder, holding each pressure point for 30 seconds.** Then slowly lift your arm straight up 1 to 3 times, stopping as needed at the most sensitive angles.

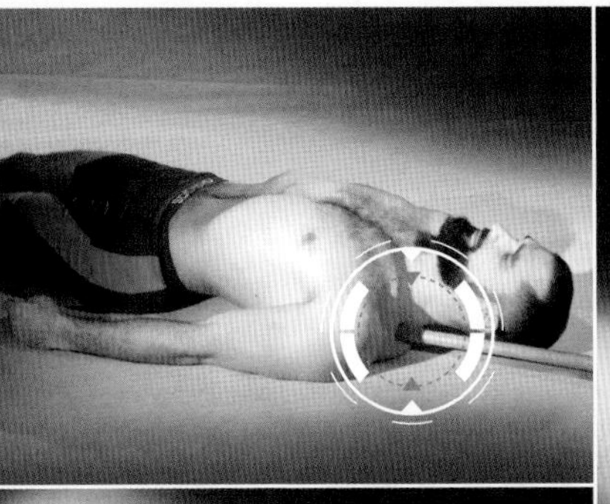

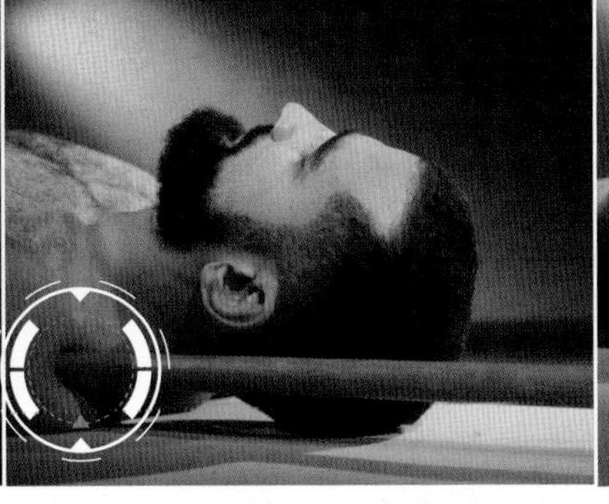

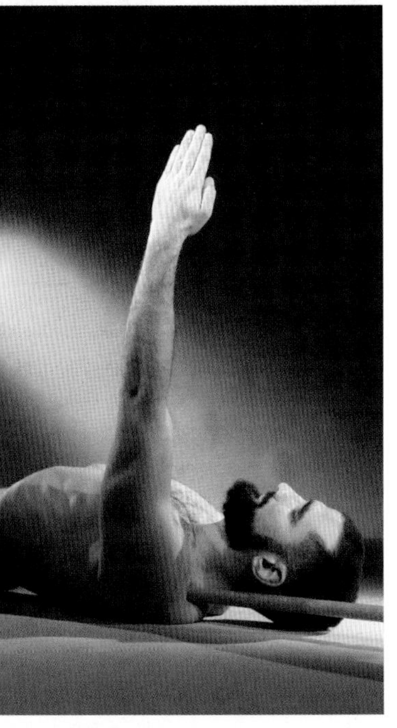

H8. TRAPEZIUS MASSAGE USING A BAND AND A BALL

Stand with your shoulder in a neutral position. Tie the band around your shoulder and place the massage ball on the trapezius muscle. The ball is held in place by the band. Apply strong pressure using the band and massage ball. **Perform 1 to 3 sets of 10 top-to-bottom rolls, 10 left-to-right rolls, and 10 circular rolls per shoulder.** Then slowly lift your arm straight in front of you 10 times. Repeat 1 to 3 times, stopping as needed at the most sensitive angles.

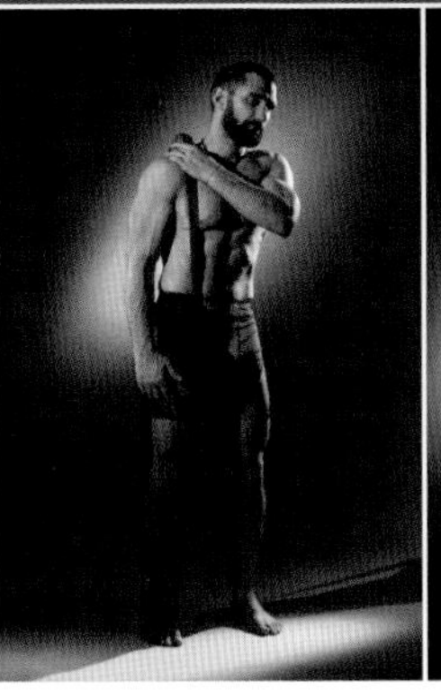

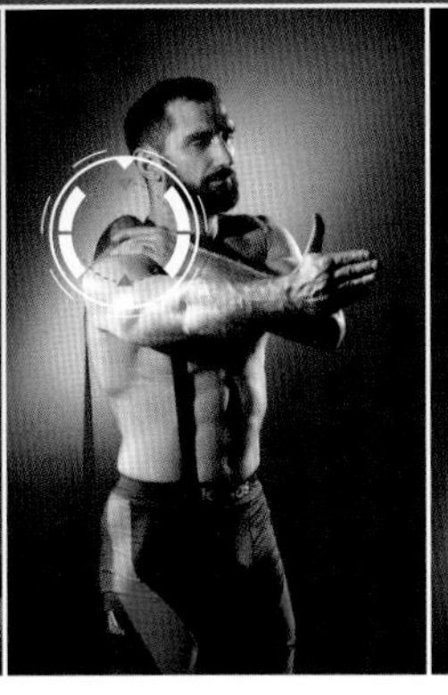

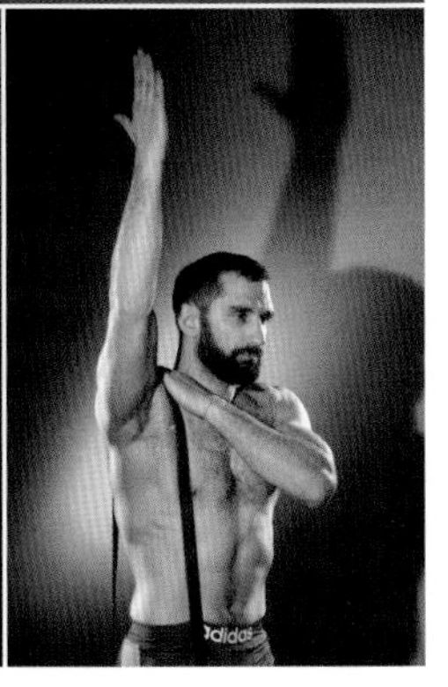

H9. LATERAL STRETCH USING A RESISTANCE BAND

Tie the band around your shoulder and anchor it to the floor, keeping it vertical. Adopt a forward lunge position with the leg opposite of the band in front. Allow your shoulder to relax downward. From this initial position, stretch your neck to the side, possibly adding weight with the opposite hand.

Perform 1 to 3 sets, holding for 30 seconds.

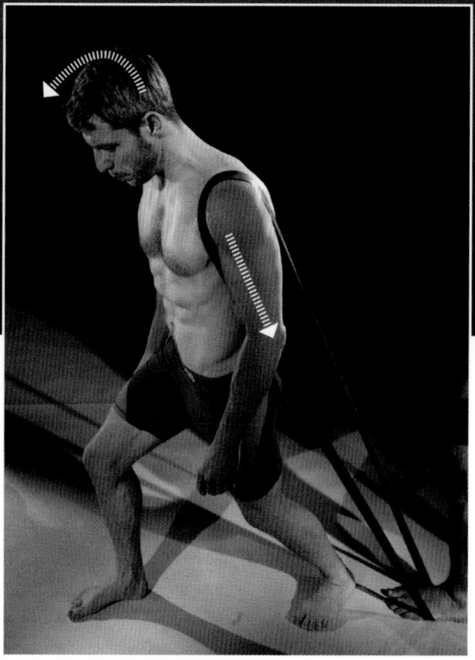

H10. PROPRIOCEPTION USING AN EXERCISE BALL

Hold the ball with your hands at first then without your hands as you progress. Without rounding your back, place the ball between your head and a wall.

Close your eyes and roll 6 times from top to bottom, 6 times from left to right, and 6 times in a circular motion.

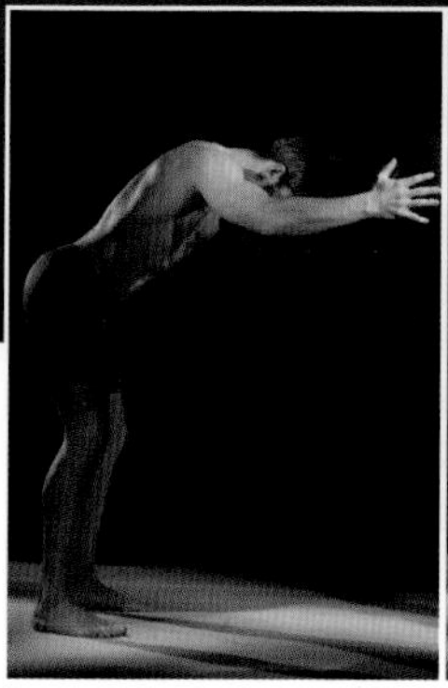

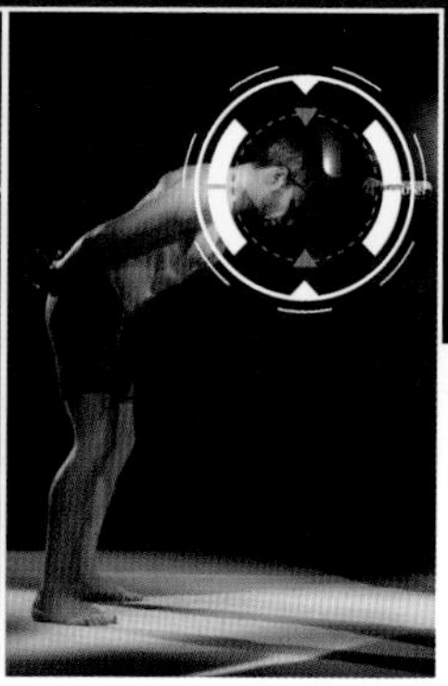

Sample 3-week mobility program targeting the neck (including exercises for neighboring areas)

MONDAY	TUESDAY	WEDNESDAY	THURSDAY	FRIDAY	SATURDAY	SUNDAY
H1*, H2, H4, H5	H3, H1, H4, H6	B2, B3, B4, B6	H1, H5, H7, H9, H10	E1, E2, E3, E4, E7	H3, H5, H8, H9, H10	B2, B3, E3, E6, E4

*These letter/number combinations refer to the exercises and techniques found on pages 26 through 76.

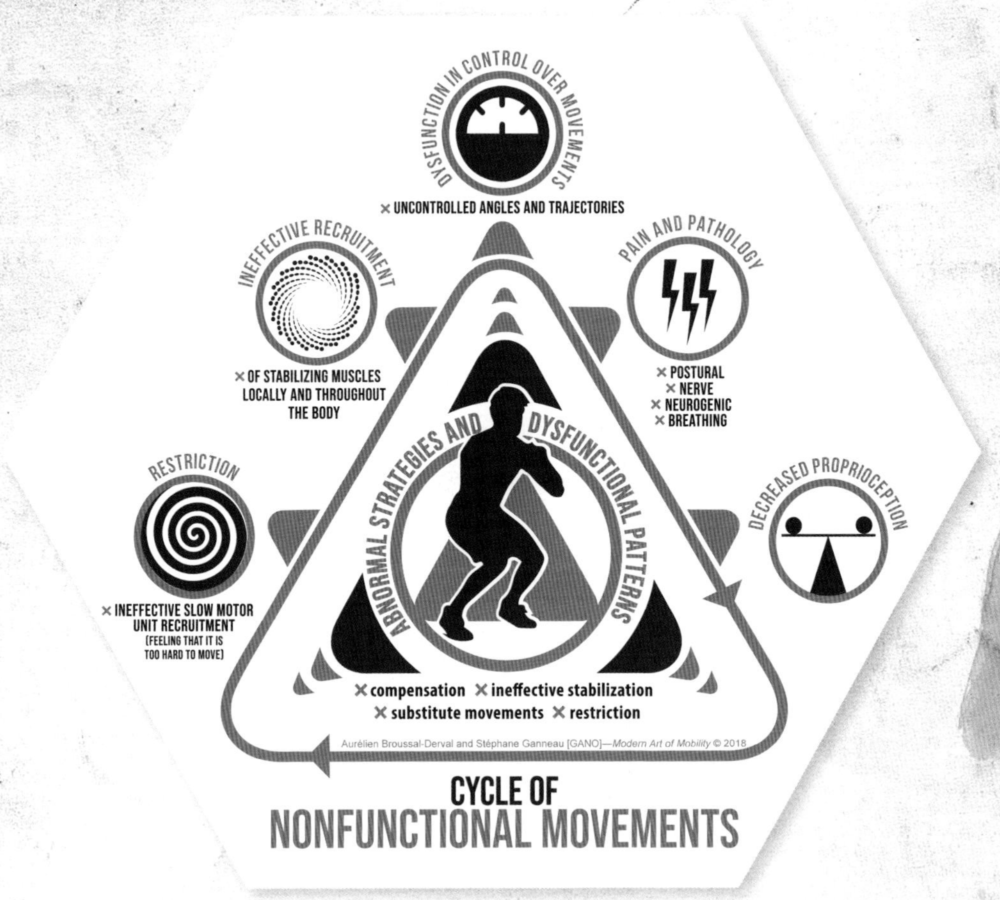

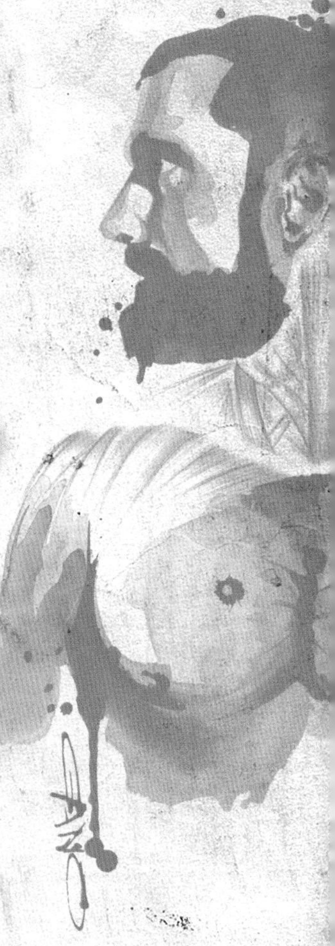

Conclusion

Pain is a daily struggle; you can only eliminate pain if you devote enough time to it. Never skip an opportunity to address the pain, whether you are in the office, in the car, or at home. If you continually chase the pain away, it will gradually recede and then disappear. But remember that stretching is also very important; self-massage on its own is only a modest short-term solution.

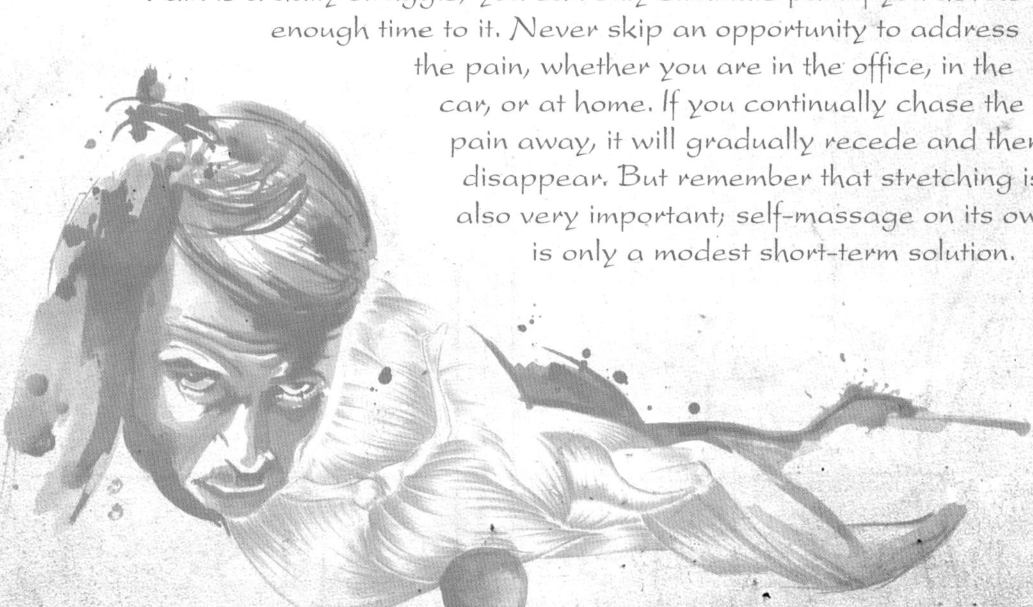

PART II

BREATHING

Unlike a computer, you can never fully switch off the human body. It constantly oscillates between different levels of alertness, continually using cognitive resources and energy systems.

Every day, we use dozens of automated systems within our bodies that do not require thought. This is the case when it comes to breathing. If we are alive, we are breathing. Or rather, we breathe to keep us alive.

Breathing is not any different from other automatic functions. It can be active, mechanically (and therefore voluntarily) controlled, and adapted to any situation. Breathing is also not immune to problems. As with other basic automated systems, such as walking or controlling your posture, breathing can be affected by intense situations such as stress, anxiety, or intense physical exercise.

20,000 OPPORTUNITIES TO BREATHE BETTER EVERY DAY

On average, we breathe 20,000 times per day. If these breaths are affected by stress and are not taken properly (partial breaths, mainly thoracic breaths, breaths taken too frequently, etc.), postural problems, impaired performance, record levels of stress, and even training plateaus can occur. Therefore, this vital element must be taken very seriously; you must learn, maintain, and train yourself to breathe.

Breathing when you are stressed or exhausted predominantly uses the chest and rib cage. These areas are stronger and are more adapted to performance. Conversely, breathing with your diaphragm requires much less energy.

Life puts strain on our automatic and instinctive design. Intense work and exercise environments overwhelm our systems by inducing chronic stress and anxiety. As a result, our bodies begin to use clavicular and thoracic breathing more often than necessary and sometimes, in the most extreme cases, exclusively. Prolonged sitting, anxiety, and intense or unsuitable exercise enhance this phenomenon.

Breathing

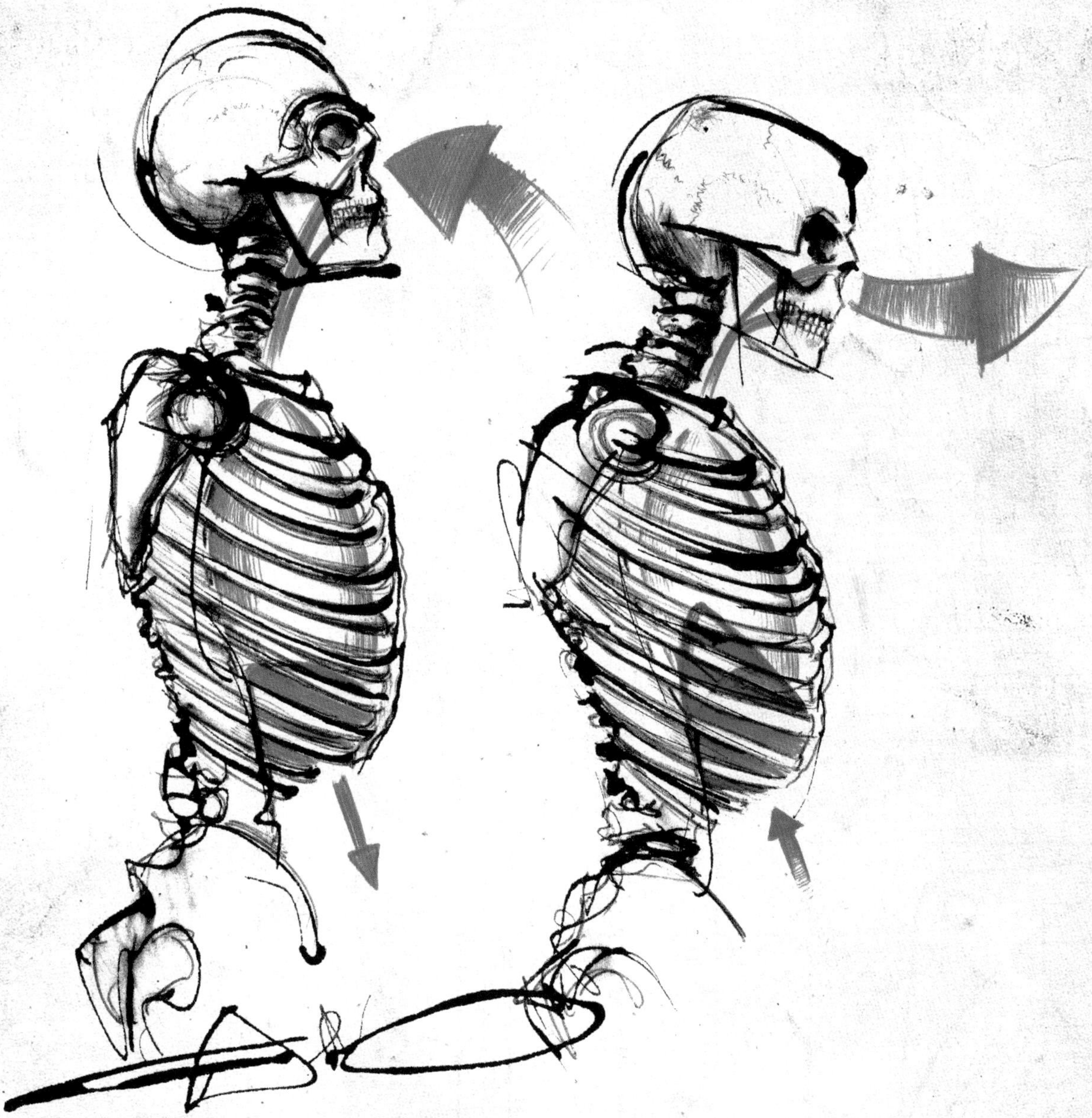

On average, we breathe 20,000 times per day. If these breaths are affected by stress and are not taken properly (partial breaths, mainly thoracic breaths, breaths taken too frequently, etc.), postural problems, impaired performance, record levels of stress, and even training plateaus can occur. Therefore, this vital element must be taken very seriously; you must learn, maintain, and train yourself to breathe.

01 THE RELATIONSHIP BETWEEN STRESS AND BREATHING

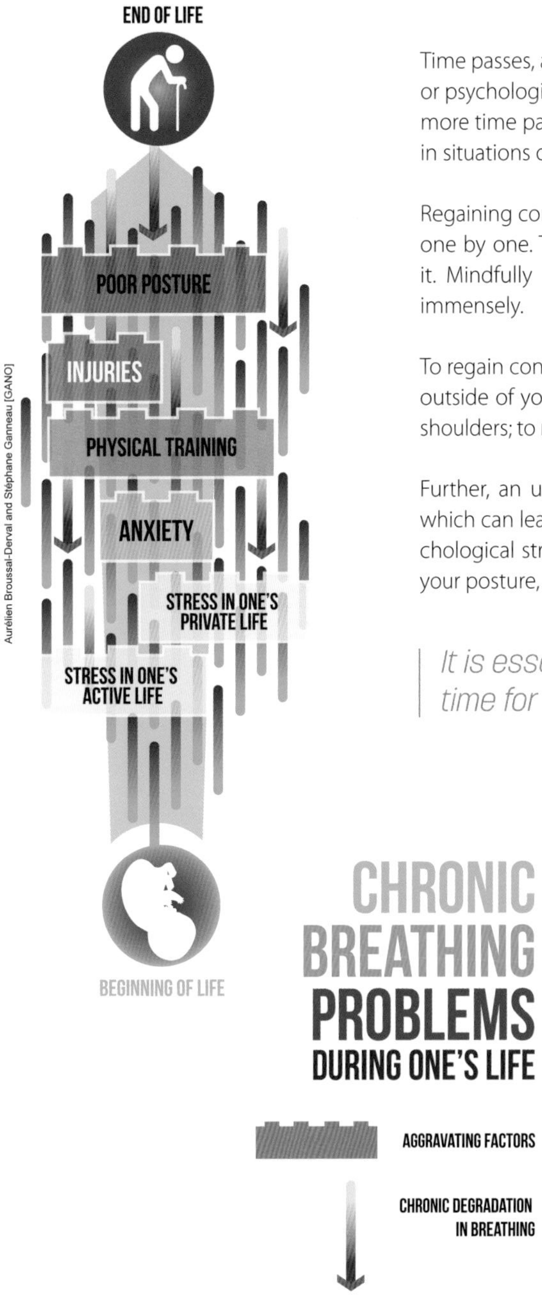

Time passes, and life happens. Disappointments, pressures, anxiety, and physical or psychological injuries can aggravate both your physical and mental health. As more time passes, issues can pile up, like heavy blocks of concrete, and put you in situations of increasingly high and chronic stress (see diagram).

Regaining control of your breathing will help you remove these concrete blocks one by one. Take the time to work on each issue to reduce or even eradicate it. Mindfully practicing the techniques described in this book will help you immensely.

To regain control, you must stop each issue from growing so that it remains well outside of your chronic stress zone. You must be aware of the weight on your shoulders; to manage this weight, you need to use techniques to eliminate stress.

Further, an unreasonable increase in stress inevitably leads to chronic stress, which can lead to breathing problems and even more intense physical and psychological stress. When breathing is affected in the long term, it will influence your posture, add stress, and cause injuries.

> *It is essential to take time for yourself.*

COMFORT ZONE AND STRESS ZONE 02

Normally, we find ourselves in a comfort zone between *diaphragm breathing* (relaxed) and *thoracic breathing* (active), depending on the situation.

Following a very intense, temporary period of stress (isolated period of anxiety, training session, etc.), the body's breathing mechanism goes into action mode and leaves the comfort zone behind to remain effective. This is not a problem; this situation is temporary and necessary.

However, chronically disordered breathing due to overly frequent and prolonged exposure to stress causes a decreased use and reduced volume of diaphragm breathing. Instead, the thoracic zone is used for all moderate breathing, and its trigger threshold becomes instant and automatic.

A vicious cycle begins: The muscles used for thoracic breathing are overused, and the diaphragm becomes less sensitive and begins to atrophy. Now is the time to take back control.

STRESS AND POSTURE

The physical and psychological sources of stress are particularly varied in our society. The human body memorizes stressful situations and creates self-protective reflexes. The more regular (or even permanent) a stressful situation becomes, the more the body adapts by adopting a defensive posture and breathing more using the chest and shoulders (thoracic breathing). This is especially harmful to good posture (Hamaoui et al. 2010).
The most well-known postural reflex is the *withdrawal reflex*: When an individual perceives excessive psychological or physical stress (physical or verbal attack, professional pressure, great physical effort, etc.), the shoulders roll forward, contracting the chest and rounding the back. The hip flexors activate, and the head retreats into the shoulders. If this posture is adopted too often or maintained for a long time, the body adapts, causing muscle compensations such as deactivation, atrophy of certain muscles, imbalances, stiffness, and muscular fragility. In the long term, these will limit mobility.

03 THE MUSCULAR SYSTEM AND BREATHING

Improper breathing affects numerous psychological and physical aspects of the body.

Improper breathing affects numerous psychological and physical aspects of the body. Quick and jerky breathing can disrupt digestion, cause headaches, increase hunger, and cause a general state of fatigue. In this section, we will mainly focus on the physical effects of breathing on your muscles, on which exercise has the most impact.

EFFECTS OF POOR BREATHING ON PERFORMANCE

Improper breathing impacts performance by reducing the amount of time in which the body can take in oxygen. The body's cells have less time to extract oxygen, so there is less oxygen available for the body to work. This significantly limits endurance since the aerobic energy production system relies completely on the use of oxygen. In extreme cases, this ineffectiveness could cause the body to switch to producing energy anaerobically (which does not use oxygen) during less-than-maximum effort, a change that normally only occurs during much more intense work. Highly stressed people will also see a decrease or even an inability to maintain normal levels of effort; they are literally restricted by their respiratory system.

This negative "loop" keeps itself going: The body's failure to rely on the aerobic system to produce energy can lead to *respiratory alkalosis* (problems balancing the blood's acid level due to respiratory issues, characterized by an increase in pH), which also causes anxiety. Movement then becomes affected because muscles become less effective when in an anxious state. As a result, posture suffers (rounded back, lowered head, hunched shoulders, etc.), breathing is negatively affected, less oxygen is available for the body, and so on.

TAKE CONTROL OF YOUR BREATHING

Poor breathing decreases an individual's tolerance to pain (Bordoni et al. 2016). One of the keys to effective movement and posture is the eradication of pain, so it is clear why it is important to regain control of our breathing.

At the same time, relaxation goes hand in hand with regaining control of your breathing. Each of these two elements supports the other, and both should be tackled together (in the same session or through focused sessions) to maximize your results.

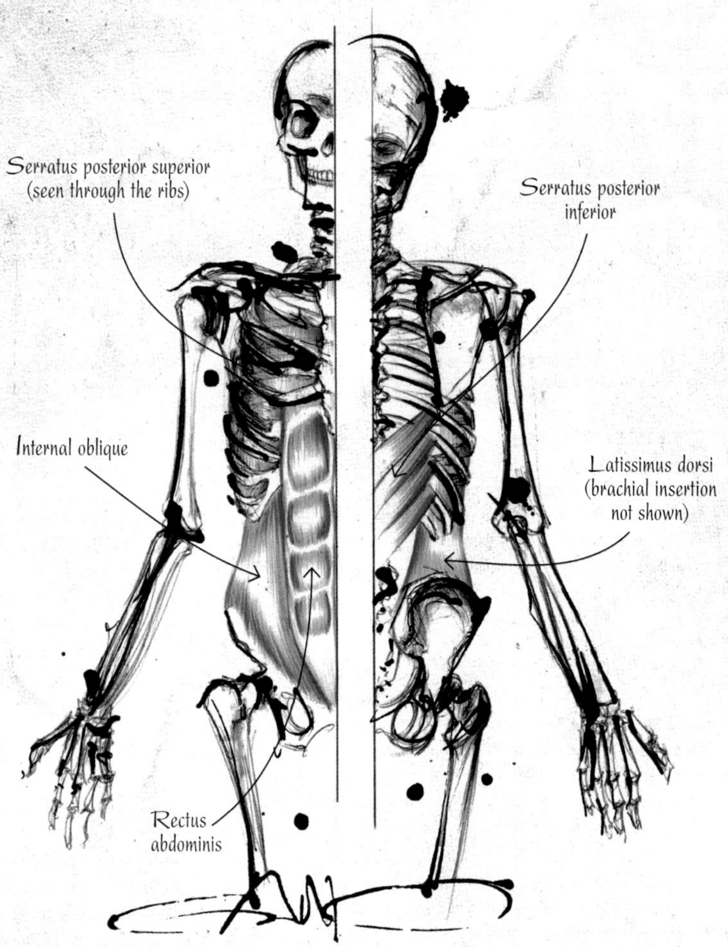

The ribs are the framework for breathing. If this frame becomes too rigid or not flexible enough, then the whole torso, from the shoulders to the spine, experiences excessive tension. For example, when poor breathing techniques cause the upper ribs to rise, their cartilage and intercostal muscles become sensitive.

This problem in the ribs also affects the function of the spine, causing a loss of stability and mobility in the thoracic region. Breathing becomes painful and uncomfortable.

Overuse of and extreme tension in the deltoids, latissimus dorsi, and neck muscles near the upper back (sternocleidomastoid, scalene, and upper trapezius) will make this breathing problem worse and affect posture and movement through

→ stiffness in the neck,
→ loss of mobility and shoulder stability,
→ increased likelihood of spasms,
→ increased likelihood of cramps, and
→ increased tension in the ribs, back, and chest.

The effects of a breathing problem are not limited to the thoracic region and can spread directly to the center of the body—to the very sensitive hinge between the torso and the legs—by disturbing two muscles that are essential for movement and posture: the iliopsoas and the quadratus lumborum. Both muscles are connected to the diaphragm muscle via the spine, where they insert, and via the fasciae and ligaments. The diaphragm is an impressive muscle that has multiple insertions on the spinal column (T12, L1, L2, and L3), thereby directly linking posture to breathing (in particular, stiffness in the spine as described by Shirley et al. 2003).

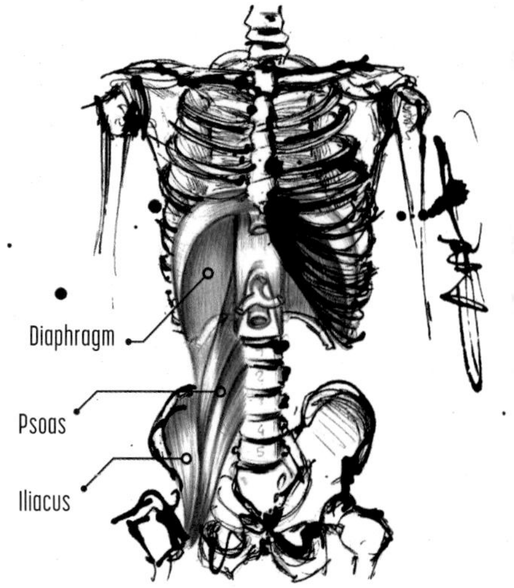

Thus, a respiratory problem can cause (Hamaoui et al. 2002)

1. back pain (Smith et al. 2009),
2. a decrease in stability, and
3. the loss of mobility in the hips or lower back.

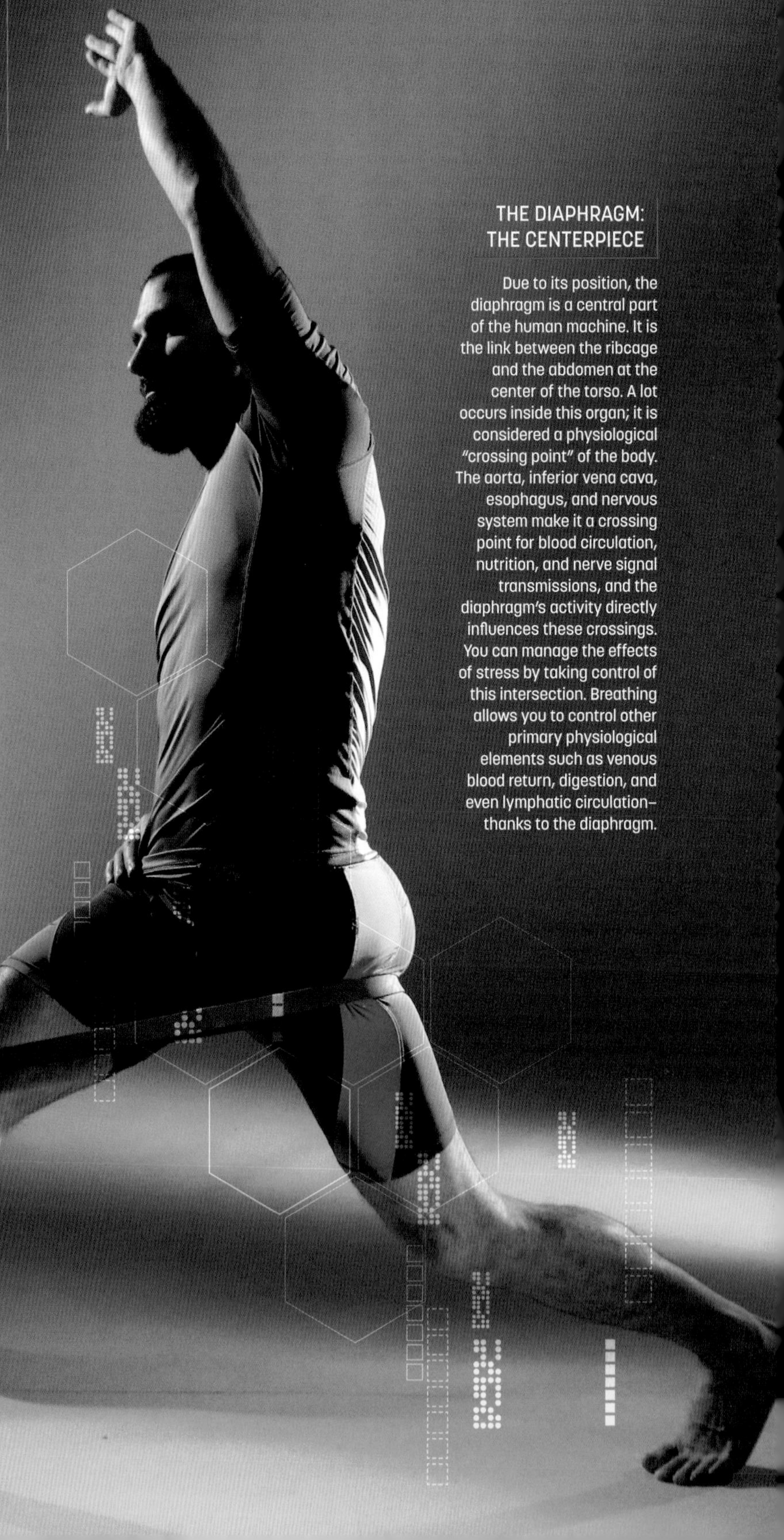

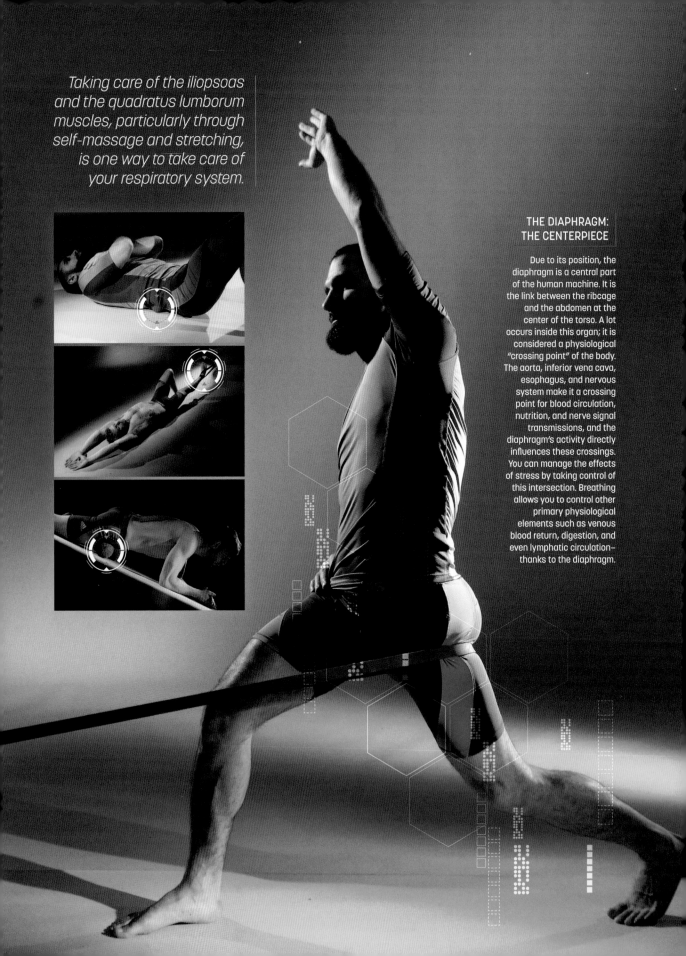

Taking care of the iliopsoas and the quadratus lumborum muscles, particularly through self-massage and stretching, is one way to take care of your respiratory system.

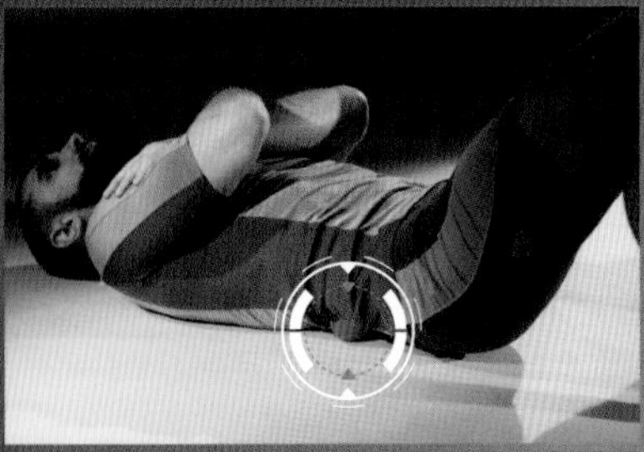

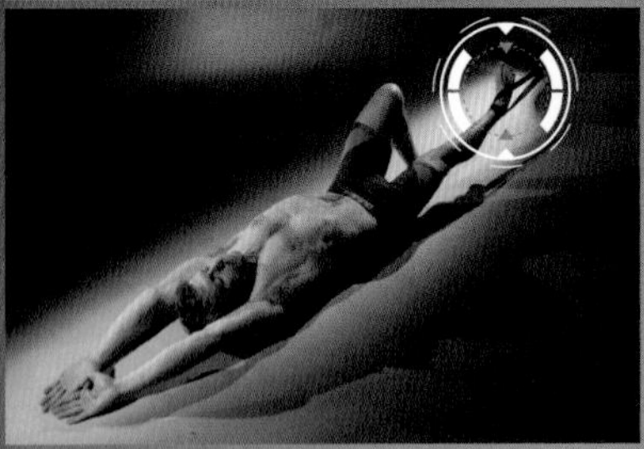

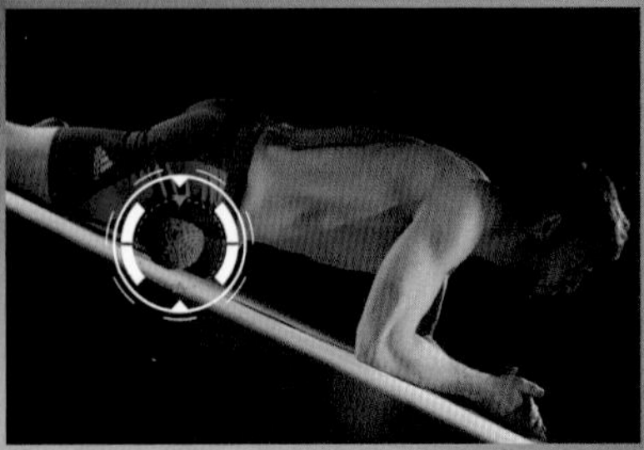

THE DIAPHRAGM: THE CENTERPIECE

Due to its position, the diaphragm is a central part of the human machine. It is the link between the ribcage and the abdomen at the center of the torso. A lot occurs inside this organ; it is considered a physiological "crossing point" of the body. The aorta, inferior vena cava, esophagus, and nervous system make it a crossing point for blood circulation, nutrition, and nerve signal transmissions, and the diaphragm's activity directly influences these crossings. You can manage the effects of stress by taking control of this intersection. Breathing allows you to control other primary physiological elements such as venous blood return, digestion, and even lymphatic circulation—thanks to the diaphragm.

From both a semantic and functional point of view, resistance training consists of dynamically strengthening a system and protecting it with supple and adaptable muscles. Although the diaphragm is typically not considered a muscle that is the target of a resistance training program, it still is a muscle. Its role is to boost and reinforce the body's complex stability from the spine to the pelvis. The internal activation of the diaphragm is part of a complex abdominal support system that includes the pelvic floor (which is also under tension) and the spine (that benefits from the support of the intervertebral muscles).

To improve your stability, you must learn to control your breathing.

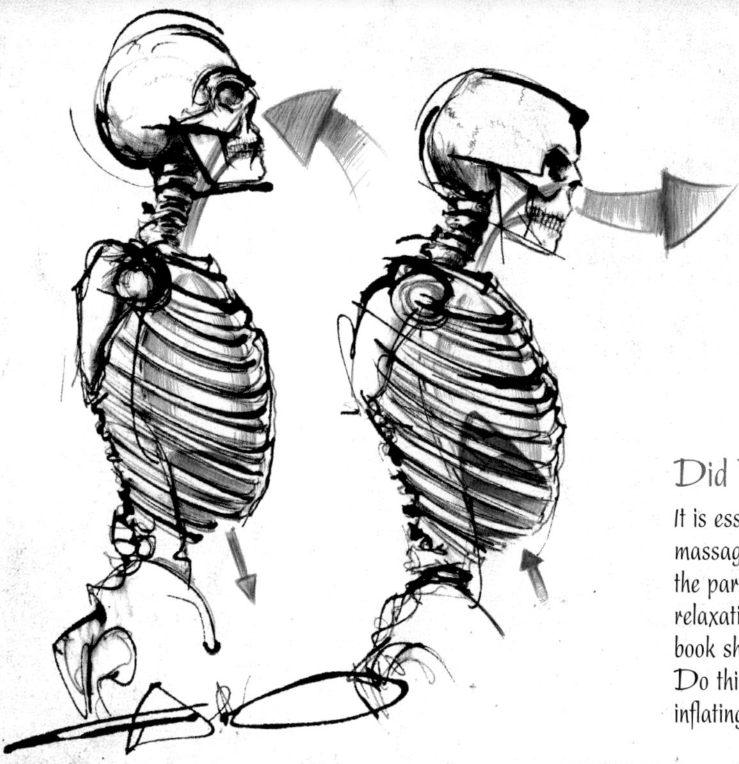

Let's discuss internal stability: When you are breathing properly, your diaphragm moves down as you inhale, increasing the intra-abdominal pressure by pushing the organs downward. This means that all the powerful abdominal muscles are under tension, from the deepest layers (transverse abdominis) to the most visible layers (the obliques and the rectus abdominis muscles) that we usually—incorrectly—focus our efforts on.

Did You Know?

It is essential to breathe using the diaphragm during self-massage. This breathing technique allows you to boost the parasympathetic nervous system, which is ideal for relaxation. All self-massage exercises presented in this book should be practiced using diaphragm breathing. Do this by breathing slowly through your nose, inflating your abdomen, and then exhaling calmly.

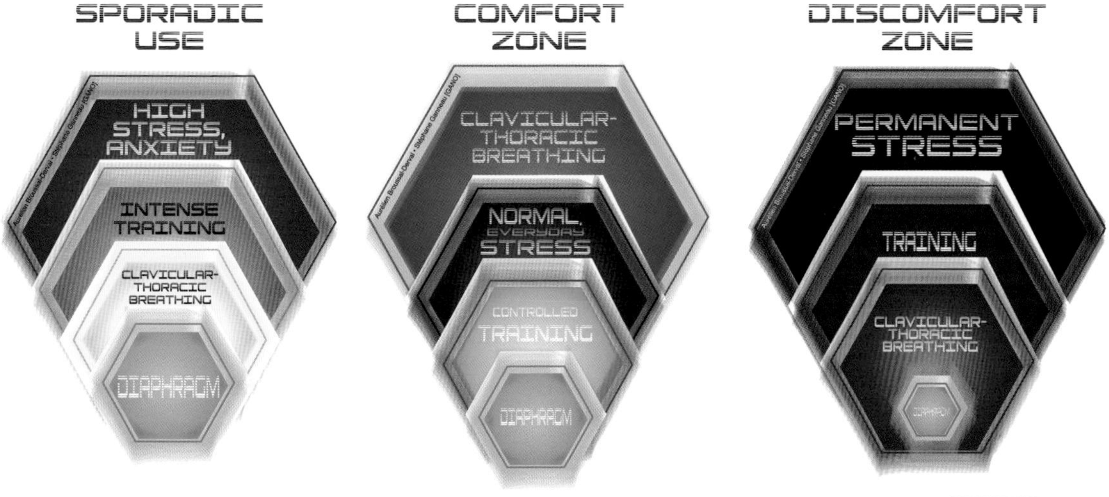
SPORADIC USE
HIGH STRESS, ANXIETY
INTENSE TRAINING
CLAVICULAR-THORACIC BREATHING
DIAPHRAGM
COMFORT ZONE
CLAVICULAR-THORACIC BREATHING
NORMAL, EVERYDAY STRESS
CONTROLLED TRAINING
DIAPHRAGM
DISCOMFORT ZONE
PERMANENT STRESS
TRAINING
CLAVICULAR-THORACIC BREATHING

04 RETRAINING THE DIAPHRAGM

Learning how to breathe properly again can take time, depending on how badly and how long you have been experiencing problems. In some cases, even the diaphragm muscle itself may need to be retrained to function differently.

We must remember that the diaphragm, like any muscle, can retract, contract, develop adhesions, and lose elasticity and even effectiveness. If this happens, the diaphragm tends to move up inside the chest cavity.

We must prioritize ourselves.

EXERCISE TO REGAIN CONTROL OF YOUR DIAPHRAGM (LYING ON YOUR BACK)

This basic exercise requires you to be self-aware and, over time, actively practice it during normal breathing. Lie on your back with your knees flexed and your feet on the floor. Place your hands at the base of your abdomen. As you breathe in, inflate your abdomen to move your hands up. Your chest should not inflate at all; allow the flow of air to pass directly to your abdomen. Try to inflate your abdomen from the lower section as much as possible. Inhale through your nose and exhale calmly and gradually through your mouth.

When you are comfortable with this exercise, try to depress your abdomen down as much as possible with each exhale by flattening it against the spine. In doing so, you will activate the transverse abdominis muscle.

Next, use all your internal supporting muscles to breathe. At the end of your exhale, take a short and intense breath in, without allowing air to enter (you can manually block your airways to help you by closing your throat). Try to move your abdomen up and under the ribs and "lock down" your abdominal muscles on your pelvic floor.

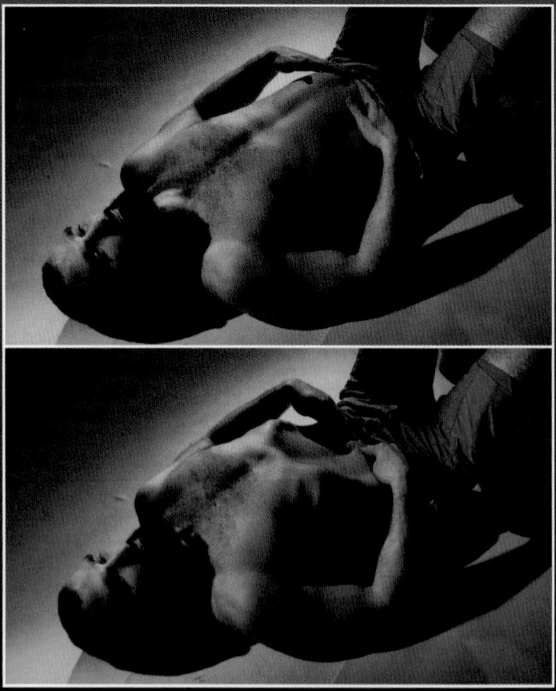

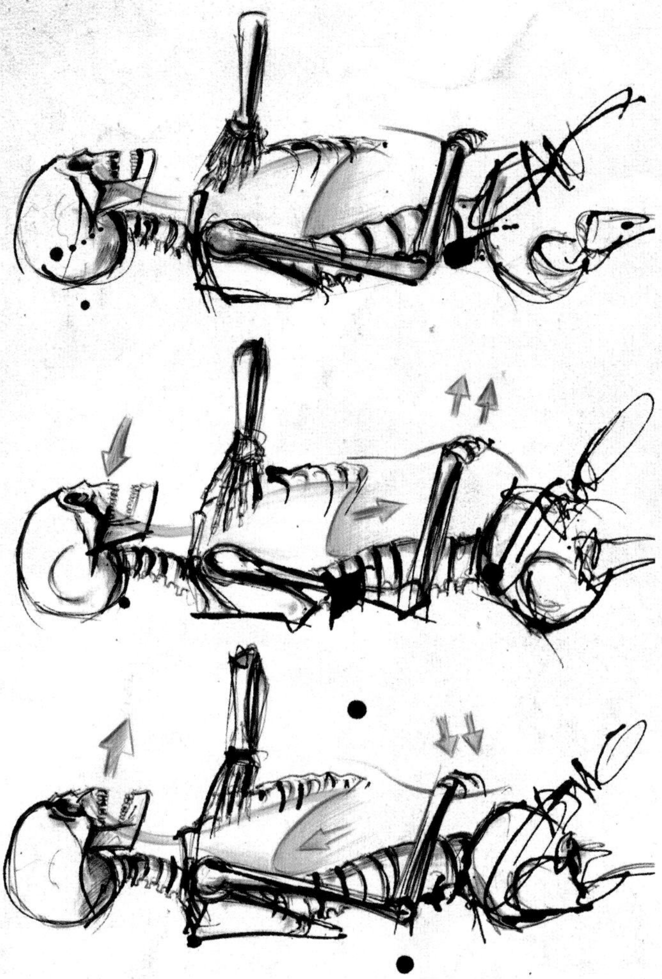

EXERCISE TO REGAIN CONTROL OF YOUR DIAPHRAGM (LYING ON YOUR BACK, ARMS ANCHORED USING A BAND)

This exercise requires you to internally sense the activation of the diaphragm because your hands are no longer placed on your abdomen but are anchored overhead by a band.

Lie on your back with your knees flexed and feet on the floor. As you breathe in, inflate your abdomen. Your chest should not inflate at all; allow the flow of air to pass directly to your abdomen. Try to inflate your abdomen from the lower section as much as possible. Inhale through your nose and exhale calmly and gradually through your mouth.

Resting your head on the floor significantly reduces tension in the neck muscles, allowing you to concentrate more on your diaphragm.

When you are comfortable with this exercise, try to depress your abdomen down as much as possible with each exhale by flattening it against the spine. In doing so, you will activate the transverse abdominis muscle.

Next, use all your internal supporting muscles to breathe. At the end of your exhale, take a short and intense breath in, without allowing air to enter (you can manually block your airways to help you by closing your throat). Try to move your abdomen up and under the ribs and "lock down" your abdominal muscles on your pelvic floor.

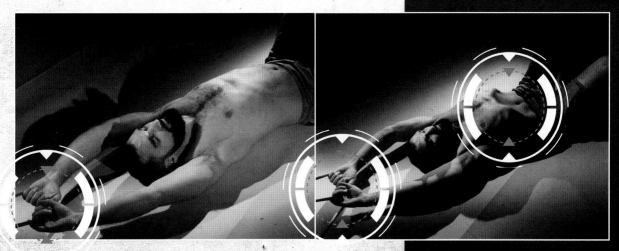

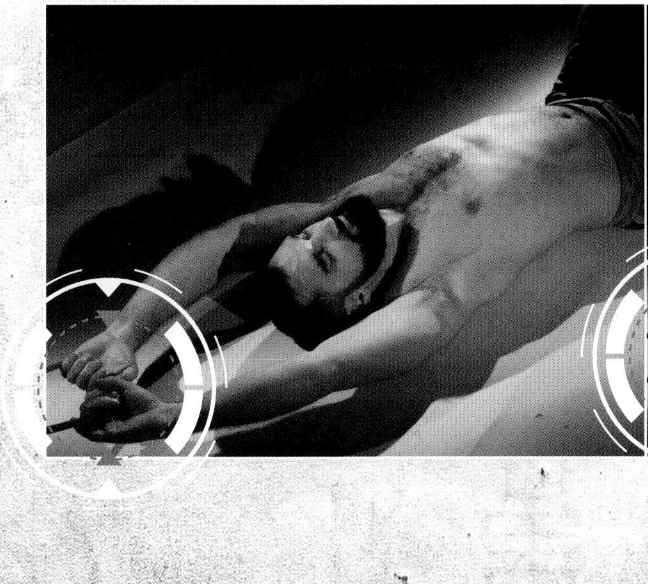

DIAPHRAGM SELF-MASSAGE

Once you become aware of your breathing potential, you must learn to relax your diaphragm, which is often strained due to long-term stress. As with any other muscle, this relaxation can be achieved through self-massage. In the case of the diaphragm, the results can be felt throughout your entire body and in your psyche (Bordoni et al. 2016).

The diaphragm is not used to being massaged so be prepared for some discomfort. In the most extreme cases, some people use the diaphragm so little that it stays fixed under the ribs and is therefore difficult to reach. Start sitting in a kneeing position with your hands on your thighs. Lean forward and slide your fingers under your ribs as far as you can starting at the outside of your ribs and gradually upward toward the *solar plexus* (the upper, center part of your torso behind your stomach).

Once you have mastered the first two exercises, this exercise will become the first exercise.

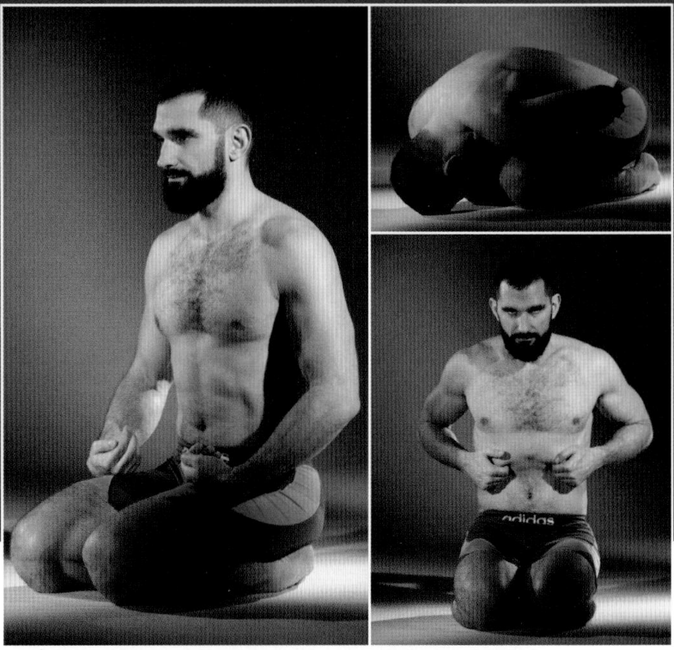

SITTING WITH YOUR LEGS EXTENDED AGAINST A WALL, ARMS STRETCHED USING A BAND

This exercise activates shoulder stability, which automatically reduces thoracic breathing. The whole neck and chest area also relaxes, allowing the diaphragm to more freely move.

Extend your legs up against a wall, bringing your buttocks as close to the wall as much as the flexibility of the back of your legs will allow. Flex your feet to press your heels against the wall and wrap a thinner (lower intensity) resistance band around the back of your upper thighs. Stretch the band by pressing your arms over your head.

Begin to gently move your abdomen out when inhaling. Your chest should not inflate at all; allow the flow of air to pass directly to your abdomen. Try to inflate your abdomen from the lower section as much as possible. Inhale through your nose and exhale calmly and gradually through your mouth.

Resting your head on the floor significantly reduces tension in the neck muscles, allowing you to concentrate more on your diaphragm.

When you are comfortable with this exercise, try to depress your abdomen down as much as possible with each exhale by flattening it against the spine. In doing so, you will activate the transverse abdominis muscle.

Next, use all your internal supporting muscles to breathe. At the end of your exhale, take a short and intense breath in, without allowing air to enter (you can manually block your airways to help you by closing your throat). Try to move your abdomen up and under the ribs and "lock down" your abdominal muscles on your pelvic floor.

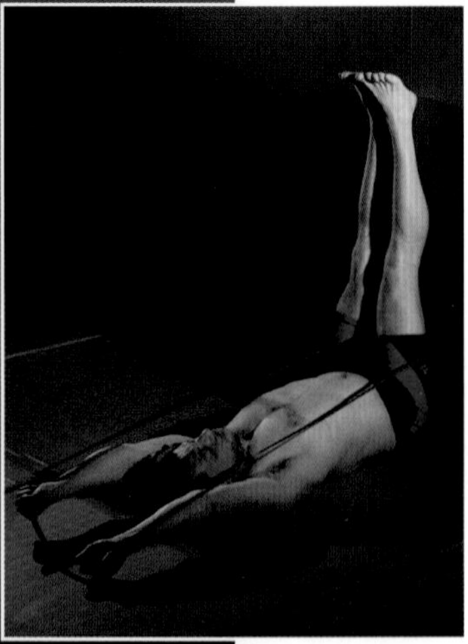

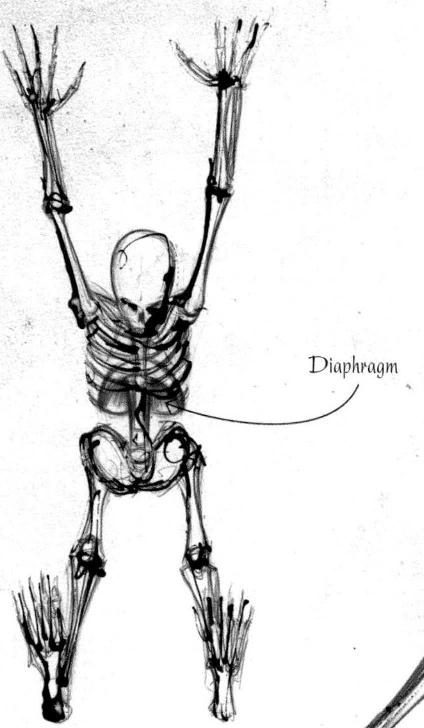

Did You Know?

Due to the effects of gravity, the diaphragm is positioned differently depending on the body's position. In 2017, Hellyer and his team showed that the diaphragm is wider when sitting down than when standing. In 1994, Bouisset and his team stated that the body's balance is affected more when the individual is sitting. Therefore, the body should be placed in different positions during diaphragm training sessions.

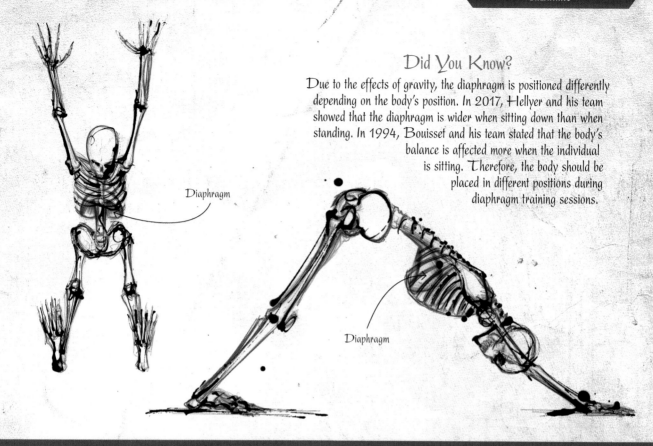

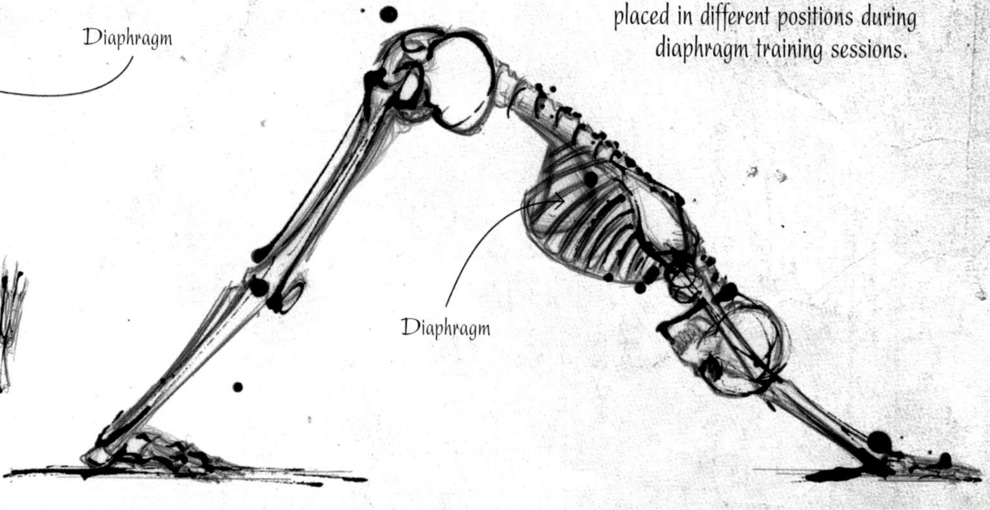

DOWNWARD FACING DOG (ADHO MUKHA SVANASANA)

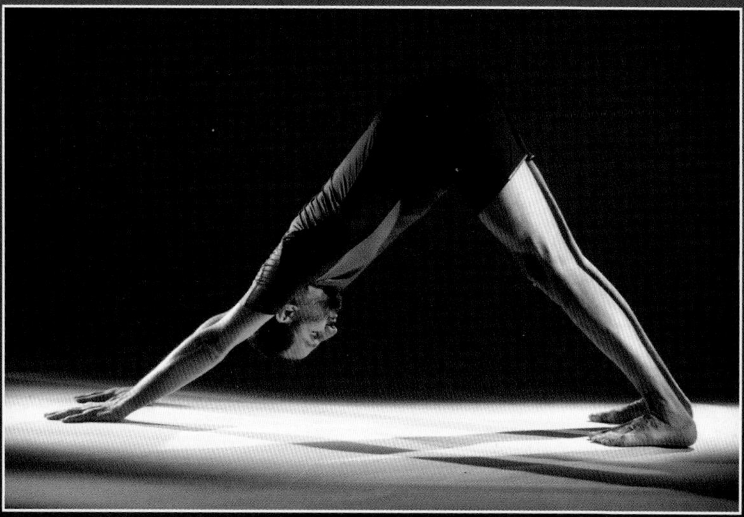

This exercise effectively inhibits the scalene muscles and activates the deep neck muscles, which allow the other neck muscles to relax. Since the diaphragm is wider when you are sitting down (Hellyer et al. 2017; see "Did You Know" above), that position is more comfortable. Overall, by using calm and controlled breathing, chest breathing is decreased in favor of abdominal breathing (Hudson et al. 2016).

Move onto all fours. Raise your buttocks as much as possible by pushing your arms into the floor while keeping your knees and elbows fully extended and your head in line with your torso. Your back must remain straight. In this position, inhale deeply and slowly as you inflate your abdomen then exhale completely through your mouth.

HOLDING ON TO THE SUSPENSION TRAINER, LEGS BENT

This exercise uses shortened suspension trainer straps on rings or a stationary bar with an adjustable height. Grab the handles and, keeping your arms straight, allow yourself to hang freely. Only your grip requires any force. Adjust the strap so that your feet are vertically in line with your knees.

This suspension exercise lengthens the latissimus dorsi and the pectoralis minor while activating the iliopsoas for stability. Your shoulders will regain some mobility and your pelvis and lower back will gain stability. This overall relaxation exercise allows you to easily concentrate on the diaphragm without being completely at rest, as in the previous exercises.

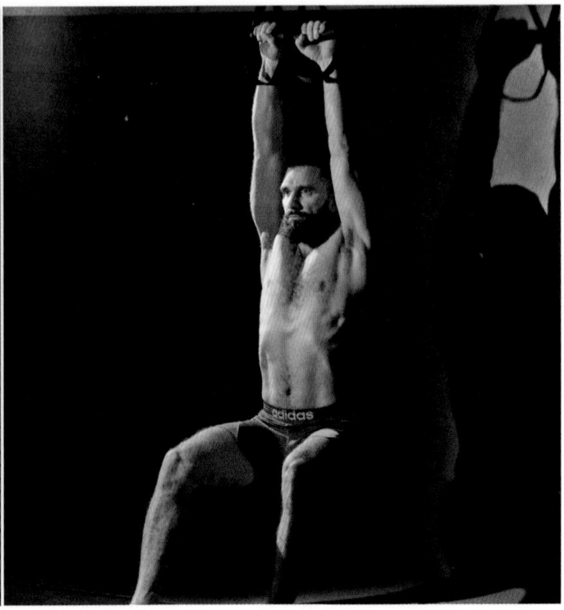

DAILY EXERCISES

Each morning or evening, perform 3 to 5 self-massages and 5 to 10 inhales and exhales for 3 exercises of your choice. If you have sufficient time, you can do a full session by performing 3 sets of each exercise in this section.

Practice breathing using your diaphragm while sitting or lying down as often as possible throughout the day.

DURING RECOVERY

During resistance or speed training, practice diaphragm breathing without trying to achieve total relaxation (because you need to maintain a level of activation and there is insufficient recovery).

During aerobic training, practice diaphragm breathing only if recovery is long enough to allow you to return to a normal breathing rate.

BEFORE WARMING UP

Before starting intense training, perform 3 to 5 self-massages and 5 inhales and exhales in 1 exercise of your choice as a lead-in to the warm-up.

The Allure of a Flat Abdomen

A flat abdomen has been worshipped for many years. Abdominal fat increases with each decade of life despite the fact that people increasingly try to hold in the bulge. During the 1990s, the functional solution of holding in your abdomen was discovered to be an effective way (when practiced correctly) to activate the transverse abdominis muscles and increase core stability. A completely flat abdomen reduces the activation of the diaphragm, however.

To effectively retain the diaphragm, it is important to learn how to pull the abdomen in, how to flatten it, and even how to raise it toward the ribs.

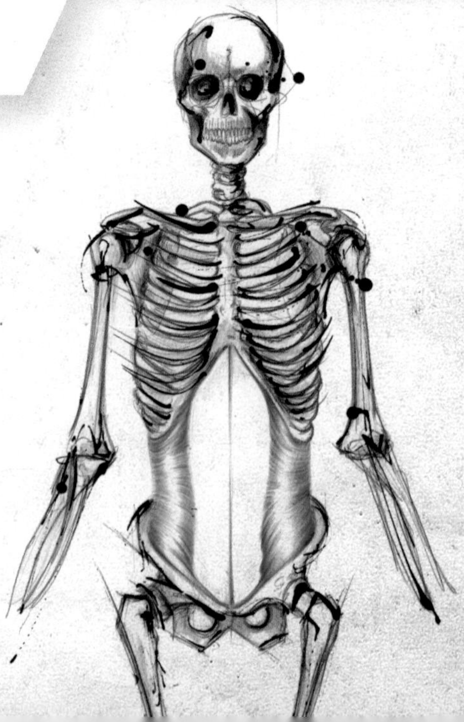

TRAINING THE RESPIRATORY SYSTEM 05

All the breathing exercises described in the previous section will help to develop the muscles of your respiratory system. Strengthening the core muscles and taking care to activate the diaphragm and the transverse abdominis muscles also play an important role.

Specifically training the muscles for inhaling and exhaling will allow us to improve our respiratory potential.

The muscles we use for breathing are permanently activated (they never fully rest) and have all the qualities of endurance muscles (see Arend et al. 2016). They are full of slow-twitch fibers, so they are especially resistant to fatigue (an adult's diaphragm has barely 20 percent fast-twitch fibers (see the Muscle Fiber Types and Movement section on page 256 for more information). Even if they are properly made to withstand continuous contraction and relaxation cycles, long-term stress or strain (Carrio 2010, 2017) can eventually exhaust these muscles, which limits the human body's performance.

Fortunately, you can train the inhalation system and the exhalation system to work together for proper breathing.

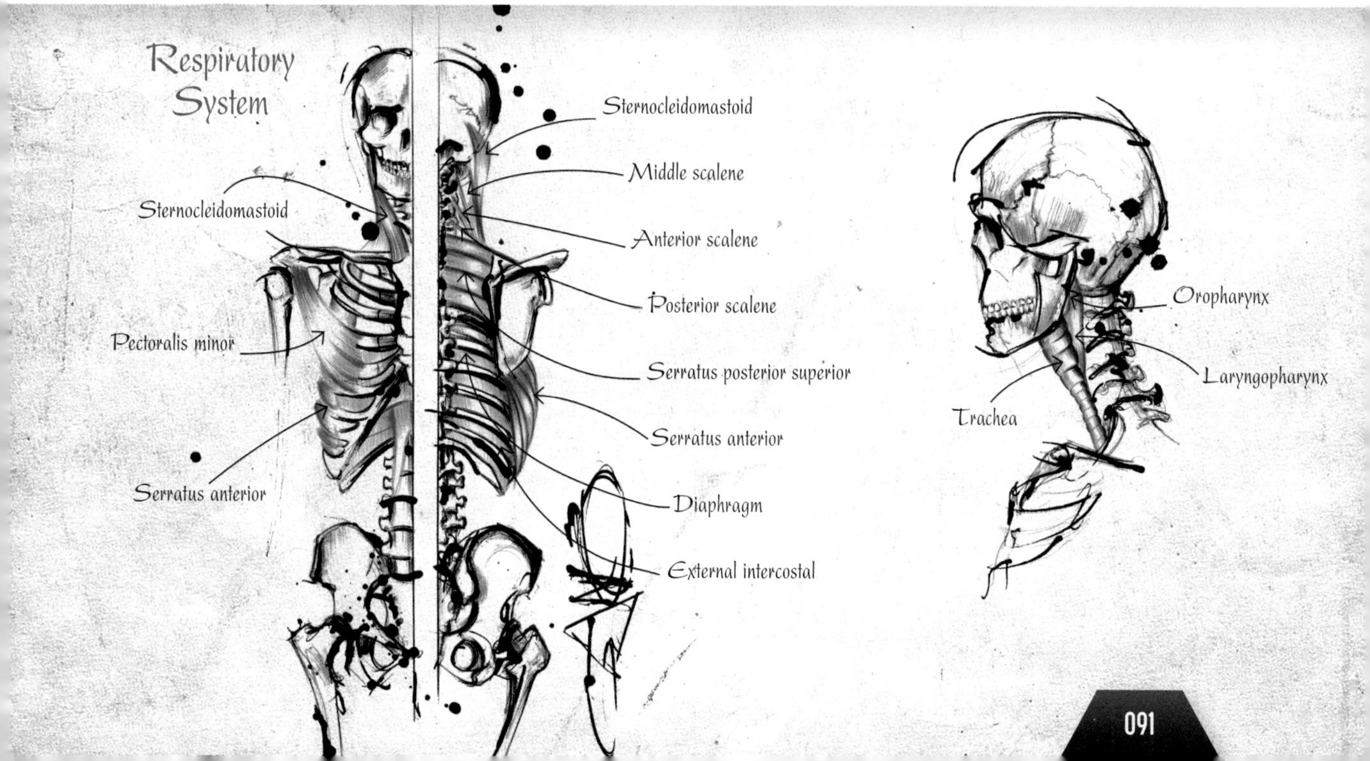

When tools for training the inspiratory muscles were developed in the early 2000s, there were many questions regarding their effectiveness (Hart et al. 2001).

Tools such as the POWERbreathe, Threshold, and PowerLung inspiratory muscle trainers were later developed that scientifically showed their effectiveness for training and the ability to measure progress. Like any other muscle group, the inspiratory muscles can be trained to be stronger and more powerful with increased endurance during activity and at rest.

In 2011, Kellens' team sought to determine the effectiveness of a POWERbreathe training session during leisure sports. Within 8 weeks, 22 percent of the tested group made progress in inhalation and 18 percent in exhalation. Keeping this in mind, we recommend using the following training program.

POWERbreathe Training Program
Perform 5 sets of 6 full inhalations with 45 seconds of recovery between each set. Do this twice a day at 85 percent of maximum inspiratory pressure, taking at least 30 minutes to recover between the 2 groups of 30 inhalations.

RESPIRATORY SYSTEM

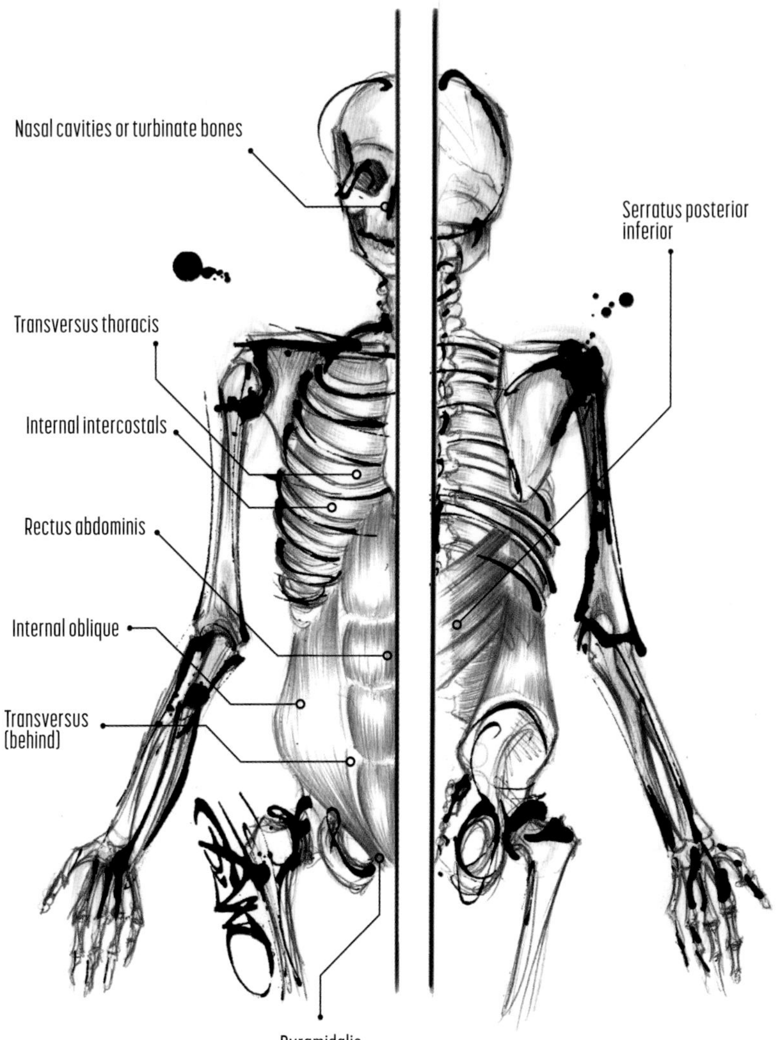

Adjust resistance as your maximum inspiratory pressure increases.

This type of exercise is also aided by a warm-up. In 2016, Arend and his team showed that activation of the inhalation muscles significantly increased after they had been warmed up, and they suggest using the following approach.

POWERbreathe Warm-Up Program
Perform 2 sets of 12 inhalations at 60 percent of maximum inspiratory pressure or perform 2 sets of 30 inhalations at 40 percent of maximum inspiratory pressure.

MANAGING YOUR DAY 06

Stressful and tiring situations are not permanent and can be managed using different techniques. Sometimes you might find yourself being too relaxed, and so you might need a little boost in your breathing.

The *sympathetic nervous system* is in charge of the fight or flight responses.

It is this system that is most sensitive to stress. Conversely, the *parasympathetic nervous system* regulates your basic vital functions and maximizes recovery; it is the system most sensitive to rest.

The respiratory system is directly connected to the parasympathetic system. If you are fully aware and in control of this system, it will have a positive effect on your nervous and hormonal systems. On the other hand, if you begin to lose control due to chronic stress or different emotional states, you can regain it by managing your sympathetic nervous system. It is common to alternate back and forth between these two systems in our increasingly stressful lives. Therefore, alternating between activation and relaxation respiratory exercises throughout the day is an effective way to maintain balance. We suggest alternating between sessions of inhalation, holding your breath, and exhalation—all at different tempos.

In the two following programs, we will provide you with simple techniques for the most common situations. Remember the following general principles:

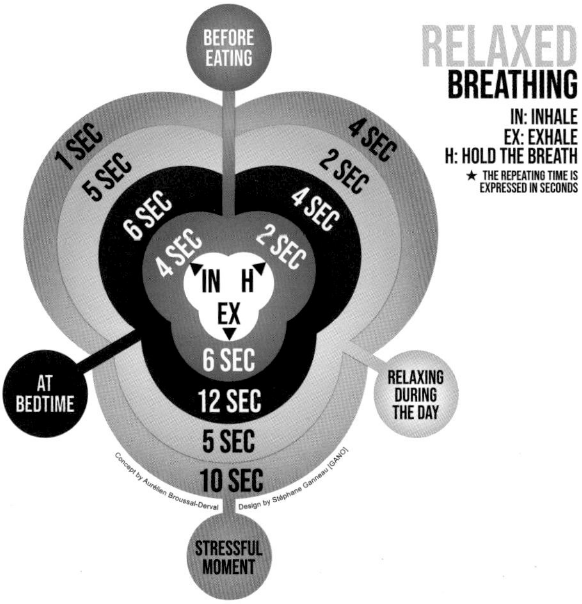

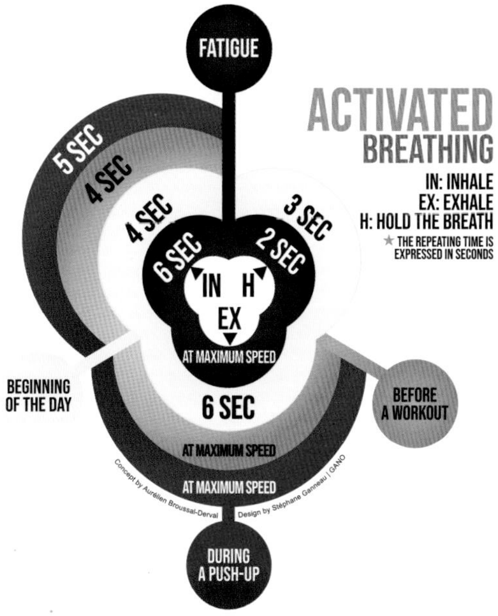

Understanding Movement

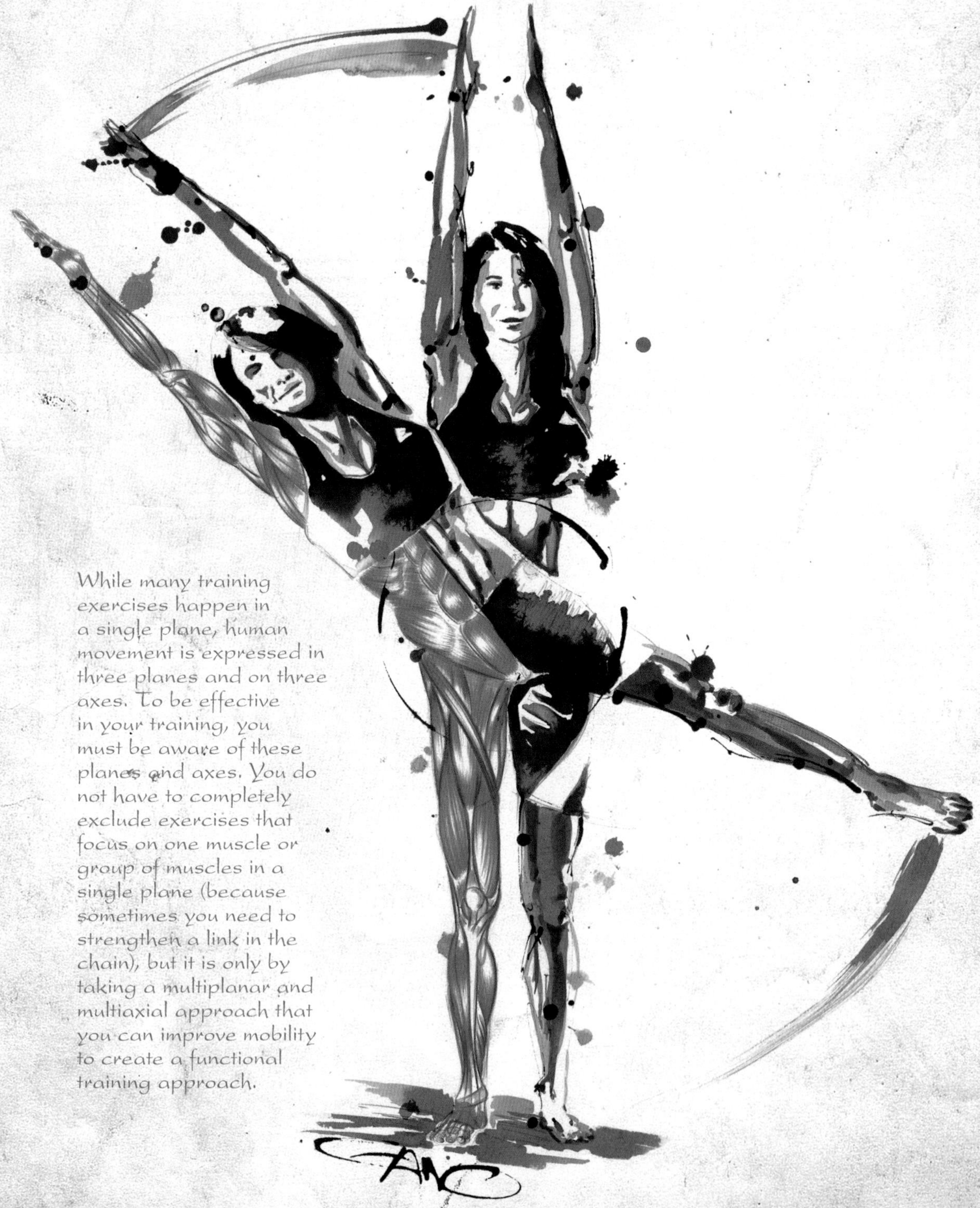

While many training exercises happen in a single plane, human movement is expressed in three planes and on three axes. To be effective in your training, you must be aware of these planes and axes. You do not have to completely exclude exercises that focus on one muscle or group of muscles in a single plane (because sometimes you need to strengthen a link in the chain), but it is only by taking a multiplanar and multiaxial approach that you can improve mobility to create a functional training approach.

PART III MOVEMENT

There is no excuse for not understanding the richness of movement.

While many training exercises happen in a single plane, human movement is expressed in three planes and on three axes. To be effective in your training, you must be aware of these planes and axes. You do not have to completely exclude exercises that focus on one muscle or group of muscles in a single plane (because sometimes you need to strengthen a link in the chain), but it is only by taking a multiplanar and multiaxial approach that you can improve mobility to create a functional training approach.

THE HUMAN MACHINE MOVING IN SPACE

To completely grasp the possibilities of the human body's movement, we need to describe the three planes of movement and three axes of rotation:

Sagittal plane

Frontal plane

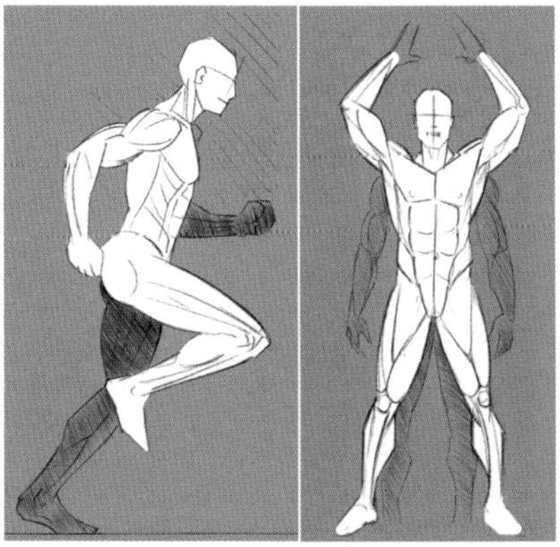

Horizontal plane

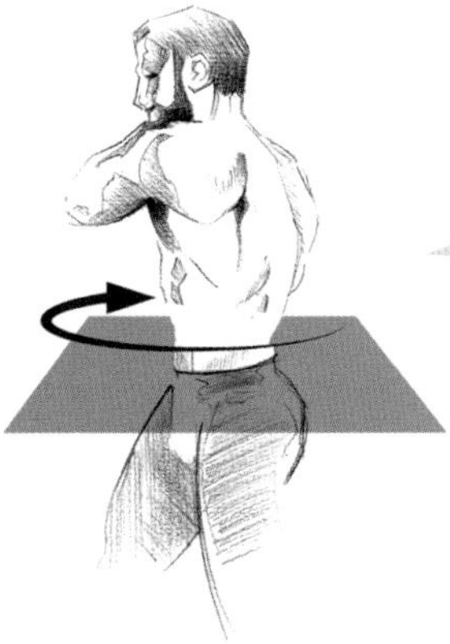

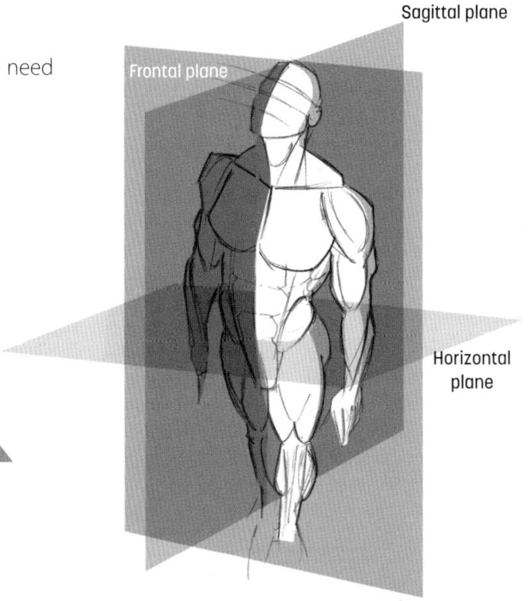

SAGITTAL PLANE

The *sagittal plane* divides the body into right and left parts. It includes all motions where the limbs move up and down in front of or behind the body (like your legs do when you march in place). In this plane, we run, walk, or jump. Movements such as *flexion* (bending a joint) and *extension* (straightening a joint) take place in the sagittal plane.

FRONTAL PLANE

The *frontal plane* divides the body into front and back parts. It includes all motions where the body parts move away from or closer to the central axis. In this plane, for example, we lift the arms away from or closer to the sides of the body (like a bird flapping its wings up and down) or spread the legs apart and bring them together (like playing hopscotch). *Adduction* (toward the body) and *abduction* (away from the body) are movements that occur in the frontal plane.

HORIZONTAL PLANE

The *horizontal plane* divides the body into top and bottom parts. It includes all motions with rotation. In this plane, we swing, twist, and play racket sports. Some sources call this plane the *transverse plane*.

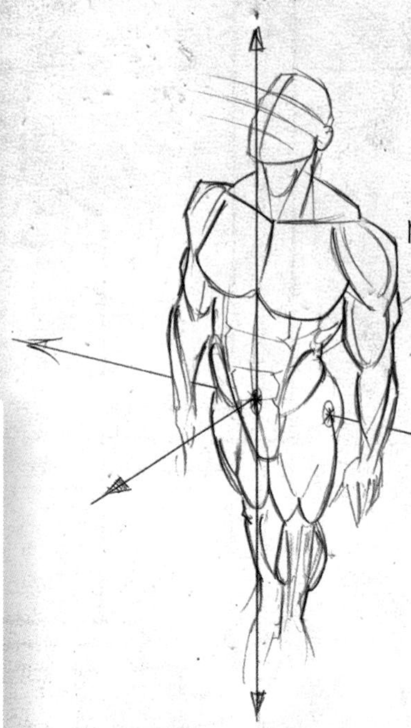

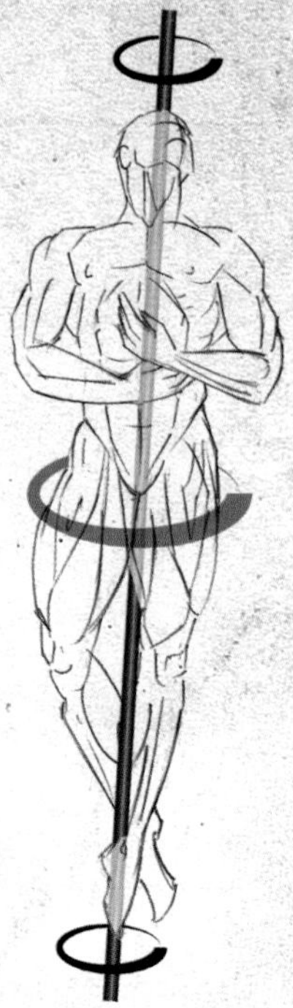

These three planes are supplemented by axes around which we move. These are the axes of rotation. The three axes are represented by the intersections of different planes:

- The **vertical axis** is at the intersection of the frontal and sagittal planes and is perpendicular to the horizontal plane. It crosses the body vertically from the head to the toes. It is on this axis (and through the horizontal plane) that the human body rotates during an axel jump when ice skating, for example.
- The **anterior-posterior axis** is at the intersection of the sagittal and horizontal planes and passes horizontally from the back to the front of the body. It only allows movement in the frontal plane.
- The **frontal axis** is at the intersection of the frontal and horizontal planes, crossing the body horizontally from left to right. It is the axis used to do somersaults, for example, in the sagittal plane.

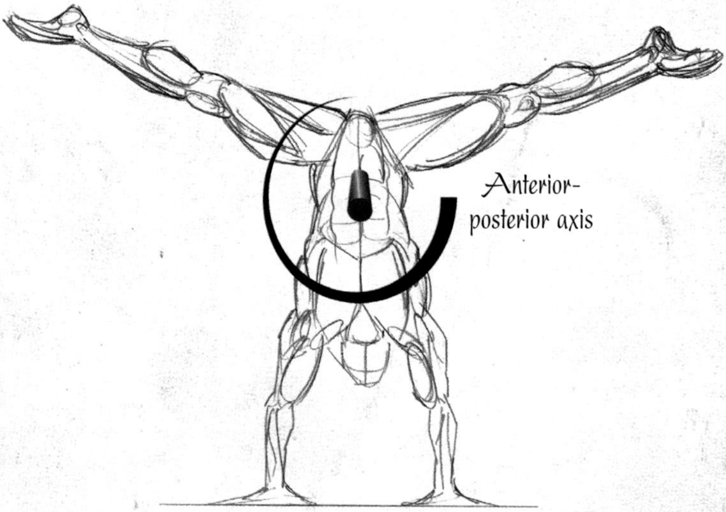

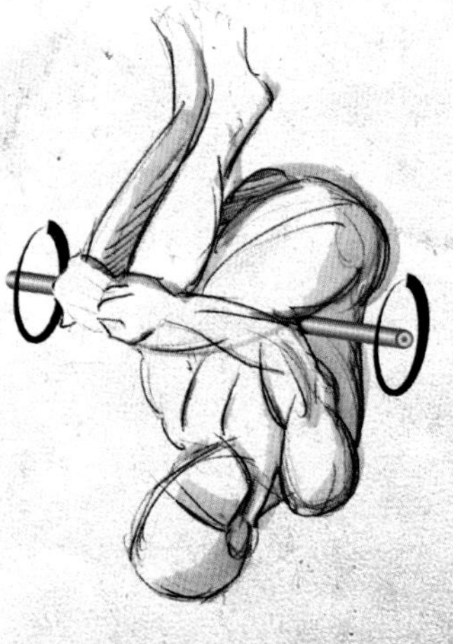

> *Because we move in complex ways, training should not be limited to a set of exercises within a singular plane or axis.*

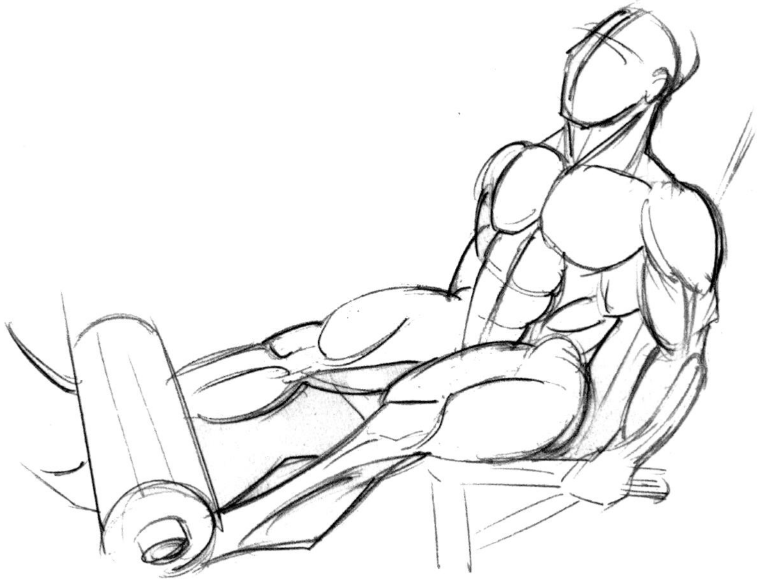

In many gyms, machines are often limited to one plane. Often, the horizontal plane is missing.

Training a single joint, limited in its planes and axes of movement, is still important for strengthening a weak link in a muscle chain. However, this only one part of the many complex movements that need to be trained to maximize athletic performance.

> *A multiplanar, multiaxial approach should be widely used in training programs.*

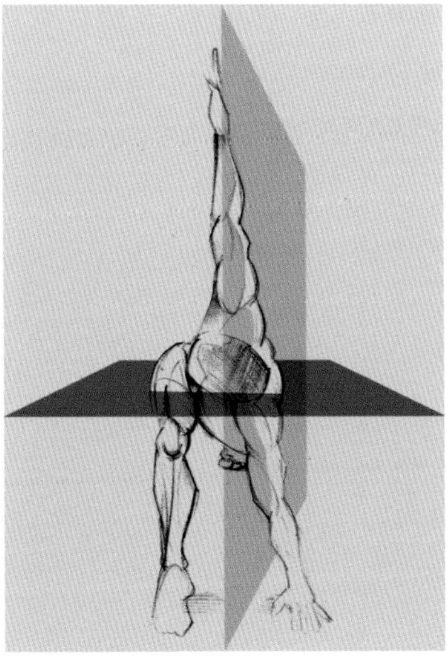

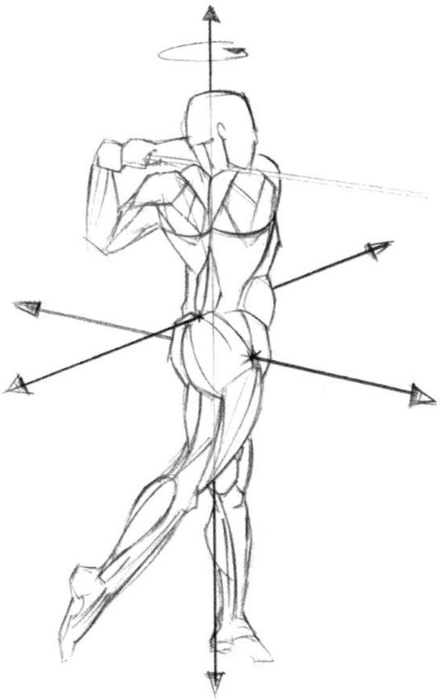

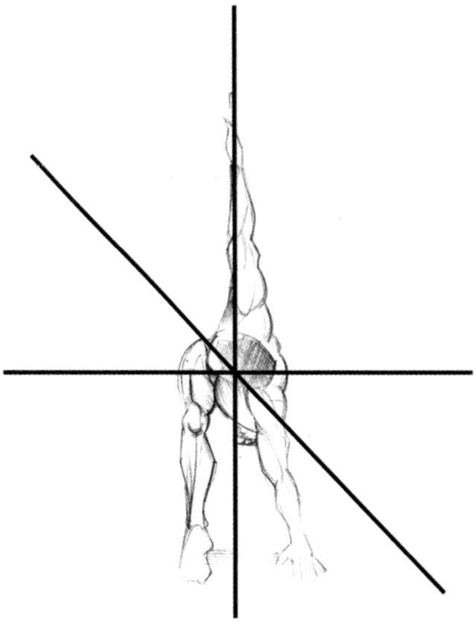

01 MUSCLE CHAINS

The movement system involves a coordination of the joint, myofascial, and muscle systems along with the nervous, psychosocial, and physiological systems. Analyzing movement relies on a complex and systemic approach.

As in everything that deals with a functional training approach, it is important to develop a comprehensive training program. Isolating a muscle only makes sense for strengthening an isolated link in the chain. It is crucial to design your training program using more comprehensive exercises.

Even theoretical approaches, which are necessary to understand human anatomy, are very standardized. This simplification is necessary but completely artificial. For example, although the four tissues of the body (connective, epithelial, nervous, and muscular) are traditionally studied one at a time, it is important to know that they are all intermixed within the body.

THE MYOFASCIAL NETWORK

As part of the connective tissue system, the *fasciae*, which are fibroelastic membranes that cover or envelop a joint structure, are what keep the skin attached to the muscle.

THE FOUR TYPES OF TISSUE IN THE HUMAN BODY

- Connective tissue supports all tissues in a functional manner. It is involved in many functions including support and protection, nutrition and repair of tissues, growth, immune response, connectivity, and even storage. For example, the *periosteum* surrounds bones and provides a connective border for ligaments and tendons. Cartilage protects the joints, and the visceral and parietal fascia hold and position the internal organs. The blood is a liquid connective tissue that allows the body's molecules to be transported between the storage and usage areas. Connective tissue makes up two-thirds of the total volume of the human body.
- Epithelial tissue has the primary function of covering the border between another tissue (usually connective tissue) and a cavity or surrounding air. It has a protective chemical and mechanical role and enables cellular movement and exchanges. Furthermore, it has a glandular function and is involved in secreting substances required by the body.
- Nervous tissue is responsible for controlling and transmitting information. It chemically or electrically transmits messages to and from the brain from all over the body.
- Muscular tissue has the primary function of contraction to maintain proper posture and create movement.

DIFFERENT TYPES OF FASCIA

Bichat first introduced the different types of fascia in his "Treatise on Membranes" in 1816. These structures of connective tissue, which are visible with the naked eye, are divided into five categories:

- The **superficial fascia** is subcutaneous. It is the deep layer of the skin made up of loose connective tissue.
- More deeply, we find the **deep fascia**, a fibrous muscle structure of dense connective tissue. The superficial fascia lies on top of it. It separates superficial muscles and subcutaneous tissue.
- The muscles are also surrounded by fasciae (**muscular fascia**) made up of dense connective tissue.
- **Fasciae made up of loose connective tissue** also exist between certain internal organs.
- The **visceral fascia**, which envelops some organs, is made up of dense connective tissue.

Organized in a network, the fasciae ensure that stresses caused by muscular activity or forces outside the body are properly transmitted. Very rich in collagen fibers, the fasciae are even capable of contracting and can affect muscle mechanics (Schleip 2005). Since nerves connect to them, fasciae also play a role in helping us be conscious of the position and movement of our bodies (Willard 2012), also called *proprioceptive awareness*.

The human machine is not just a collection of parts. The fasciae surround the muscles, certainly, but they also penetrate them, as well as the bones, the blood vessels, the nerves, and even the organs. The myofascial network is a continuously connected structure and is present throughout the entire body in all planes. To be clear: Fasciae are everywhere. Historically, people have thought about muscles in an isolated manner and have divided muscle training in the same way. However, muscles are a link in a more global chain, organized in a network with a layer of fasciae. This is why we call it the *myofascial network*.

Proper understanding of the myofascial network is essential to comprehend the multiple planes as part of overall movement.

The myofascial network is the basis for muscle chains. Identifying it precisely allows you to

- understand the logic behind complex movements presented in this book,
- choose the exercises that best fit your movement needs (whether they are specific to a sport or to everyday life), and
- treat areas of localized stiffness or pain through stretching and self-massage of the whole chain.

Within this vast myofascial network, we identify lines of connection. The deep fasciae link the muscles to one another, and they are sometimes connected to each other by one or several bones. This is what we call a *muscle chain*. Tom Myers proposed the following representation of these muscle chains, which he calls *anatomy lines*, within the myofascial network (Myers 2013).

DID YOU KNOW?

Fasciae are not just structurally important; they are also involved in scar formation, immune function, and transmitting information (Willard 2012). Stretching and self-massage are at the heart of both retraining and preventive therapy. Further, fasciae should be properly warmed up to facilitate fluid and effective movement.

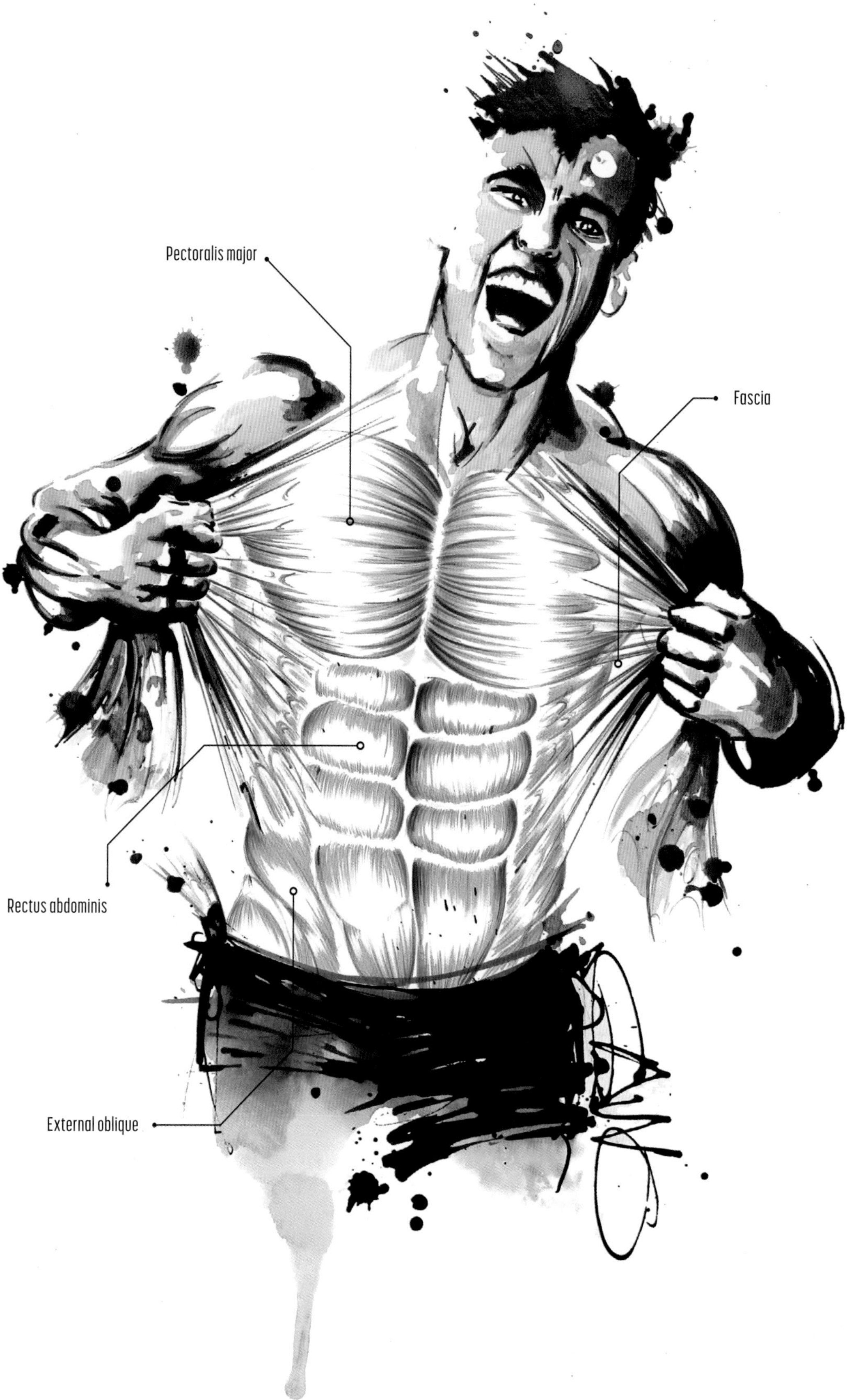
Pectoralis major
Fascia
Rectus abdominis
External oblique

The Body's Muscle Chains

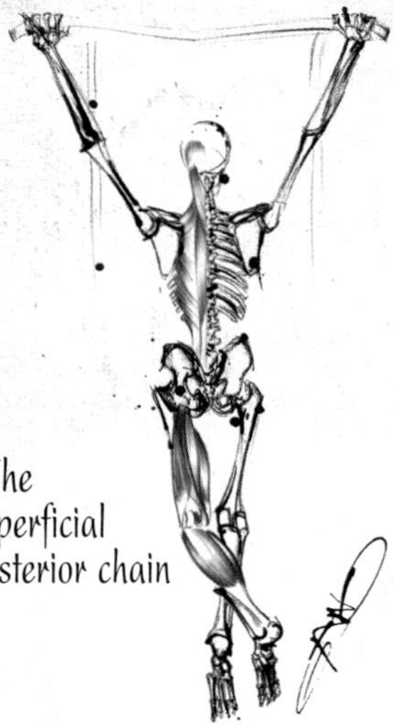

The superficial posterior chain

The superficial anterior chain

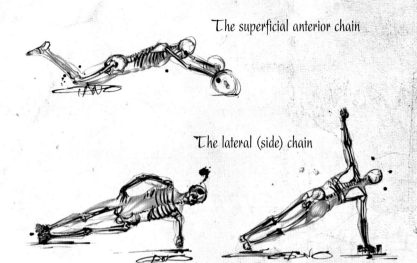

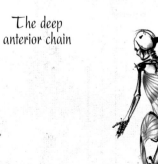

The lateral (side) chain

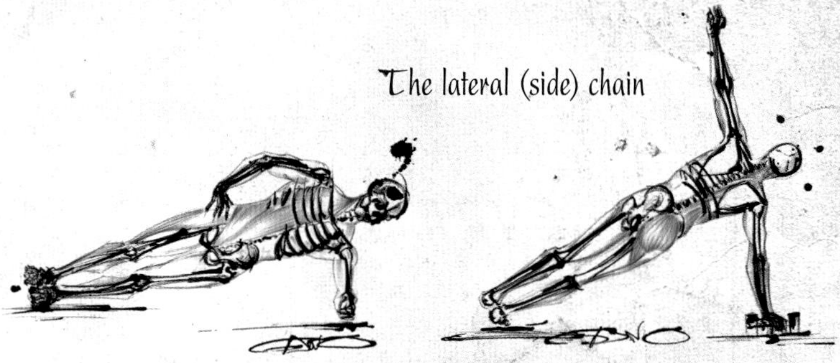

The spiral chain

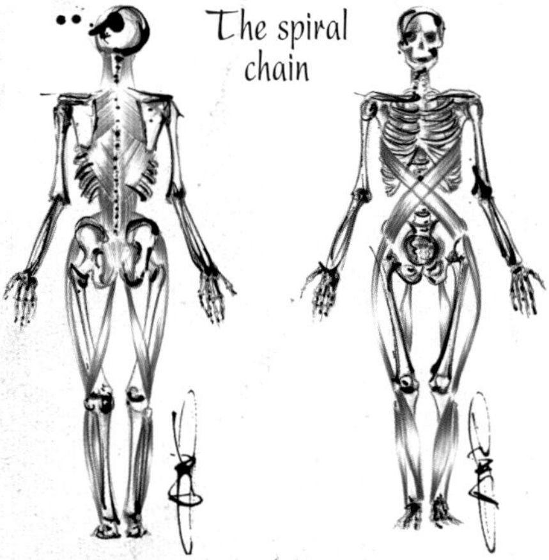

The anterior arm chains

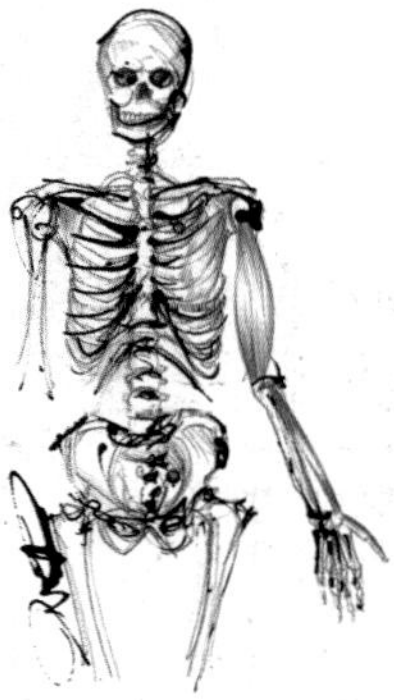

The posterior arm chains

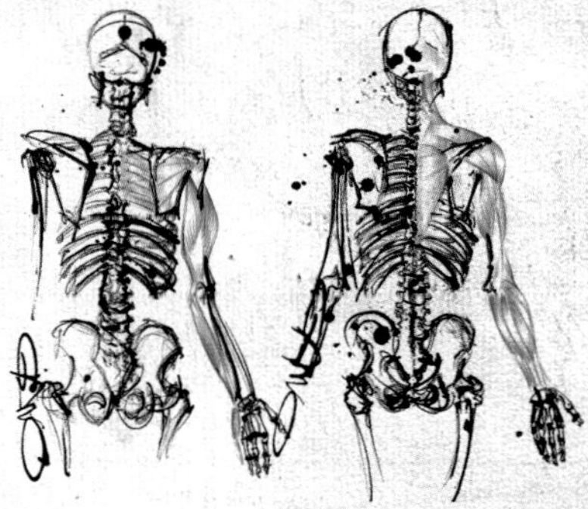

The deep anterior chain

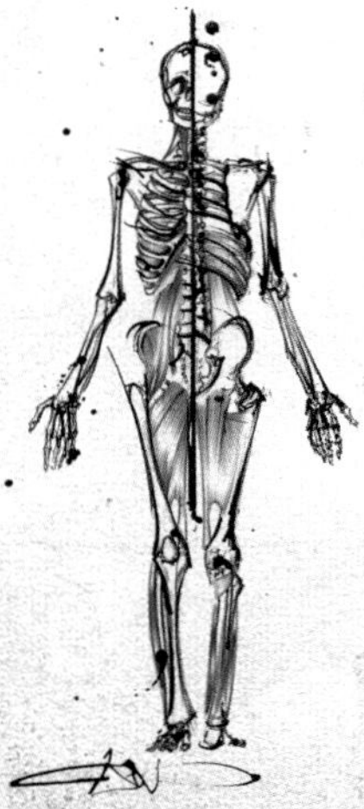

The posterior and anterior functional chains

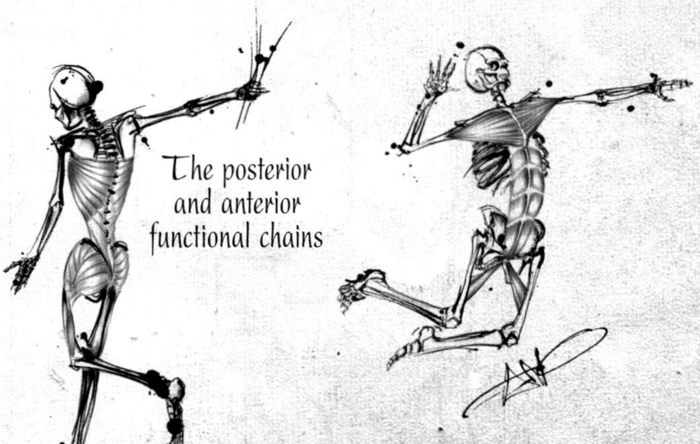

THE AGONIST, ANTAGONIST, SYNERGIST, AND NEUTRALIZER MUSCLES

You can avoid the training mistake of solely isolating muscles by being aware that the diversity and complexity of movement allows the different muscle chains to interact with each other. Though we can try to partially isolate them during training to accelerate development, muscle chains must often work together during movement, even in the most common exercises.

Let's explore agonist and antagonist muscles.

Each muscle system that drives movement (*agonist*) is paired with a braking system (*antagonist*).

Their synergy allows for precise control of movement, as in a knee extension: The quadriceps create movement, and the hamstrings stop it. Any malfunction in this system could reduce the knee's functionality or even cause injury.

This is not the only interaction that exists between muscle chains. The agonist muscles are assisted by auxiliary muscles, which we call *synergists*. For example, this is how some deep layers in the abdomen are activated during movements such as walking: The synergists control rotation and balance of the torso so that the agonist-antagonist muscle pair can work to the best of its ability.

Poor training, an injury, over-repetition, or automation of an incorrect or even dangerous movement—or even using an unsuitable weight—could cause a muscle to stop performing its proper role and start performing another role for which it is not well suited. The antagonist, for example, could contract at the same time as the agonist or the synergist, producing a co-contraction that limits its proper movement; this muscle is no longer playing its antagonist role, so it becomes a *neutralizing muscle*.

Apart from a comprehensive training approach, optimizing your movement to become functional can be done through balanced strengthening of the functional agonistic-antagonistic-synergist axis and reprogramming the neutralizing muscles.

STRAIGHT TO THE POINT

A muscle chain is made up of many links. Even though some individuals or companies recommend an exclusive or "trademarked" approach to train those links, it is important to understand that a comprehensive, multi-joint, functional approach to training cannot happen without a precise, single-joint analysis. Moreover, attention can be given to the muscles that would benefit from self-massage, stretching, strengthening, or activation. Often, overly tight and often shortened (*hypertonic*) muscles or, conversely, overly relaxed, nonreactive (*hyperphasic*) muscles need special care. If you want to get straight to the point to analyze your muscle chains, you can start your journey on the next page.

PRESTRESSING

The concept of prestressing is essential in the preventative approach of manual therapists. Julien Cramet, a physiotherapist for French weightlifting teams, often reminds me how essential this principle is for physical preparation.

In a muscle chain, some tissues (like muscles or ligaments) are stiffer than others. Just like different exercise bands with varying levels of elasticity, the muscle chain is not homogenous throughout its structure. Because of this, these tissues are already tense or prestressed when resting, like they are when they are pulling. Any additional stress on these tissues, like carrying a weight or making a very wide movement, exposes them to damage or injury. Studying the different areas of tension, the restrictions, and the *kinetic* (meaning movement or effort) chains experienced by our body allows us to anticipate and prevent some injuries.

The Superficial Posterior Chain

Sole of the foot: arch, quadratus plantae, flexor digitorum brevis, plantar fascia

Calves: gastrocnemius, soleus, Achilles tendon

Hamstrings: semitendinosus, semimembranosus, biceps femoris

Erector spinae: iliocostalis, longissimus, spinalis

Suboccipital: obliquus capitis, rectus capitis, occipitalis

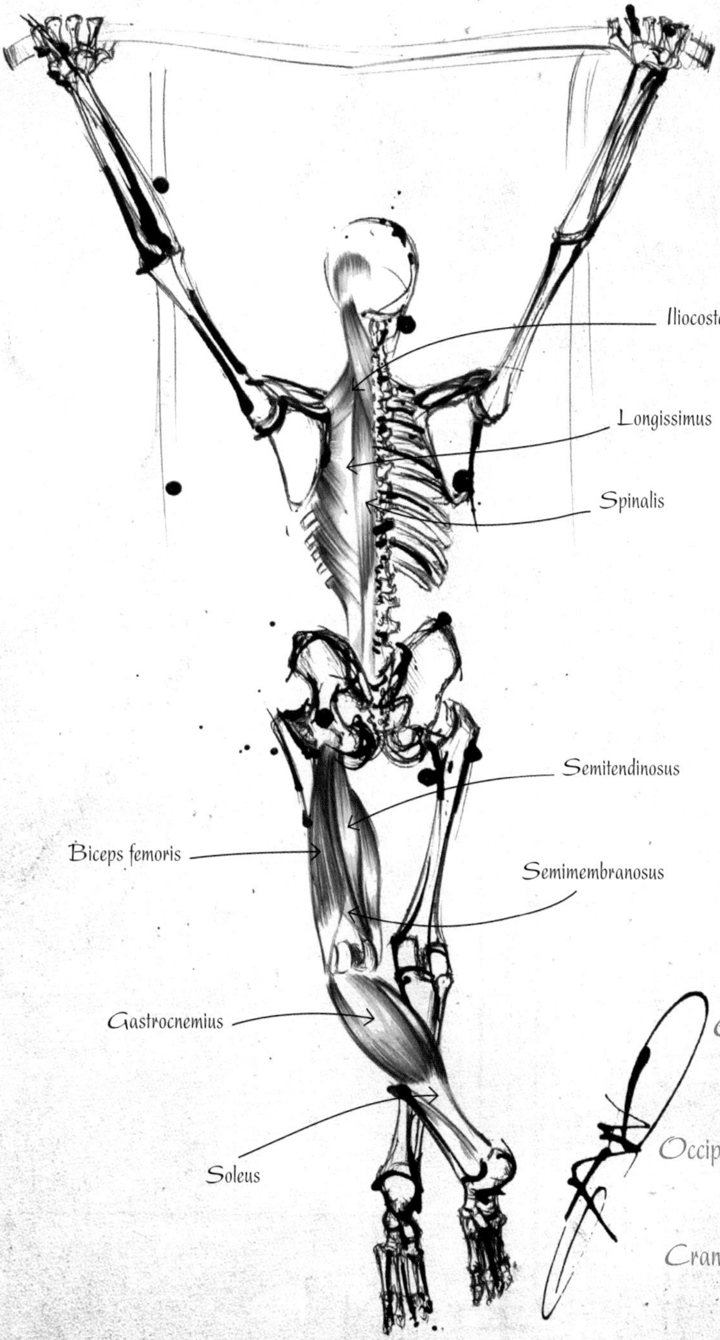

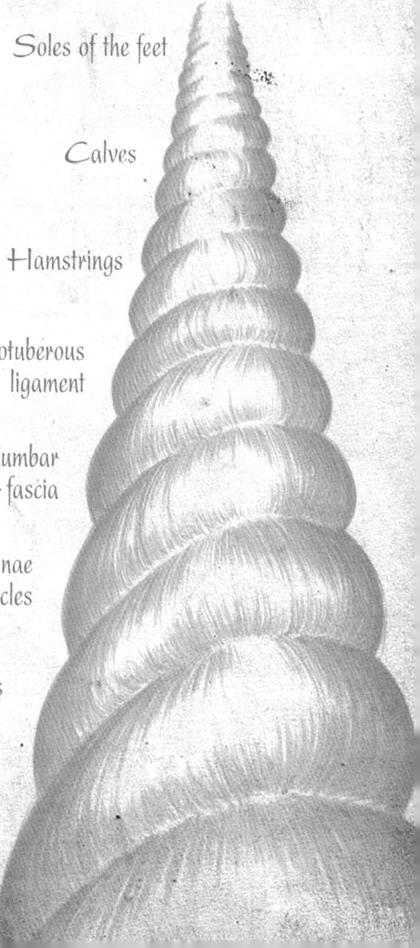

The superficial posterior chain is essential for our posture. It is responsible for keeping the body straight and vertical, both when standing still and when moving.

The postural function of this chain is why it is particularly resilient. Most of the muscles it contains are made up of slow and not very powerful fibers, which is why you should develop them carefully and gradually. The hamstrings are worthy of special mention in this chain; in some people, they are not very resilient or strong. They are very sinewy muscles that are not supplied with a lot of blood. Thus, they have limited energy reserves, so they are fragile and can become easily fatigued. If not trained properly, they will become stiff, weak, and unbalanced. Strengthening them methodically and regularly is essential for this muscle chain to function properly. Here are three exercises to achieve this:

01. ARABESQUE

Start with your feet close together and parallel with your arms next to your torso and thumbs pointing forward. Slightly shift your weight to your left leg and hinge your left hip to move your torso forward while simultaneously reaching your arms ahead of your body and extending your right leg backward with the toes of the right foot pointing toward the floor. Your torso and right leg should move at the same time and your left knee and both elbows should be fully extended. (Be sure not to compensate by rotating your torso to open your right hip outward.) Your left knee should be very slightly flexed to create a stable base throughout the movement. Perform 3 to 5 sets of 6 to 10 reps per leg with 30 seconds to 1 minute of recovery.

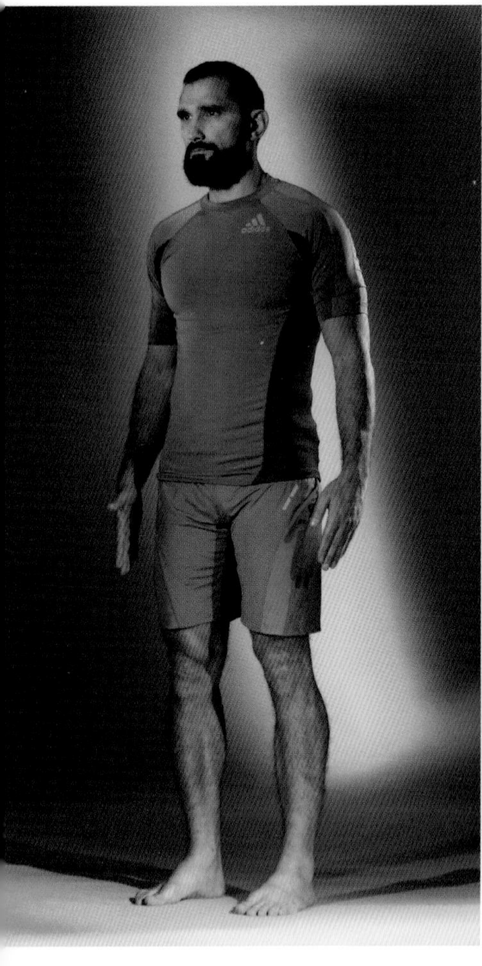

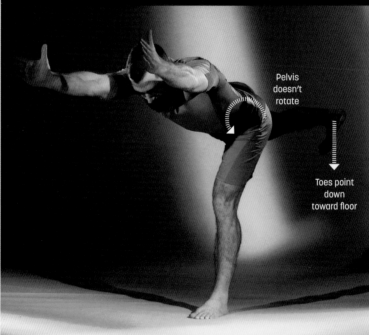

02. STRENGTHENING THE BACK WITH SMALL HEEL STEPS

From a bridge position with your hips fully extended, step your feet forward and then back to the starting position. This exercise is all about core stability, so your hips must stay completely extended throughout the exercise and your abdomen should be flat. Be careful not to exaggerate your lumbar curve. Use your breathing to control your diaphragm. **Perform 3 or 4 sets of 5 reps with 30 seconds to 1 minute of recovery.**

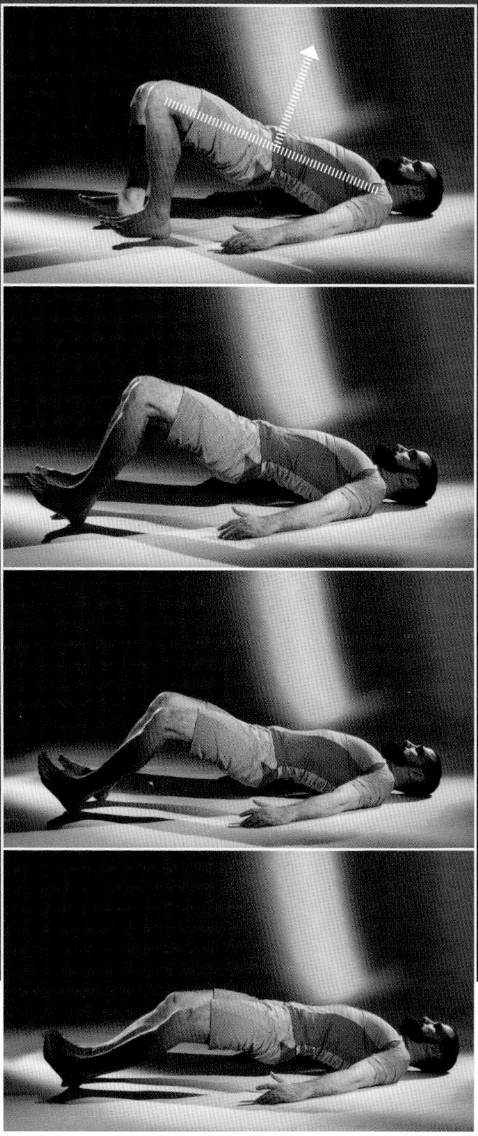

03. STRAIGHT-LEG BRIDGE

From the same starting position as the previous exercise, follow the same principles of core strengthening. Straighten the knee of one of your legs and hold the extended position (while keeping the leg in line with your torso) for 3 to 5 seconds. **Perform 3 or 4 sets of 4 reps per leg with no recovery.**

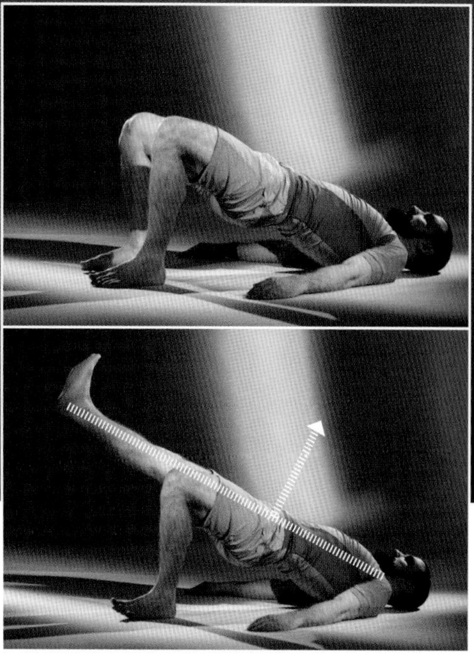

The muscles of the calves have a high endurance capacity; they are used nearly as much during walking as they are when you are standing still.

Despite their small volume, the calves are made up of particularly strong muscles that are capable of supporting and balancing the entire body from ankle level. Thus, it is important to strengthen them using heavy weights and long sets. Here are two particularly effective exercises:

01. STRENGTHENING THE CALVES USING A LEG PRESS AND MAXIMUM WEIGHT

Use the maximum weight for five reps, after a suitable warm-up. Place the balls of your feet on the bottom edge of the leg press platform and straighten—but do not lock out—your knees. Allow the platform to push your toes back for three seconds and then point your toes for one second. **Perform 3 or 4 sets of 4 reps with 3 minutes of recovery.**

02. STANDING FRONT-BACK TILT USING A BAR ON YOUR SHOULDERS

Stand fully erect with a bar on your shoulders. Shift your weight back on to your heels and lift your toes off the floor, then slowly transfer your weight toward the balls of your feet and point your toes to lift your heels off the floor. Strive for the maximum range of motion at both ends of the movement.
Perform 4 sets of 5 to 20 reps with less than 1 minute of recovery.

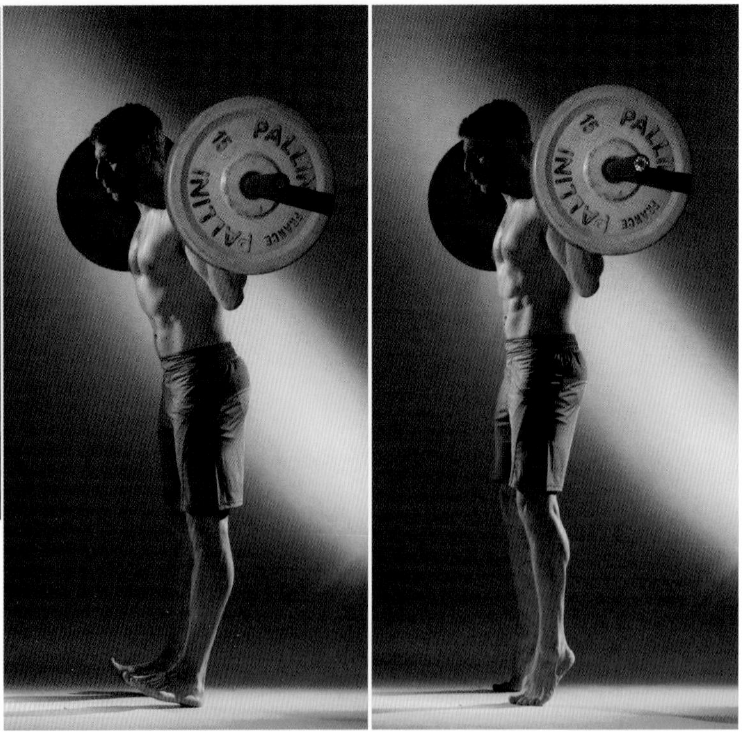

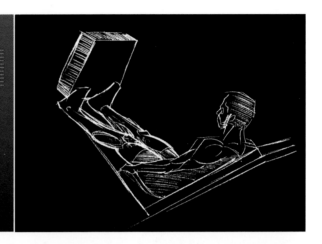

Sitting Breaks the Chain

We spend too much time in a position that breaks the superficial posterior chain. The hamstrings insert on both sides of the knee; the semitendinosus and the semimembranosus connect to the inside of the tibia, while the biceps femoris inserts on the head of the fibula. This system only allows for continuity in the superficial posterior chain when the knee is extended; sitting breaks the chain. A simple, everyday solution to strengthen the posterior chain is to mobilize it, which will maintain proper posture and allow for better movement. When training and when resting, it is best to sit on an exercise ball. The ball should be big enough so that your knees are not flexed more than ninety degrees while sitting down; if they flex more than that, the deeper muscles would take over to provide active support as compensation for the break in the chain. You should only sit on a bench when doing exercises for maximum strength and power; we always recommend doing these types of exercises in a standing position when possible.

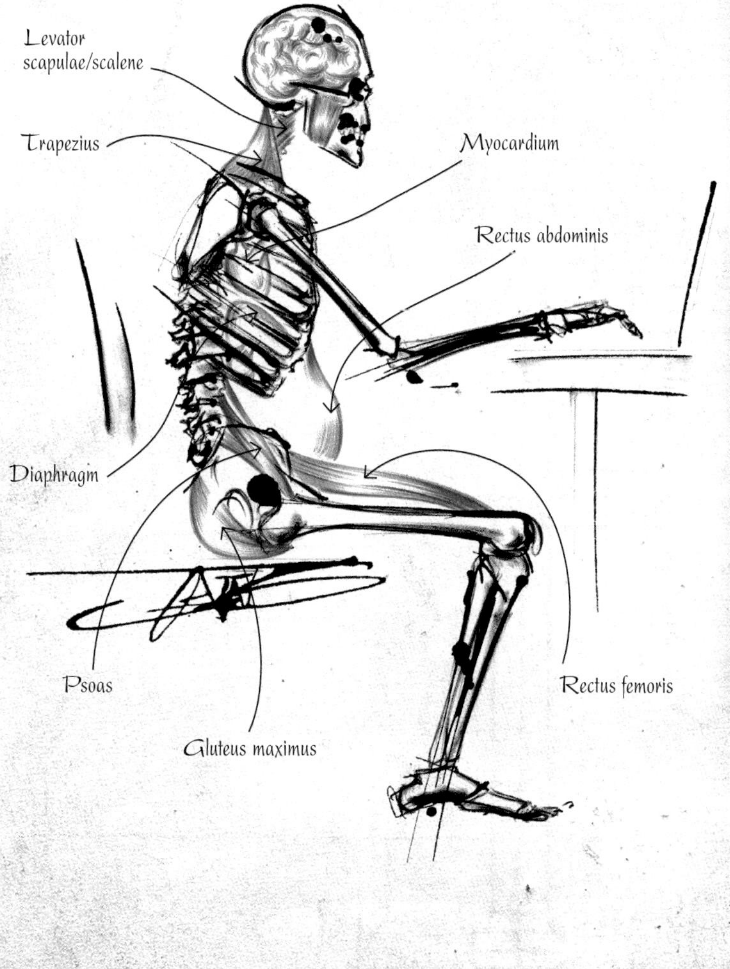

Possible Malfunctions in the Superficial Posterior Chain

- When all or part of the muscle chain is lengthened for a long time or too regularly, the muscles involved are not working hard enough to maintain sufficient strength or levels of endurance to ensure effective posture or movement. This happens, for example, if you lie comfortably on a couch for several hours every day.
- Conversely, sudden, intense, or repetitive movements can lead to an overdevelopment of strength or endurance in all or part of the links in the muscle chain and create imbalances. The areas of lower strength expose your human machine to problems within that muscle chain or between muscle chains.

KILLER MOVES
TO DEVELOP THE POSTERIOR CHAIN

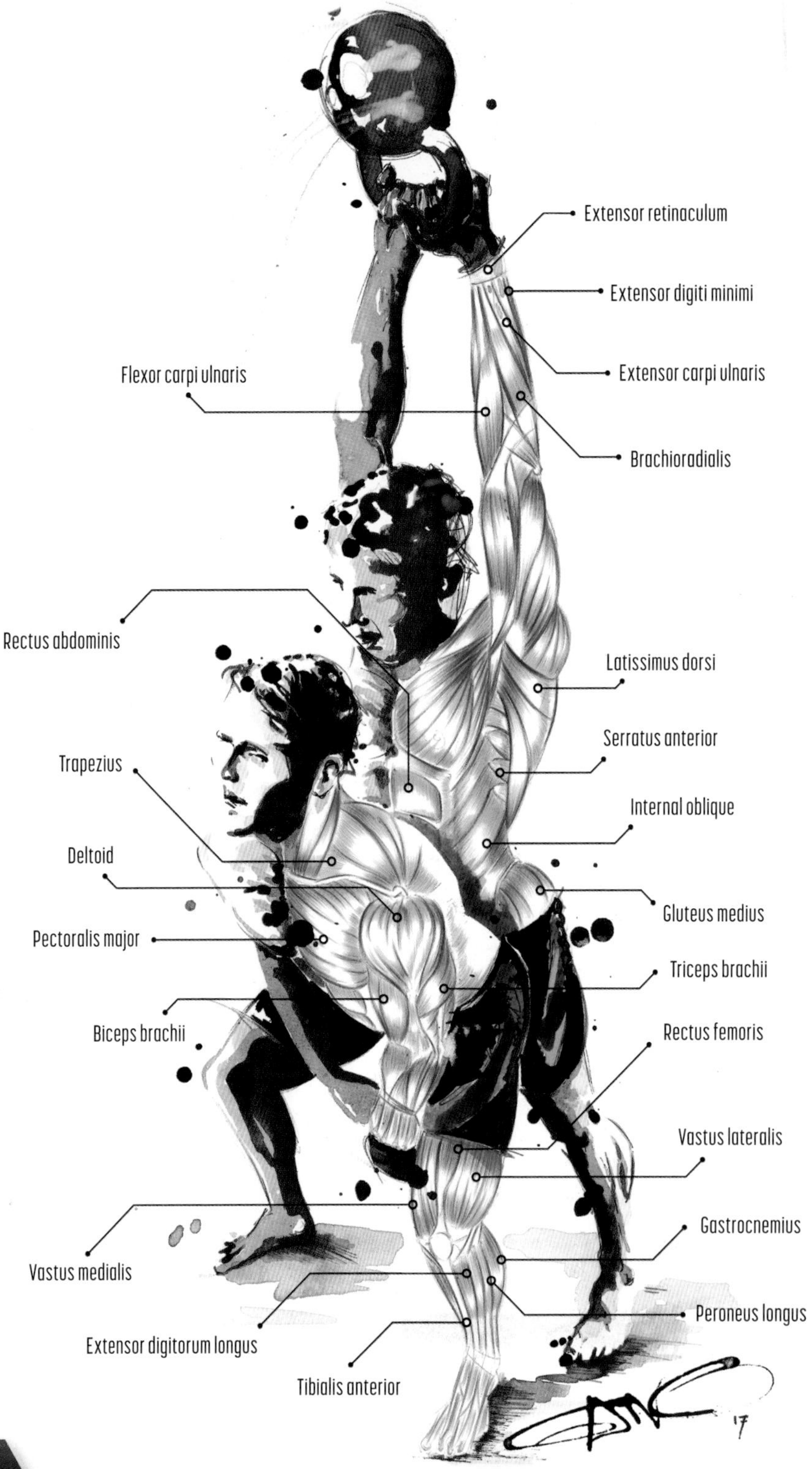

01. KETTLEBELL SWING

Place your feet slightly more than shoulder-width apart, keeping a natural opening of the toes (parallel or facing slightly outward but always symmetrical and flat). Start with the kettlebell between your legs. Push your chest out, keep your shoulders down and back, and place your head in a neutral position by looking at a point slightly above the horizon (look "through your eyebrows"). Activate your gluteal muscles and hamstrings and drive the kettlebell up and forward with straight arms just after an energetic inhale. Continue the move by exhaling rapidly as you extend your hips and knees to straighten up to standing and lift the kettlebell to your chest or even your forehead. In some versions, you lift the kettlebell above your head. Note: your shoulders are not responsible for propelling the kettlebell; the extension of your hips causes your torso to rise. This means the kettlebell does not rise any higher than is permitted by the force of your hip extension. Keep your back in a neutral position (without exaggerating any of its natural curves) throughout the exercise. Do not extend your hips beyond the line between the shoulders and ankles.

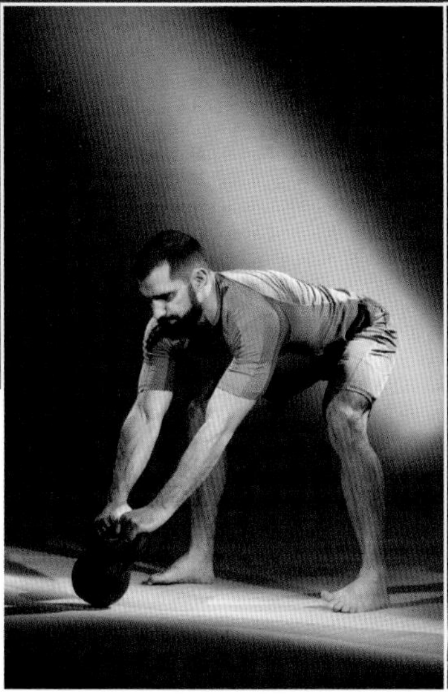

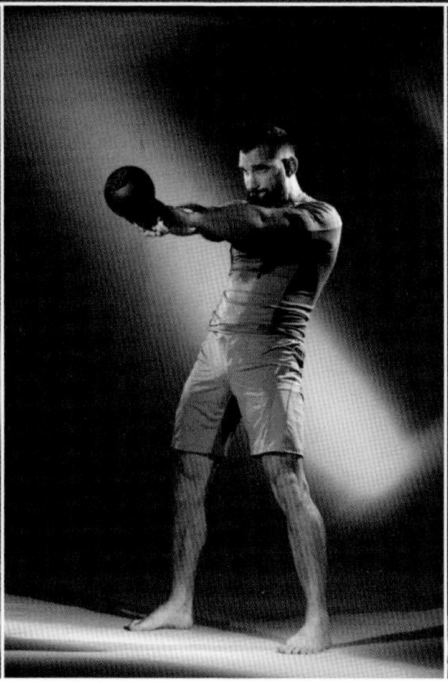

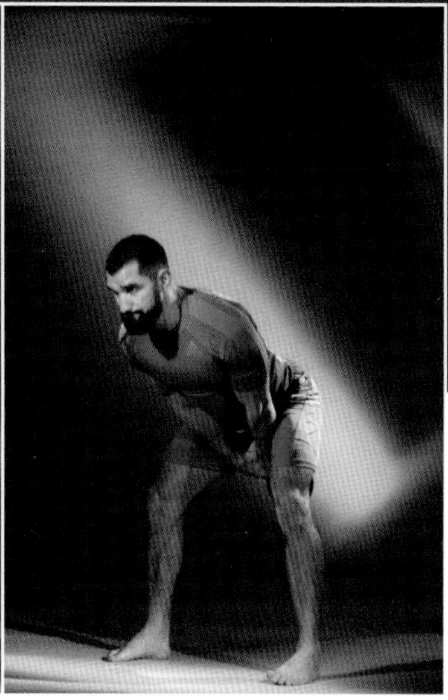

02. ARABESQUE

Start with your feet close together and parallel with your arms next to your torso and thumbs pointing forward. Slightly shift your weight to your left leg and hinge your left hip to move your torso forward while simultaneously reaching your arms ahead of your body and extending your right leg backward with the toes of the right foot pointing toward the floor (see page 104). Your torso and right leg should move at the same time and your left knee and both elbows should be fully extended. (Be sure not to compensate by rotating your torso to open your right hip outward.) Your left knee should be very slightly flexed to create a stable base throughout the movement. If this exercise becomes too easy, you can make it harder by holding a weight in your right hand with your right arm hanging perpendicular to the floor. As an alternative (not seen in the photo), you can change the load on the posterior chain by holding a weight in the hand opposite the moving leg.

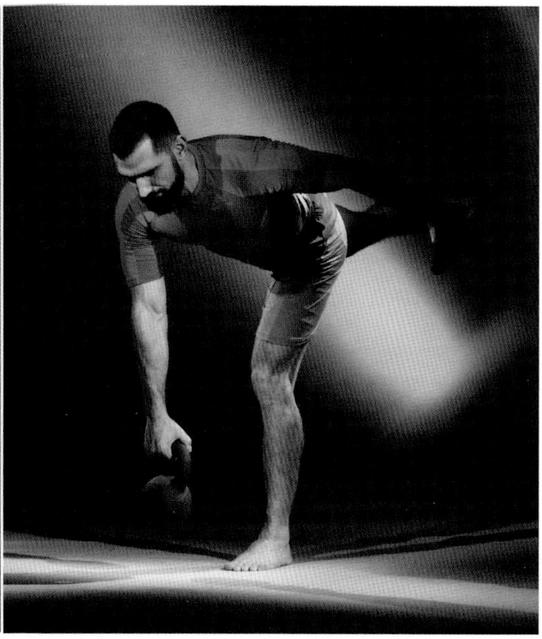

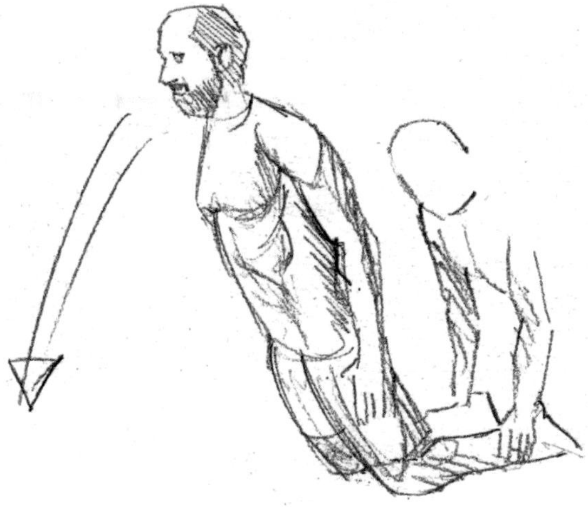

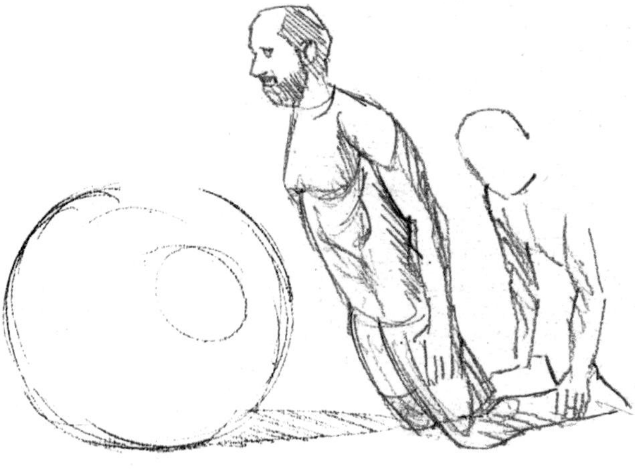

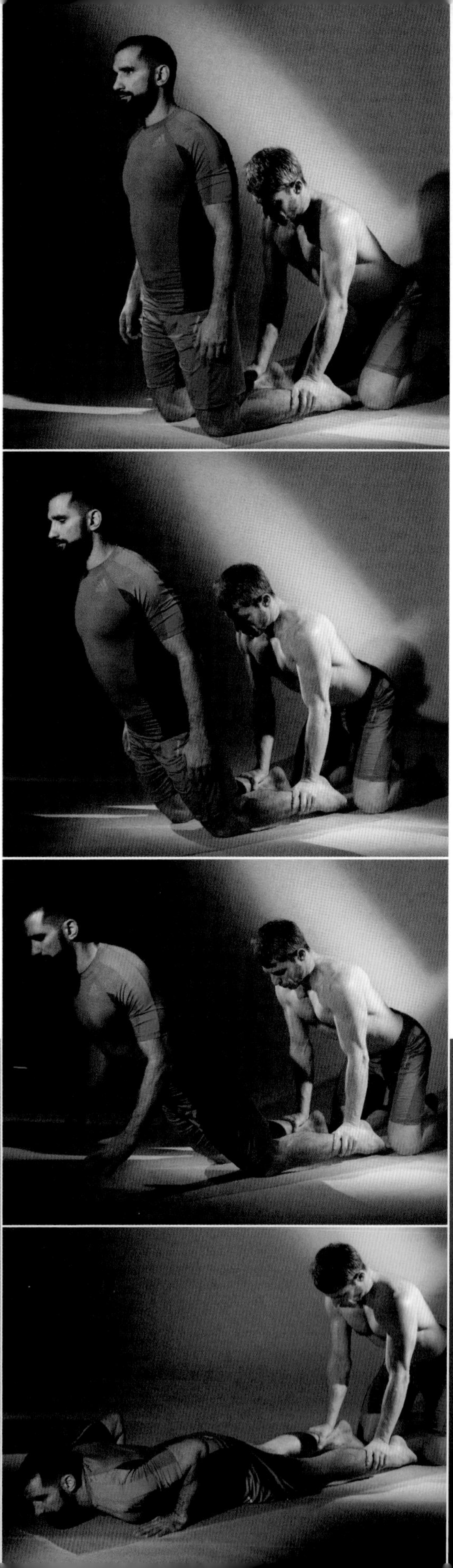

03. NORDIC HAMSTRING CURL

Kneel on a comfortable mat (not seen in the photos; one or two twice-folded yoga mats work well) and lock your lower legs under a plate-loaded bar (that is stabilized so it will not roll) or ask a partner to hold them. Activate your gluteal muscles and abdominals so that you never compromise the full extension of your pelvis. Allow yourself to fall forward but slow your descent as much as possible and land in a push-up position. Even if you gain speed at the end of the movement, keep your hips fully extended. If this exercise is too difficult, you can use an exercise ball to help you. In level 1, land with your torso on the ball. In level 2, roll the ball in front of you. Level 3 is done without the ball.

04. REVERSE HYPEREXTENSION

Lie on your abdomen on a bench or box. Bring your legs under the bench or against the box as much as possible then tighten your gluteal muscles and abdominals and straighten your legs by pushing your heels back. Do not arch your back to raise the legs more than necessary. Focus on aligning the different sections of your body and fully extending your knees. You can separate your legs to make the exercise more lateral, or you can tilt the bench to make the exercise harder. In that case, keep your legs straight throughout the exercise.

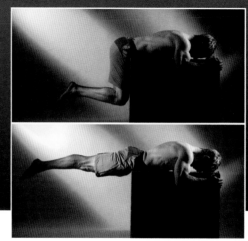

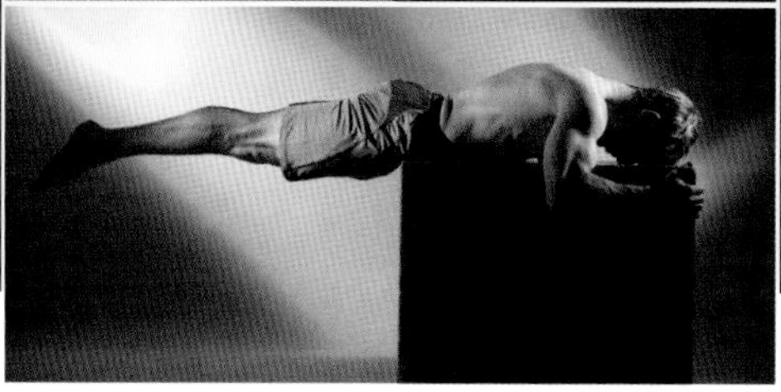

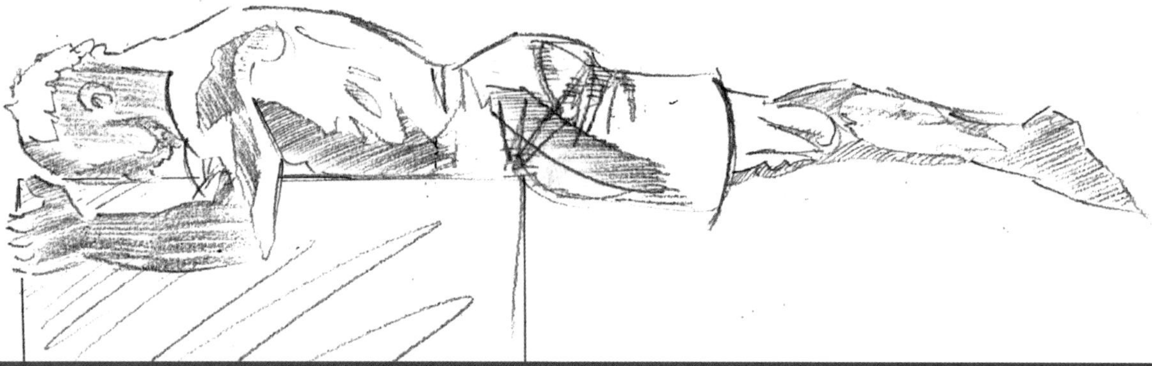

05. GLUTEAL MUSCLE BRIDGE WITH A BAR

This exercise should first be mastered without the bar. In its basic version, it is possible to add a bar while keeping your shoulder blades on the floor. The more advanced version involves supporting your back on a bench. Specifically focused on the hip extensors, this is a powerful exercise to help you squat and deadlift better, but it also allows you to lower and lift your body more easily in everyday life. This exercise really works the hamstrings and gluteals. Lie on your back with your legs straight. Roll the bar over your legs and hips to place it in the required bridge position. Flex your knees and hips to place your feet flat on the floor. Place the bar about two inches (five centimeters) below your hip bones and hold the bar with a wide grip. Keep the bar in position by keeping your arms straight and pushing down. With your feet flat on the floor, lift the bar explosively by fully extending your hips, exhaling at the end of the move. Keep steady as you come back down. If you cannot fully extend your hips, the bar is too heavy. For comfort, you can use a roller pad or something similar to cushion the weight of the bar on the hips.

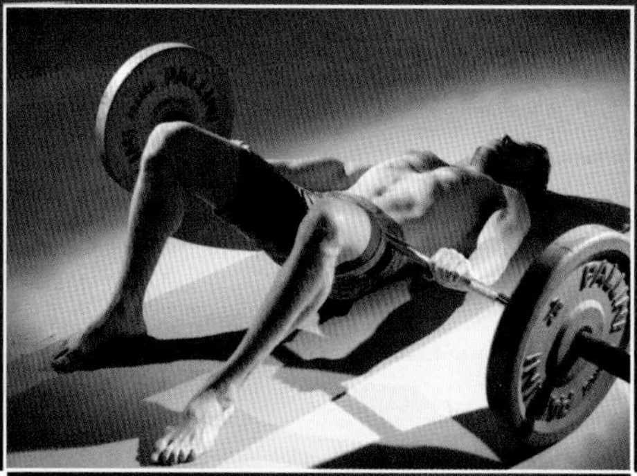

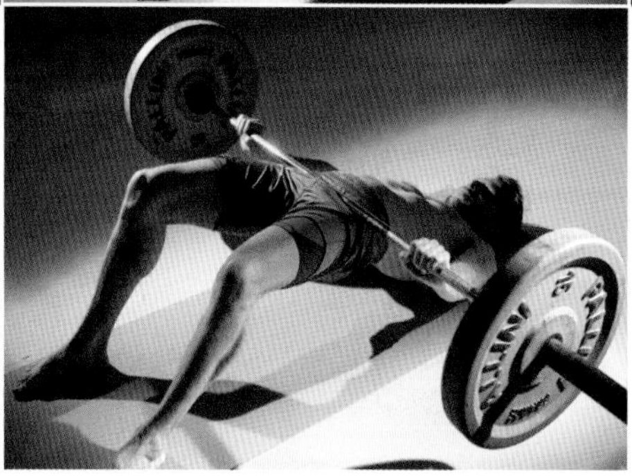

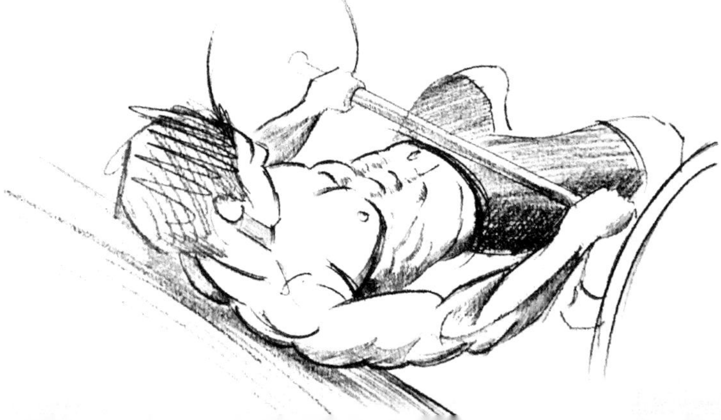

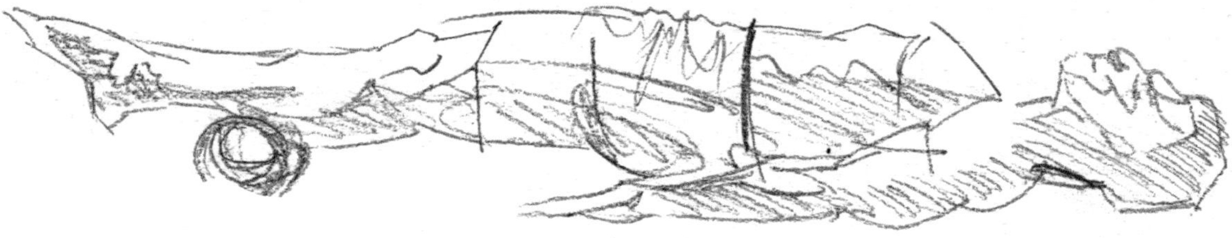

06. LEG CURL

Lie on your back. Pull your abdomen in, squeeze your gluteal muscles, and extend your hips. In the most accessible version of this exercise, we recommend using a simple massage roller that you roll from front to back by flexing and extending your knees. As you progress, you can use an exercise ball. Trap the ball with your toes to activate the muscle chains all the way to your toes. The most advanced version of this exercise can be done with suspension trainer straps. Each version of this exercise can be done with one or two legs.

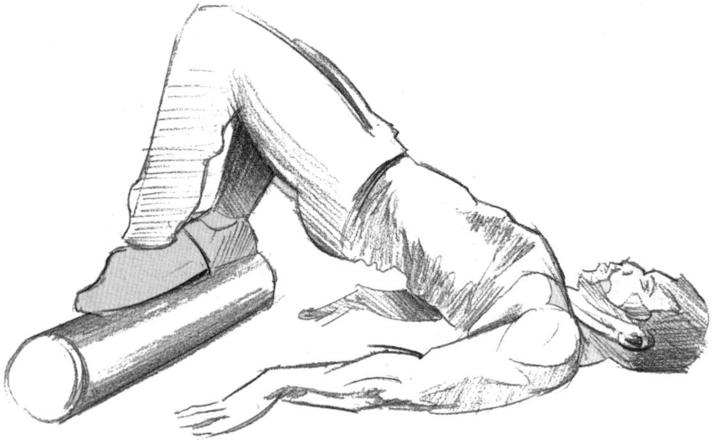

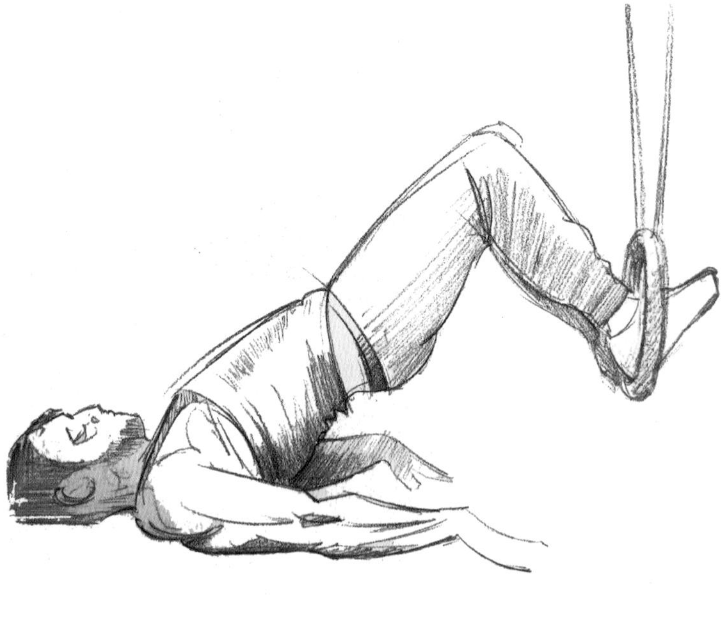

The Superficial Anterior Chain

Front of the foot: front of the shin, extensor digitorum brevis, extensor digitorum longus

Shin: Patellofemoral ligament, patellar tendon

Thigh: rectus femoris

Torso: rectus abdominis (connected to the pubic tubercle), ribs, sternum

Neck: sternocleidomastoid muscles

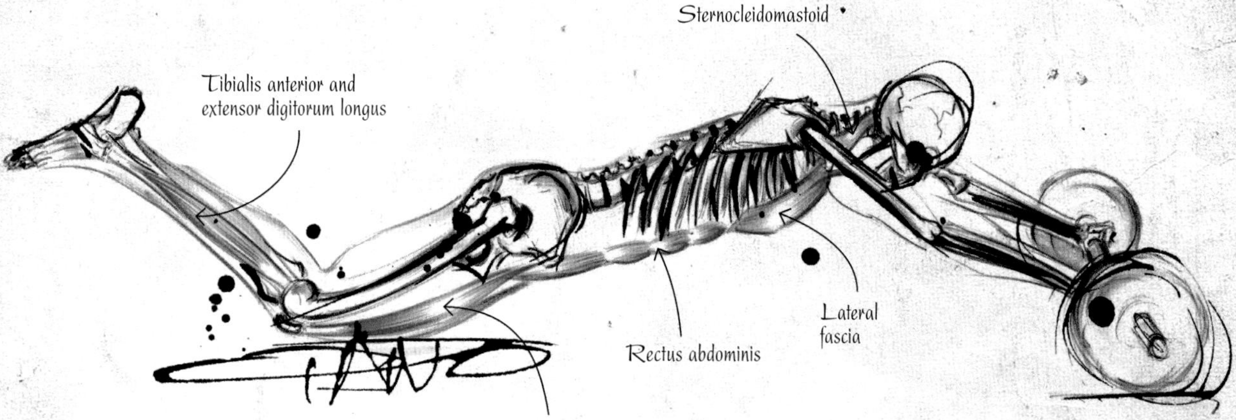

The superficial anterior chain controls balance in the sagittal plane. Functionally, it works together with the superficial posterior chain, acting as its antagonist. When the posterior chain stretches as the torso moves forward or flexes over the legs, the anterior chain contracts. Conversely, when the posterior chain contracts during a back extension, the anterior chain stretches. Therefore, this chain is said to be reactive: It is at the heart of our adaptation behaviors and compensating strategies.

These two chains must be balanced and synchronized to keep the body vertical when resting and moving as well as for proper movement when walking or running. This synergy is continuously evolving. The superficial anterior chain contracts or stretches quickly to adapt to the angle of the torso. This muscle chain does not have a large mass, and the muscles it contains are generally strong with low endurance.

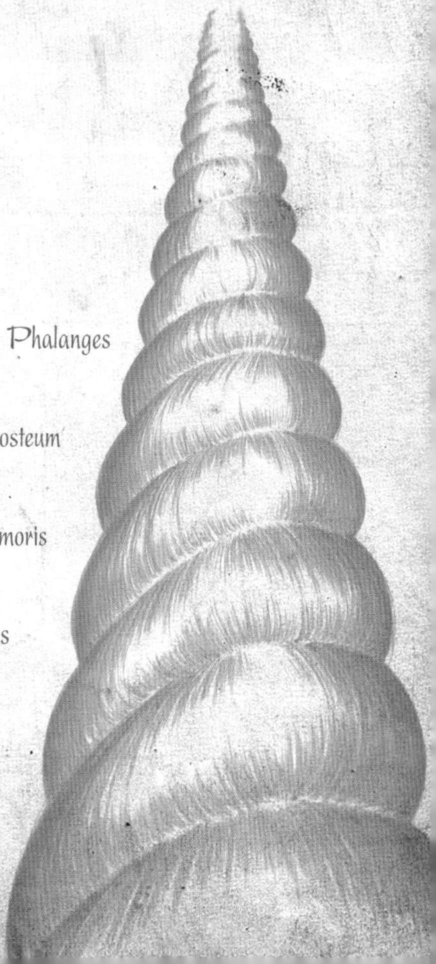

Possible Malfunctions in the Superficial Anterior Chain

AN ESSENTIAL MUSCLE CHAIN FOR BALANCE

Since the superficial anterior chain ends at the sternocleidomastoid muscles close to the inner ear, it is greatly involved in the body's balance.

- Using an unbalanced weight with the posterior muscle chain often leads to structural imbalances between the superficial anterior and superficial posterior chains. Some sports cause the anterior chain to become dominant, overdeveloping it to the point that it can affect posture, cause pain due to weakness (which causes other muscles to compensate), or even cause injury. This is exactly what happens when the abdominal muscles are overworked. A one-to-one ratio should always be observed: If you follow a training program that focuses on the anterior chain, be sure to give enough attention to training the posterior chain. For example, if you do a set of crunches, alternate with a set of hyperextensions.
- If some links in this chain are too weak or lack endurance, other muscles could begin to compensate, which triggers a vicious cycle of compensation that alters movement and posture and ultimately makes the weak links even weaker. These compensations often happen in the iliopsoas, crossing both the anterior and posterior chains. Make it a priority to relax the iliopsoas through self-massage and stretching before and after any exercise that involves the anterior chain. Here are four exercises to help relax the iliopsoas:

01. PSOAS MASSAGE USING A ROLLER

Lie on your abdomen and place the massage roller under your hip. Slowly roll from front to back about a dozen times and tilt from left to right about a dozen times to complete one set. Perform 3 times per side without resting (since you are changing sides, the exercise time is equal to the recovery time; when one side is working, the other is resting).

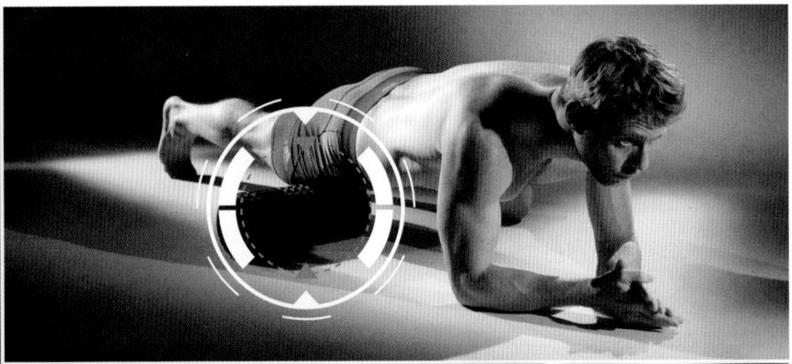

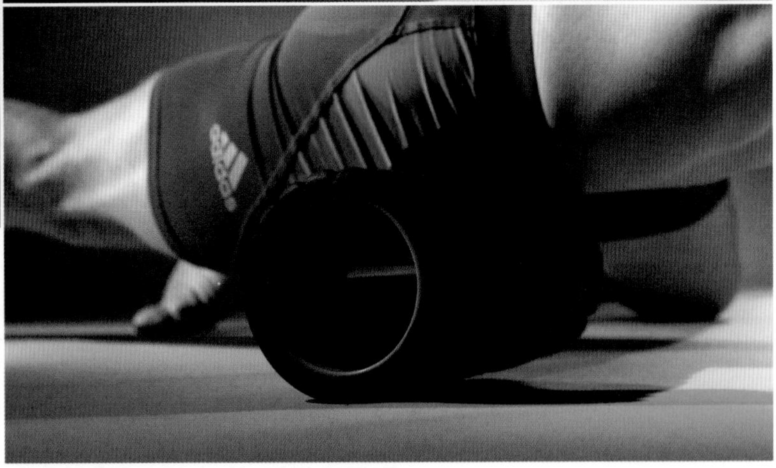

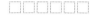

02. ILIAC MASSAGE USING YOUR HAND

Lie on your side and push your fingers firmly into the fold of your hip. Tilt onto your side, using your forearm as a lever.

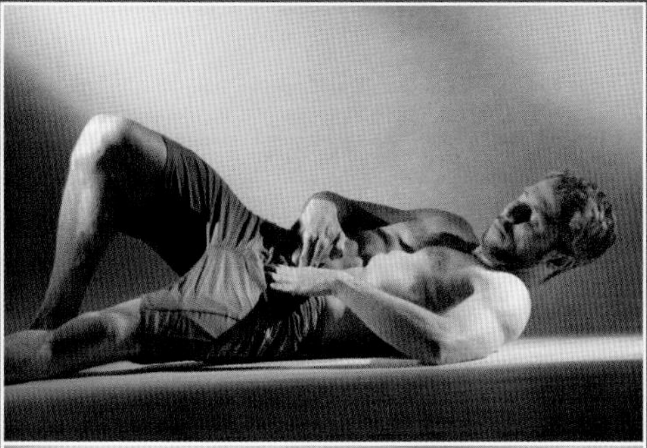

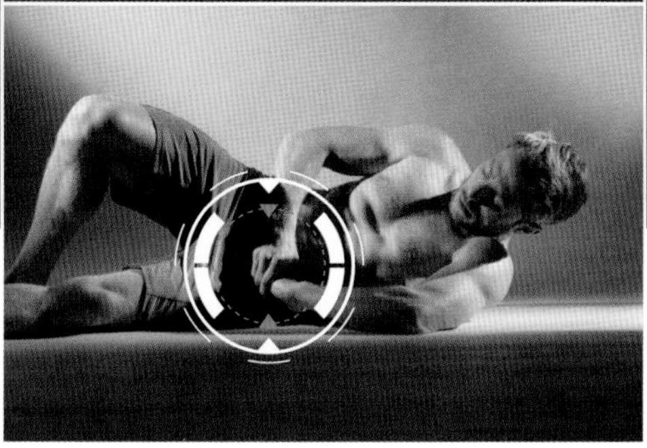

03. STRETCHING THE ILIOPSOAS

Get into a long forward lunge position and lower your body down until you feel a stretch in the hip flexors of your rear leg. Reach forward with the arm opposite your front leg, reach back with the arm opposite your rear leg, turn your torso away from the rear leg, and hold this position for 20 seconds. Perform 3 times per side without resting (since you are changing sides, the exercise time is equal to the recovery time; when one side is working, the other is resting).

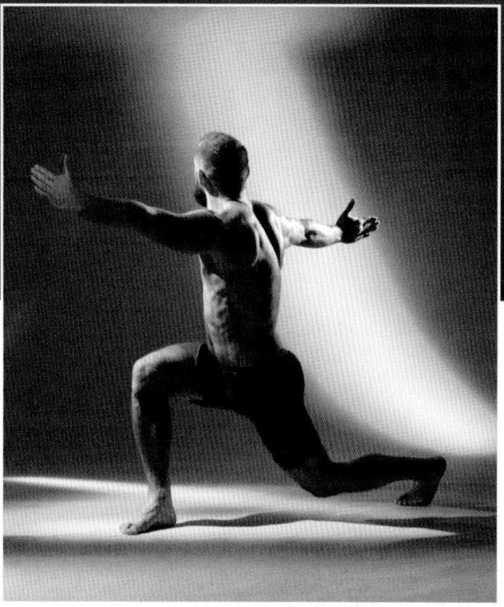

04. STRETCH TO REALIGN THE HEAD OF THE FEMUR

Place your hips through the loop of a resistance band that is stretched horizontally. Move into a forward lunge position to feel the stretch in the hip flexors of your rear leg.

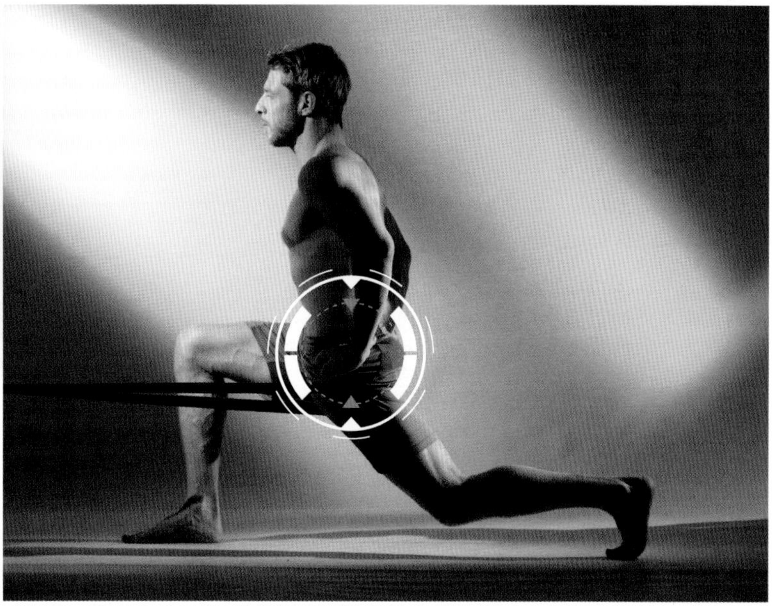

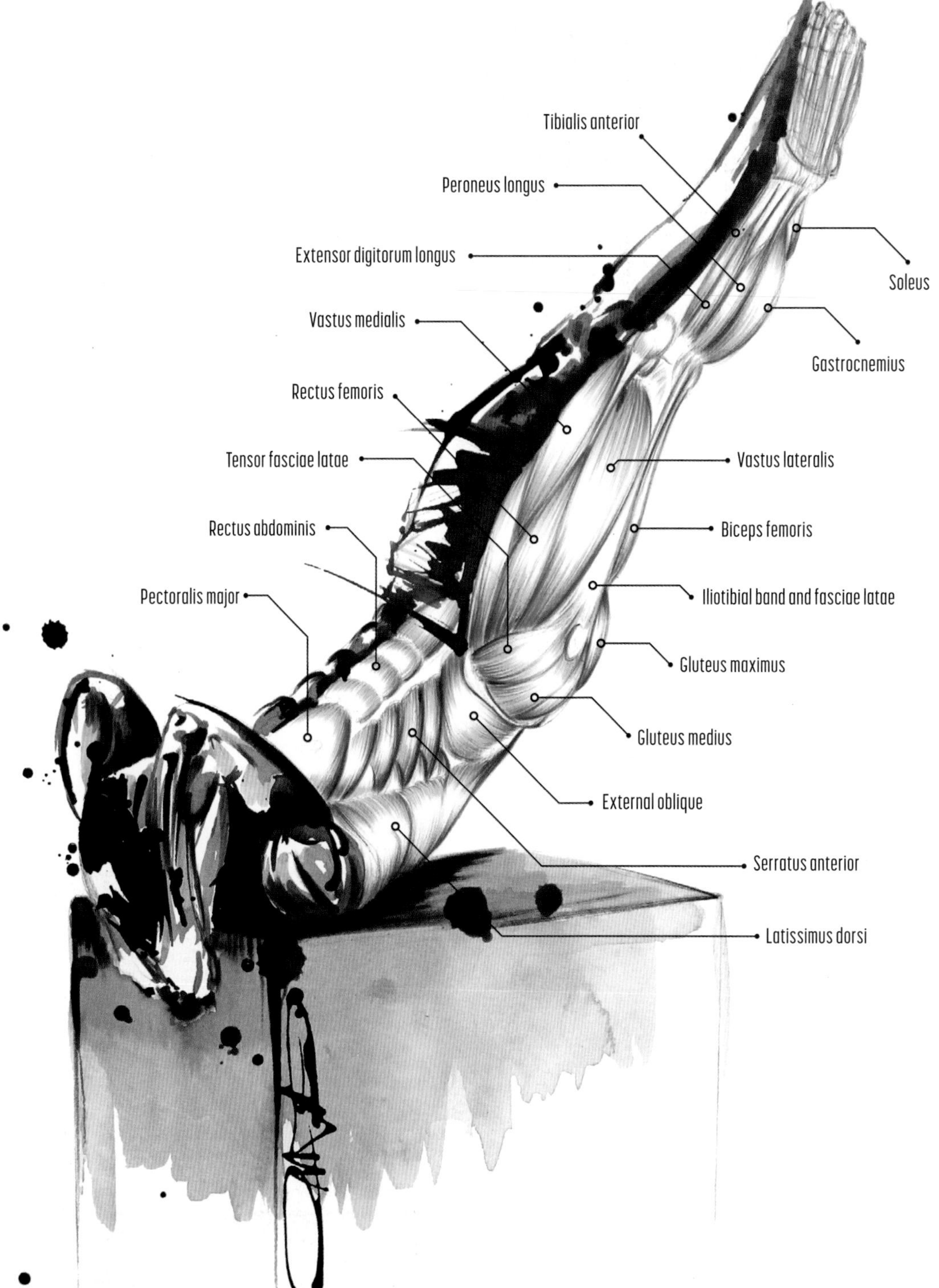

Tibialis anterior
Peroneus longus
Extensor digitorum longus
Soleus
Vastus medialis
Gastrocnemius
Rectus femoris
Tensor fasciae latae
Vastus lateralis
Rectus abdominis
Biceps femoris
Pectoralis major
Iliotibial band and fasciae latae
Gluteus maximus
Gluteus medius
External oblique
Serratus anterior
Latissimus dorsi

01. TUCK

Tucks are one of the best ways to train the anterior chain; they can be done on an exercise ball or with suspension trainer straps. Place your feet on the middle of the ball or into the stirrups of the straps. Align your posture by tilting your pelvis backward slightly to prevent your lower back from dipping. Pull your abdomen in to engage your abdominal muscles and push your chest out as you lower your shoulders to prevent your spine from curving forward. Finally, maximize the force generated by your shoulders and their stability by screwing your hands into the floor; do this by slightly opening your arms outward and, most importantly, rotating your elbows inward. Once you have the correct basic posture, bring your knees to your chest then return to the starting position, keeping your movements controlled.

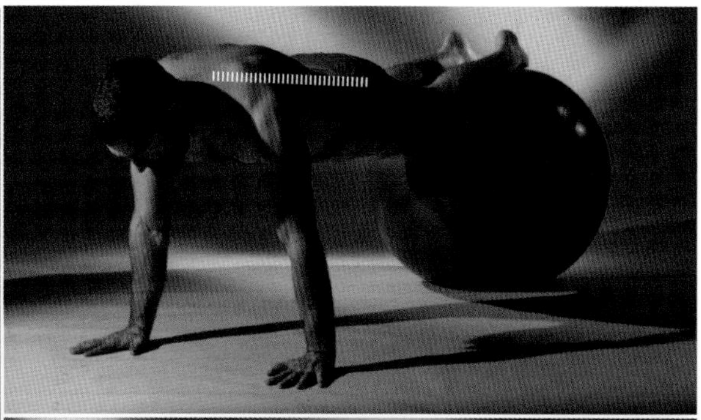

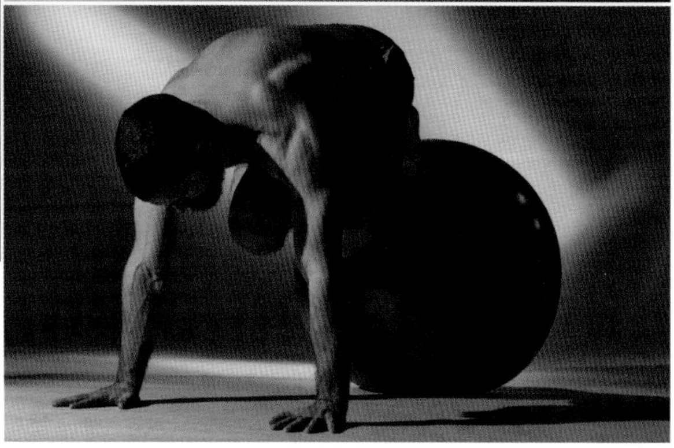

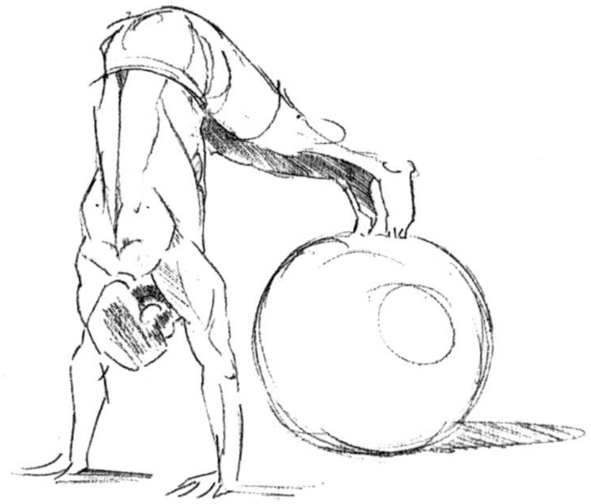

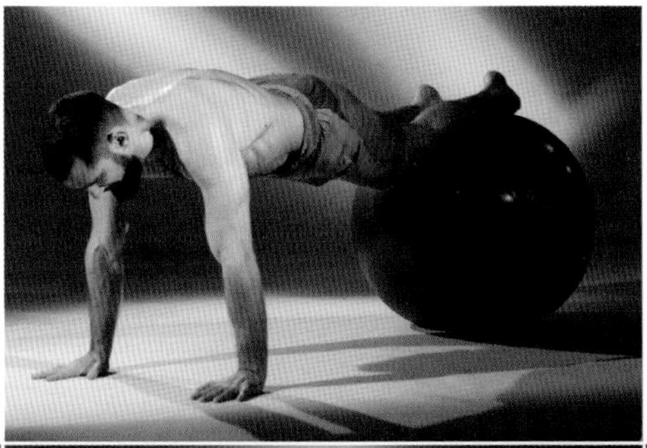

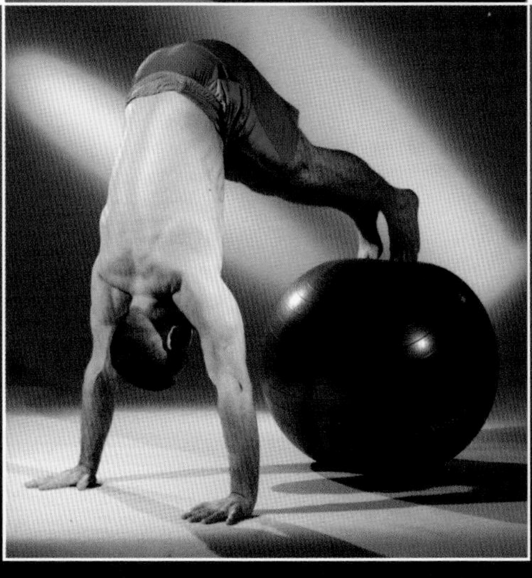

02. EXERCISE BALL OR SUSPENSION TRAINER PIKE

With your feet on the center of the ball or in the straps, align your posture by tilting your pelvis backward slightly to prevent your lower back from dipping. Pull your abdomen in to engage your abdominal muscles and push your chest out as you lower your shoulders to prevent your spine from curving forward. Maximize the force and stability of your shoulders by screwing your hands into the floor. Without jeopardizing this basic position, activate your abdominal muscles and your gluteal muscles then close your hips to lift your buttocks. Keep your arms straight and try to make your back as straight as possible. If your mobility allows it, try to align your straight arms with your chest vertically, like a handstand. Control your return to the starting position and do not round your back at the end of the movement.

03. SUPERMAN ON THE SUSPENSION TRAINER

Leaning forward, keep your back straight, chest out, and shoulders down. Support yourself using the suspension trainer and screw your hands inward by internally rotating your arms. Activate your abdominal muscles and pull your abdomen in. Allow the handles to slide forward as your body gradually extends. With your arms above your head, move your body into a full extension by extending your knees and hips before gradually returning to the starting position. You can make this exercise harder by pausing when your body is extended.

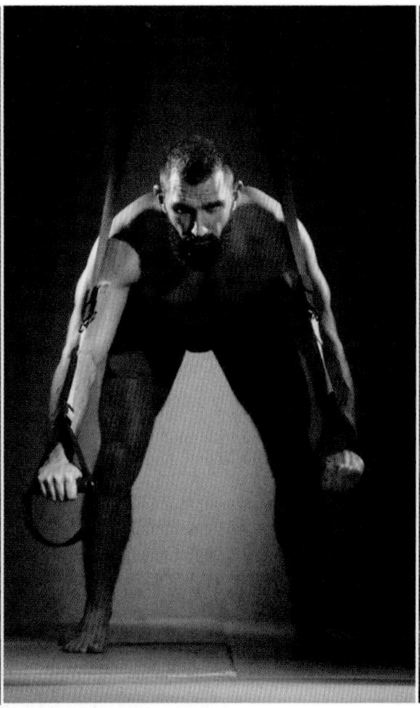

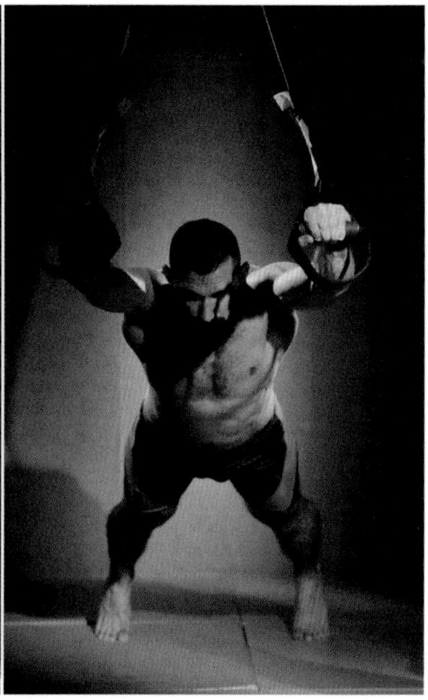

04. KNEELING ROLL OUT

On your knees, straighten your arms and grab the bar with a wide grip in front of you (alternatively, you can support yourself using suspension straps). Push out your chest and pull your abdomen in by tightly squeezing your gluteal muscles. Roll the bar forward. The challenge in returning to the starting position is losing control of the lower back. If you curve the lower back too much because your pelvis is tilting forward, your anterior chain is broken. Do not push too far or exceed this working angle. The aim is to align your arms, torso, and legs as much as possible while keeping your head between both outstretched arms. If you are in really good shape, you could even start from your feet instead of your knees.

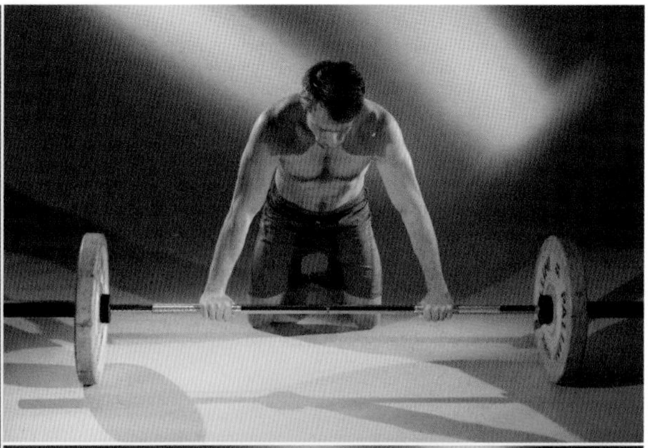

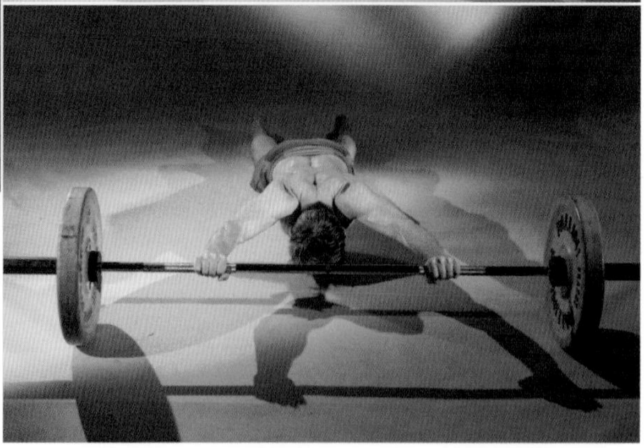

05. LEG RAISES ON A STATIONARY BAR

Your grip in this exercise is very important; use a *pronated* (palms facing forward) grip that is slightly wider than your shoulders. Start in a suspended position with your arms straight. Your shoulders begin the pendulum movement, allowing you to alternate between flexing your torso (when lifting your feet to the bar) and arching your back (when lowering down to a hanging position).

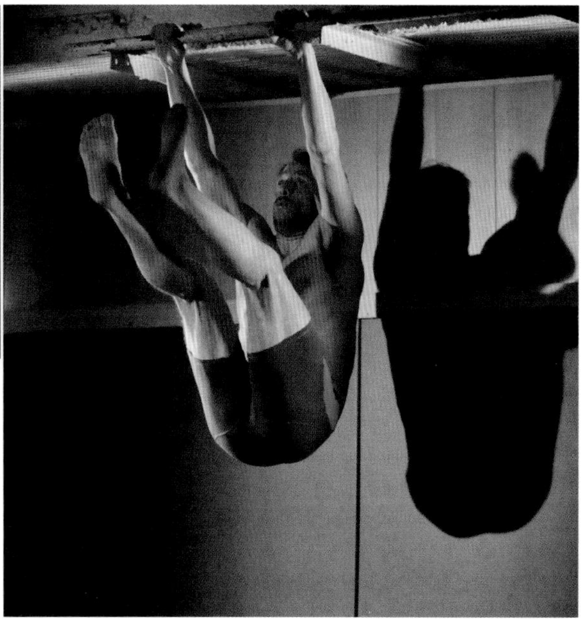

06. DRAGON FLAG

This exercise was made popular by Bruce Lee and is one of the most intense moves for the anterior chain. Hold on to an anchor point behind your head (e.g., a gym ladder or bench). Raise your body vertically while keeping it straight (a position also referred to as the *candle pose* or *shoulder stand* although those movements typically do not involve holding on to an anchor point), then return to the starting position. Try to avoid the common pitfalls of hyperextending or arching your back. Common modifications include getting into the candle pose with only one leg extended or raising the hips with your knees tucked in next to your torso.

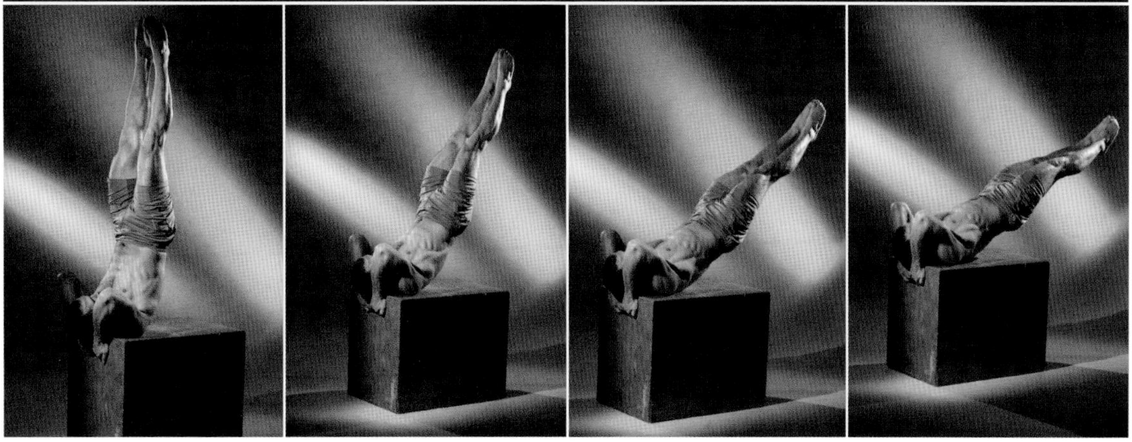

The Lateral (Side) Chain

Side of the foot: peroneus longus

Tibia section: peroneus longus, anterior cruciate ligament

Thigh: IT band, gluteus maximus, tensor fascia latae

Abdomen: quadratus lumborum, obliques, intercostal muscles

Head: sternocleidomastoid, splenius capitis, splenius cervicis, iliocostalis cervicis

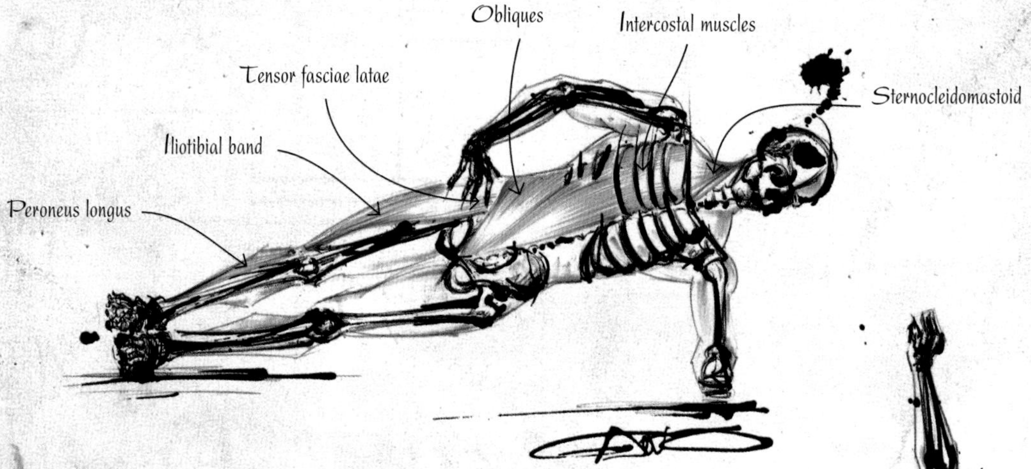

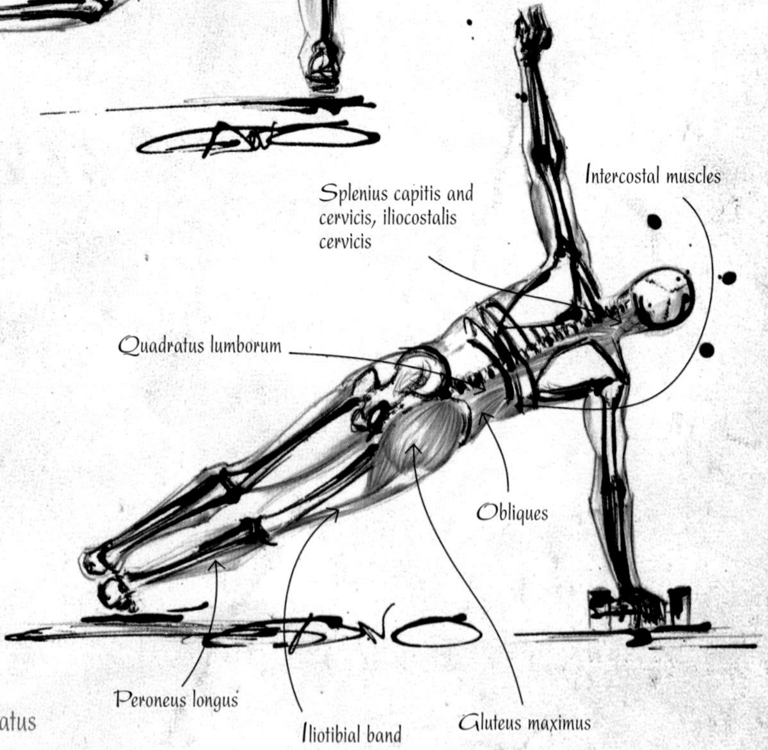

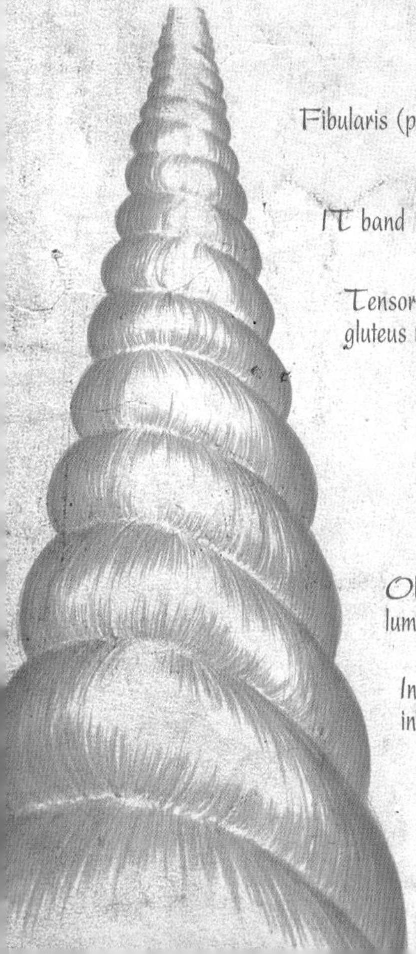

> *The lateral (side) chain controls balance in the lateral plane and contributes to stability in the frontal plane. Like the anterior chain, it ends very close to the inner ear and contributes to the body's balance.*

However, this muscle chain, laterally and deeply, also connects to the superficial anterior and posterior chains. If you neglect lateral flexion and extension exercises and focus only on the anterior and posterior chains or if your sport does not specifically involve lateral movement, you risk diminishing the quality of the collaboration between the anterior and posterior chains, possibly leading to muscle compensation in the lateral chain.

This chain's distinctive quality of being somewhere between an endurance chain and a strength chain gives it a mixed profile, capable of producing great strength and having excellent stamina at the same time.

Possible Malfunctions in the Lateral (Side) Chain

- Physical activities cause the body to become laterally unbalanced quickly and for a long time. Adaptations can take the form of stiffness, lack of strength, and loss of motor control before transforming into pain or injury. When you become aware of these imbalances or the activities causing them, you should begin to stretch and strengthen the injured side while also maintaining its mobility. When training for mobility as a way to protect and train the body, it is a good idea to work on both sides equally.
- The second type of dysfunction involves the muscles in this chain that are compensating because of a failure in either the superficial anterior or posterior chain. In this case, the anterior or posterior chain must be treated first to ensure it is functioning optimally before working on the lateral chain.

KILLER MOVES
TO DEVELOP THE LATERAL (SIDE) CHAIN

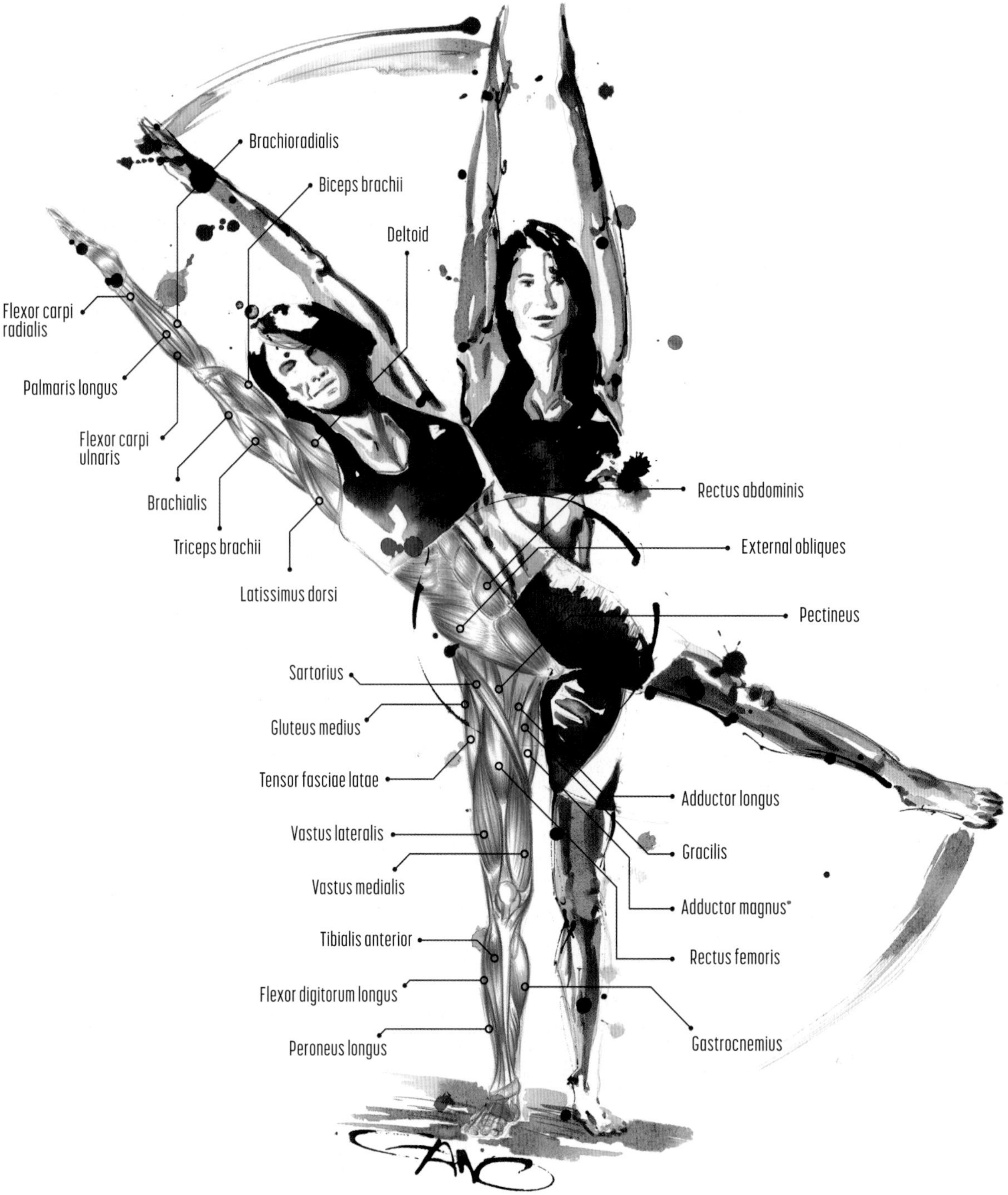

01. STANDING OBLIQUE CRUNCH USING A SUSPENSION TRAINER

With the straps in a shortened position, hold your arms above your head. Stand perpendicular to the anchor point of the straps. Pull your abdomen in and squeeze your gluteal muscles before allowing yourself to drop to the side in a lateral bend of the hips and torso. This stretch can help not only with a shortened or overactive chain as you bend your body, but it can also strengthen a weak chain as you straighten back up. Pay attention to how you are feeling to discover what your body needs most. If it hurts to stay in a low stretched position, this is a sign of stiffness. If you find it difficult to come back up to the starting position, this is a sign of weakness. When in doubt, perform both exercises.

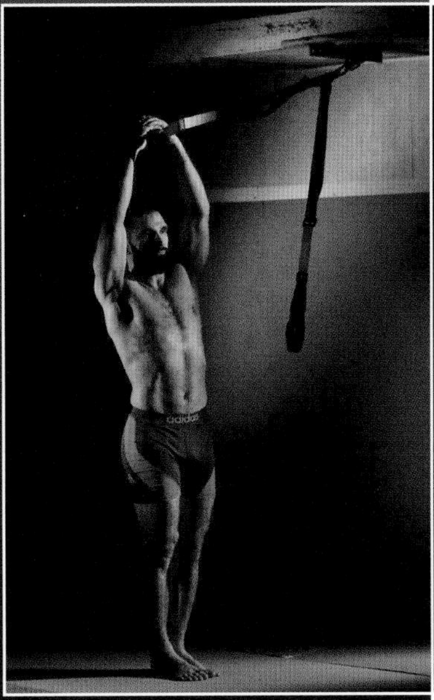

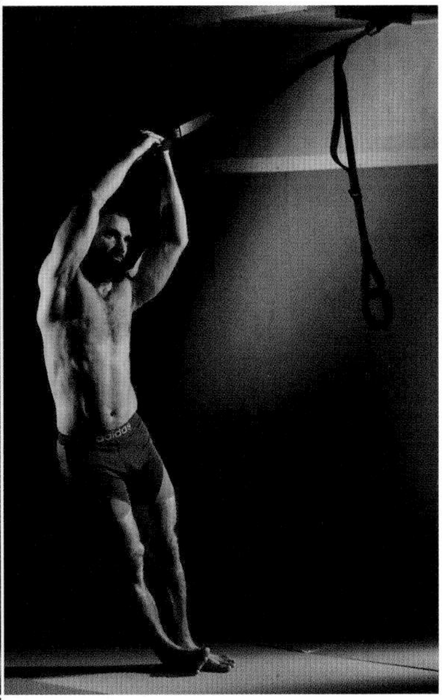

02. LATERAL HIP RAISE USING A SUSPENSION TRAINER

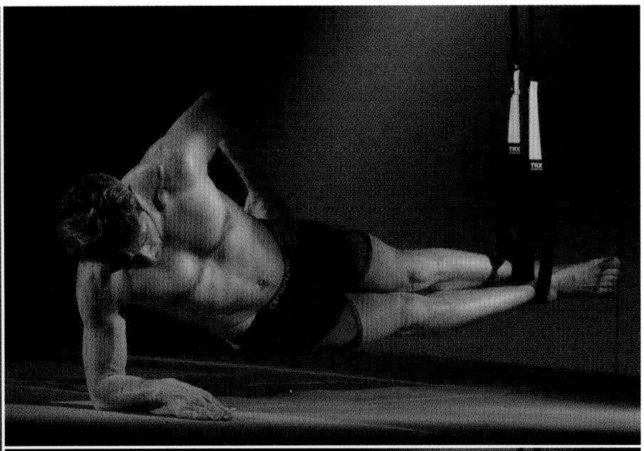

Support yourself on one elbow on the floor and place your feet into a suspension trainer stirrup that is at head level. Pull your abdomen in, squeeze your gluteal muscles, and try to keep your pelvis neutral (do not tilt it backward or forward). Keeping your head aligned, raise and lower your hips as high and as low as possible without moving your hips forward or backward. Do not allow your shoulders to move out of line. Any muscle compensation must be avoided; keep the head of the humerus as centered as possible. This stretch can help not only with a shortened or overactive chain as you lower your body down, but it can also strengthen a weak chain as you come back up. Pay attention to how you are feeling to discover what your body needs most. If it hurts to stay in a low stretched position, this is a sign of stiffness. If you find it difficult to come back up to the starting position, this is a sign of weakness. When in doubt, perform both exercises.

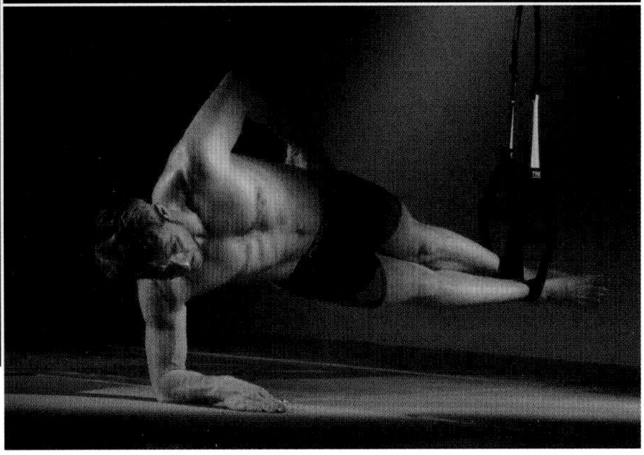

03. SIDE CRUNCH ON AN EXERCISE BALL WITH FEET ON THE WALL

With one side of your hips on top of the exercise ball, put your legs into a lunge position and block your feet in the corner of a room. Place your hands behind your head and then lower your upper body so the side of your torso contacts the ball. Reverse the direction of movement to raise your upper body up to side-crunch your torso as far as you can go. To maintain proper alignment during the exercise, keep your abdomen pulled in with your shoulders back and chest out as much as possible.

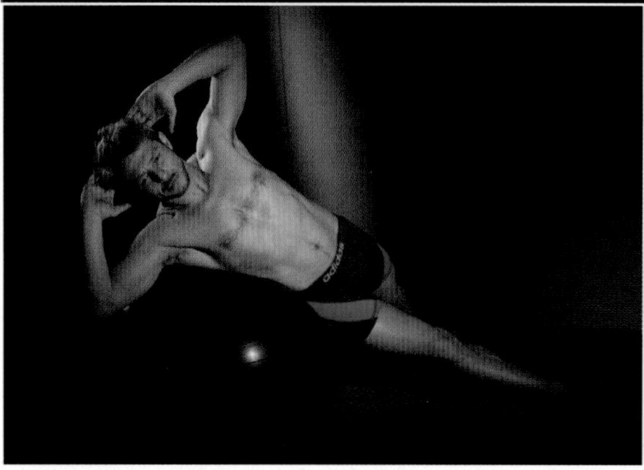

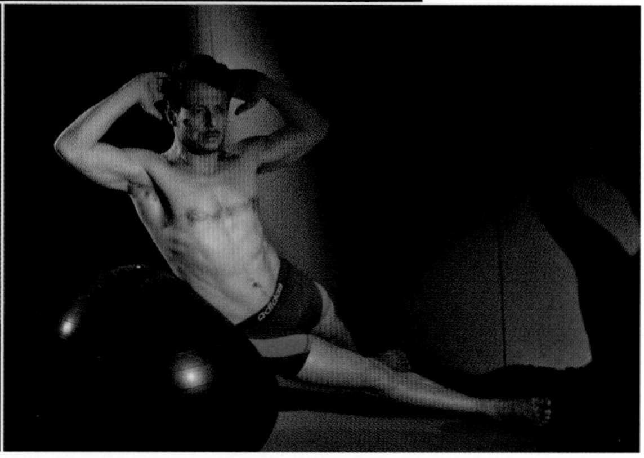

04. STANDING STAR

This exercise is a functional and dynamic core stability exercise that activates the lateral chain just like a balance exercise. Stand with your feet together and straighten your arms above your head with palms facing each other. Squeeze your gluteal muscles, make your abdomen flat, and tilt your body weight gently toward the supporting foot as your raise your other leg to the side. Throughout this exercise, try to lengthen your body through your head and fingers without losing your balance or leaning forward or backward. (If you need help with balance, raise your top arm up to be perpendicular to your torso.)

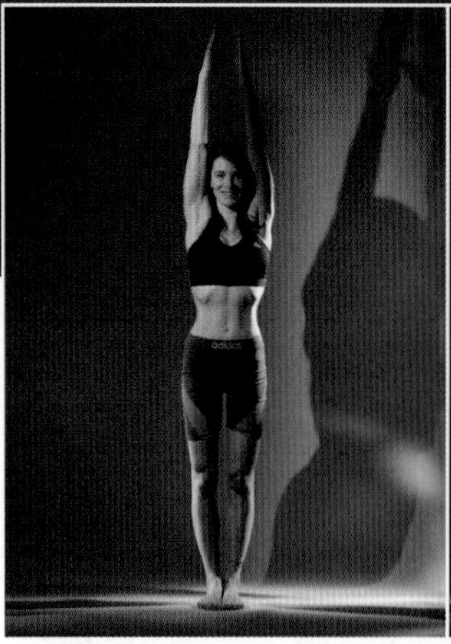

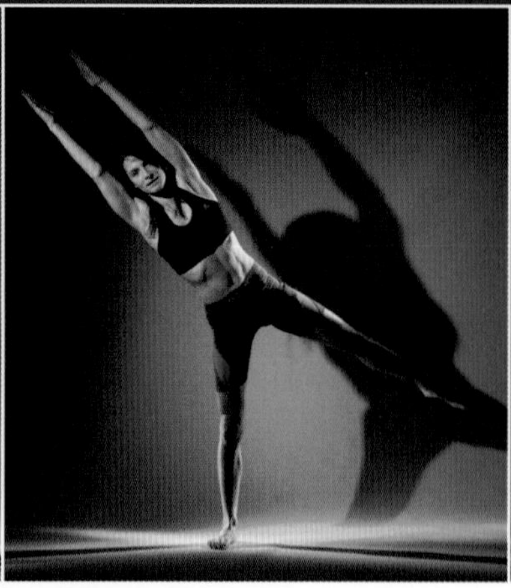

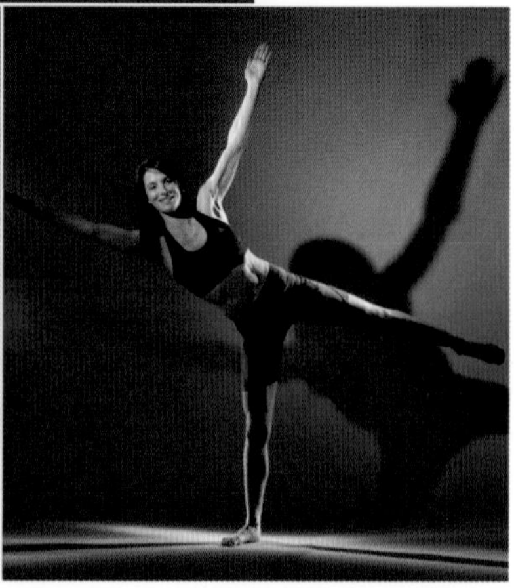

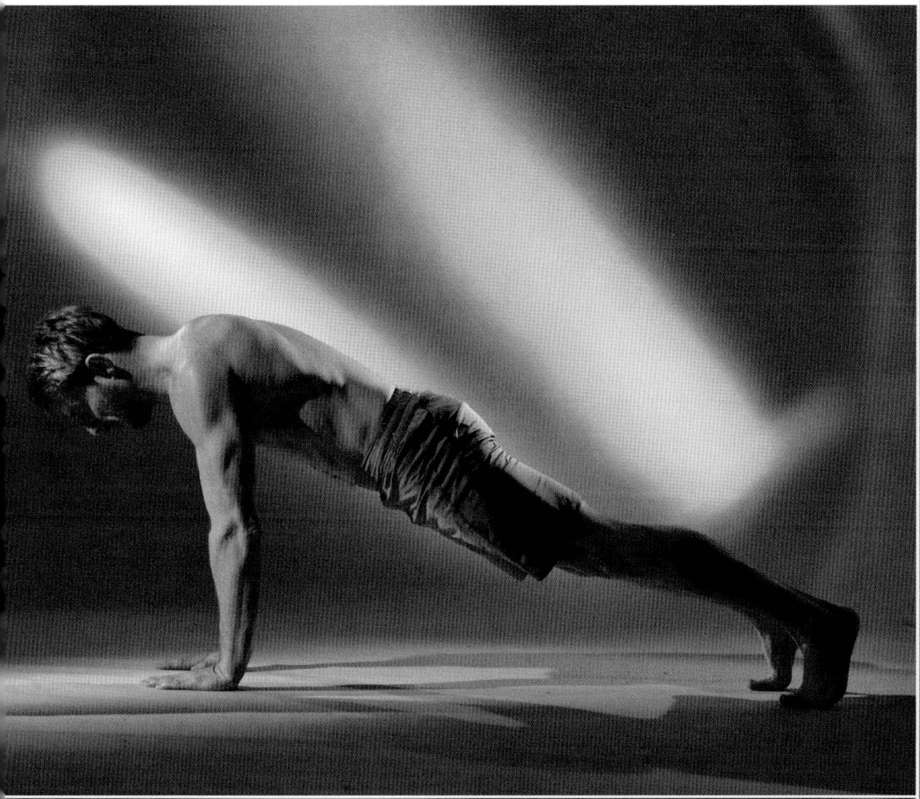

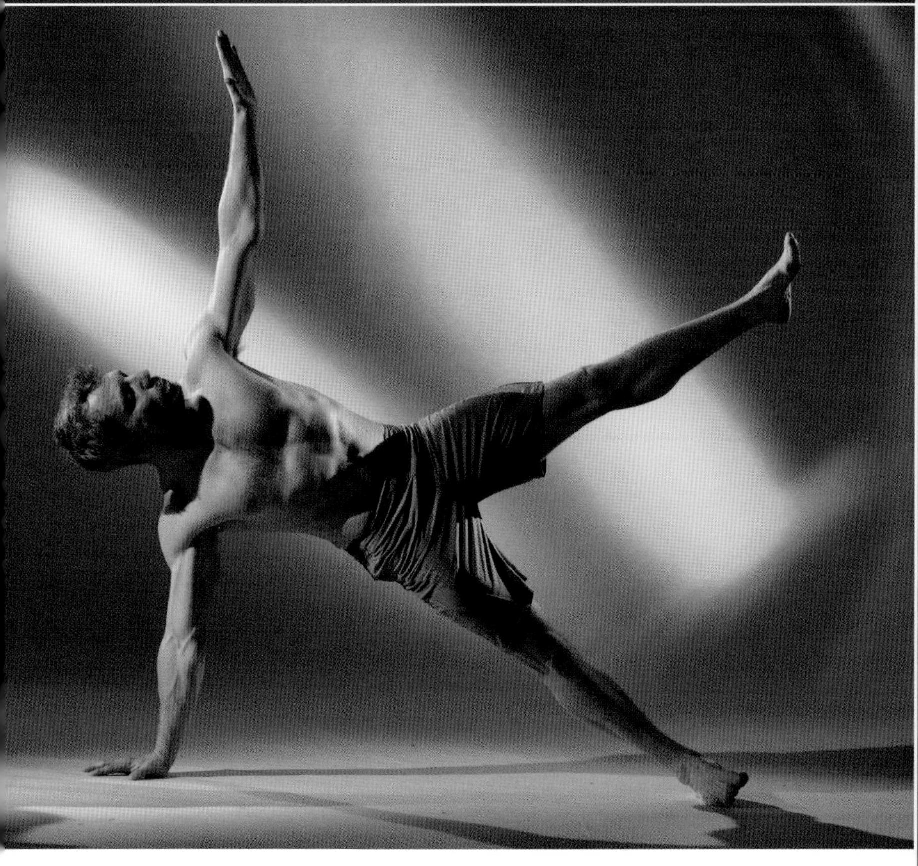

05. STAR ON THE FLOOR

This floor version makes the star exercise more difficult, intensifying both balance and core strength work. Start in a plank position, then open one hip and rotate your body (pivoting your bottom foot from the toes to the outside edge) to support yourself on one hand while raising your top arm to be perpendicular to your torso and your top leg as high as possible above your bottom leg.

The Spiral Chain

Pelvis: both spirals originate at the anterior superior iliac spine

Leg: tensor fasciae latae, IT band, tibialis anterior (going one way), peroneus longus, biceps femoris (head of the fibula to the ischium, going the other way)

Foot: first metatarsal, big toe

Abdomen: internal oblique, linea alba (abdomen), external oblique (opposite side)

Shoulder girdle: serratus anterior, rhomboids

Neck and head: splenius capitis, splenius cervicis, erector spinae, sacrum, sacrotuberous ligament, lumbosacral fascia

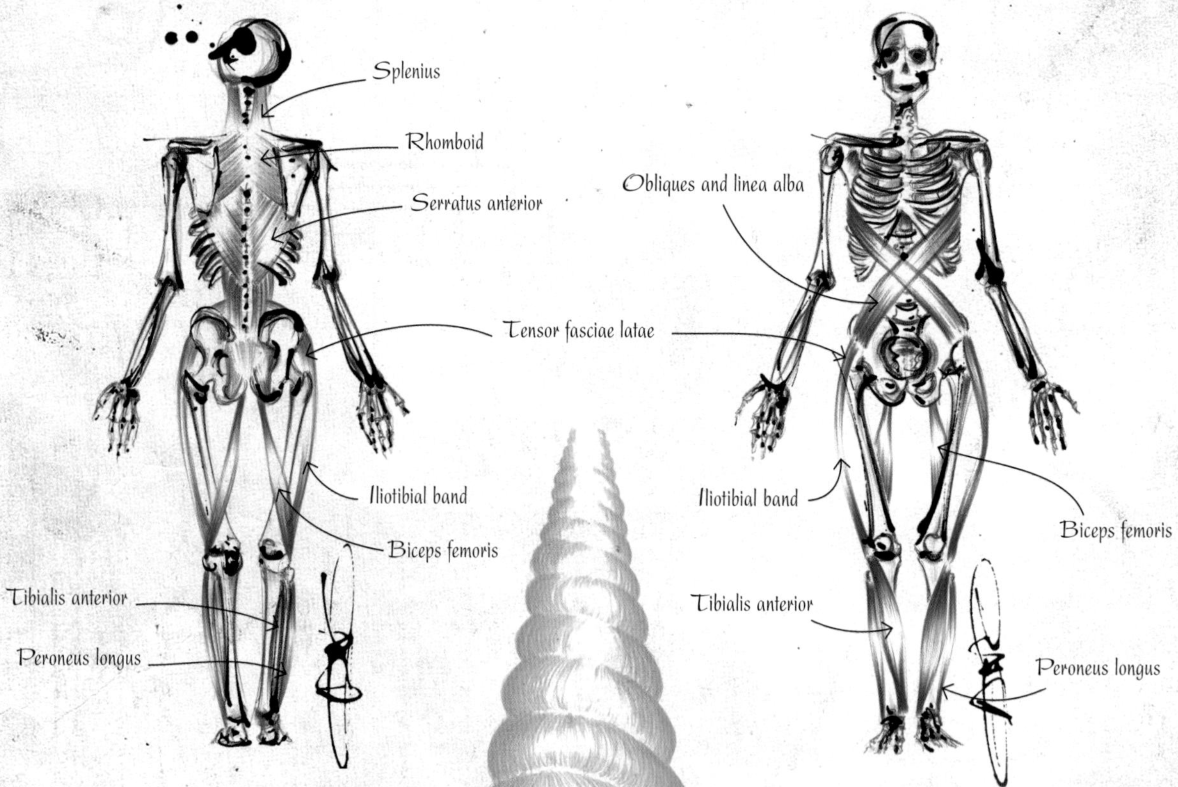

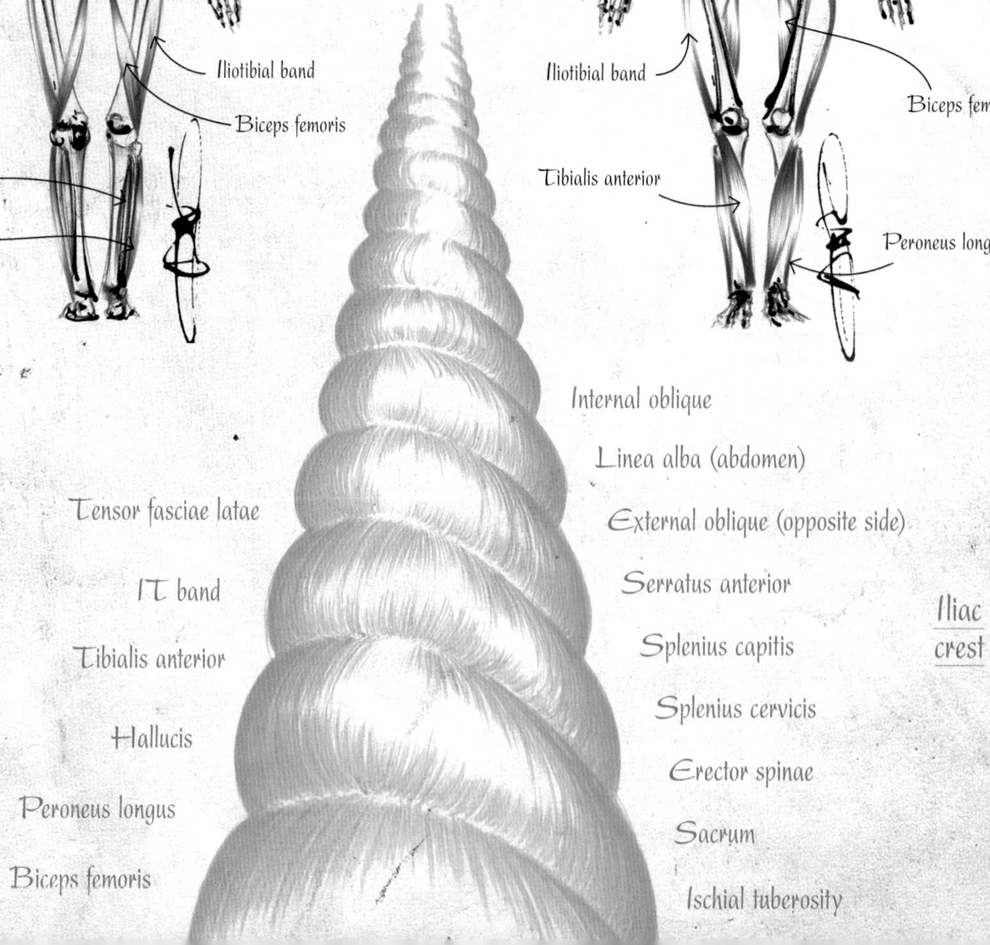

Essential for the functional plane, the spiral chain is also called the rotation chain *or the* double chain.

The spiral chain effectively forms a double "straight jacket" and is divided into two opposing chains: one going from the iliac ridge downward and the other from the iliac ridge upward. Moving along the body, it connects with the anterior chain and the posterior chain. Its effectiveness is directly linked to physical activity or sport. The muscles it contains contribute to postural balance as well as correct motor function.

Possible Malfunctions in the Spiral Chain

Most problems are caused by training in only one plane such as focusing on doing single-joint exercises with no exercises for rotation:

- Not doing any type of rotational movement as you train will weaken the spiral chain. If your sport requires rotation, you will not make any progress unless you specifically focus on the spiral chain.
- Using an incomplete program will have the same effect. Even if you do not use these rotation movements in your daily or sporting activities, some muscles belonging to this chain, which are useful in other planes (in both movement and posture), can become ineffective if they are underused.

CONNECTING THE DOTS

The first myofascial spiral found in the lower limbs forms a structure that connects the movement of the pelvis to the arch of the foot. This means that a collapsing arch in the foot may be due to the pelvis tilting forward. Conversely, massaging the arch of the foot with a ball can return mobility to the pelvis.

DISCOVER THE LIMITATIONS OF THE SPIRAL CHAIN

This chain is particularly complex and is exposed to numerous and various limitations. **It is unrealistic to try to treat everything immediately; you must begin with the simplest and worst problems, often linked to the cervical spine.**

1. Determine if there are any limitations in the rotation of the cervical spine by doing the following test: Sit on a chair or a box with your knees together and cross your arms over your chest. Try to keep your buttocks in the starting position as you turn to each side as far as you possibly can. Observe the differences when turning to the right and to the left.

2. Isolate the limitations that are directly linked to the cervical spine by using a version of the previous test. This time, do not move your shoulders and try to turn your head as far as possible to the right and to the left. A complete, optimal program for the spiral chain often involves neck exercises.

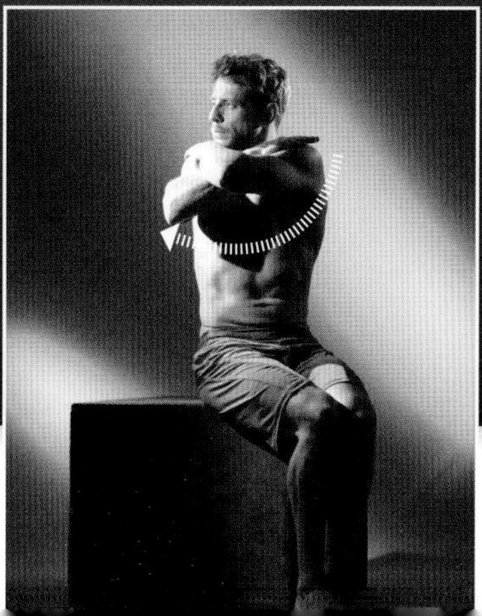

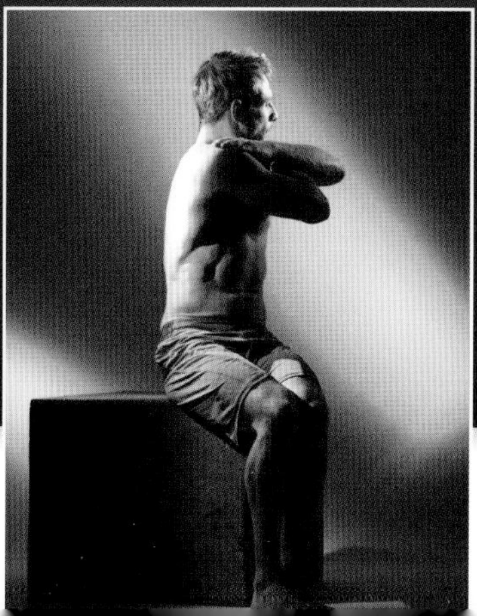

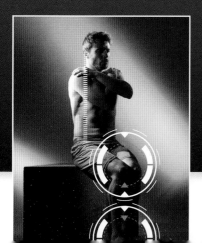

3. Expand the test by involving your lower limbs. Stand up with your feet together, arms abducted directly out to the sides at about 35 degrees, and the palms of your hands facing forward. In the same way, try to turn as far as possible to each side while keeping the same arm position.

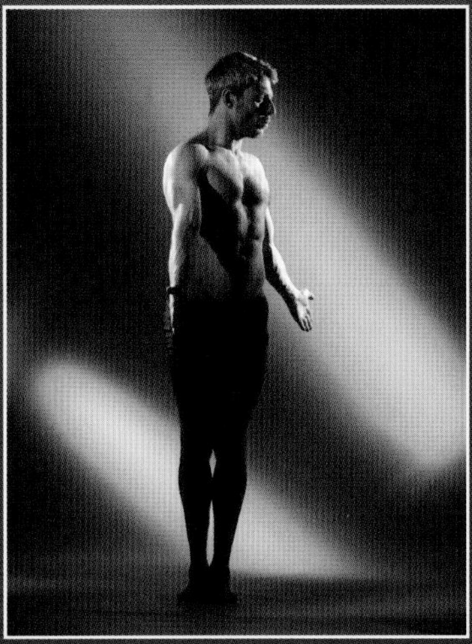

4. Take into consideration the limitations of the entire chain in a more complex movement and determine which segments are compensating, particularly when you are turning. The tripod exercise is perfect for this: Get into a long forward lunge position and lower your body down until you feel a stretch in the hip flexors of your rear leg. Place the hand of the arm opposite your front leg on the floor parallel to your front foot and in line with your rear foot, rotate your torso away from your rear leg, and reach directly up with the arm opposite your rear leg.

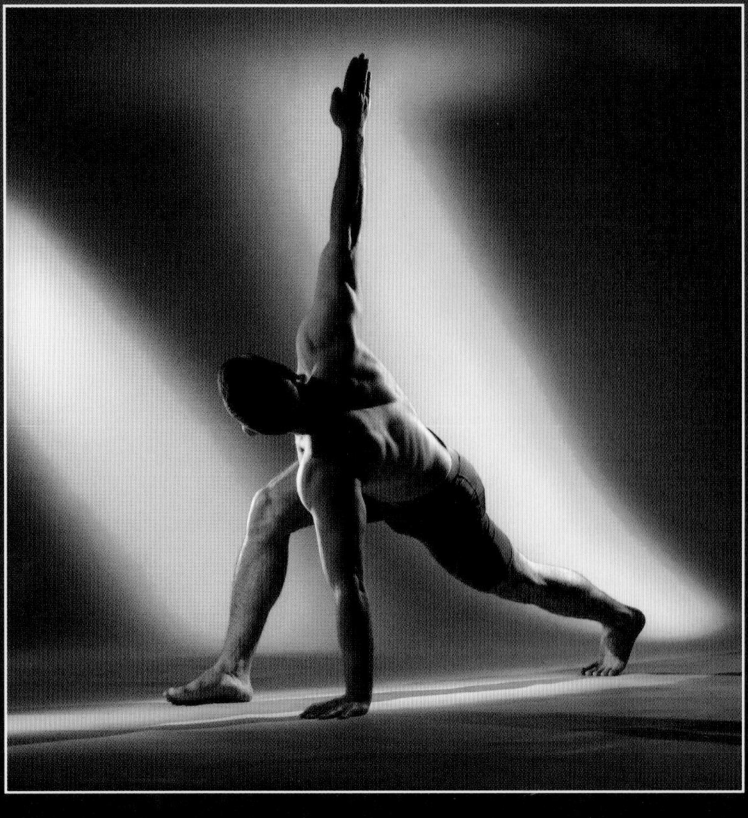

IN CONCLUSION

These four steps allow you to identify problematic areas before you begin to perform more complex movements.

Does it hurt? If it is not pathological, solve the problem using the section in this book dedicated to treating pain area by area.

Is it stiff? Or is there any restriction of movement? You need to read the section dedicated to rediscovering mobility. Listen to your body; you know it better than anyone.

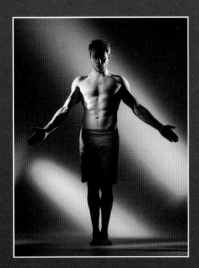

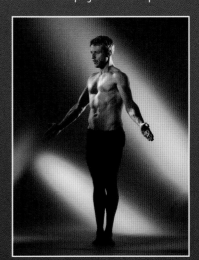

KILLER MOVES
TO DEVELOP THE SPIRAL CHAIN

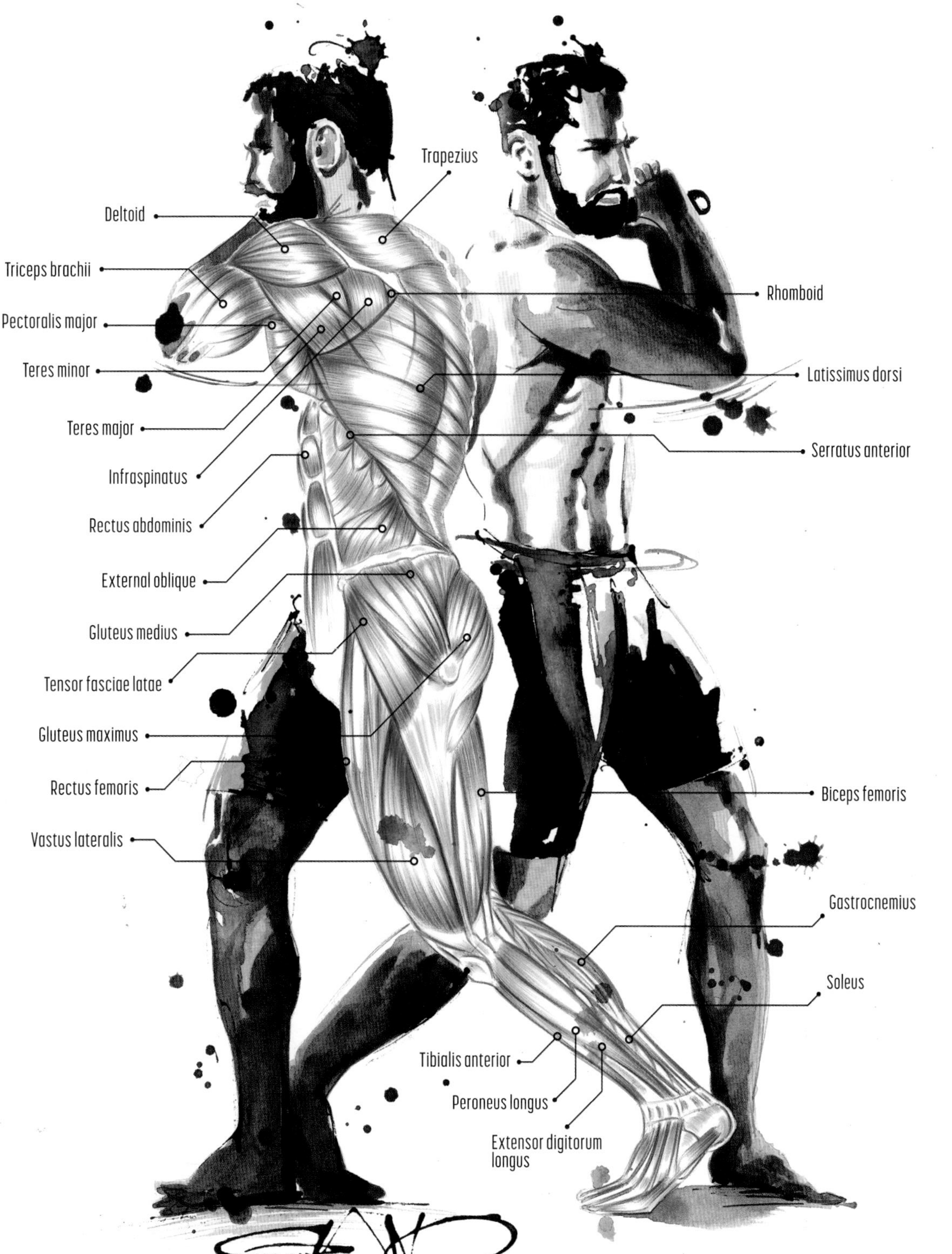

01. WINDSHIELD WIPER LEG KICK ON AN EXERCISE BALL

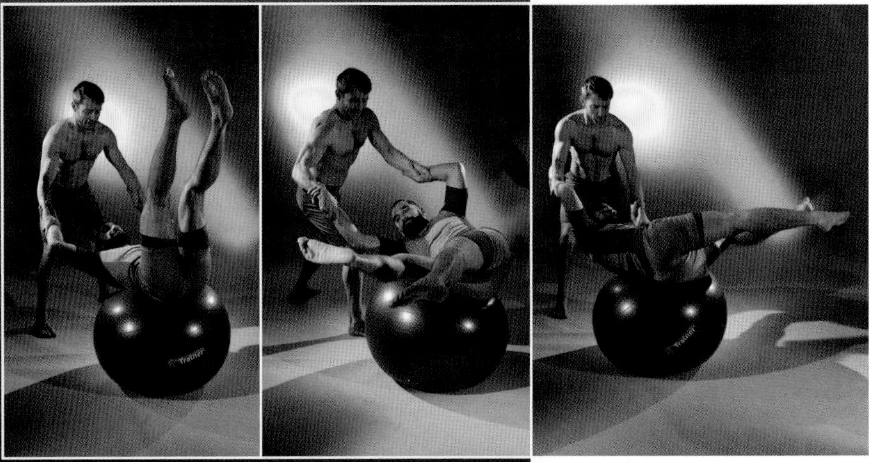

Lie face-up on the exercise ball with your back aligned to raise your awareness of the position of your spine and pelvis; in this position, do not allow your back to arch over the ball (when you move laterally, you must keep your spine supported). Hold on to a gym ladder or bench or ask a partner to support you. Lift your legs up to be perpendicular to the floor, then kick your legs as you pivot your hips from right to left (while continuing to kick your legs). Throughout the exercise, keep your abdomen as flat as possible, tilt your pelvis slightly forward, and lock down your pelvic floor.

02. SKI KETTLEBELL SWING

Stand erect with your feet and knees together and hold one kettlebell in both hands. Flex your knees slightly and move the kettlebell once to the right and once to the left of your body like a pendulum. Keep your back straight, your chest out, and your shoulders pulled back throughout the exercise. Lift the kettlebell in front by strongly pushing your lower limbs to generate the movement (see the third photo). Your upper body should only follow the movement; it does not initiate it. Depending on the version, the kettlebell will stop at your forehead or go all the way above your head. Be very careful throughout this exercise to not bend your knees inward or to the side. Your kneecaps should always follow the line of your toes, and the knees should remain parallel.

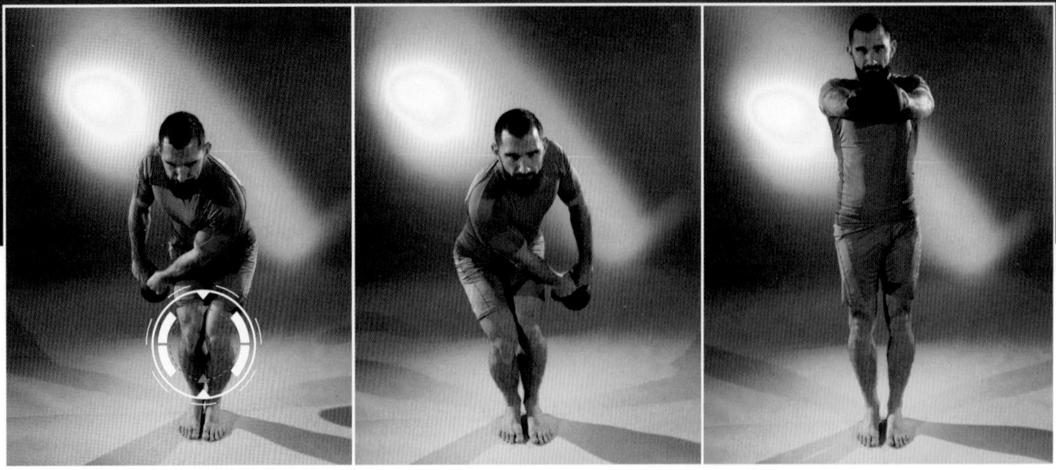

03. ROTARY KETTLEBELL SWING

Start in a neutral position with your feet positioned between hip- and shoulder-width apart. Do not lock out your knees and hips. Hold the kettlebell with both hands and bring it to one shoulder. Flex your knees and keep your feet parallel and in line with the kettlebell. Pull your shoulders back, keep your back straight, and push your chest out. Swing the kettlebell laterally toward your other shoulder, trying to keep it as horizontal as possible. Do not let the kettlebell swing out from your body. As you swing, pivot your feet, knees, and hips to follow the kettlebell. Control the trajectory of the kettlebell with your hips and slightly tighten your grip to cushion its contact with your opposite shoulder and arm.

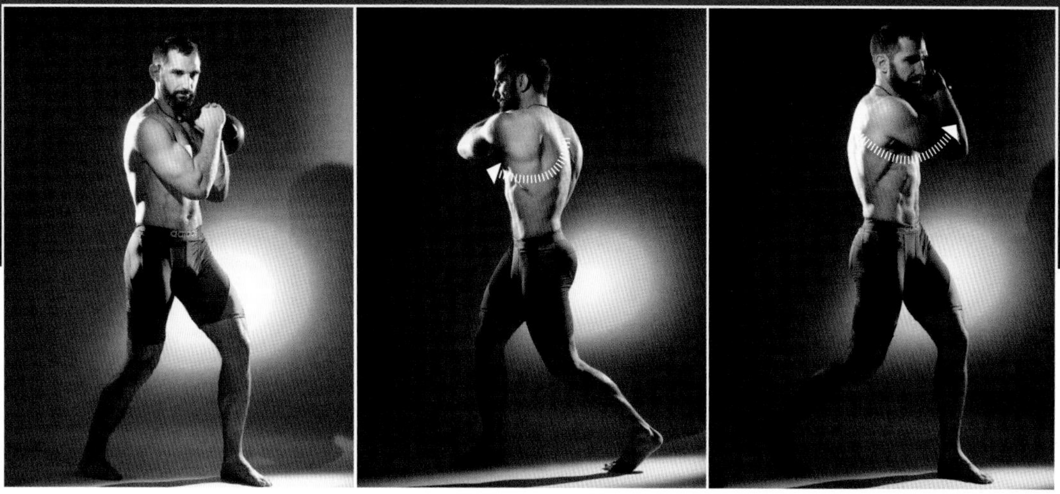

04. KNEE ROTATION USING AN EXERCISE BALL

In this mobility exercise, there is no measurable increase in weight or repetition. The only indicators you should be noticing are the fluidity of movement and the speed of execution.

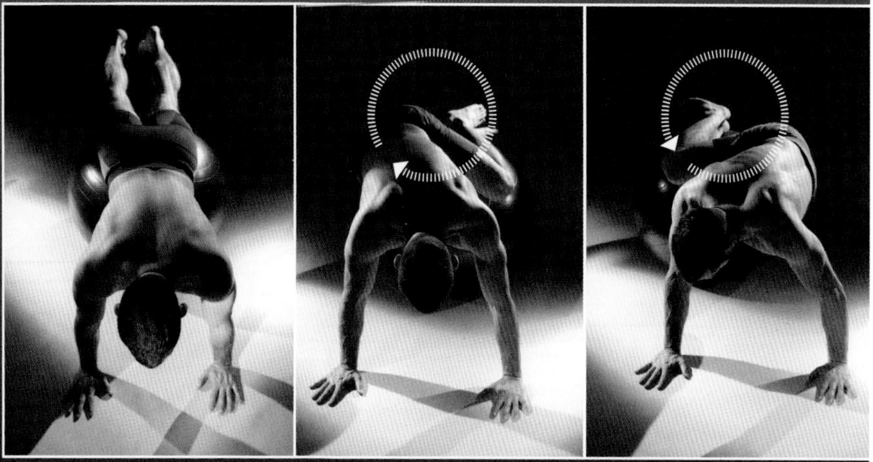

Lie face-down with your lower hips/upper thighs on the top of an exercise ball. Place your hands on the floor and fully extend your arms to get in a push-up position. Keeping your feet together throughout the exercise, pivot your hips to the side as you bring your knees toward your chest. Turn your hips in line with the ball to tuck your knees under your chest. Pivot your hips in the other direction and drive your knees toward the other side of the ball as they extend. Throughout the movement, the ball draws a circle on the floor. Repeat this exercise with as much fluidity as possible, then as fast as possible.

05. SUPER SCORPION

In this mobility exercise, there is no measurable increase in weight or repetition. The only indicators you should be noticing are the fluidity of movement and the speed of execution.

Lie face-down with your lower hips/upper thighs on the top of an exercise ball. Place your hands on the floor and fully extend your arms to get in a push-up position. Pivot your hips to the side and swing one slightly flexed leg as far across as possible. Allow the leg to hang and move farther before reversing this position. Try to slowly progress in range of motion by pausing for a moment to control and even emphasize each hip rotation.

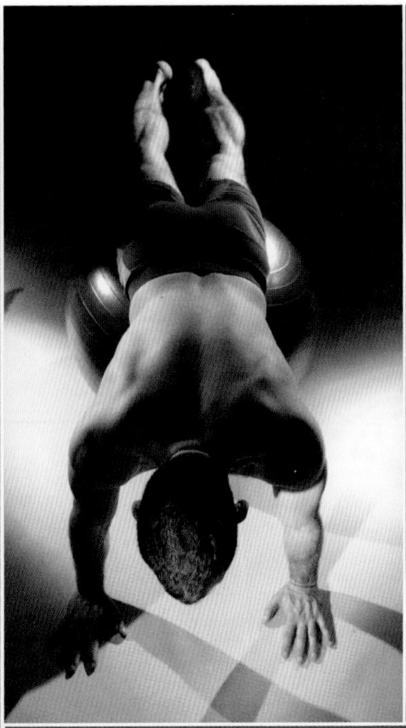

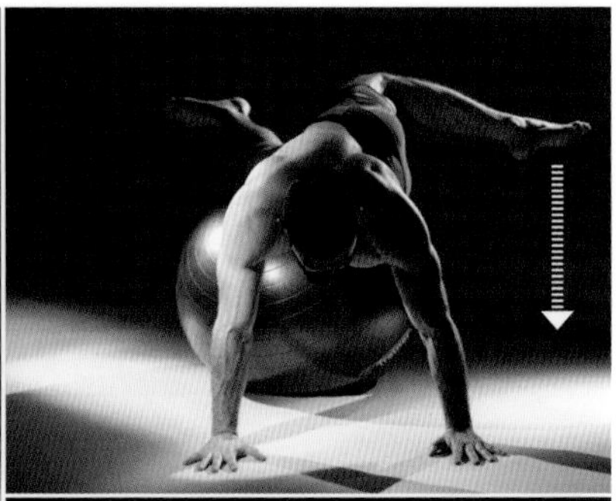

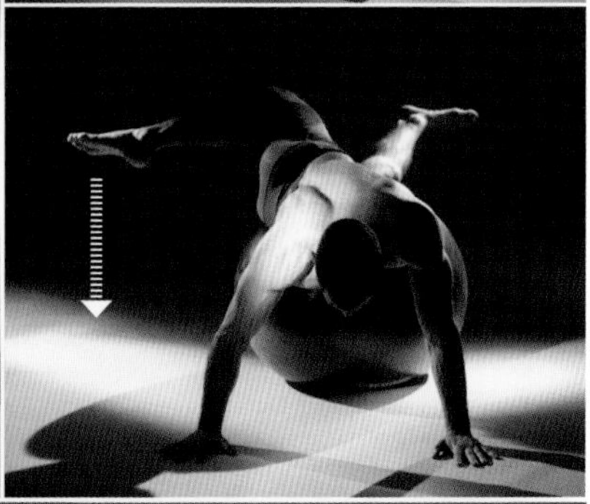

Once you have sufficient range of motion, increase the challenge of the exercise by bringing your hips back as quickly as possible. Relax and be as fluid as possible as you move.

06. STANDING WOOD CHOP USING A CABLE OR A BAND

Using a band or high pulley with a cable, place your feet in a staggered stance with one side of your body facing the anchor point of the band or the machine. Pull your abdomen in, tighten your abs and gluteal muscles as much as possible, and pull the band or cable diagonally with both hands by rotating your torso. Do not tilt forward; you should be in control of your balance throughout the whole exercise. Be sure to keep your back fully erect (do not round your shoulders), chest out, and elbows fully extended throughout the exercise.

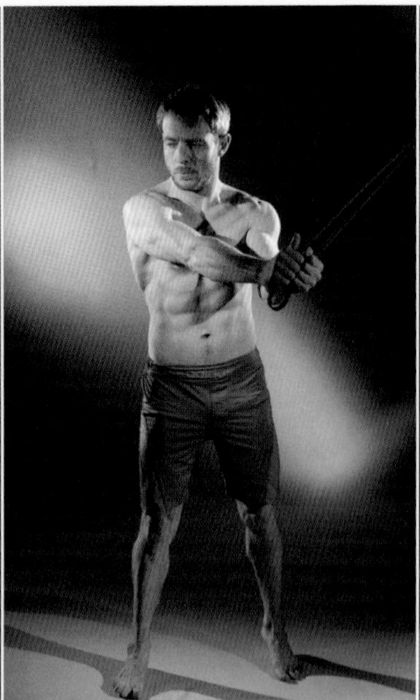

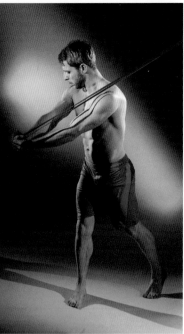

The Anterior Arm Chains

Sternum: starting point of the chain, with insertions on the pectoralis major

Ribs: pectoralis minor insertions

Shoulder blade: coracoid process toward the biceps brachii in direction of the radius

Humerus: latissimus dorsi and biceps brachii insertions; prolongation of the medial epicondyle of the ulna toward the flexor digitorum profundus

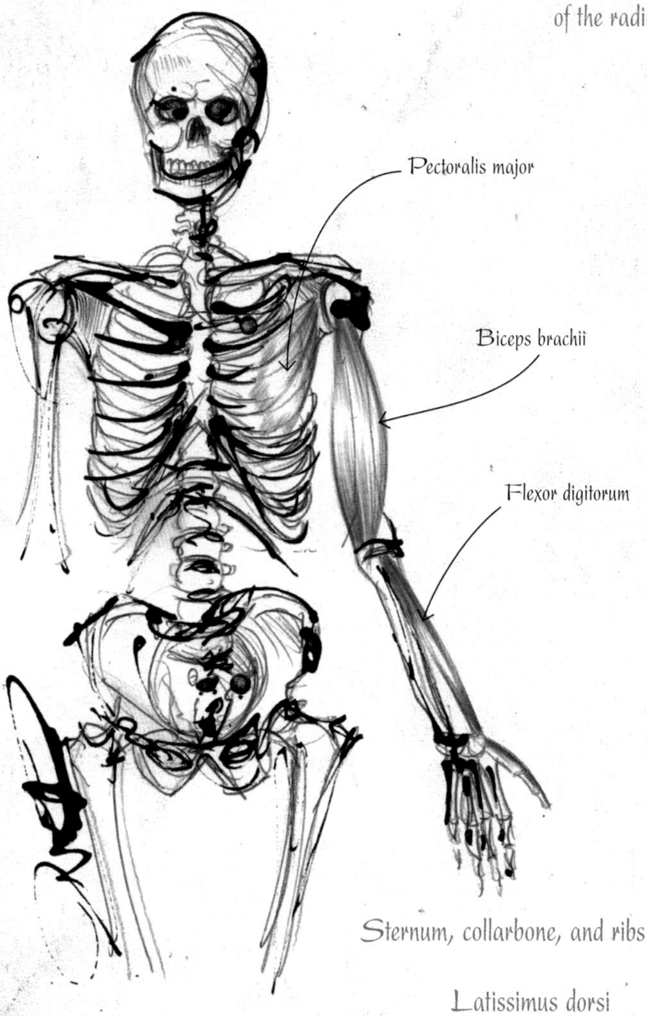

Superficial anterior arm chain

Sternum, collarbone, and ribs

Latissimus dorsi

Teres major, teres minor, and pectoralis major

Intermuscular membrane of the arms

Medial epicondyle of the humerus

Flexor digitorum profundus

Palm of the hand and fingers

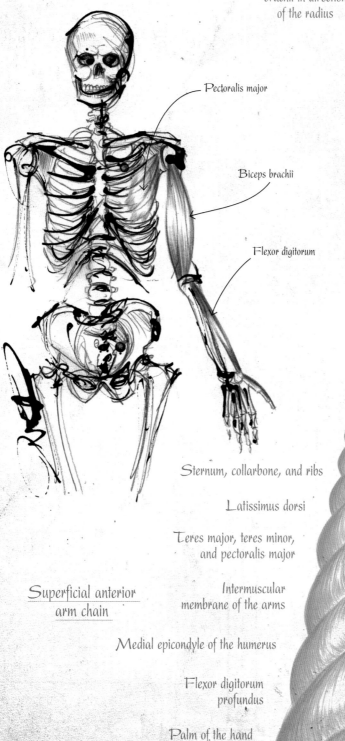

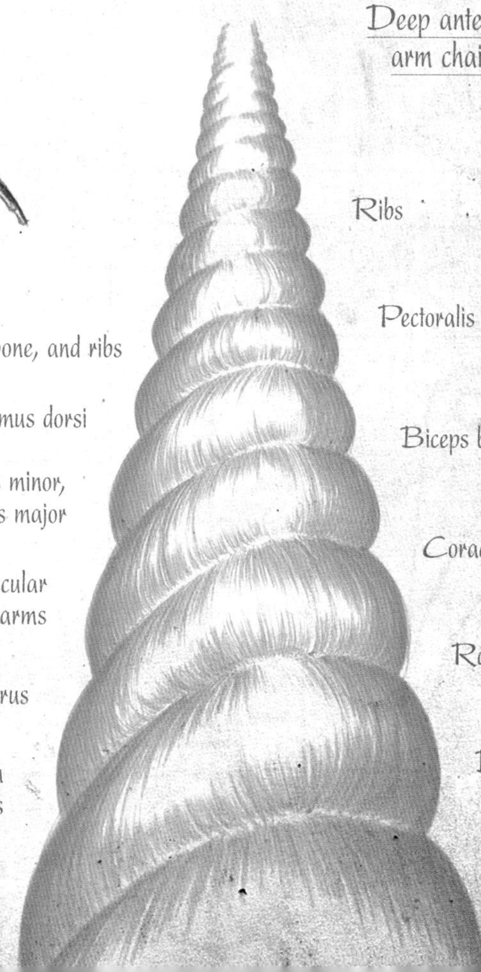

Deep anterior arm chain

Ribs

Pectoralis minor

Biceps brachii (short head)

Coracobrachialis

Radius

Base of the thumb

Continuing from the superficial and deep anterior chains, there are also two anterior arm chains: a superficial one and a deep one. Like the superficial anterior chain, the superficial and deep anterior arm chains are reactive and are involved in various postural and motor adaptations and compensations.

The superficial anterior arm chain goes from the sternum, ribs, and collarbone to the insertions of the pectoralis major and then to the nearby insertions on the humerus, to the latissimus dorsi, and to the long head of the biceps brachii. Here, there is an intermuscular partition that extends through the medial epicondyle of the ulna to the flexor digitorum profundus. The chain continues through the carpal tunnel to finish at the palmar face of the fingers.

The deep anterior arm chain has fewer links but also connects to the ribs (only to the third, fourth, and fifth ribs), as well as to the pectoralis minor. It continues toward the short head of the biceps brachii, passing through the coracoid process in the shoulder blade before rejoining the radius. The chain comes to an end at the periosteum at the anterior base of the thumb, just before the scaphoid.

Possible Malfunctions in the Anterior Arm Chains

Often overworked in weightlifting programs, the muscles in the anterior arm chains are not treated often enough with self-massage and mobilization. Any postural problems will result in major consequences for the anterior arm chains. In addition to localized tension, the imbalances caused by these postural problems can produce or sustain issues in the chest, shoulders, and neck.

KILLER MOVES
TO DEVELOP THE ANTERIOR ARM CHAINS

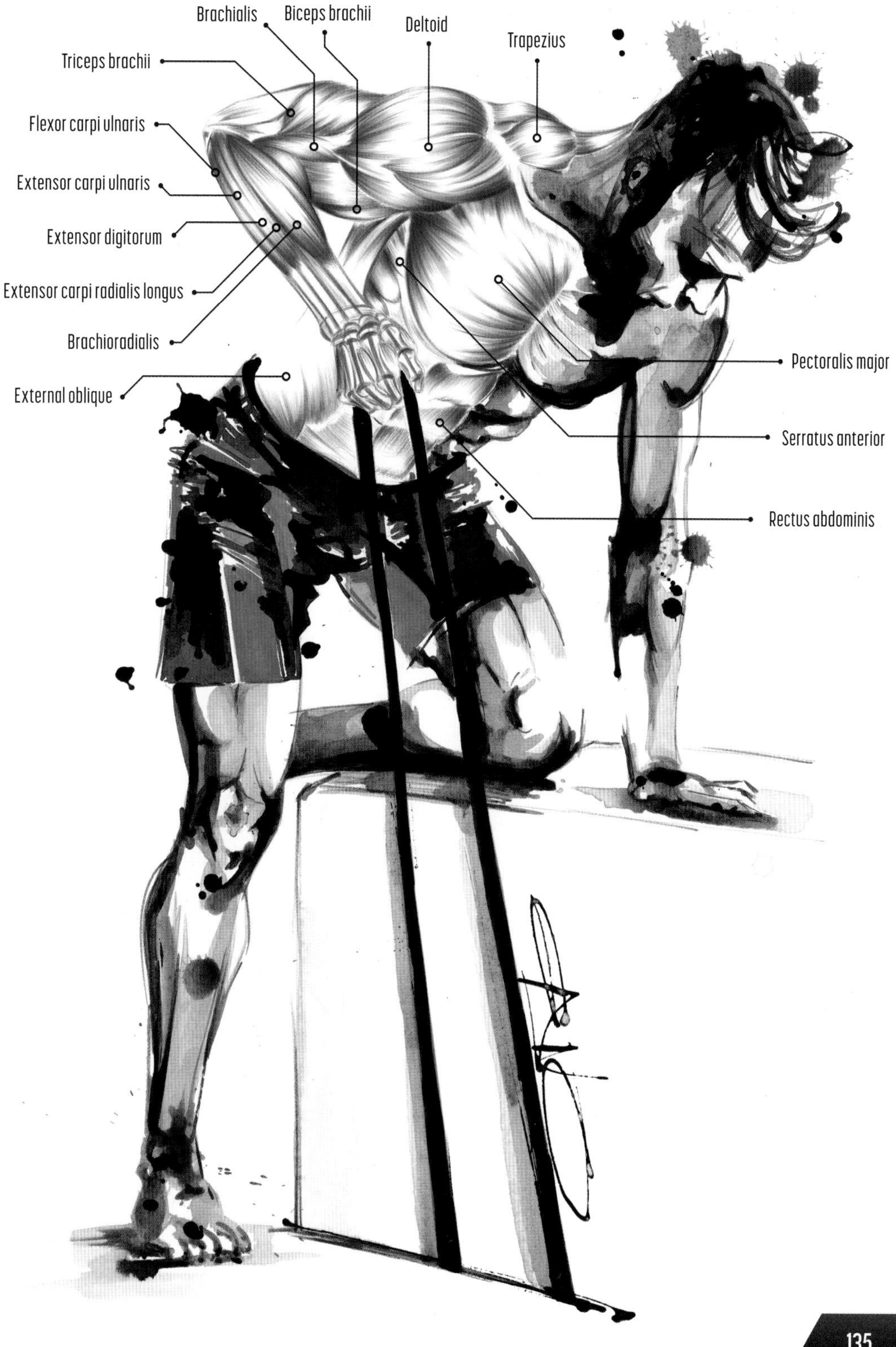

01. PULL-UP

When done correctly, this classic exercise can be a particularly formidable way to develop the anterior arm chains. There are many versions of this exercise; let's start with the standard version. Hold on to a stationary bar (your palms can face in either direction) or a high fixed ledge with a space between your hands that is slightly wider than shoulder width. Allow yourself to hang with straight arms. Push your chest out and start your set by trying, without arching your back, to bring your shoulder blades close to one another and then finish the upward movement by pulling your chest up to the bar or ledge. When lowering to the starting position, be careful not to let yourself fall suddenly.

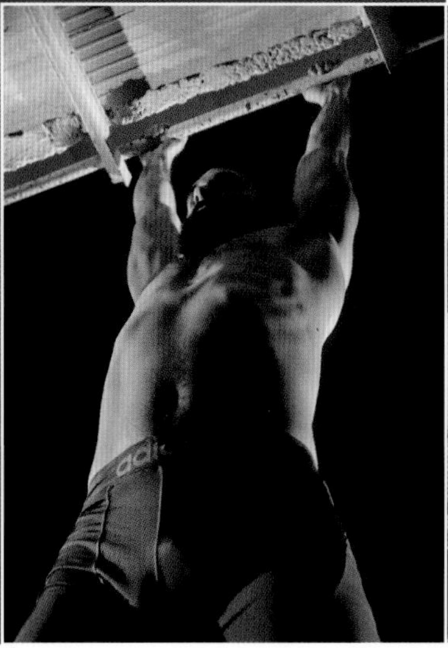

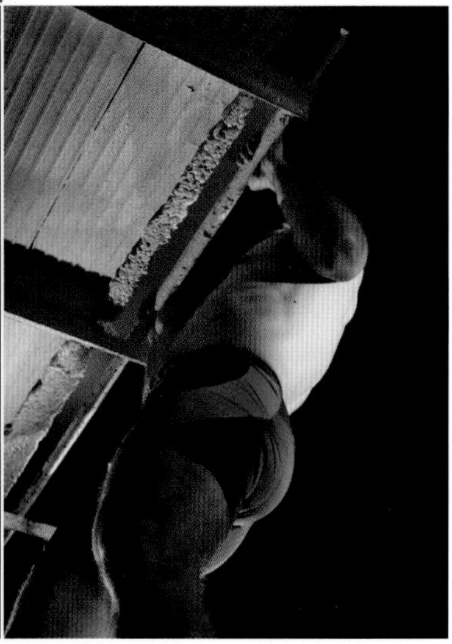

02. HIGH PULLEY ROW

This exercise is most often done using a high pulley machine, but a resistance band can also be used. Grab the bar or band with a space between your hands that is slightly less than shoulder-width apart. Sit on the floor (or the seat, if the machine has one) with your back straight, your chest out, and your shoulders lowered and pulled back. (If you sit on the floor, find a position in relation to the high pulley or band anchor position that, when the exercise is performed, will not strain your shoulders or hyperextend your back.) Tighten your abs and pull the bar or band toward your chest by flexing your arms and then straightening them back to the starting position.

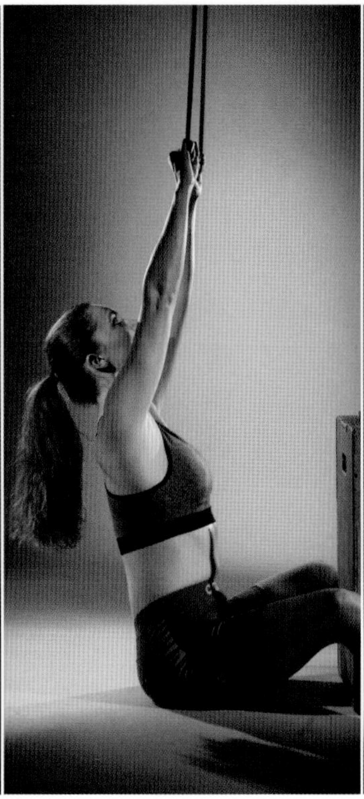

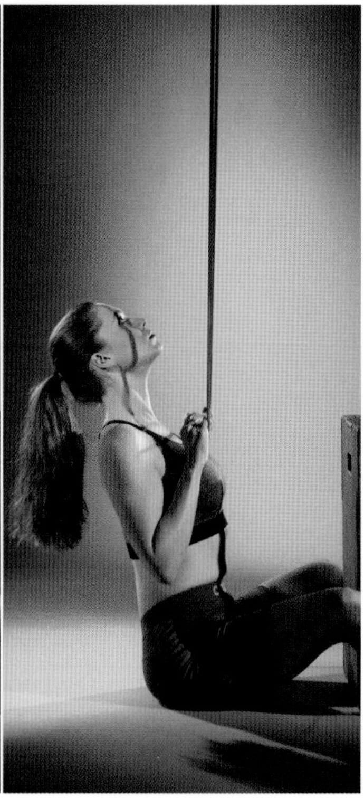

03. ONE-ARM ROW

Stand to the right side of a box, anchor a band under the inside edge of the box, and place your left knee on the top of the box. Lean forward and place your left hand ahead of your left knee with your right foot on the floor parallel to the inside edge of the box. Grasp the band with your right hand, slightly flex your right knee, and adjust the position of your left knee and hand to create a stable body position with your back as straight as possible. On the pulling (right) side, move your shoulder blade as close as possible to your spine, pull your shoulder back, and then finish the upward movement by pulling the band up to hip level. Reverse the movement to return to the starting position.

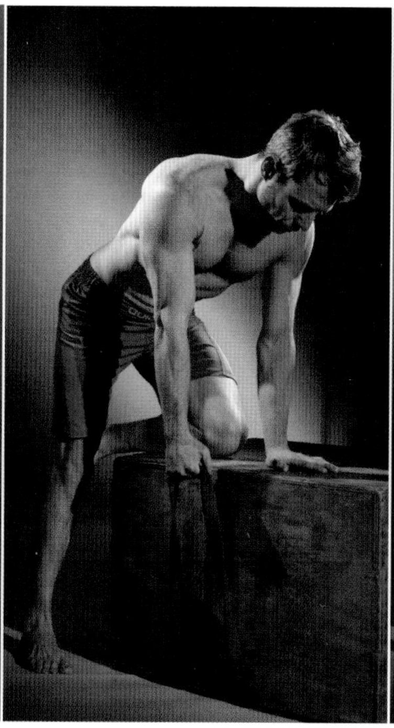

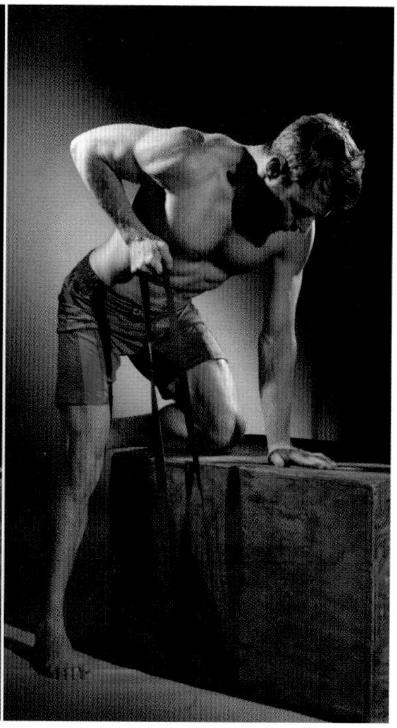

04. REVERSE PULL USING A SUSPENSION TRAINER

With the suspension trainer straps at a middle height, stand under the anchor point. Keeping your body in a straight line, rock back on your heels until your arms are fully extended away from your torso and your palms are facing the floor. Begin by bringing your shoulders back, pushing your chest out, and squeezing your shoulder blades together. Pull your body up by bringing your elbows as close to your ribs as possible and then finish the pulling movement by rotating your forearms so your hands finish close to your ribs with the palms facing each other. Reverse the movement to return to the starting position.

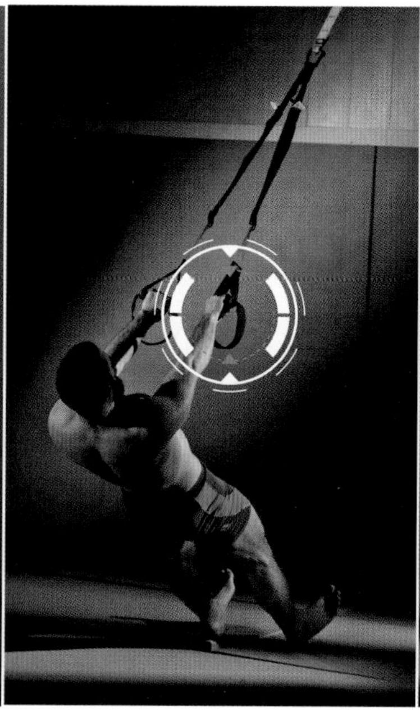

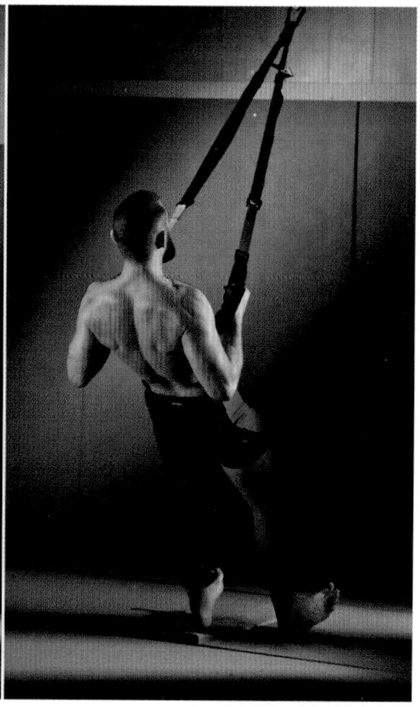

05. POWER PULL USING A SUSPENSION TRAINER

With the suspension trainer straps at a middle height, place yourself in a stable position. Stand on your heels, hanging from the strap with straight arms and palms toward the floor. Grab one handle with one hand. Straighten your other arm and keep it in line with your other arm and handle. Begin by bringing your shoulders back, pushing your chest out, and squeezing your shoulder blades together. Pull your body up by bringing the elbow of the arm holding the strap toward your ribs. Bend your other arm and bring your hand in toward your ribs to mimic the arm holding the strap. Reverse the movement to return to the starting position and complete one rep.

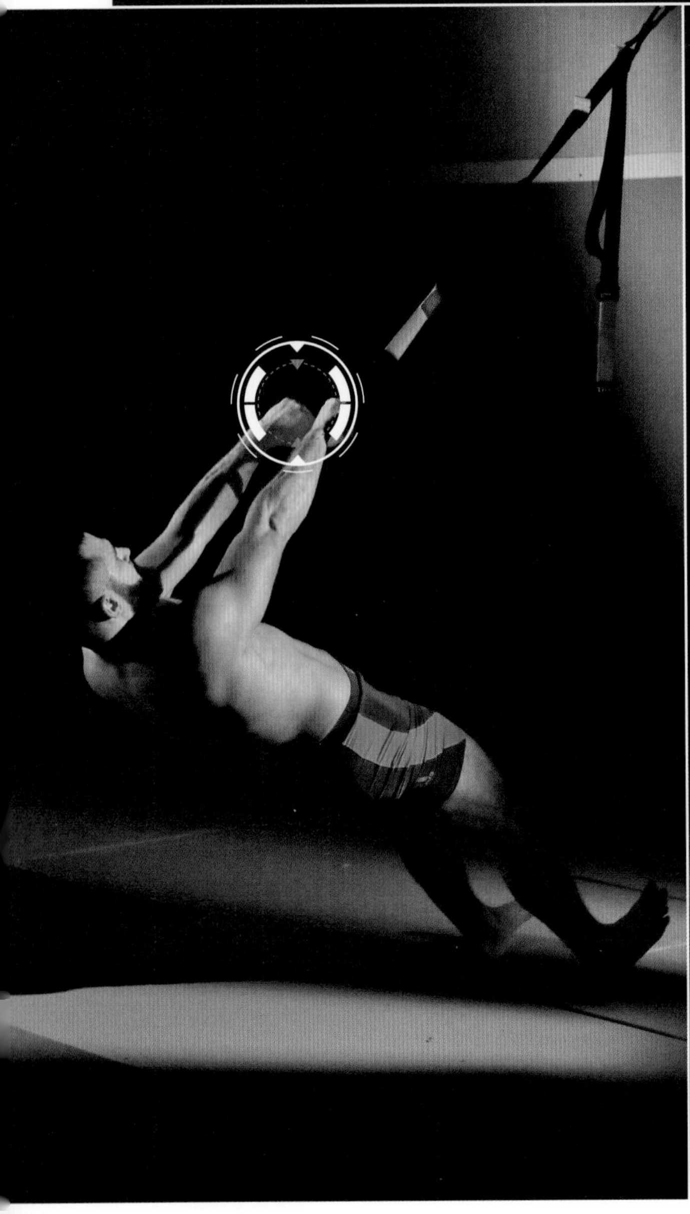

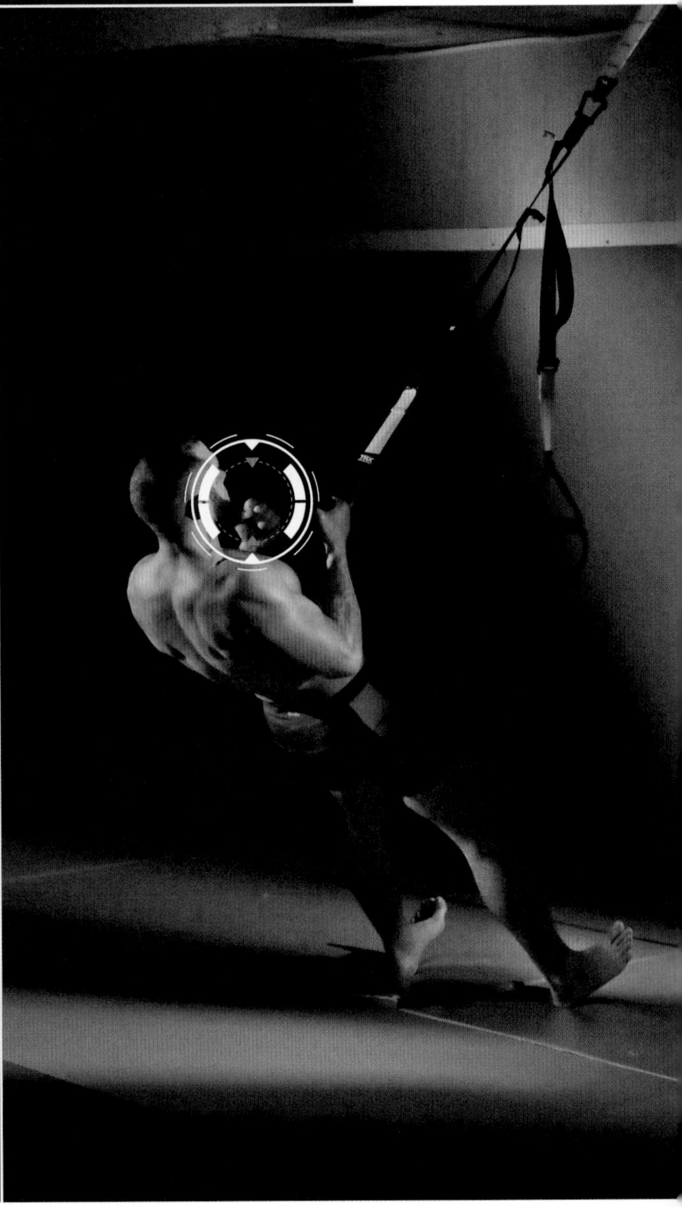

The Posterior Arm Chains

Back of the head: insertion of the trapezius to the vertebrae through the spinal processes

Shoulder: convergence of the trapezius fibers toward the scapular spine, extension in the shoulder through the deltoid

Arm: path continues through the deltoids toward the humerus then along the humerus through the external intermuscular partition

Forearm: from the lateral epicondyle of the humerus to the extensor digitorum toward the wrist

Hand: completes this chain by inserting on the phalanges and carpals

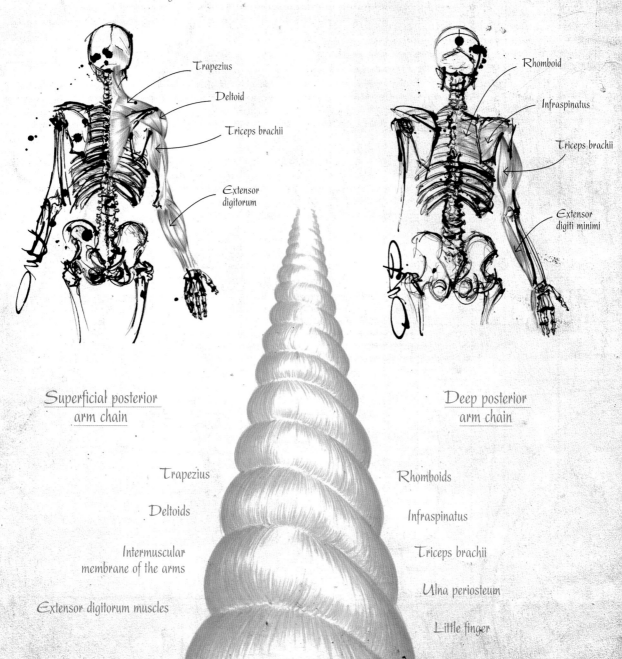

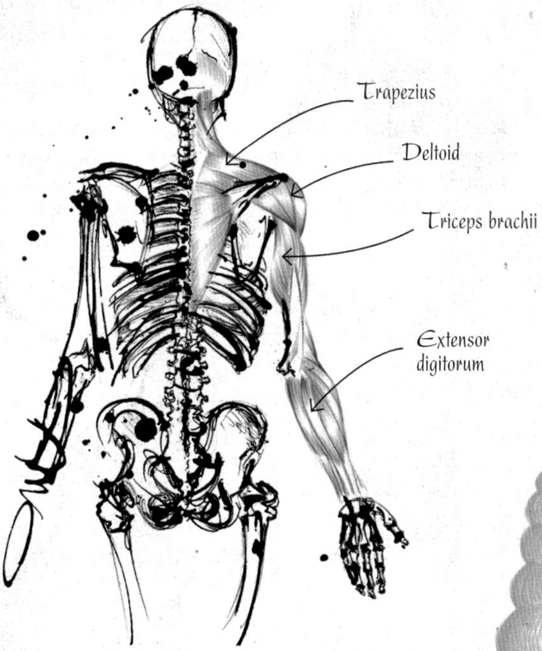

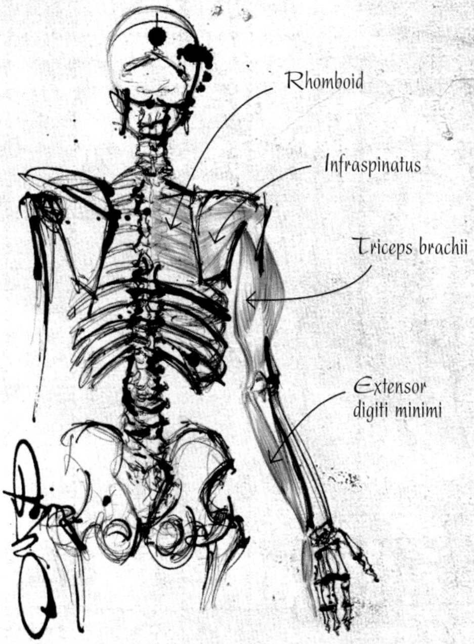

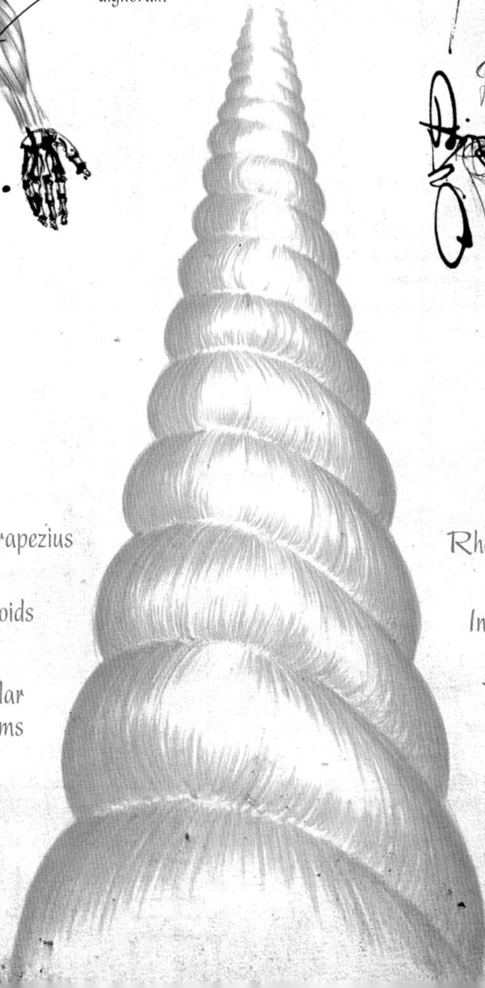

Superficial posterior arm chain

Trapezius

Deltoids

Intermuscular membrane of the arms

Extensor digitorum muscles

Deep posterior arm chain

Rhomboids

Infraspinatus

Triceps brachii

Ulna periosteum

Little finger

> *These postural chains are essential in many programs for correcting posture.*

Preventative treatment of a posterior chain—whether we are talking about a large chain like the superficial posterior chain or a smaller chain like the superficial or deep posterior arm chain—can help prevent imbalances in the anterior chain, especially in the arms. Strengthening the superficial or deep posterior arm chain is part of this principle and is therefore a fundamental part of postural training.

Possible Malfunctions in the Posterior Arm Chains

Often overworked in weightlifting programs, the muscles in the posterior arm chains are not treated often enough with self-massage and mobilization. Any postural problems will result in major consequences for the posterior arm chains. In addition to localized tension, the imbalances caused by these postural problems can produce or sustain issues in the chest, shoulders, and neck.

KILLER MOVES
TO DEVELOP THE POSTERIOR ARM CHAINS

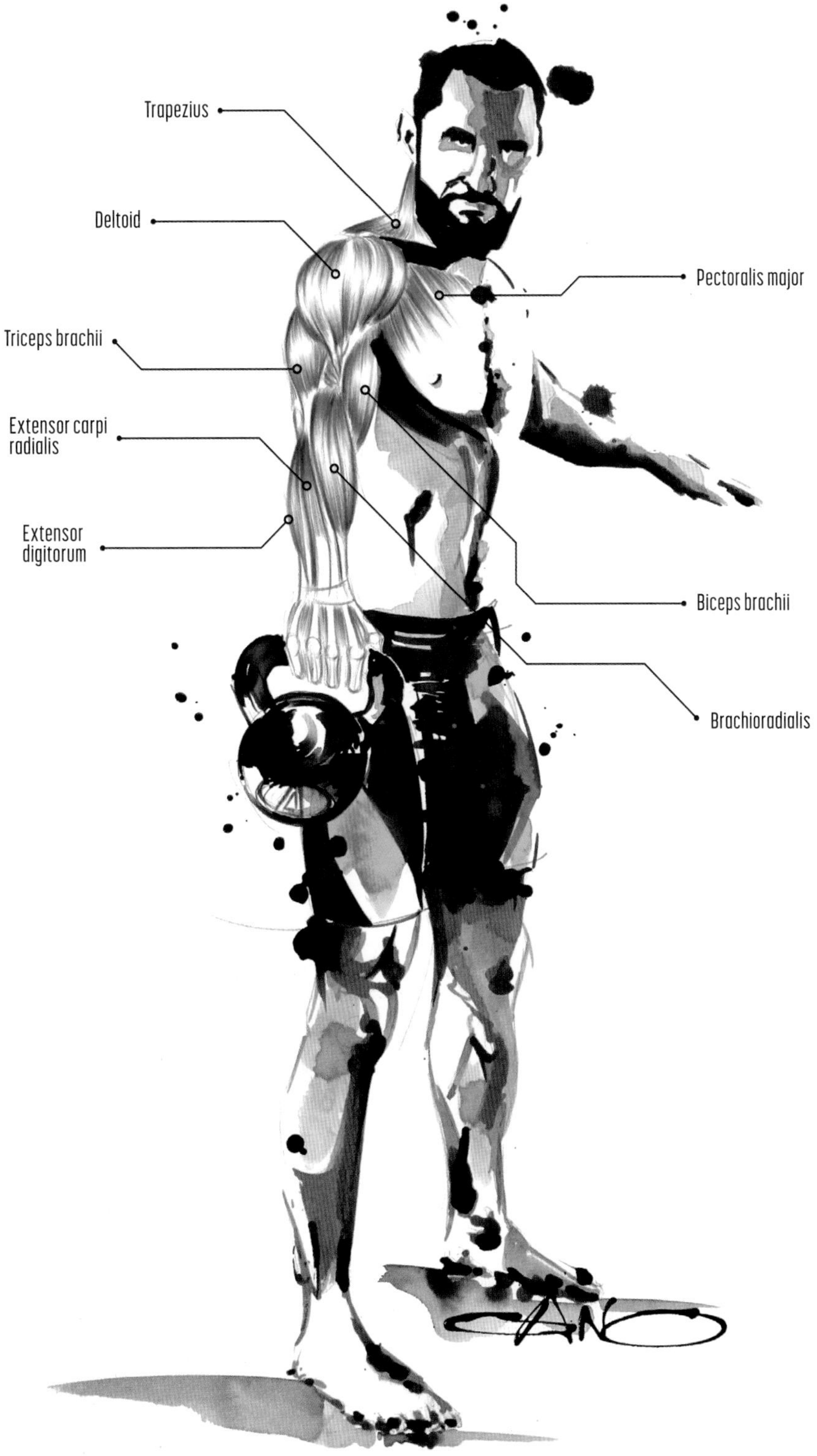

01. PALLOF PRESS

This exercise combines strengthening and activation of the posterior arm chains. Stand perpendicular to (and in a location away from) the anchor point or machine so that there is tension in the band, cable, or strap. Begin by holding the band or handle with both hands in front of your body with your shoulders low and elbows near your sides. Pull your abdomen in and squeeze your gluteal muscles and keep this position as you extend your arms out in front without disturbing the posture of your back or pivoting your hips or chest toward the anchor point. Perform a set on each side of the body.

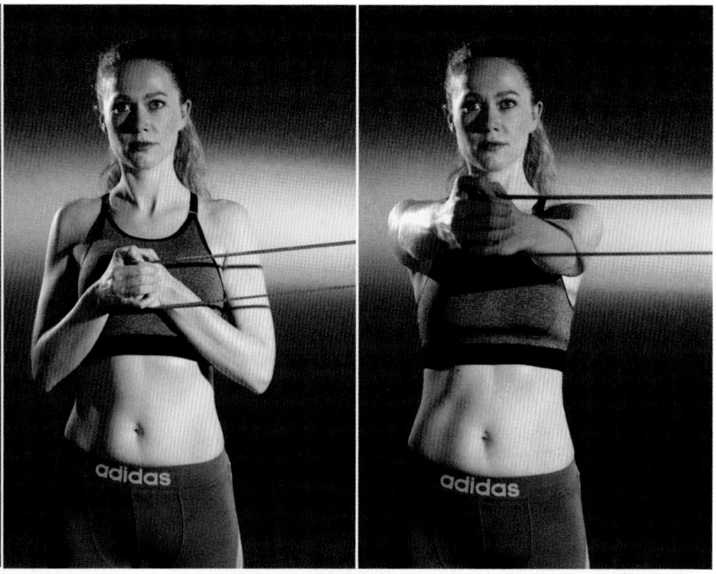

02. PIKE PUSH-UP

Adopt a classic push-up position but with your hands closer together and feet farther apart. In the bottom position, your elbows should be close to your body with your chest out and abs and gluteal muscles engaged. Push up with your arms as you lead with your gluteals and close your hips.

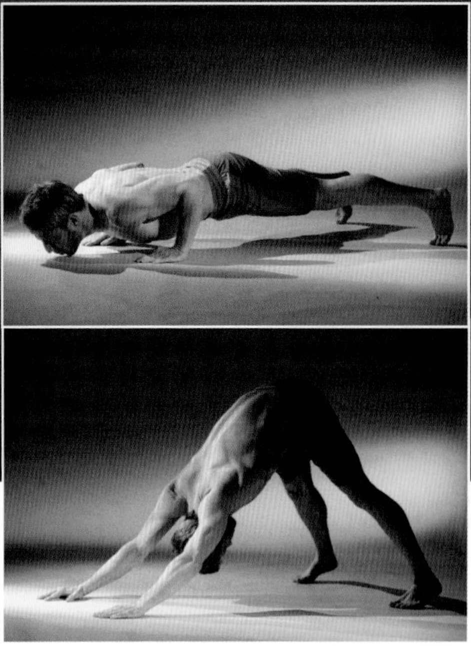

03. TRICEPS EXTENSION USING A SUSPENSION TRAINER

With your back to the suspension trainer, grab both handles and lean forward while straightening your body as much as possible by fully extending your knees, pulling your abdomen in, and squeezing your gluteal muscles. Position your upper arms next to your head with your elbows fully flexed and palms facing forward. Perform the exercise by fully extending your elbows while keeping them in line with your torso and next to your head. Try not to spread your elbows wide; keep your arms parallel to each other during the entire movement.

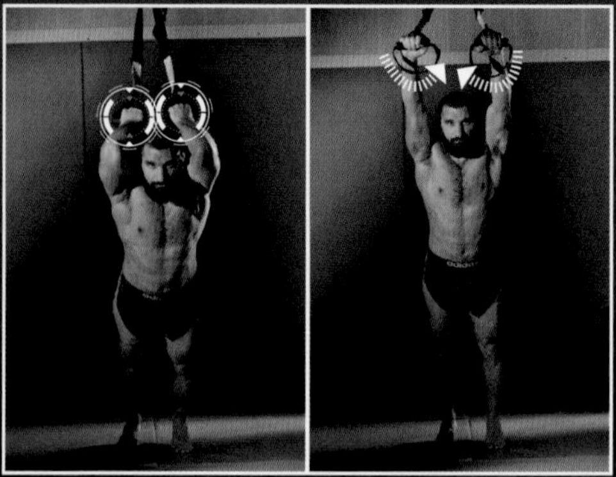

04. OI ZUKI

In karate, this technique brings the power of both legs to the arms. In its complete form, this exercise goes far beyond the posterior arm chains to involve the spiral chains. By adopting a deep, steady lunge position and using the shoulder blades in dynamic strengthening work, this exercise becomes a killer move for the posterior arm chains. Hook a resistance band onto a gym ladder. Grab it with one hand and face away from the ladder. With your other hand, lift a kettlebell above your head with your elbow fully extended (the arm extended overhead is on the same side as your front leg). Push out your chest and drive the arm holding the band forward with a closed fist, palm toward the floor, as if you were throwing a punch.

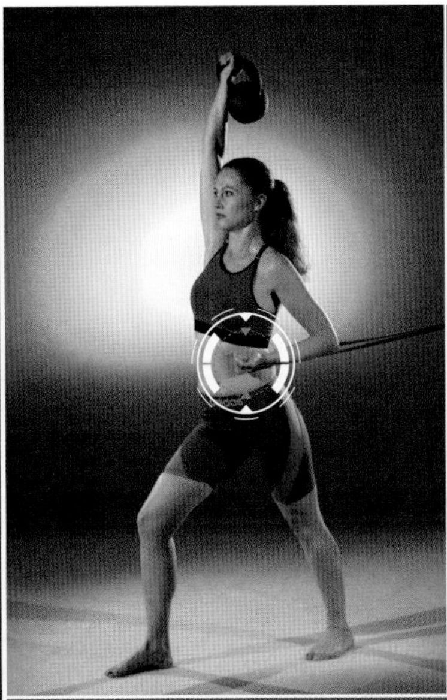

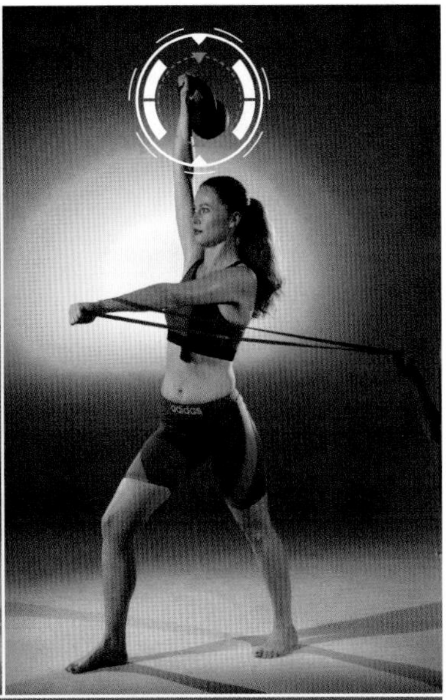

Oi zuki can also be carried out in reverse by pulling on the band; this is a killer move for the anterior arm chains.

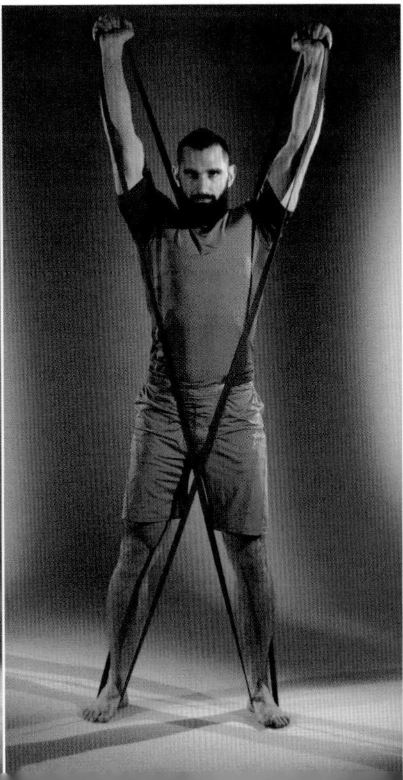

05. EXPANDED CROSS USING A BAND

Use two resistance bands, one under each foot, and cross them diagonally in front of your body. Hold a band in each hand with your hands facing each other and then extend your elbows to press the bands toward the ceiling without altering your back posture (be careful not to arch).

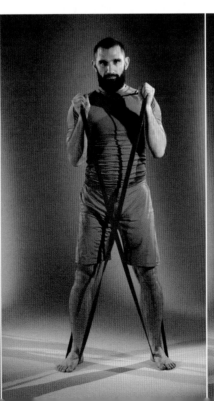

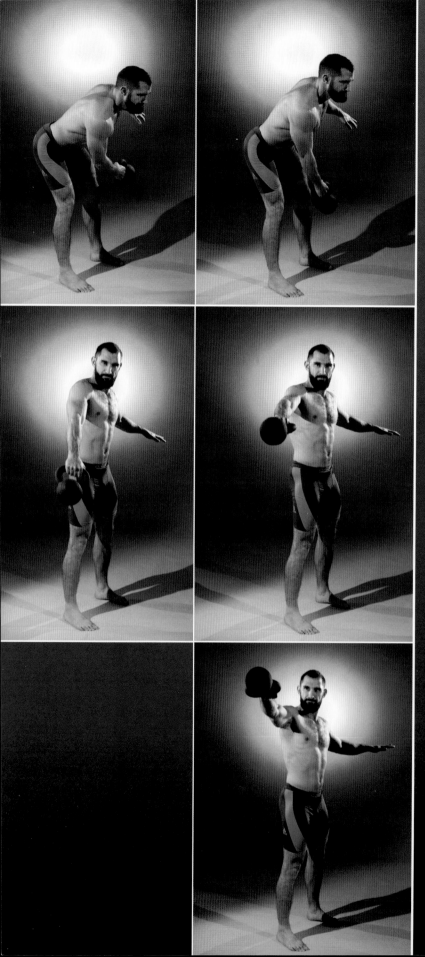

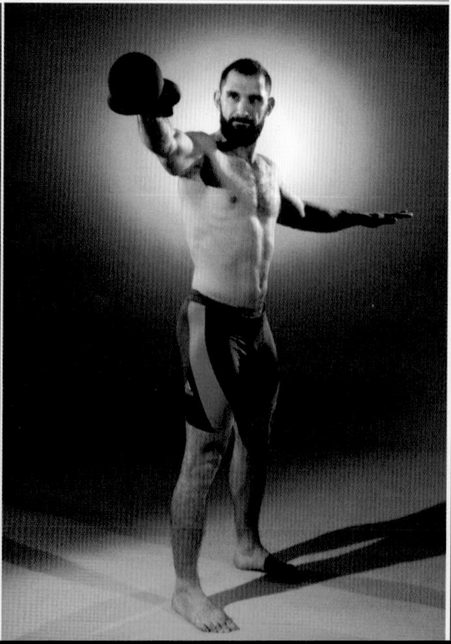

06. LATERAL KETTLEBELL SWING

Lean your body forward as you would in a traditional one-handed swing. Begin the pendulum from your feet, transferring your body weight from left to right. As the kettlebell passes your knees, extend through your knees and hips to stand up. As you gain speed, the kettlebell will move higher. When the kettlebell reaches chest height, you can begin to rotate the arm out until your palm is facing the floor. Always keep your hips extended in a lateral rotating movement. Engage the hip on the side where you are swinging the kettlebell. As your weight moves to the front foot and the back foot becomes free, allow your heel to lift as both feet pivot in the direction of movement (not seen in the photos).

The Deep Anterior Chain

Foot: flexor digitorum longus, tibialis posterior and tibialis anterior, peroneus longus

Leg and hip: popliteal fossa, adductors

Pelvis: pelvic floor

Torso: quadratus lumborum, iliolumbar ligament, iliopsoas, diaphragm, pericardium, posterior aspect of the sternum, pharynx, scalene muscles, anterior longitudinal ligament, longus colli, longus capitis

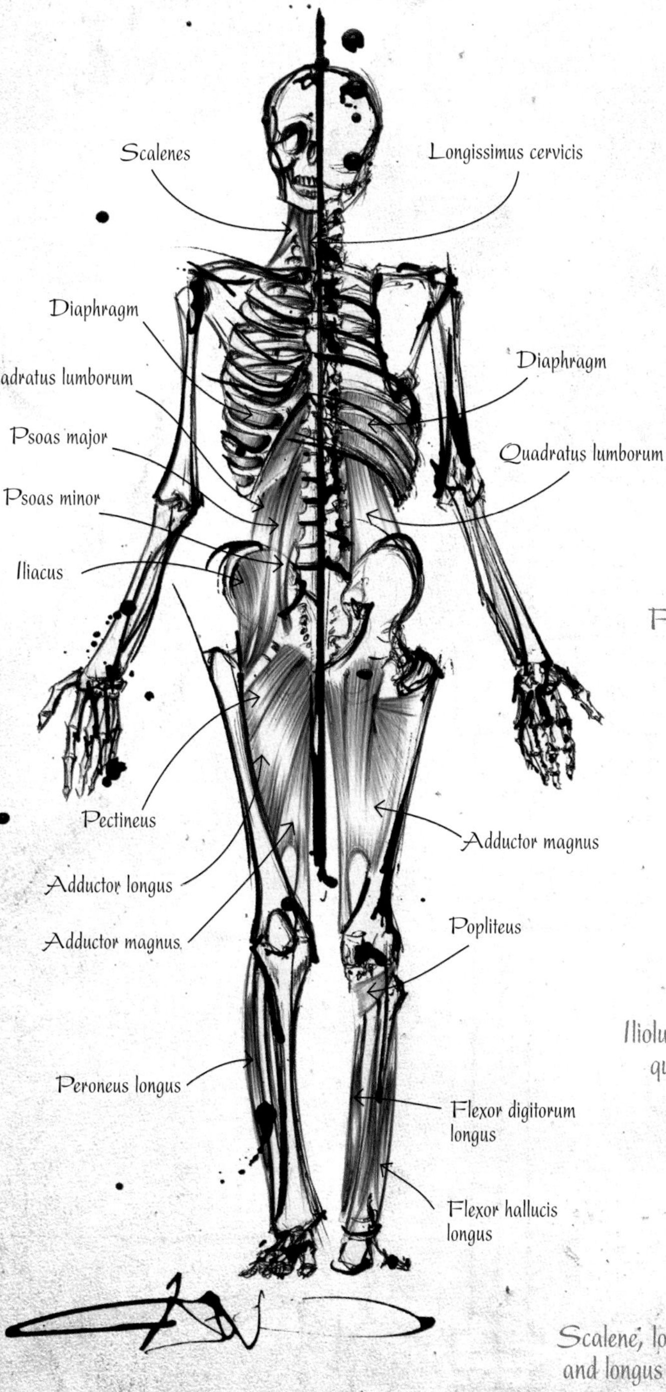

Scalenes
Longissimus cervicis
Diaphragm
Quadratus lumborum
Psoas major
Psoas minor
Iliacus
Diaphragm
Quadratus lumborum
Pectineus
Adductor longus
Adductor magnus
Adductor magnus
Popliteus
Peroneus longus
Flexor digitorum longus
Flexor hallucis longus

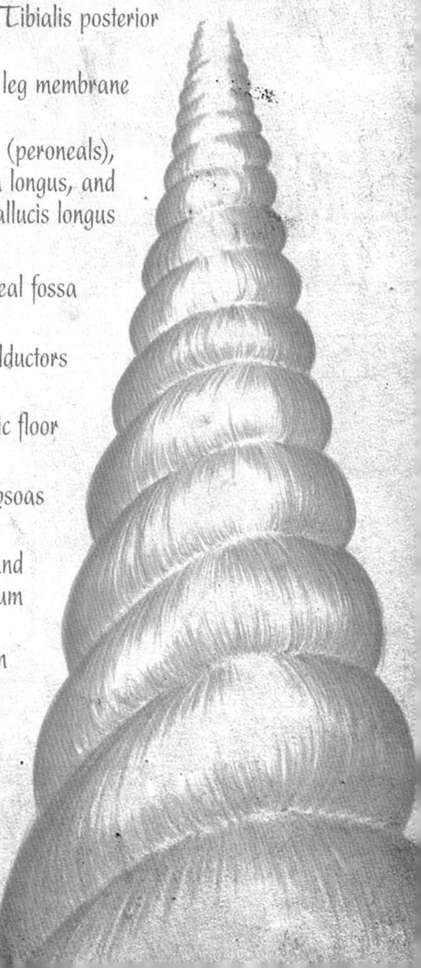

Tibialis posterior
Interosseous leg membrane
Fibularis muscles (peroneals), flexor digitorum longus, and flexor hallucis longus
Popliteal fossa
Adductors
Pelvic floor
Iliopsoas
Iliolumbar ligament and quadratus lumborum
Diaphragm
Pericardium
Pharynx
Scalene, longus capitis, and longus colli muscles

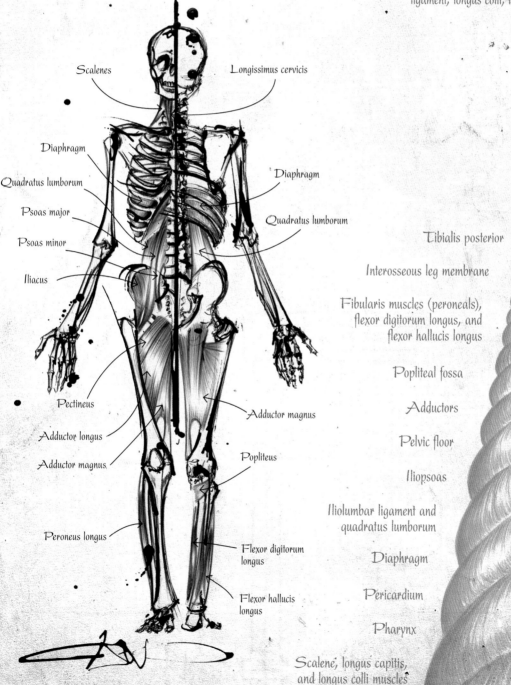

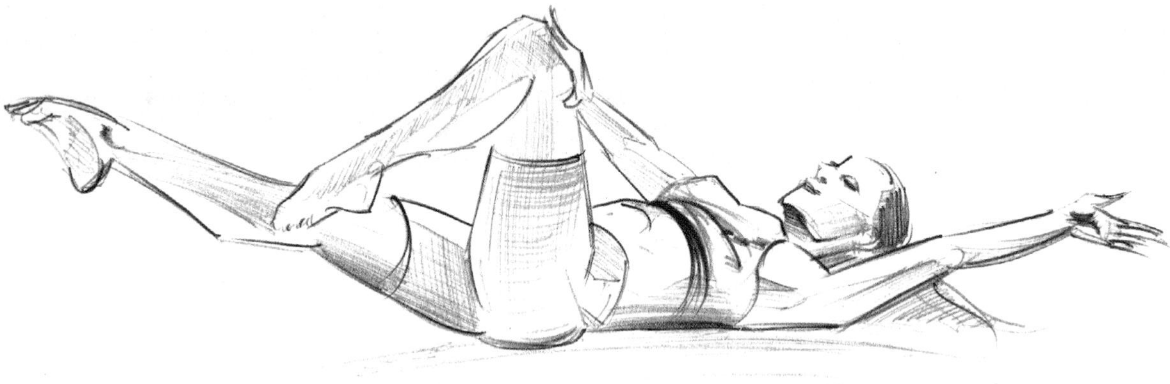

The deep anterior chain is the muscle chain for core stability and is also essential for balance.

Strengthening this chain is essential for working in synergy with other chains to ensure functional stability and transfers of strength. It is the deepest postural connection of muscle and fascia for balance in the body. It is the key to proper functioning throughout the human machine.

Breathing plays a major role in the deep anterior chain (see page 78). Respiratory problems cause stiffness in the neck, often because of overuse and tension in the scalene muscles. Breathing problems also cause stiffness in the hip flexors and adductors.

Possible Malfunctions in the Deep Anterior Chain

- Breathing is an integral part of functional balance. When breathing is disturbed, it can lead to a loss of mobility in the tongue, jaw, throat, or scalene muscles. Breathing's association with desynchronization of the longus colli and longus capitis muscles means that the support for the neck and head is also compromised, which can affect the balance of the entire body.
- Continuous activation of this chain can sometimes wear out one or several of its links because they have low levels of endurance. This is when other muscles can intervene and cause harmful compensations or even suffer tension themselves by doing work they are not supposed to do. This is the case for the psoas, for example; it is a muscle that is used more often than it needs to be.

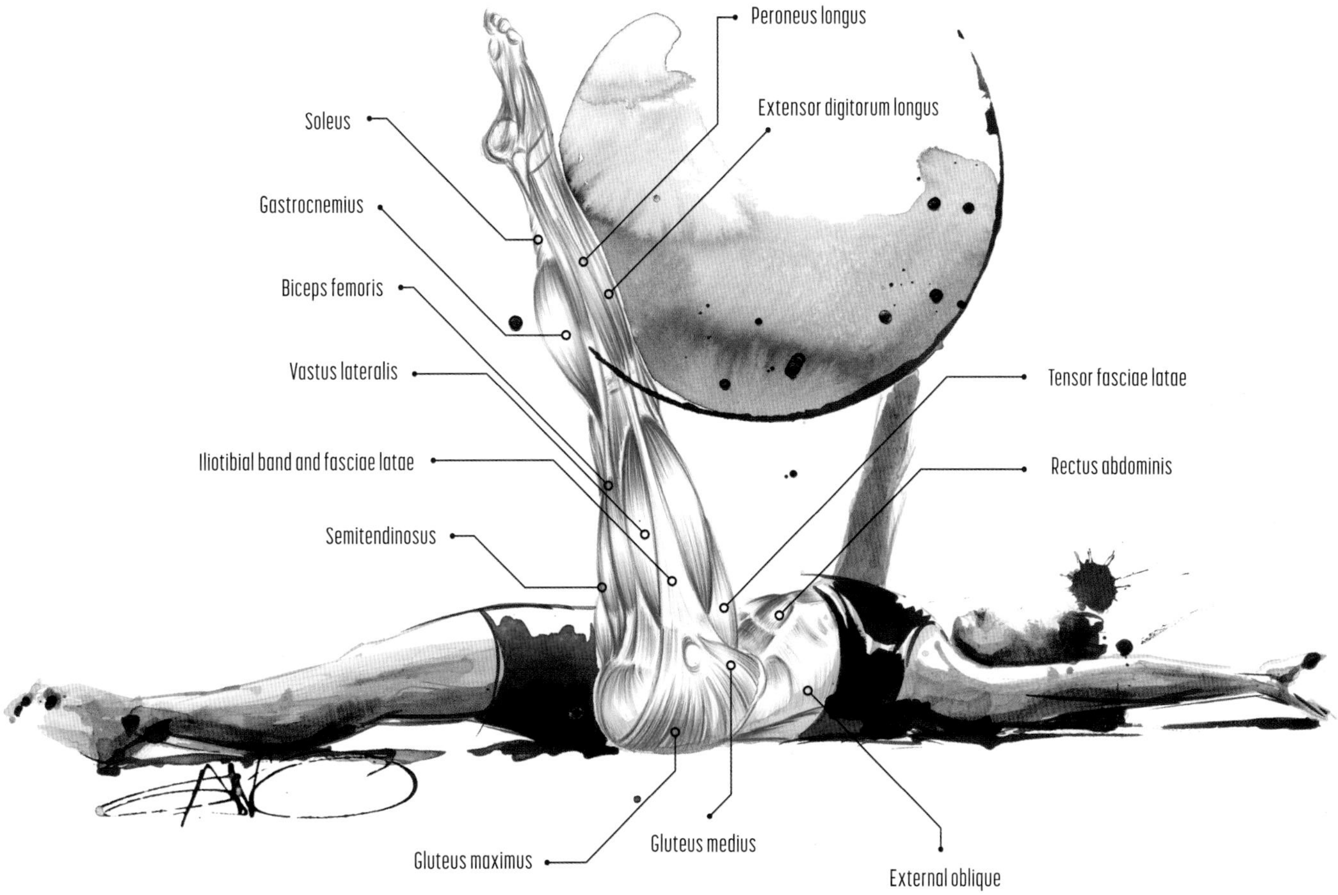

Peroneus longus
Extensor digitorum longus
Soleus
Gastrocnemius
Biceps femoris
Vastus lateralis
Iliotibial band and fasciae latae
Semitendinosus
Tensor fasciae latae
Rectus abdominis
Gluteus maximus
Gluteus medius
External oblique

01. HORIZONTAL SEAT

Start on all fours with your knees lifted, shins parallel to the floor, and an exercise ball between your buttocks and the wall. Pull your abdomen in as much as possible while straightening your back and locking your pelvic floor. Try to squish the ball as much as possible. A more advanced version of this exercise is to lift one straight arm in front of you in line with your torso.

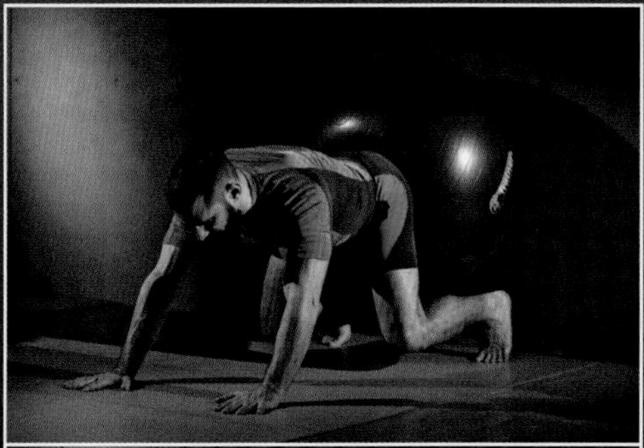

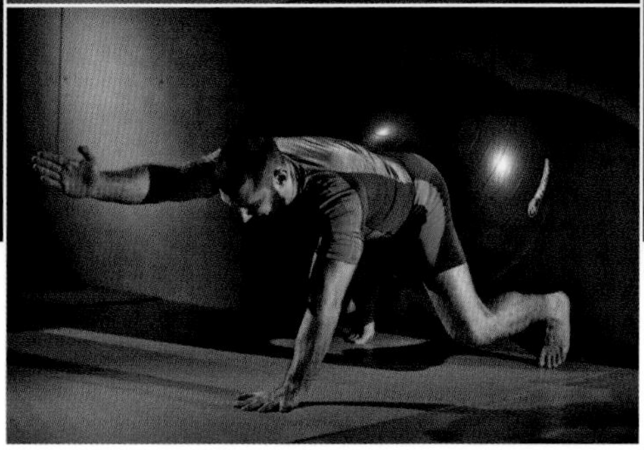

02. STRENGTHEN THE FRONTAL PLANE USING AN EXERCISE BALL

Support yourself on your elbows or hands on an exercise ball. Pull your abdomen in and tilt your pelvis back slightly to activate your gluteal and rectus abdominis muscles. Tighten your pelvic floor and pull your abdomen in to activate the transverse abdominis muscles. Alternate between supporting yourself on your elbows and then on your hands for a more advanced option.

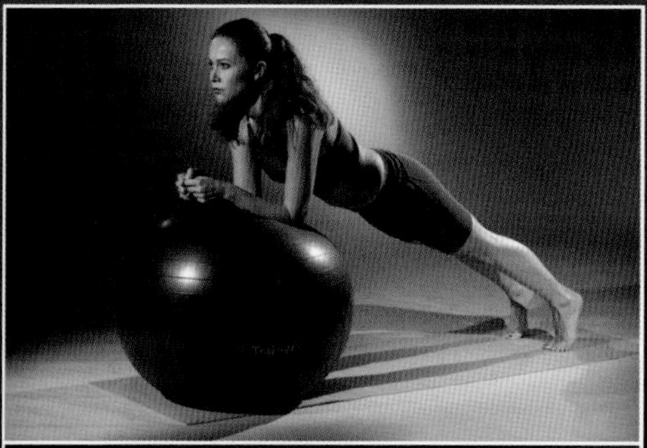

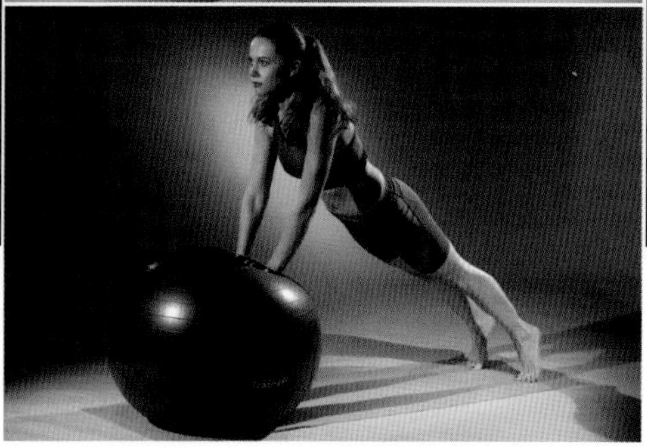

03. FLATTEN AN EXERCISE BALL WITH OPPOSITE HAND AND FOOT

Lie down with your lower back flat on the floor. Pull your abdomen in as much as possible and tighten your pelvic floor. Place an exercise ball between one leg and the opposite arm. If you are flexible, do this exercise with one leg extended and the other knee bent.

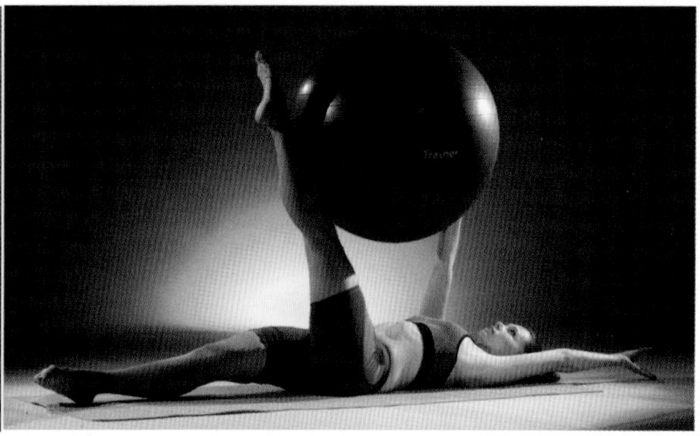

04. STRAIGHT LEG RAISE ON AN EXERCISE BALL

Lie on an exercise ball and hold on to a gym ladder or a partner. Allow the ball to mold into the shape of the curve in your lower back. Once your abdomen is as flat as possible, tighten your pelvic floor and raise your straight legs until they are vertical. Gently and slightly extend your hips. When you feel your abdominal muscles activate as you are bringing your legs down, hold that position. Perform rapid flutter kicks using a small range of motion for a more advanced option.

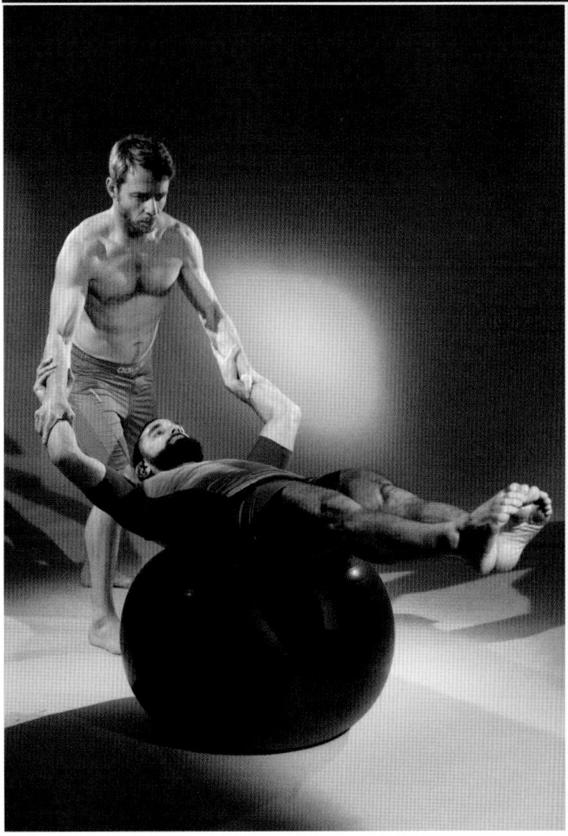

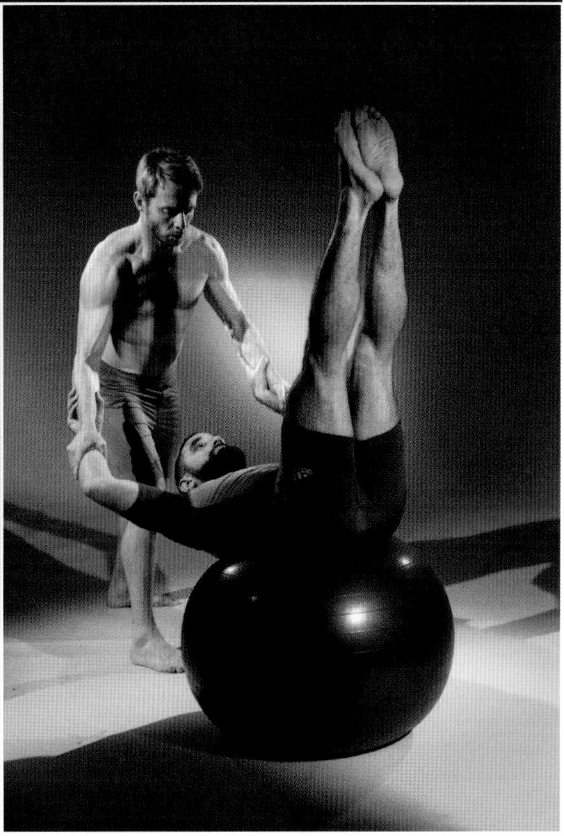

05. OPPOSITE ARM-KNEE CRUNCH WITH A STRAIGHT ARM

Lie on your back with one arm extended overhead. Keep your abdomen flat and tilt your pelvis back slightly. Push the hand of your other arm against the opposite leg. Your other leg should remain straight and slightly raised. Push your hand against your knee (and vice versa) as much as possible. Your heels should never touch the floor. Lock your pelvic floor, pull your abdomen in, and flatten your lower back throughout the exercise.

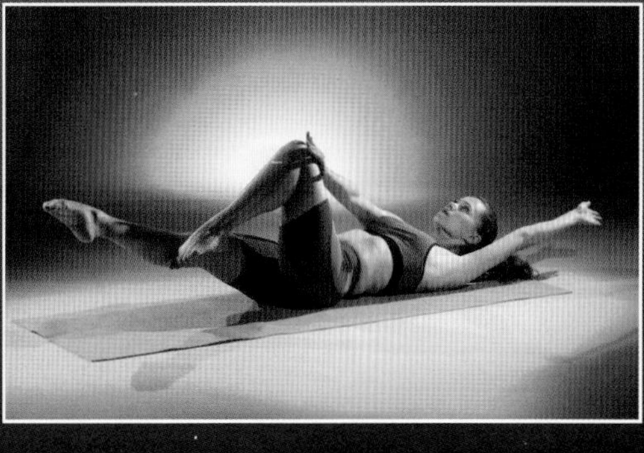

The Posterior Functional Chain

Arm: begins in the latissimus dorsi tendon

Chest: thoracolumbar fascia

Pelvis: gluteus maximus

Thigh: IT band and vastus lateralis

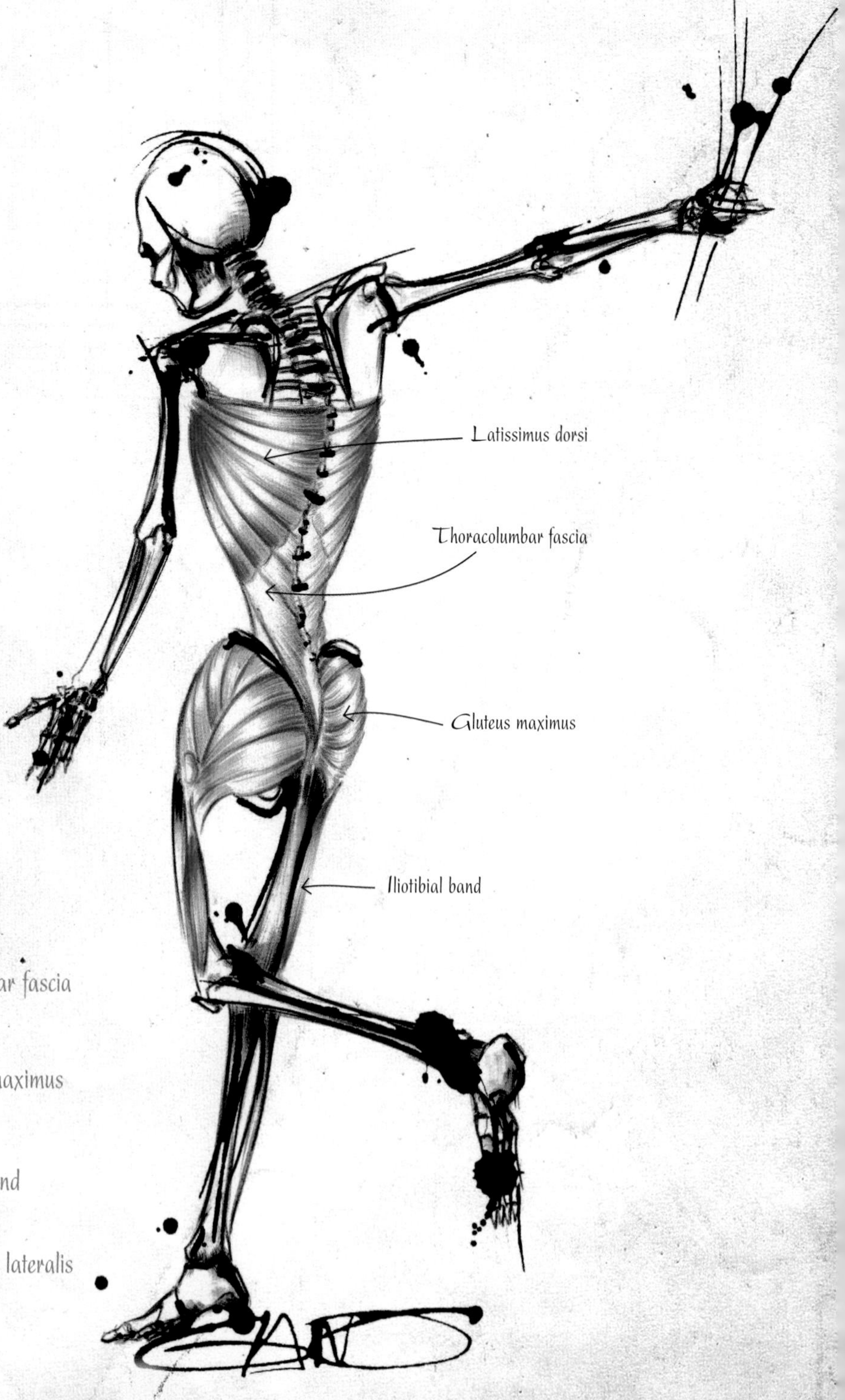

Latissimus dorsi
Thoracolumbar fascia
Gluteus maximus
Iliotibial band

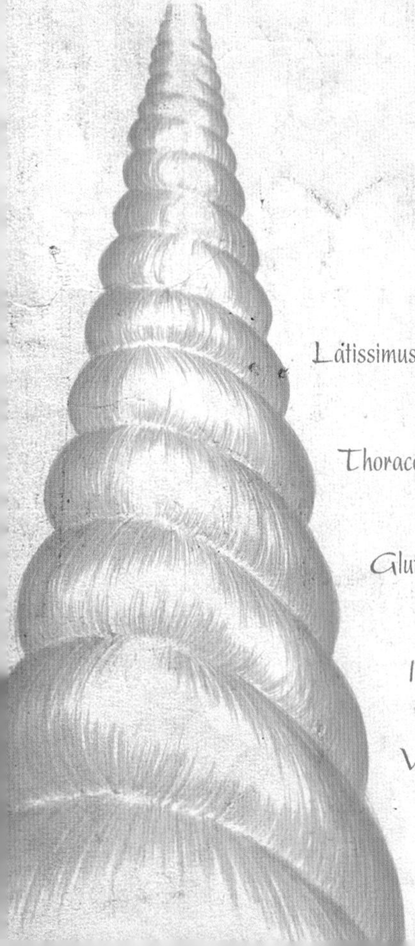

Latissimus dorsi
Thoracolumbar fascia
Gluteus maximus
IT band
Vastus lateralis

The Anterior Functional Chain

Arm: begins where the pectoralis major connects to the arm

Chest: pectoralis major, rectus abdominis, vertical abdominal cavity

Pelvis: pubic bone

Thigh: adductor magnus, internal aspect of the femur

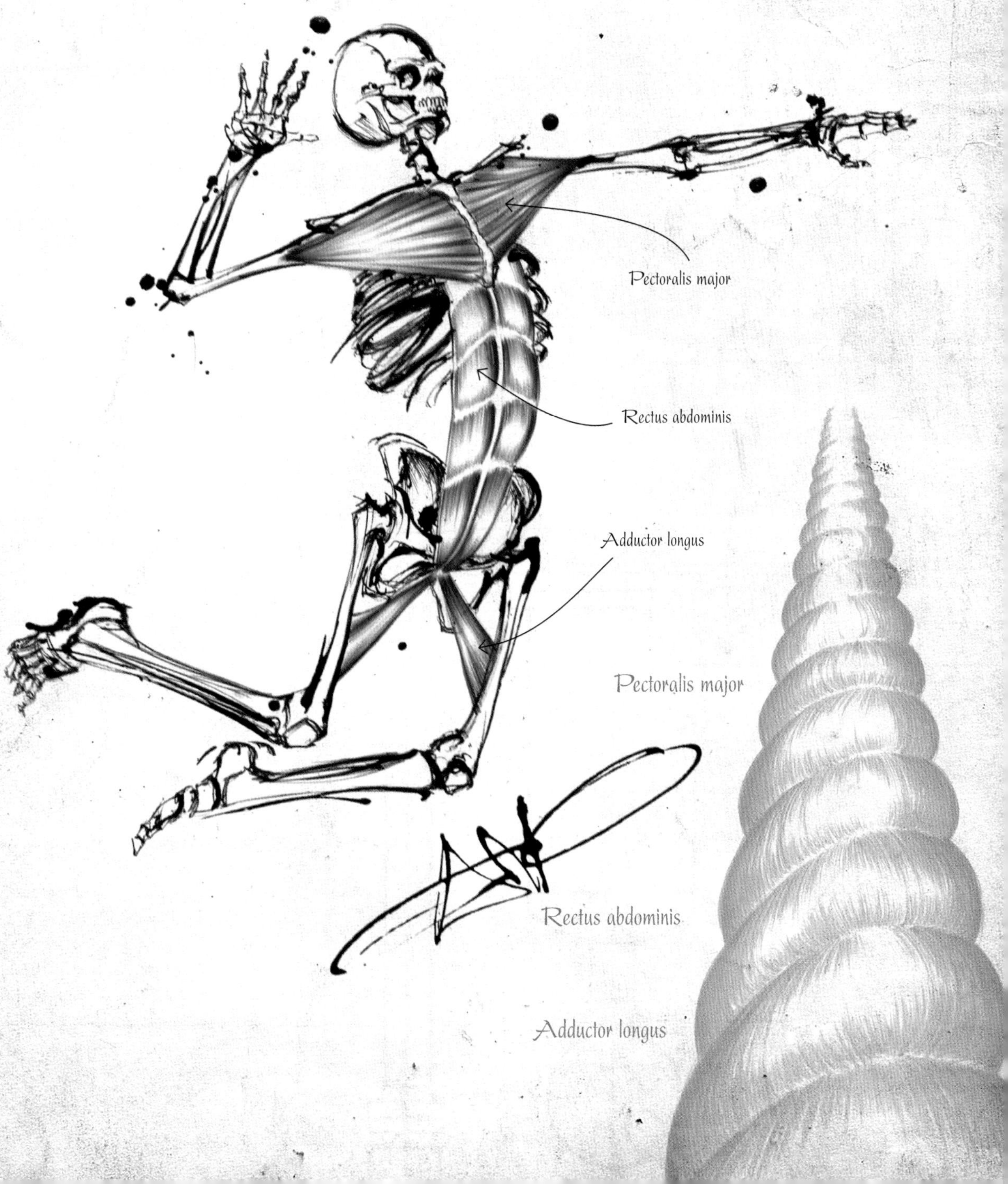

> *These muscle chains are the links that transcend the purely anatomical chains. They are an extension of the arm and leg chains, and they are responsible for effective movement in complex activities.*

If they are fully trained (and not just through isolated strengthening of the individual links), the anterior and posterior functional chains use cross-linking—by coordinating inverse use of the upper and lower limbs—that allows for greater extension, greater potential for elastic energy, and a greater ability to generate power.

As a major active element in posterior movement, exercises that recruit the posterior functional chain should always be done at the beginning of a workout involving asymmetric to dominant posterior movement patterns (e.g., backhand tennis swings and rugby passes) as a preparation tool for complex functional movement training. End your workouts with these same exercises to refocus your training and reconnect all the parts of the joint and muscle chains.

As a major active element in anterior movement, exercises that recruit the anterior functional chain should always be done at the beginning of a workout involving asymmetric to dominant anterior movement patterns (e.g., tennis serves and volleyball spikes) as a preparation tool for complex functional movement training. End your workouts with these same exercises to refocus your training and reconnect all the parts of the joint and muscle chains.

Possible Malfunctions in the Functional Chains

- Lack of coordination between the upper and lower halves of the body makes it difficult or even impossible to achieve optimal activation of the functional chains.
- An absence of pelvis-shoulder dissociation allows for mobility of the hip and torso and is required for these chains to express their full power.
- Shortening of a link in the chain: There are few links, so compensations are very limited. If the gluteal muscles or the pectoral, adductor, or back muscles are too stiff or too weak, the entire functional chain is in jeopardy.

KILLER MOVES
TO DEVELOP THE FUNCTIONAL CHAINS

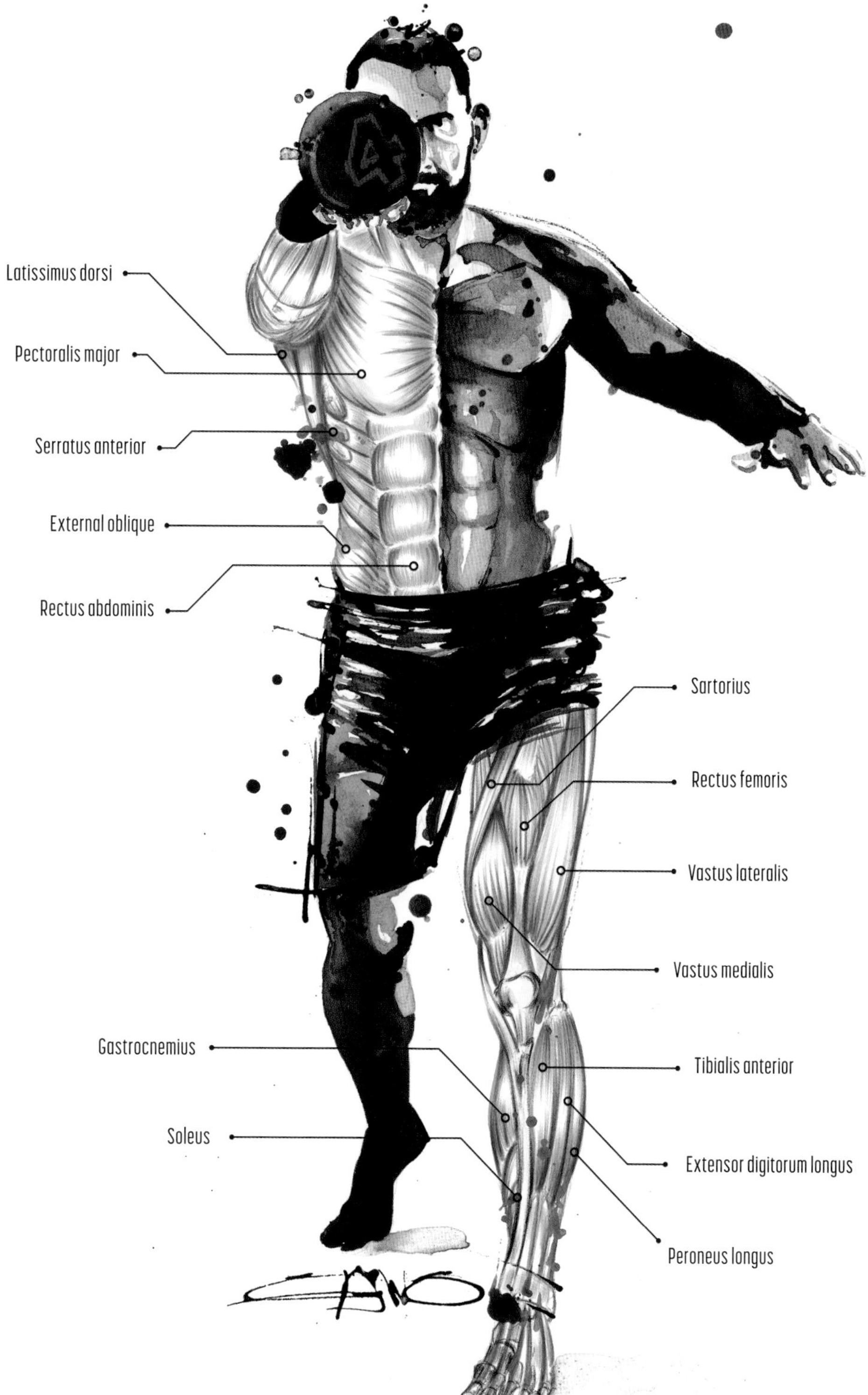

01. ATLAS SWING

Stand up straight and hold a kettlebell in two hands next to the two bases of the handle. Push your chest out and shoulders slightly back. Begin to rotate from your feet. Tilt your body weight toward the foot on the side where you will raise the kettlebell. This frees up your other foot, allowing your heel to lift off the floor for greater movement. As you rotate, both of your feet pivot at the same time in the same direction as the kettlebell. Your toes should always follow the kettlebell. Your hips begin the rotation of the body, allowing your torso to pivot perpendicularly to the starting axis. If you are doing this in a square room, start facing a wall. When your kettlebell is completely raised, you should be facing the wall that is perpendicular to the starting wall. When raising and lowering the kettlebell, point your thumbs toward the sky. The thumbs only rotate once they reach hip level so they are in the reverse position to do the exercise on the other side. The kettlebell should go as high as possible above your head when your head is between your arms. Remember, as in any swing, the drive comes from your lower limbs and is not being powered by your upper body. The pendulum movement should be fluid, with no stops, and should slow the kettlebell down as necessary from the end of the move to its reverse.

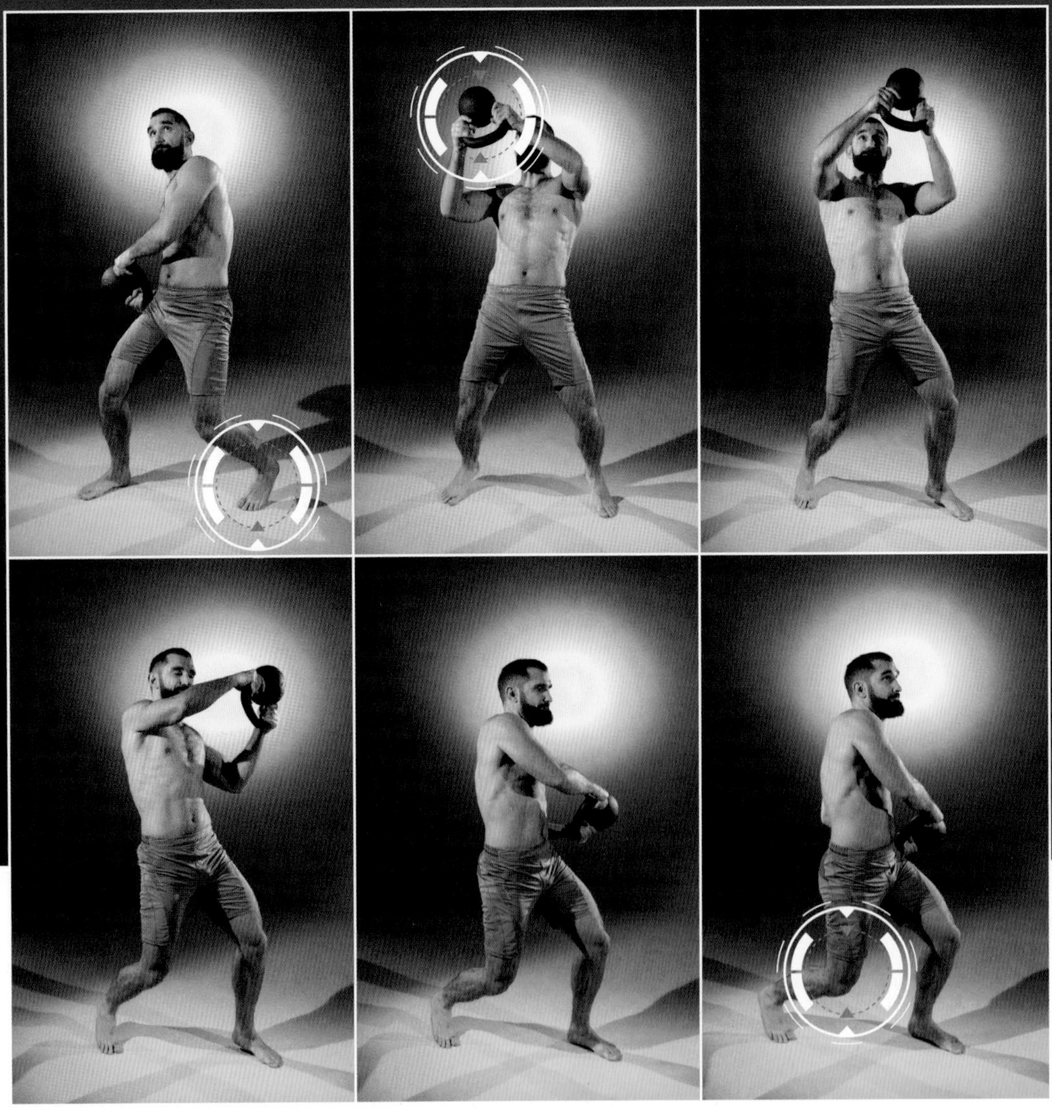

02. SIDE SWING

Place your feet shoulder-width apart and point them 45 degrees from the axis of your body. You can move your feet slightly, but they must stay in line with your knees to avoid any lateral tension in your knees and ankles.

Start the move by flexing your knees (squat one-third of the way to the floor, much deeper than in a traditional swing). Drive your legs up powerfully to propel the kettlebell forward. Keep your back straight throughout the exercise. By holding the kettlebell in both hands, you will be able to point your thumbs toward the ceiling throughout the exercise.

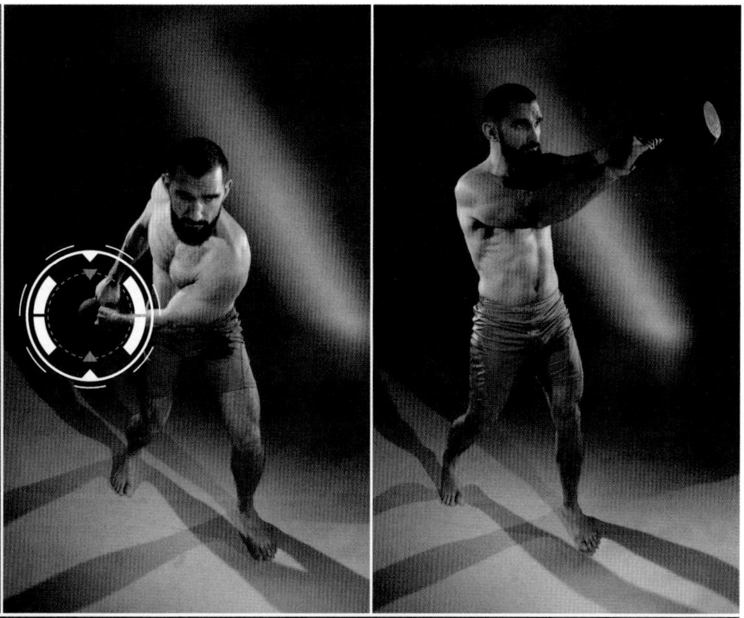

This exercise can also be done with one hand. If you do this, hold the kettlebell in your back hand. Do not alternate sides with each rep; work exclusively on one side and then the other.

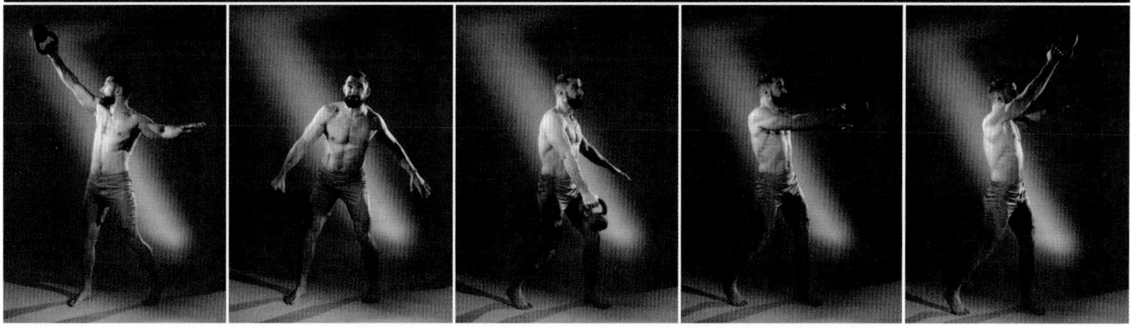

03. BENT OVER SWING

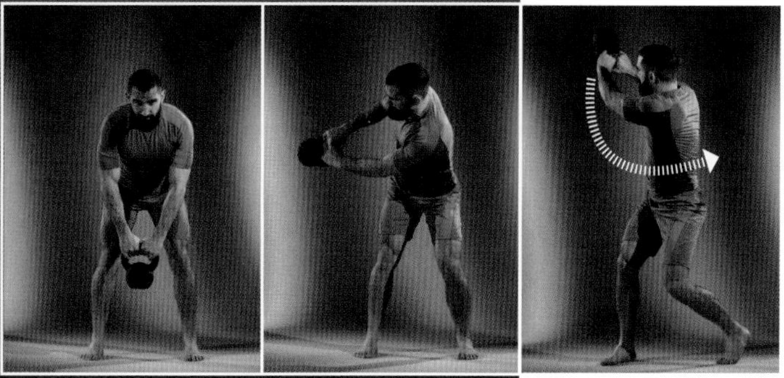

It is important to keep your feet parallel throughout this exercise. Lean forward, flex your hips and knees, and align your shoulders perpendicular to the kettlebell. Drive the kettlebell sideways without standing up too much. The kettlebell will rise diagonally up and back to align with the axis of your shoulders. At the end of the move, your shoulders, arms, and the kettlebell should all be in one line. Once the kettlebell is at the highest position, try to whip it as it moves down, using your whole body to create the acceleration. Allow the movement to slow down as you lift it to the other side to restart the exercise.

04. HIGH ROTATION

Hold the kettlebell with your hands on the sides of the handle and with your feet parallel and mobile (the toes follow the kettlebell throughout the movement). Flex your hips and knees and start with the kettlebell on your side behind your buttocks. Keep your shoulders in line with your buttocks. It is important that your front shoulder is quite high and your back shoulder is quite low so that the kettlebell is in line with them. From here, drive the kettlebell forward and up so that it almost makes a complete circle and arrives at the exact opposite position by other side of your buttocks. This circle is diagonal, not parallel, to the floor, and the kettlebell rises very high diagonally. Keep your arms partially flexed throughout this exercise.

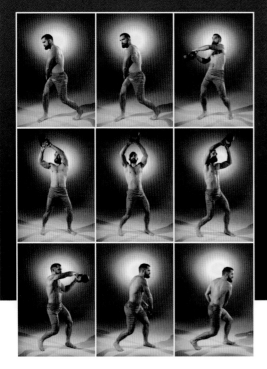

05. HORIZONTAL SWING

This exercise is done with a kettlebell in each hand. Spread your feet shoulder-width apart, keeping them as parallel as possible throughout the exercise. Drive the kettlebells from one side to the other. The kettlebells do not move simultaneously; the first is driven by the rotation of the hips and forward thrust of the legs, and the second follows the movement. Your legs are mobile and pivot at the same time to follow the direction of the body. The arms are extended throughout and do not flex at the end of the rotation. Keep your arms far apart from one another during the exercise, except at the end when your second arm wraps around the axis of your body. Note that the horizontal swing is not completely horizontal: The trajectory of the kettlebell is slightly diagonal, more in the direction of the sky than parallel to the floor. The horizontal swing can also be done with just one arm.

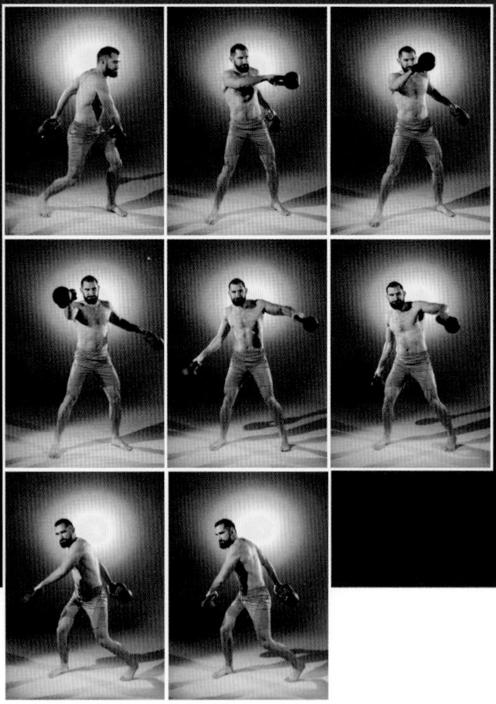

OPEN AND CLOSED KINETIC CHAINS

Muscle chains act as an open kinetic chain or a closed kinetic chain.

An *open kinetic chain* is when the distal end is free such as when throwing a punch or kicking a football. Conversely, a *closed kinetic chain* is when the distal end is stationary. This is the case when doing squats or deadlifts.

There is much debate about the exclusive use of either of the two methods in functional training to the point where the debate is often reduced to *monoarticular analytical movements* versus *polyarticular complex movements* or even *guided weightlifting exercises* versus *weightlifting exercises using free weights*. This opposition is unfounded because very often in physical training we talk about the semi-closed kinetic chain, which is when an exercise involves a free distal end moving against heavy resistance, like in cycling. Furthermore, it must be noted that a chain can be open or closed in ways apart from the simple free or guided exercise duality. Monoarticular movements can therefore be extremely functional. This is the case with the biceps curl, for example, which is completely transferable to carrying a shopping bag. Do not be fooled by this debate as, ideally, the two methods can complement each other.

Although the definitions of open and closed kinetic chains imply that they are opposites of each other, they actually can complement each other.

Recent studies on the subject (essentially based on functional reeducation, as in the Mikkelsen study in 2000 and Chatrenet's literature review in 2013) prescribe a mixed and intelligent use of these two methods, sometimes focusing on control of the weight and sometimes focusing on kinesthetic qualities.

TRAINING PROGRAMS FOR CONTRACTION

Muscles do not constantly contract when you are moving. The rhythm, speed, and tension all vary. They shorten to accelerate and produce movement. They brake by elongating to supply balance. Finally, they receive signals to coordinate movement.

Therefore, it is essential to consider training programs for contraction. During a *concentric* contraction, the muscle insertions draw close to one another, as when you stand up from a kneeling position. During an *eccentric* contraction, the muscle insertions spread apart. This happens when you decelerate from a sprint or lower the bar during the biceps curl exercise. During an *isometric* contraction, the muscle insertions do not move. This happens in static positions such as the plank exercise. All these types of muscle contractions should be used in your daily training if you want to use your human machine to the best of its ability.

Moving Better

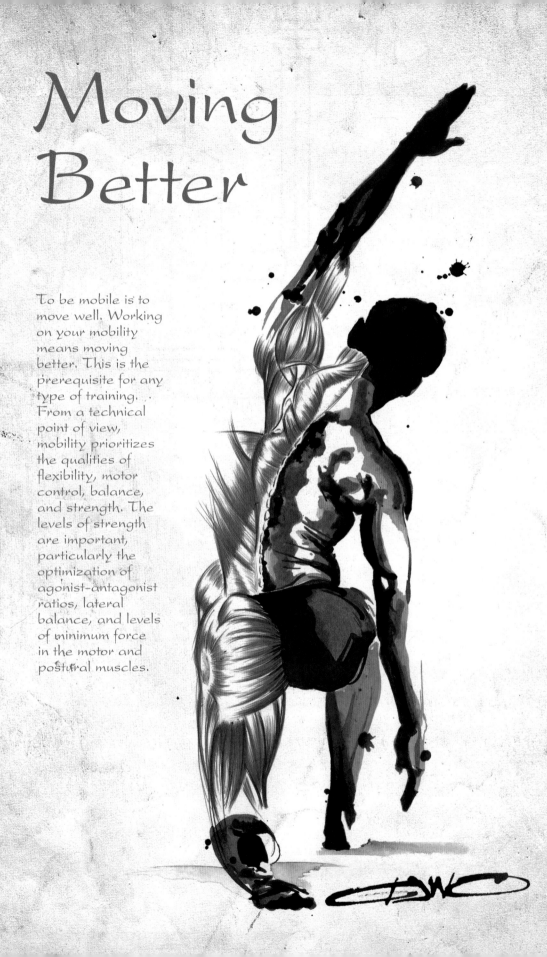

To be mobile is to move well. Working on your mobility means moving better. This is the prerequisite for any type of training. From a technical point of view, mobility prioritizes the qualities of flexibility, motor control, balance, and strength. The levels of strength are important, particularly the optimization of agonist-antagonist ratios, lateral balance, and levels of minimum force in the motor and postural muscles.

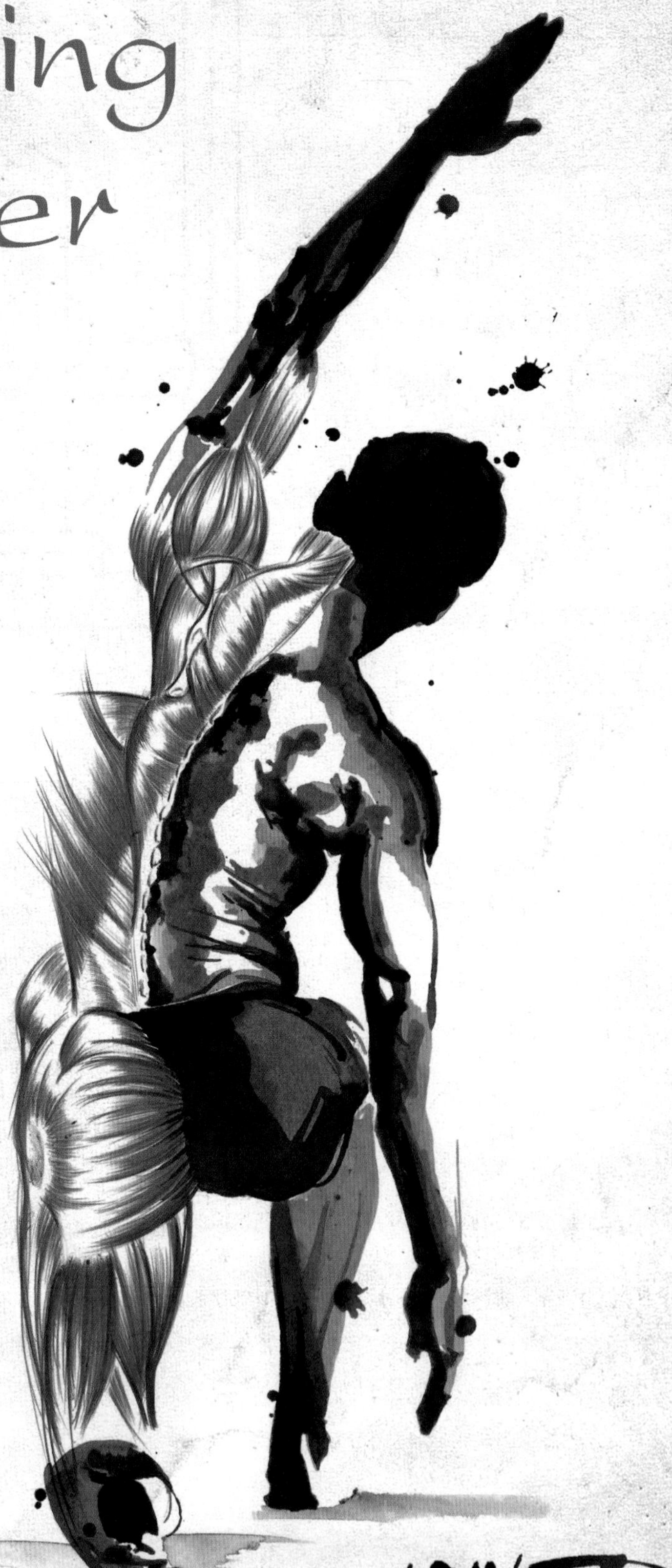

PART IV
MOBILITY

From a technical point of view, mobility prioritizes the qualities of flexibility, motor control, balance, and strength. The levels of strength are important, particularly the optimization of agonist-antagonist ratios, lateral balance, and levels of minimum force in the motor and postural muscles. When coaching people, I ask this question:

Can You Do It?

Are they able to do what I am asking them to do, before even considering the slightest additional load? Do they have the minimum ability to move and perform the exercise or pose that I am asking them to do?

FROM A TECHNICAL POINT OF VIEW, MOBILITY PRIORITIZES THE FOLLOWING QUALITIES:

FLEXIBILITY

Flexibility is simply the maximum joint range. Developing soft tissues' ability to stretch during joint movement is one of the keys to mobility.

MOTOR CONTROL

Motor control is the capacity to make dynamic postural adjustments and to direct the body and limbs when trying to do a certain movement.

BALANCE

Balance is an important physical quality. Often limited to only *proprioception* (moving all or part of the body without visual cues), an individual's ability to hold the body and maintain balance goes even further, calling on the *exteroceptive system* (responding to outside cues) and is an integral part of mobility training.

STRENGTH

In the context of mobility training, strength has nothing to do with exaggerated conventional strength, which is all about the maximum amount of force, enduring strength, or even power. Here, we are talking about the levels of minimum force required to move. The flexibility of the posterior chain may be impeccable, but if the anterior chain is not strong enough, movement will be affected.

The following levels of strength are particularly important:

- **Optimization of agonist-antagonist ratios:** Most muscles that act as an *agonist* (they shorten when the muscle contracts) have an *antagonist* that lengthens when the agonist muscle is active. Any unreasonable imbalance in the agonist-antagonist pair exposes you to injury and limits your mobility.
- **Lateral balance:** Functional lateral balance is also important. Coaches tend to be less obsessive about absolute balance today than they were in the past. In daily life, being balanced contributes to good health and is a priority when it comes to optimizing mobility.
- **Levels of minimum force in the motor muscles:** Some people are limited in their movement due to a lack of strength. This weakness is often obvious in the large motor muscles, which then must be trained so they can carry out their basic role. Strength is an essential element of functional training.
- **Levels of minimum force in the postural muscles:** Mobility is not only limited to movement; it can also malfunction when it comes to postural demands such as standing or sitting, which are often linked to weakness or stiffness in the deep muscles. Rehabilitating these muscles and strengthening them are crucial to returning to top shape.

Mobility can be described as controlled, active, polyarticular flexibility applied to movement.

EVALUATING MOBILITY

Evaluating this composite physical quality is as simple as it is complicated. We simply try to answer the question, "Can you do it?" At the same time, these capabilities are much more subjective than a physiological value like $\dot{V}O_2max$ (maximum volume of oxygen used during exercise, which is a good indication of a person's level of endurance) or a mechanical value like absolute force or absolute velocity during a muscle drive that allows for a precise evaluation of an athlete's power.

You will find effective tools in the literature such as the array of FMS® tests (Functional Movement Systems), which are excellent for quickly evaluating the motor patterns of an individual without being an expert in movement (Minick et al. 2010). This array of tests was recently increased from 21 points to 100 points, significantly increasing its precision (Butler et al. 2012). There are also the TPI® approaches (a training and certification system created in 2003, now called the Titleist Performance Institute) and Movement Matrix® (Comerford and Mottram 2012), which also provide applicable and effective solutions.

To be pragmatic and functional, we suggest using two tests for each of the major mobility development activities. In daily life, and even more in sport activities, we encounter situations that do not involve any additional weight (stooping, picking something up, sitting down, catching something, etc.) and situations with additional weight (carrying or lifting something heavy, etc.). Therefore, it is important to test both situations systematically. Furthermore, by completing our whole selection of tests, you will explore your body in its entirety, from analytical, single-joint problems to more general limitations within the whole muscle chain.

These simple tests will answer the fundamental questions:

CAN YOU DO IT?

ARE YOU FUNCTIONAL?

IF THE RESPONSE IS *NO*

Then you should make corrective adjustments within your training immediately. The goal is to regain a normal capacity for movement.

IF THE RESPONSE IS *YES*

Then these exercises will help you to maintain an already satisfactory level of mobility, and they could be spread throughout your training in a more intense or organized manner. You can also add in more intense and difficult exercises to develop your potential for movement beyond your normal level.

PLANNING FOR MOBILITY

If people are experiencing pain, they move poorly; if they move poorly, their limbs are not strong or stable. Mobility is built on movement, strength, and stability. Logically, improving mobility must be planned in the following order:

1. **Eradicate pain.**
2. **Regain minimum mobility.**
3. **Develop strength in the muscle chains.**
4. **Maintain mobility.**

Once any limitations are resolved and you reach a pain-free level of mobility, strength in the muscle chains and complex mobility must be maintained daily throughout your life. As a result, sessions to combat stiffness and pain become less urgent, but they still should be done at least weekly.

Regaining minimum mobility will no longer be a problem, but it is possible that stiffness due to age or acute or chronic injuries could push you to occasionally implement these methods again. Use this book when necessary.

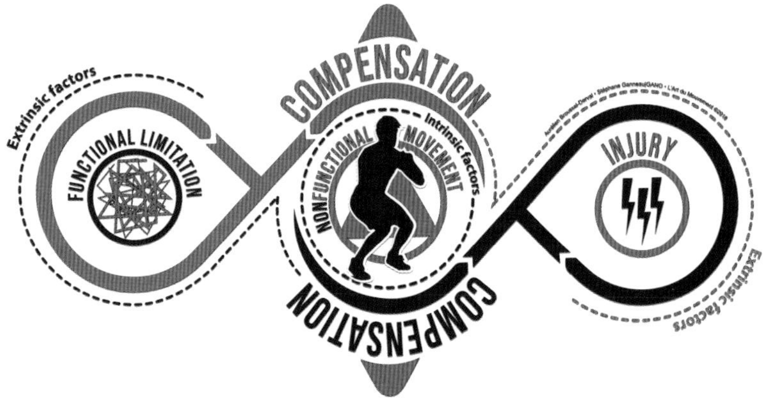

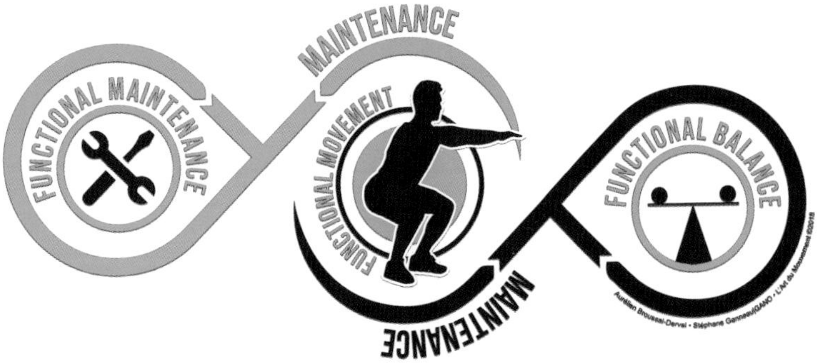

You need to create a plan to improve mobility.

REGAINING MOBILITY

The corrective method offered in this part aims to identify any lack of mobility in different movement situations. The program aims to regain minimum mobility so that your body is functional and operational, not only for training but also for a pain-free life without restrictions.

This method involves regaining optimal function during these basic movements:

- Sitting down
- Kneeling
- Lying down
- Extending
- Pulling
- Turning

Be sure to implement a corrective strategy immediately if you are unable to perform one of these basic functions or experience consistent pain when doing so.

These basic movements can be either restricted or amplified by the strong links in the muscle chains described earlier in this book and by their interactions in movement and posture. The next eight sections of the book discuss the most common mobility issues using the following titles:

- Shoulder Mobility
- Ankle Dorsiflexion
- Foot Mobility
- Stiffness in the Pelvis
- Knee Trajectory
- Restrictions in the Lower Posterior Chain
- Problems in the Upper Back
- Tension in the Lumbar Area

CORRECTIVE EXERCISES

If you notice a difficulty, a restriction, or even pain in your daily life, sporting practice, or when performing the different tests suggested in this book, you need to retrain your mobility. We recommend performing corrective exercises in three or four stages. Do these corrective exercises

- in the morning when you wake up, (Three Stages)
- in the evening before you go to bed, (Three Stages)
- during your warm-ups, and (Three Stages)
- during dedicated sessions when you can practice several exercises. In this case, you can do the fourth stage in which you add weight. (Four Stages)

THE FOUR STAGES CAN BE EXTENDED, MADE MORE INTENSE, OR BE PERFORMED SEPARATELY; HOWEVER, THEIR EFFECTIVENESS IS INCREASED BY COMBINING THEM.

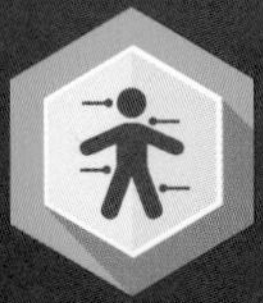

RELAX THE SOFT TISSUES

This first stage is crucial because it reduces pain and muscle tension and prepares the muscle to lengthen and move better. Self-massage is an essential first step to get the most benefit from the stretch.

INCREASE RANGE OF MOTION

Now that the muscles, tendons, and fascia are relaxed, the second stage is to change the length of these structures through stretching. All stretching techniques are designed to improve flexibility through passive poses, passive stretching by contracting and relaxing, or *ballistic* (bouncing) stretching for those who are more trained. To reprogram posture, we will also use resistance bands to re-center and open the joints during this stage.

TRANSFER TO MOVEMENT

Active flexibility, motor control, balance, and dynamic core strength are generally combined in the exercises used in this stage to enhance mobility. Since they are passive and local, increases in range of motion do not necessarily translate into movement, making this stage so important.

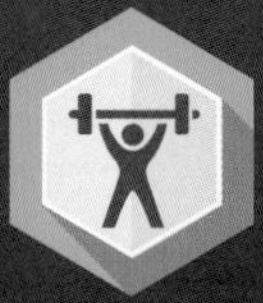

OPTIONAL: USE WEIGHT

For those who ultimately want to prepare for physical training—to benefit your daily life and to increase active flexibility—resistance training exercises using a large range of motion should be used at the end of a corrective exercise session. The correct weight must be used; we are not trying to gain strength but to increase mobility. Thus, the ideal weight varies for each person. Be sure to choose a weight that increases your range of motion without compensating your posture or the quality of the technique used to perform the exercise.

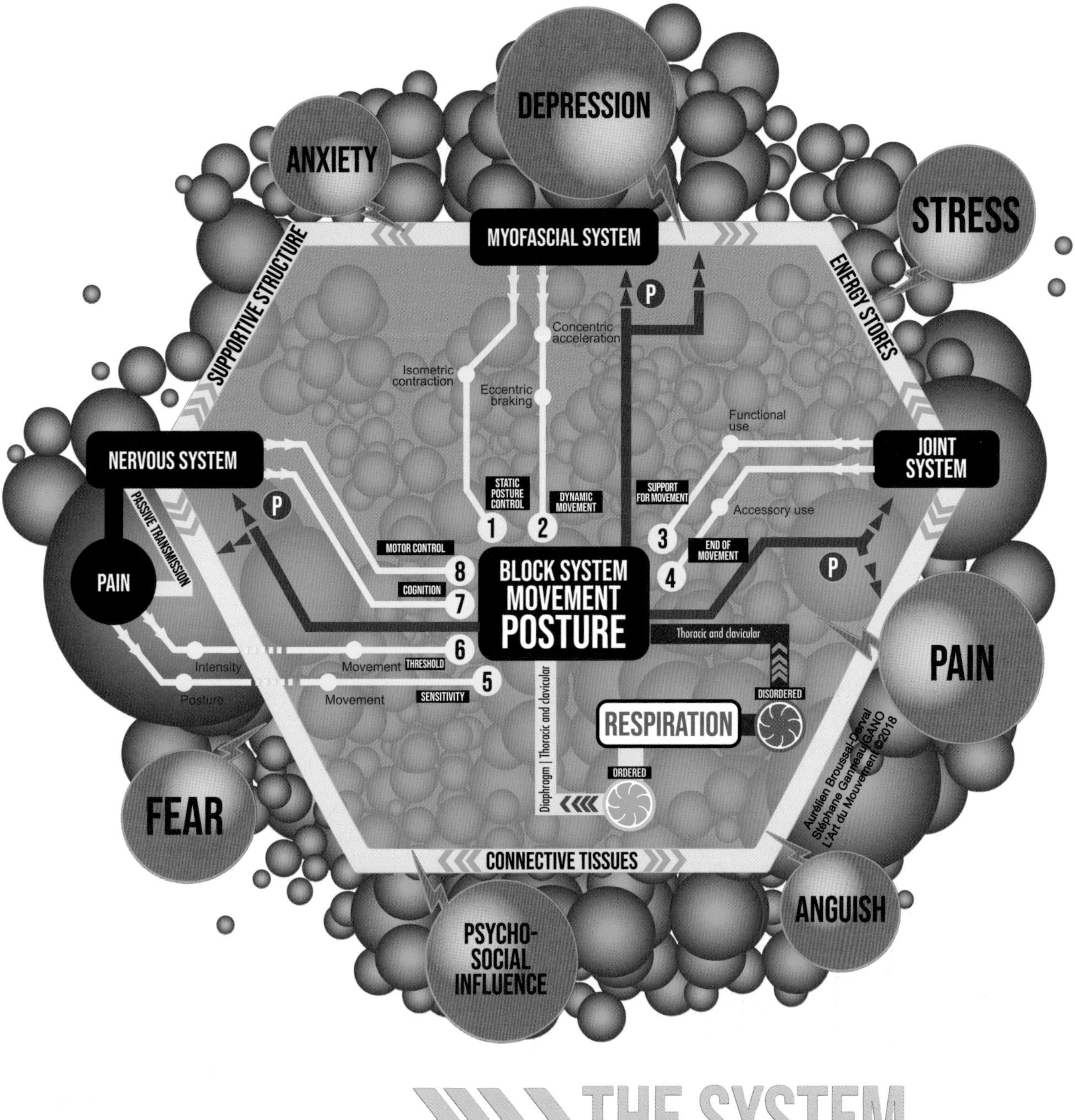

THE SYSTEM OF MOVEMENT

DISRUPTION

P PROPRIOCEPTION

DIFFERENT STRETCHING METHODS

Stretching methods are widely debated in the world of sport because they can serve many purposes. From recovery to warming up, their purposes vary; how they are used must be adjusted based on the situation. Two proven methods can be used independently during stage 2 of this method (increase range of motion).

Passive stretch: This method is generally for beginners but can be used throughout your training no matter what your level. You do risk seeing your progress plateau sooner or later, so move on to contracting and relaxing stretches when you are able.

The basic move as adapted to our method: Lengthen the muscle as much as you can without causing pain and hold the position for 20 to 30 seconds. A more advanced option for athletes who are doing purposeful flexibility training is to bounce to increase the range of motion.

Contract/relax: This method is more advanced. First, intensely contract the muscle to be stretched and then immediately perform a passive stretch for that muscle. There are several variations of this method that can be used depending on the stiffness of the area and the intensity that you wish to experience during the exercise. For example, first lengthen the target muscle then intensely contract it, either in the air (passively) or by using a band, for 3 to 10 seconds. Follow that with a 10- to 20-second stretch of the target muscle. Gradually increase your range of motion during the stretch by starting the next stretch from the position you just reached during each new contracting and relaxing cycle.

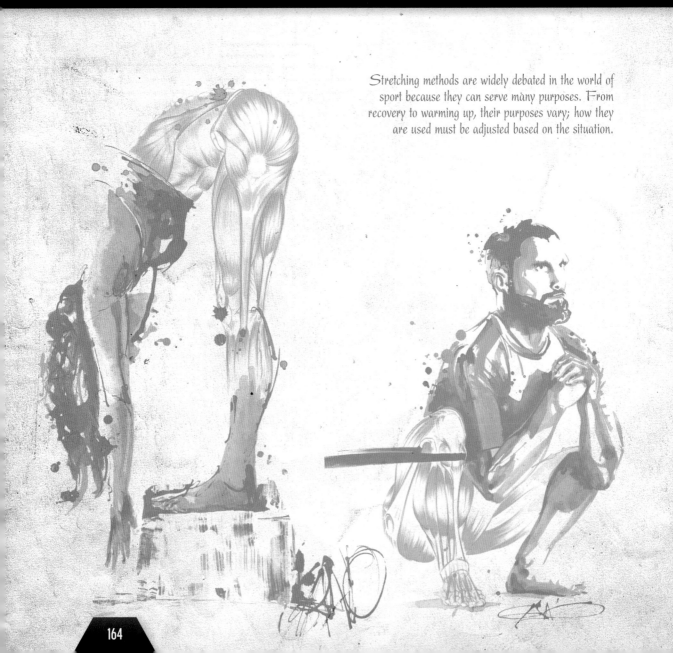

Stretching methods are widely debated in the world of sport because they can serve many purposes. From recovery to warming up, their purposes vary; how they are used must be adjusted based on the situation.

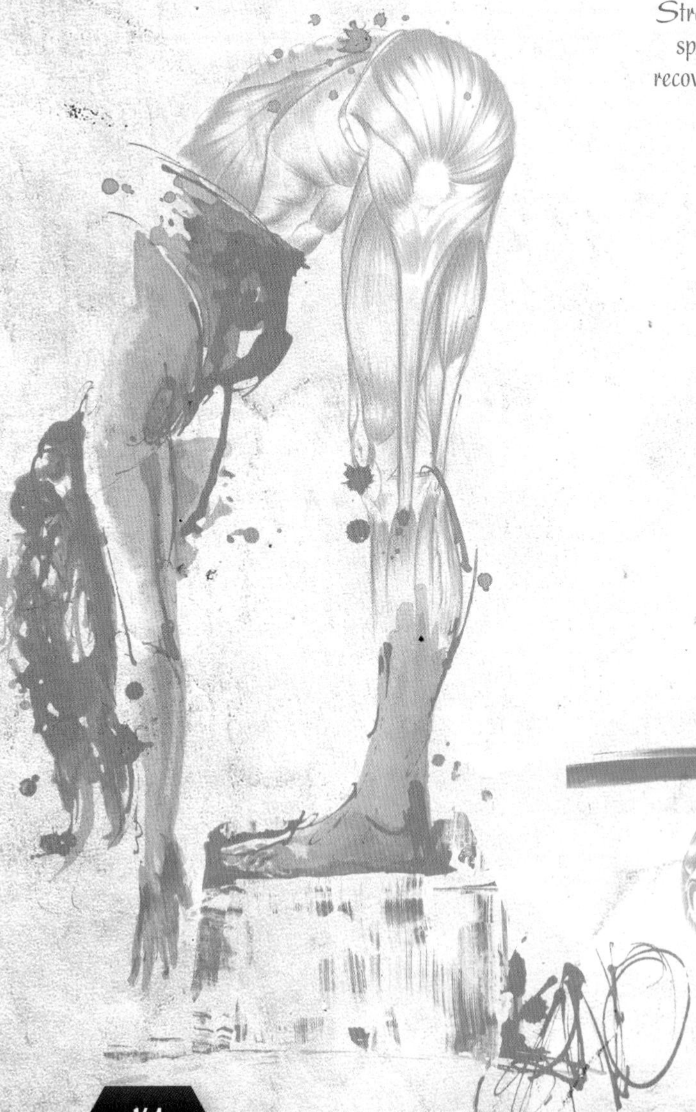

TESTS

SHOULDER MOBILITY

1

FMS Shoulder Test

Stand up and make fists with your thumbs inside. Flex your elbows and reach one arm over your shoulder and the other arm behind your back. Bring both hands as close together as possible behind your back without opening your fists. Perform the test in both directions. This test is successful if you have less than a hand-width of space between your fists.

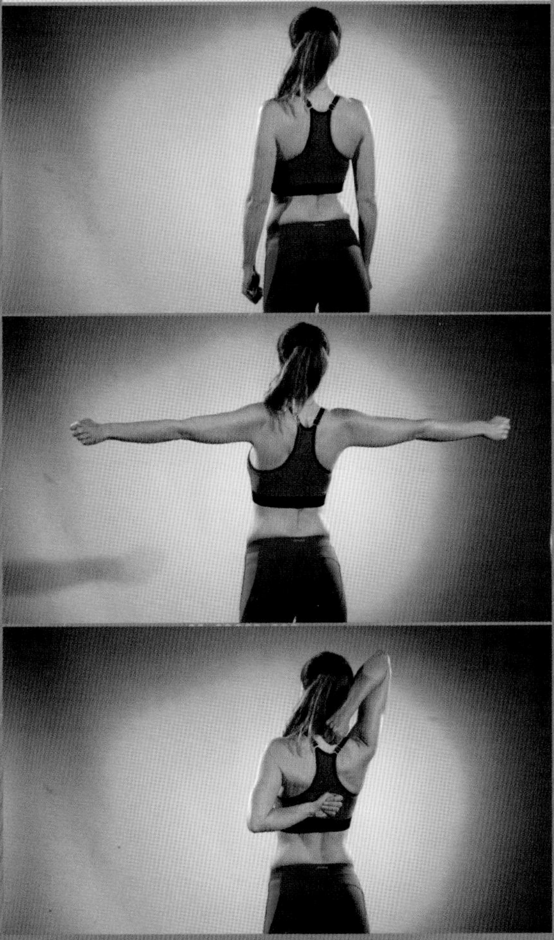

2

Dumbbell Carry Test

Stand up and hold a 20-lb (9.1-kg) dumbbell in each hand. Observe your natural position when holding them: If your chest is out, your shoulders are low and back, and the dumbbells are pointing outward, you have passed the test.

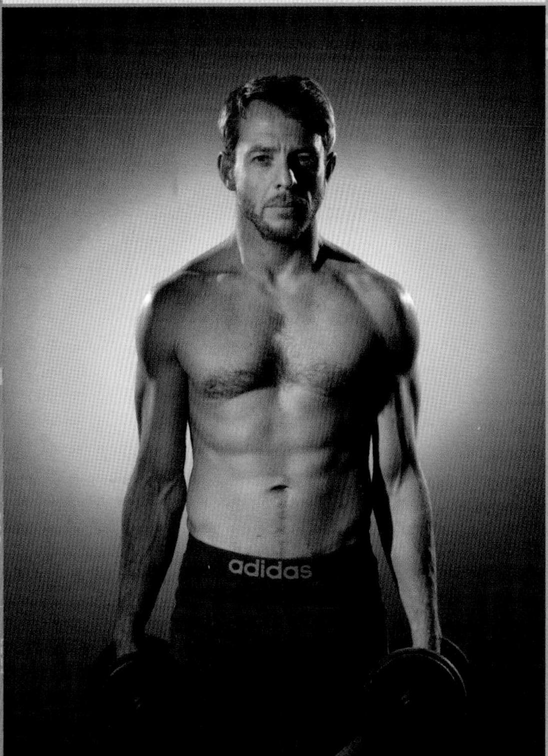

solution 01

MASSAGE STRETCHING MOBILIZATION WEIGHTS

Perform one to three sets of each of the following exercises in order on the same shoulder. Do not stop between exercises. When they are completed, go through the series again for the other shoulder.

SHOULDER MOBILITY

01. CHEST MASSAGE USING A BALL

Face a wall with one hand behind your back and place a massage ball under your collarbone on the pectoralis minor muscle. Many people can find this muscle with their fingers; it feels like a piece of rope. Block the ball between your chest and a wall. **Roll 10 times from top to bottom, 10 times from left to right, and 10 times in a circular motion on the most sensitive areas.**

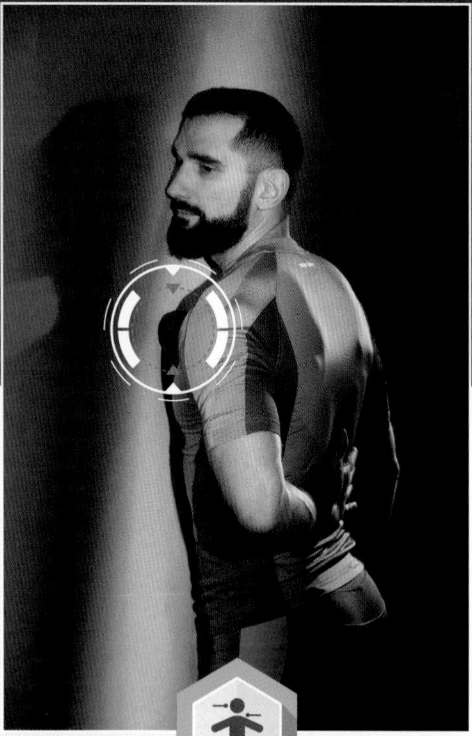

02. BAND STRETCH

Hang a resistance band from a high stationary bar. Keeping the band nearly perpendicular to the floor, put your wrist through the bottom of the loop with your hand on your back as if someone is putting you in an arm lock. Get in a lunge position with your legs (lunge with the leg opposite the arm behind your back). Without allowing your shoulder to move forward or inward, slowly lower in the lunge so the band pulls on your hand to create the stretch. Aim to lower your body to raise your hand as high as possible. **Hold the stretch for 30 seconds.**

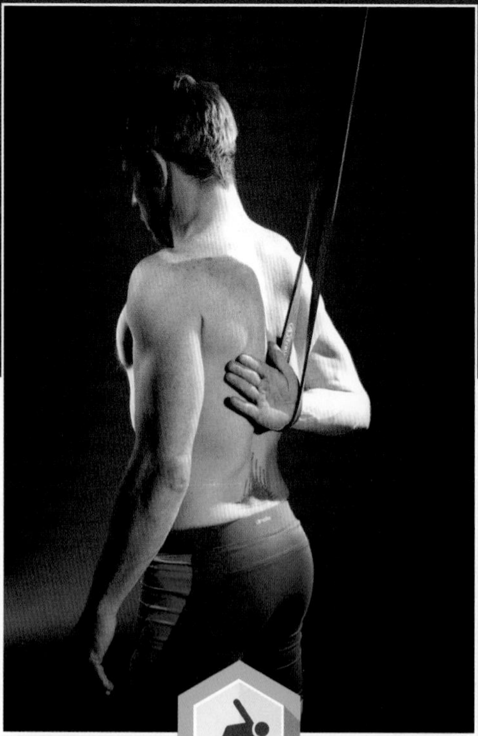

03. BLUE ANGEL

Lie on the floor on your abdomen, place a massage ball below your collarbone, and block it between your pectoralis minor and the floor. Place the arm on the side with the ball behind your back in the arm lock position and move your hand as far up your back as possible. **Repeat 10 times.**

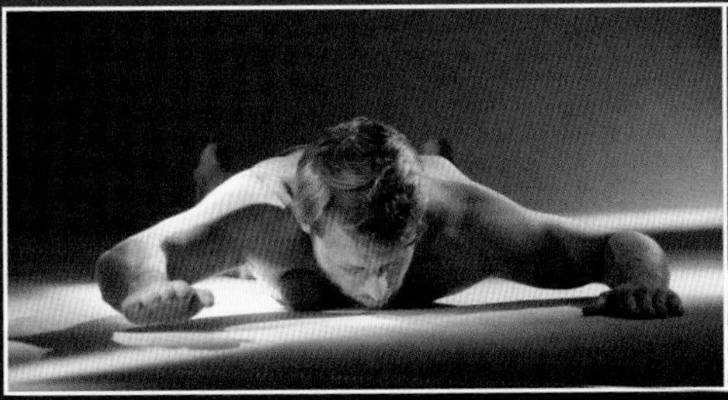

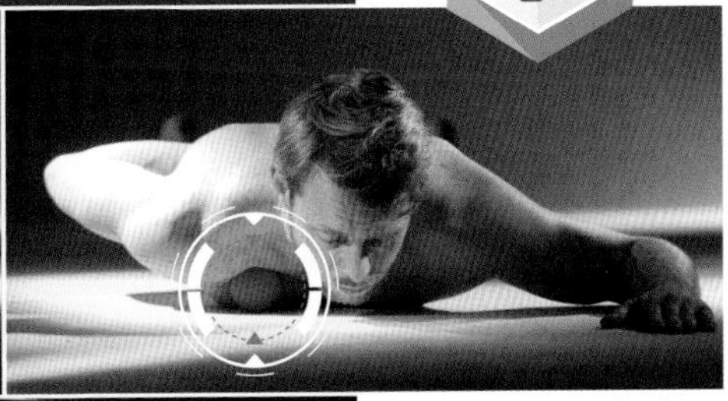

04. OPTIONAL: KETTLEBELL ARM BAR

Lie on your side in the fetal position and grab a kettlebell with both hands. Roll onto your back. Lift the kettlebell vertically with one hand. Extend your free arm above your head and flex the hip and knee of your opposite leg to place the foot flat on the floor to support yourself. Continue the lateral movement by moving the supporting leg (with the knee still flexed) across the other leg. Next, straighten both legs to a parallel position and press your hips to be flat on the floor. **Hold this pose as long as possible, at least 15 seconds.**

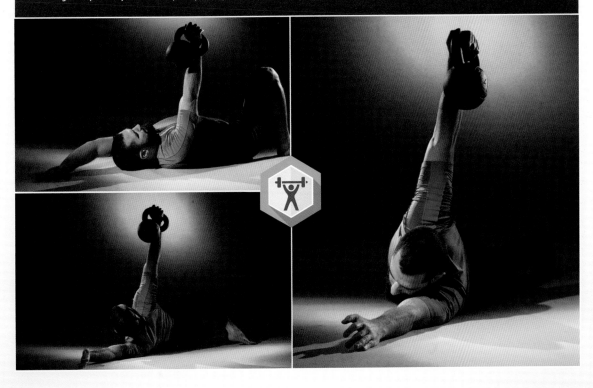

solution 02

MASSAGE · STRETCHING · MOBILIZATION · WEIGHTS

Perform one to three sets of each of the following exercises in order on the same shoulder. Do not stop between exercises. When they are completed, go through the series again for the other shoulder.

SHOULDER MOBILITY

01. MIDDLE AND POSTERIOR DELTOID MASSAGE WITH DIFFERENT ELBOW POSITIONS

Lie on your side and slide a small massage ball between the middle of the shoulder and the floor. Roll from front to back, from left to right, and in a circular motion. Keep the arm free then manually externally or internally rotate the arm. You can start the stretching stage from this position by contracting and relaxing in the externally or internally rotated position. **Perform 10 massages of each type.**

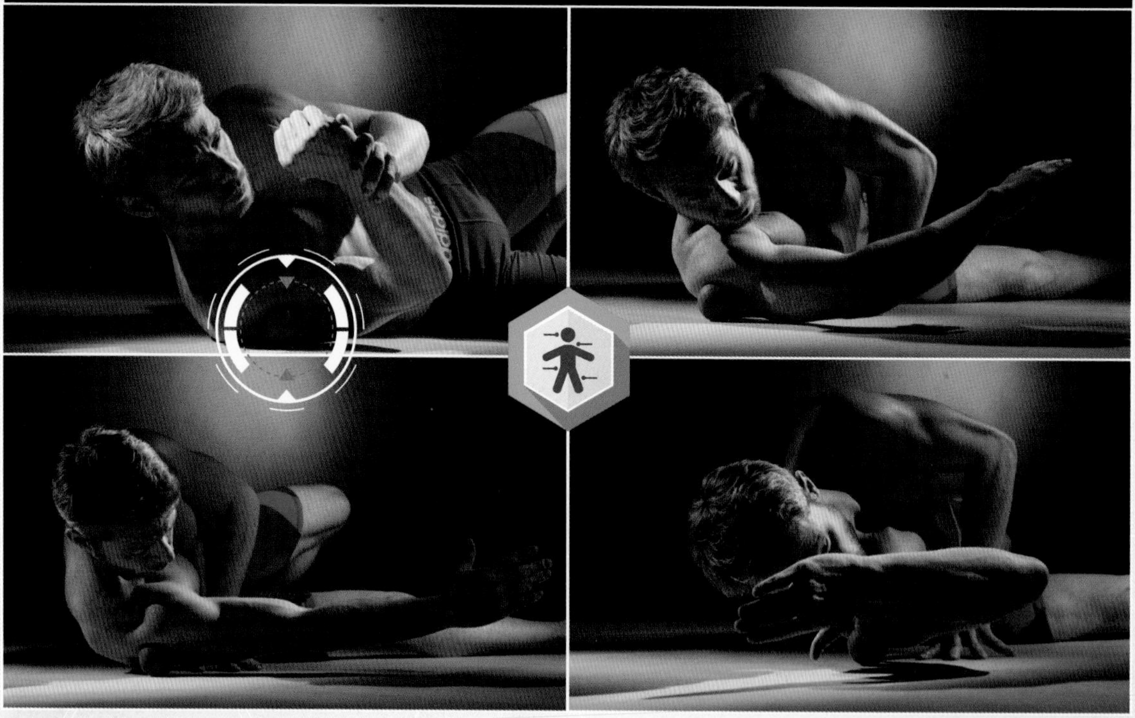

02. MIDDLE DELTOID STRETCH ON THE FLOOR

Lie flat on your abdomen (or get on all fours if you are too stiff) and cross one arm under your chest, perpendicular to your torso. Try to avoid compensating with your shoulder muscles. **Hold the stretch for 30 seconds.**

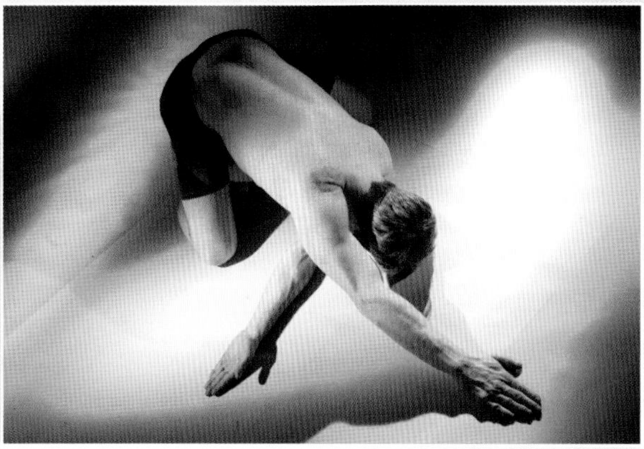

03. SHOULDER ROTATOR SMASH

Hold a ball and lie on your back with your elbow flexed and your shoulder internally rotated to 90 degrees. Slide a small massage ball under your shoulder and alternate between internal and external shoulder rotations while keeping pressure on the ball. **Perform 10 rotations.**

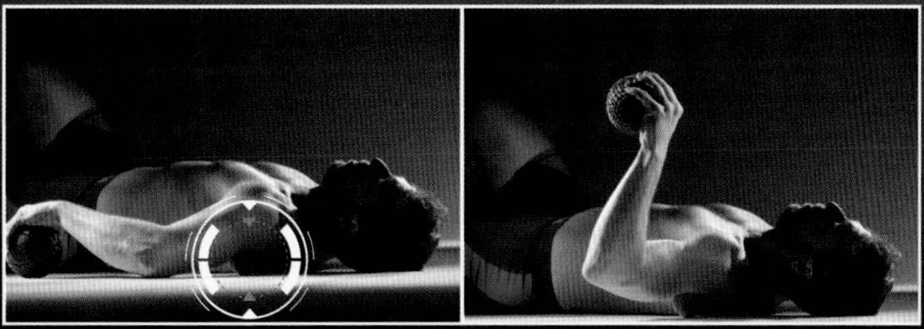

04. OPTIONAL: ROTATOR CUFF EXERCISE ON A BALL WITH A KETTLEBELL

Sit next to an exercise ball and place your elbow in the middle of the top of the ball, flattening it in the middle. Maintain pressure throughout the exercise by tilting a kettlebell from front to back using an internal or external rotation of your shoulder. Increase your range of motion on each repetition. **Perform 10 rotations.**

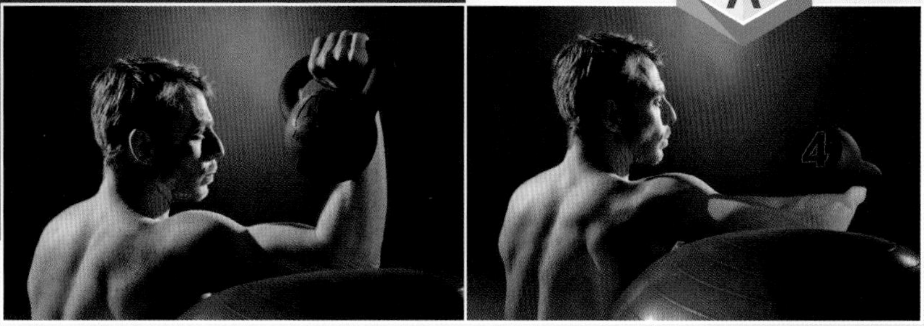

solution
03

MASSAGE | STRETCHING | MOBILIZATION | WEIGHTS

Perform one to three sets of each of the following exercises in order, alternating sides as you go along. Do not stop between exercises.

SHOULDER MOBILITY

01. POSTERIOR DELTOID MASSAGE USING A BALL

Stand with your back against a wall and place a massage ball between your shoulder and the wall (see left-hand photo). Roll from top to bottom, from bottom to top, then make circular movements. Use three different arm positions: arm behind your back, arm extended in front of you, and arm overhead. **Perform 10 massages in each position.**

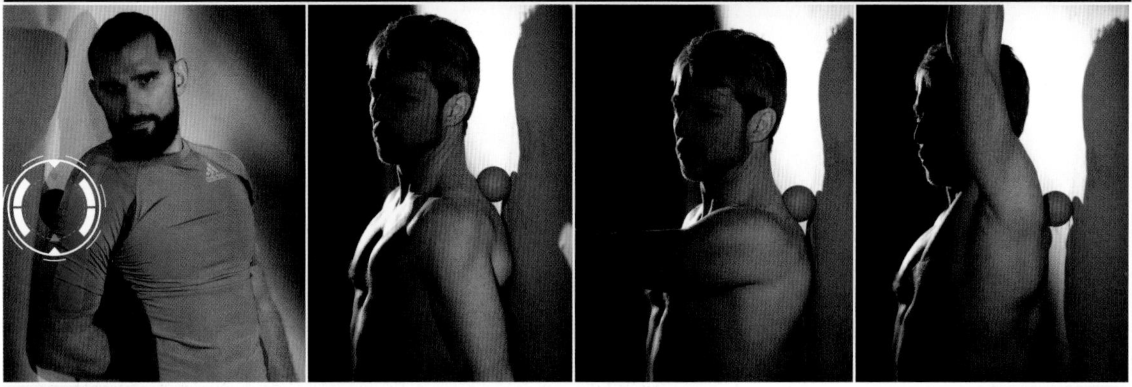

02. OVERHEAD STRETCH

Use a table for support. With your chest out and shoulders down, flex your hips and place your head between your extended arms with your chest parallel to the floor and perpendicular to your nearly straight legs and your wrists and hands on top of the table. This exercise has two variations: palms up or palms down. For a more advanced version, kneel on the floor. **Hold the stretch for 20 to 30 seconds.**

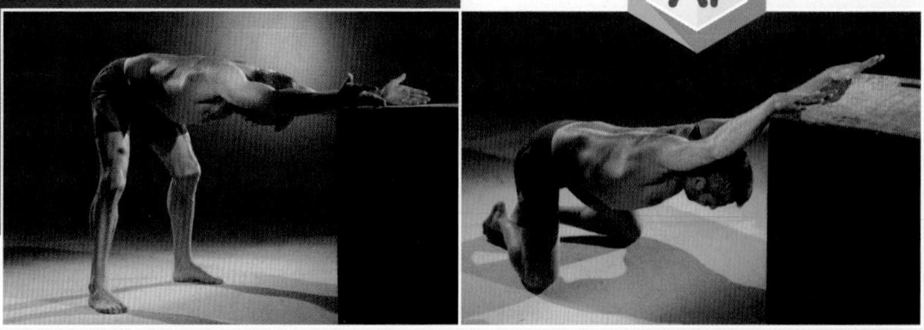

03. PRONE SWIMMING

Lie on your abdomen, extend your arms, and cross them above your head. Turn your body very slightly to the side and make a circle with the arm on the inner side, then lift your body slightly to pass the arm under your torso. The less you raise the torso, the more pressure you put on your shoulder. **Perform 3 to 4 reps on each side.**

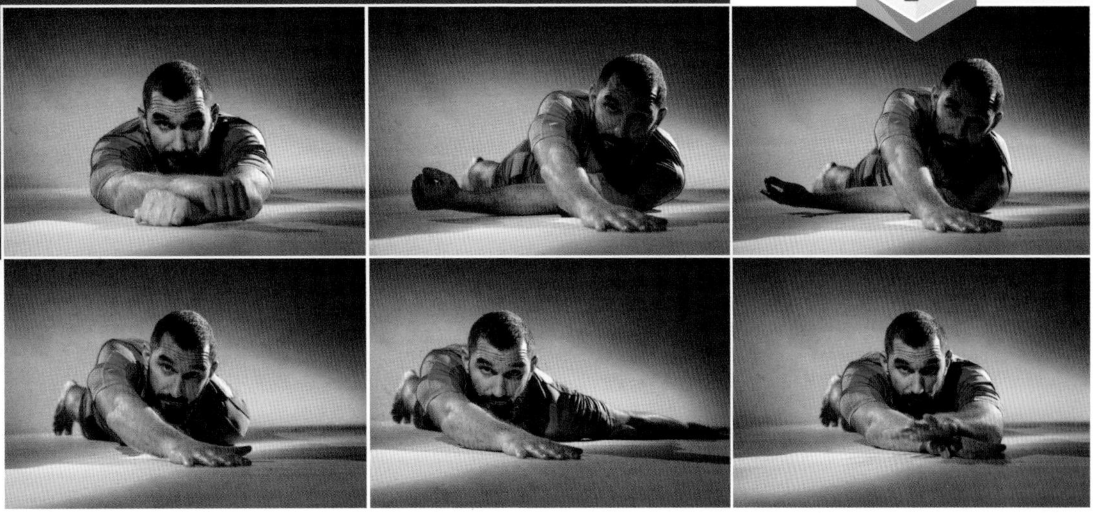

04. OPTIONAL: SHOULDER EXERCISE ON A BALL

Lie on your back on an exercise ball and support yourself on your tiptoes. Completely extend your back. Add shoulder rotations by grabbing a weight plate of 2.5 to 5 pounds (1.1 to 2.3 kg) in each hand. Lower your shoulder, keeping your little finger pointing toward your legs. As you reach hip level, rotate your hand so your thumb points down. Raise your arm with your pinky finger pointing up. Your pinky always guides the direction of movement to avoid any conflicts in the shoulder. The other arm does the same movement. **Perform 10 rotations per arm.**

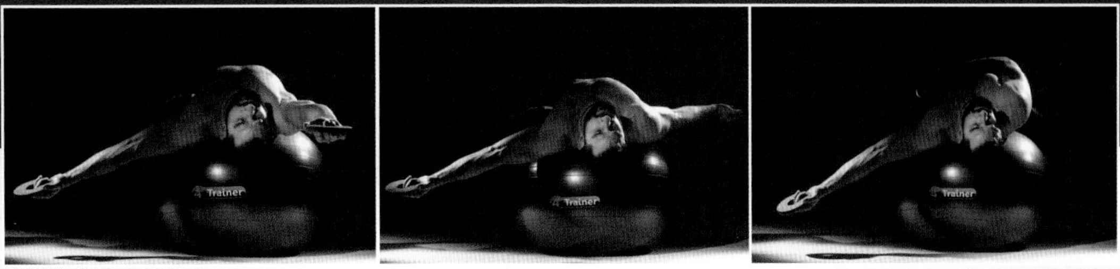

solution

04

SHOULDER MOBILITY

MASSAGE

STRETCHING

MOBILIZATION

WEIGHTS

Perform one to three sets of each of the following exercises in order on the same shoulder. Do not stop between exercises. When they are completed, go through the series again for the other shoulder.

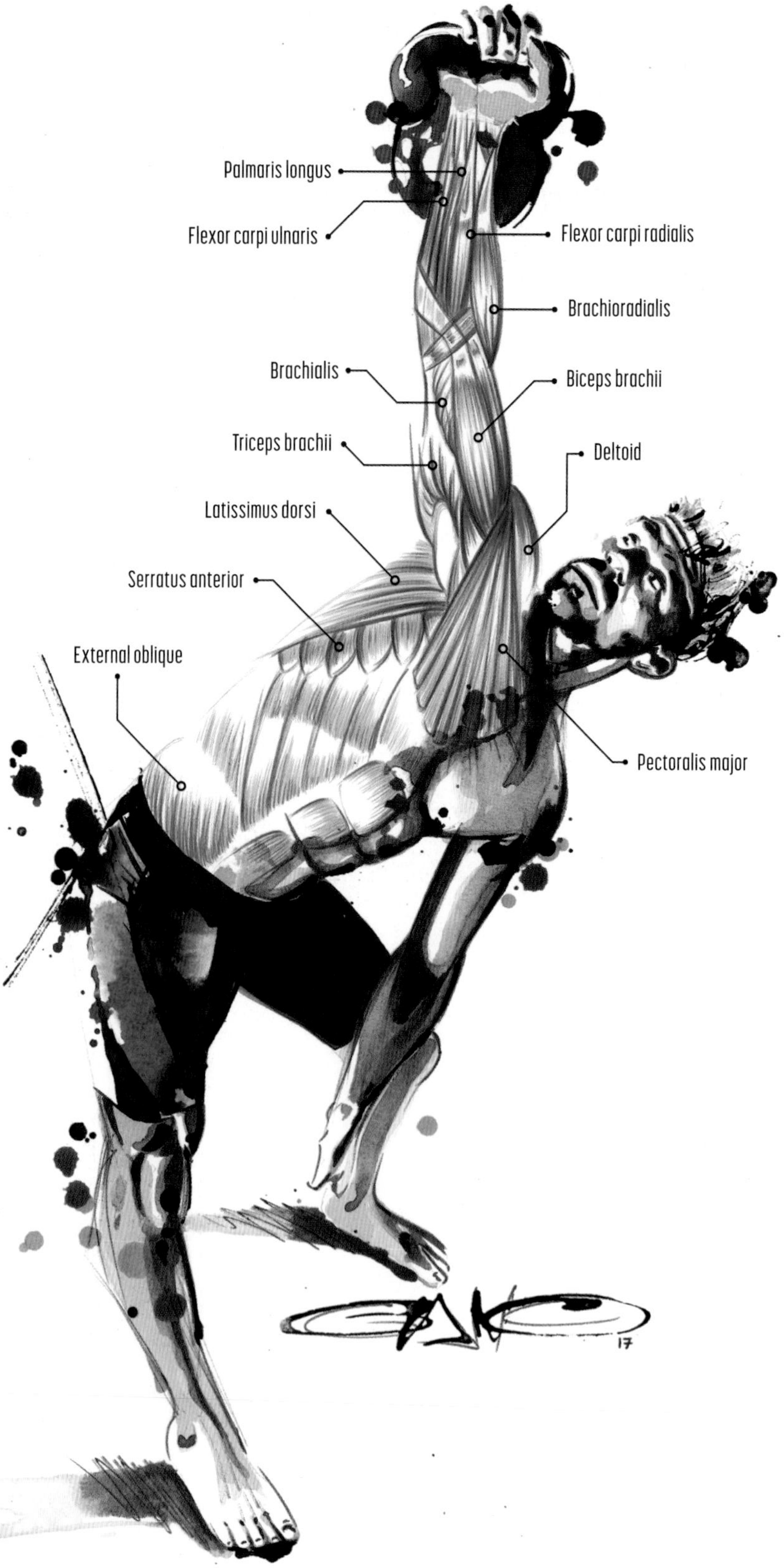

01. ANTERIOR DELTOID MASSAGE USING A BALL

Place a massage ball at the front of your shoulder, then press yourself against a wall. Roll from top to bottom, from left to right, and in a circular motion.

Perform 10 massages in each direction.

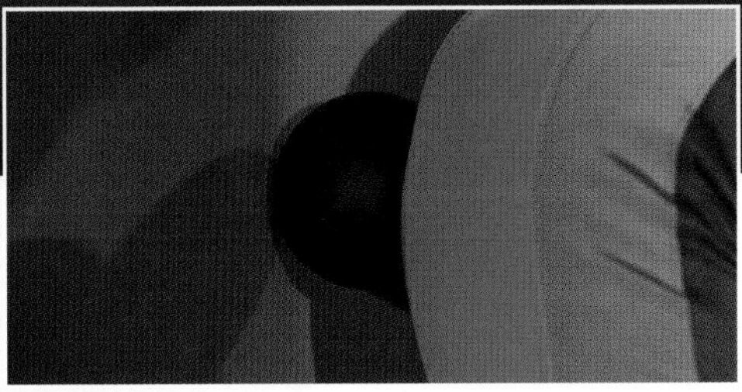

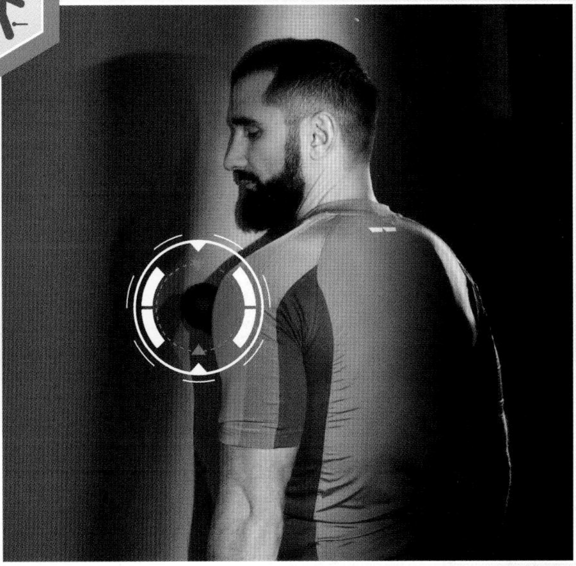

02. SUSPENSION TRAINER SHOULDER STRETCH

With the handles at middle height, flex your hips and keep your back straight. Flex your knees slightly and allow yourself to move backward as you hold on to the handles. **Hold the stretch for 20 to 30 seconds, then rotate to spend 20 to 30 seconds on each side for a greater stretch.**

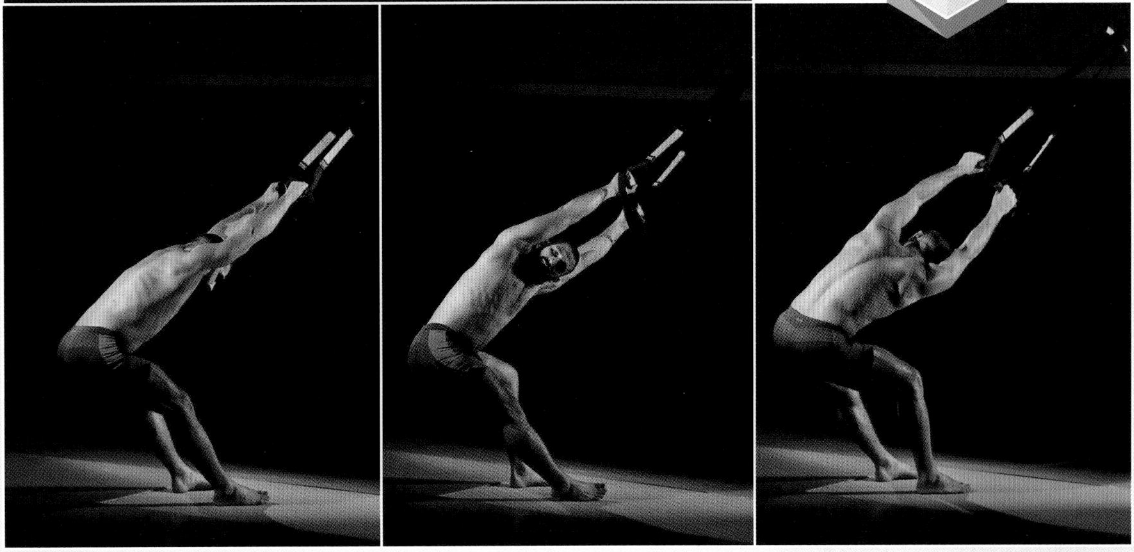

03. SUSPENSION TRAINER WALL SLIDE

With your back to the straps in their lowest position, combine a wide forward lunge with a double-arm raise overhead. Once in position, lower your elbows down to where your upper arms are parallel to the floor. Keep your elbows in line with your torso, as if your chest was leaning forward against a wall and you are trying to keep your arms from touching the wall. Do not arch your lower back when you are in the lunge position, and avoid any other postural compensations.

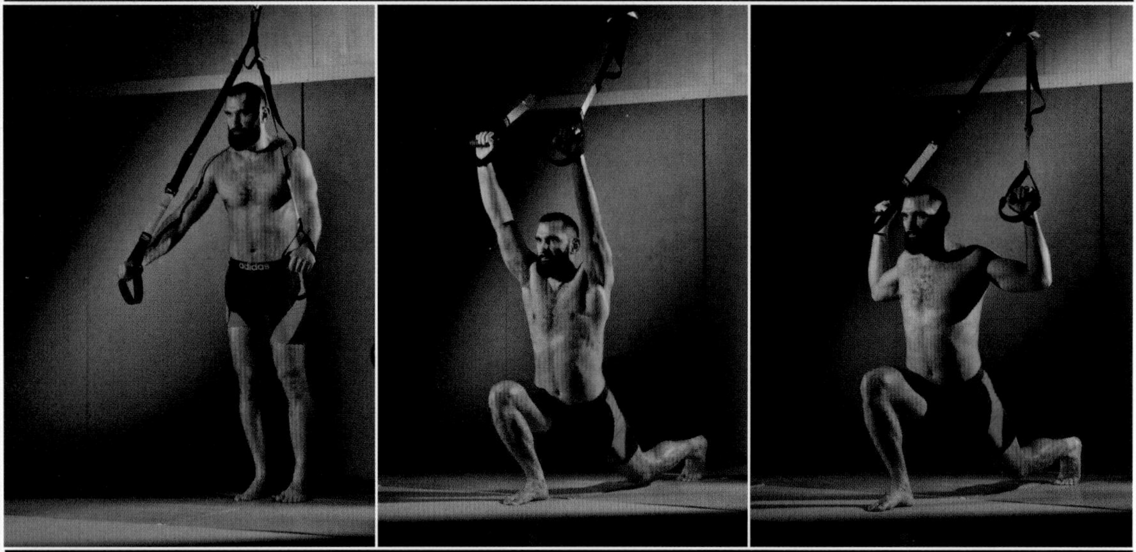

As a variation, rotate to each side when you are in the lunged and double-arm overhead position to engage your functional and spiral chains. **Perform 5 reps on each side.**

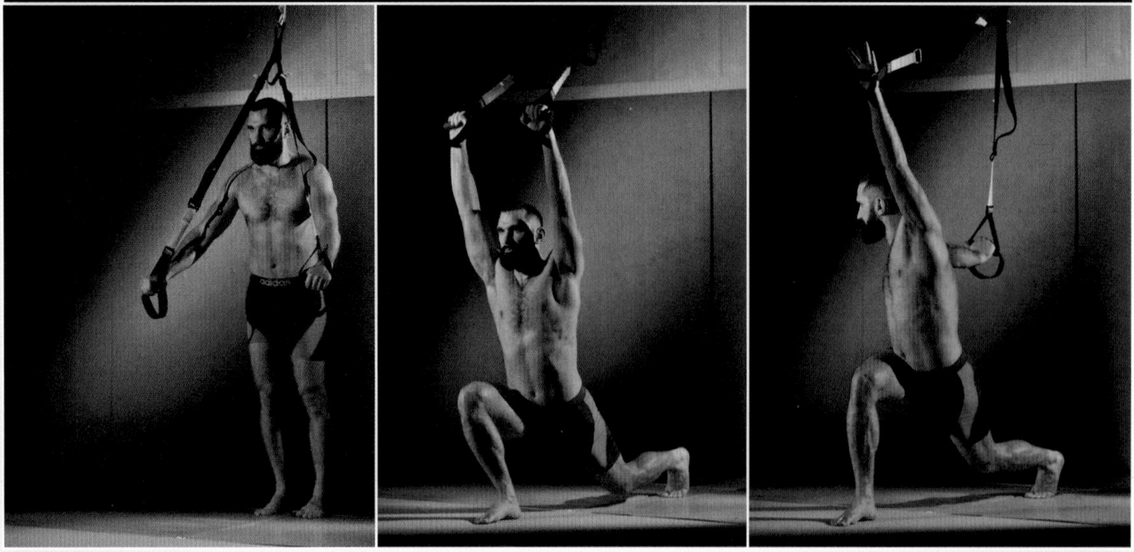

04. OPTIONAL: WINDMILL KETTLEBELL

From a standing position, hold a kettlebell above your head with a fully extended elbow. Without flexing your elbow, flex your torso forward and rotate so that your free arm slides along the leg (on the same side) until, if possible, your fingers touch the floor. Keep visual contact with your kettlebell throughout the exercise. Ideally, keep both knees extended. If you must flex one of your knees, flex the knee on the free side, which will apply an additional stretch. Move down as low as possible, then move up in the same slow and controlled manner, always keeping visual contact with the kettlebell. **Perform 10 repetitions per arm.**

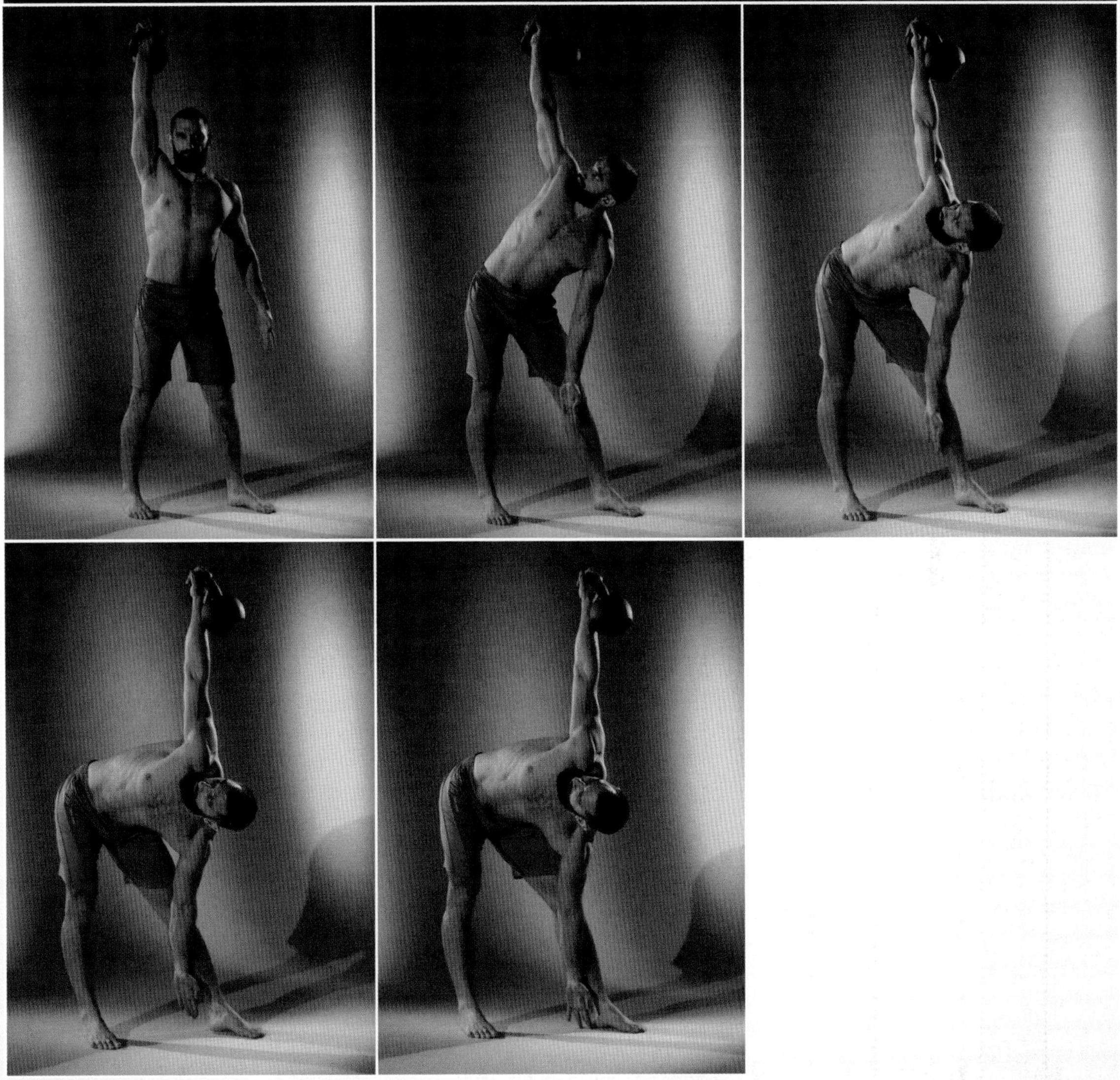

solution 05

MASSAGE | STRETCHING | MOBILIZATION | WEIGHTS

Perform one to three sets of each of the following exercises in order on the same shoulder. Do not stop between exercises. When they are completed, go through the series again for the other shoulder.

SHOULDER MOBILITY

01. TRAPEZIUS MASSAGE USING A WEIGHT BAR

In a staggered stance position, place a weight bar on top of your trapezius as shown in the middle photo. Tilt your head forward and away from the bar to lengthen the muscle. A variation is to perform the massage with the arm on the same side as the bar extended overhead. **Perform 10 times by rolling the bar up and down over the trapezius.**

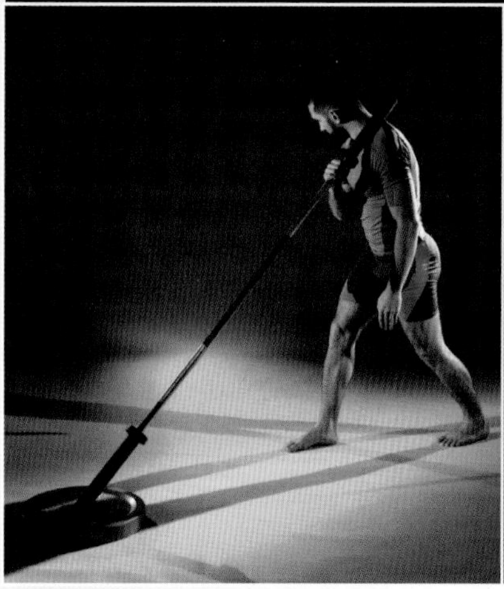

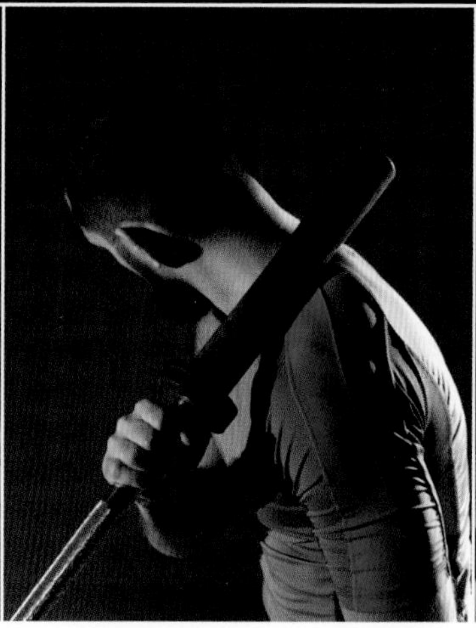

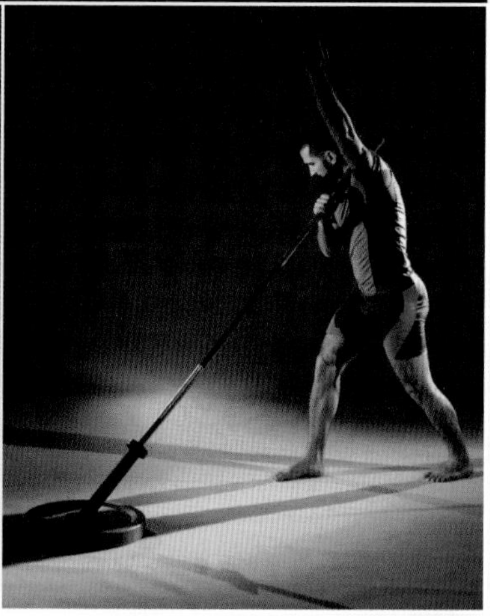

02. RESISTANCE BAND SLING STRETCH

Anchor the band to the floor and loop it over your shoulder with the anchor point behind you. Lunge forward so the band pulls your shoulder down and backward; try to relax your trapezius as much as possible. Hold the stretch for 20 seconds. Then shrug your shoulder and hold it in the elevated position for a few seconds and then relax back to the stretched position for a few seconds. Finish by making circles with your shoulder. **Hold for 20 seconds in a passive stretch. Perform 3 contracting/relaxing movements, then perform 10 circles.**

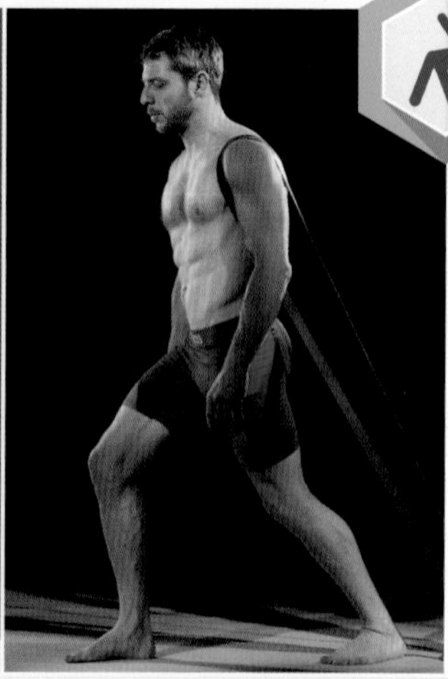

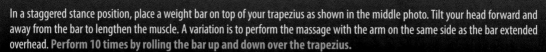

03. ARM RAISE WITH A COMPRESSION STICK

Lie on your back with a stick stuck between a wall and your trapezius. Raise your arm (on the same side as the stick) up to be perpendicular to the floor and then over your head. Keep your hand open and your palm facing in throughout the movement. **Perform 10 reps.**

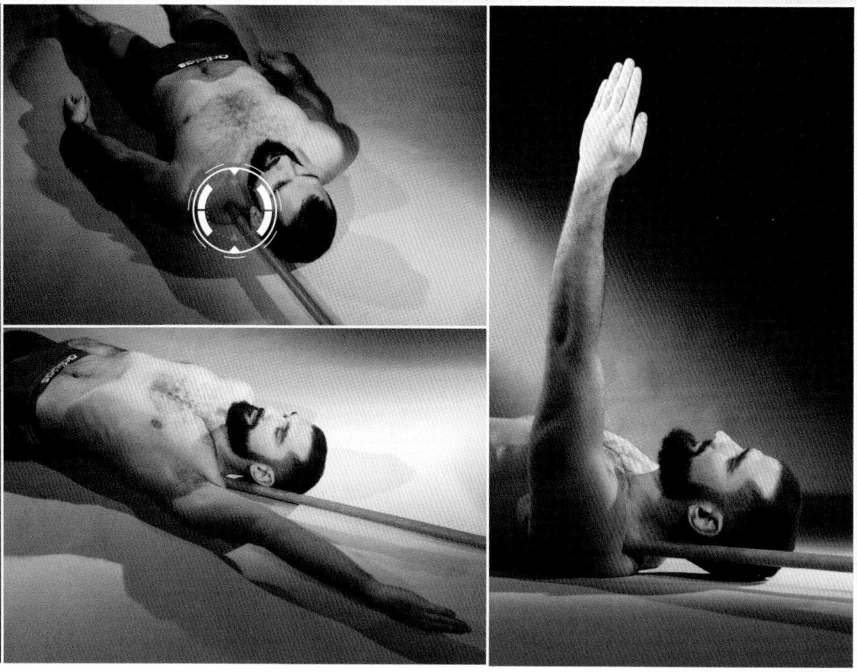

04. OPTIONAL: KETTLEBELL AND RESISTANCE BAND COMBINATION

Lie on your back and raise a kettlebell in a neutral grip above you. On that same arm, hook a resistance band around the upper arm. Have the band pull the upper arm out to (from) the side. Raise your hips in a bridge position to move the shoulder to the back of its socket. In this position, slowly rotate your shoulder in and then out. **Perform 6 reps (3 inward rotations and 3 outward rotations).**

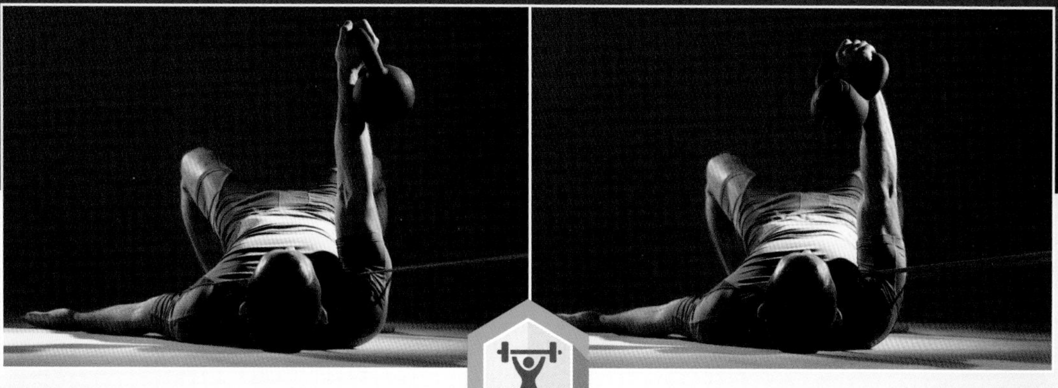

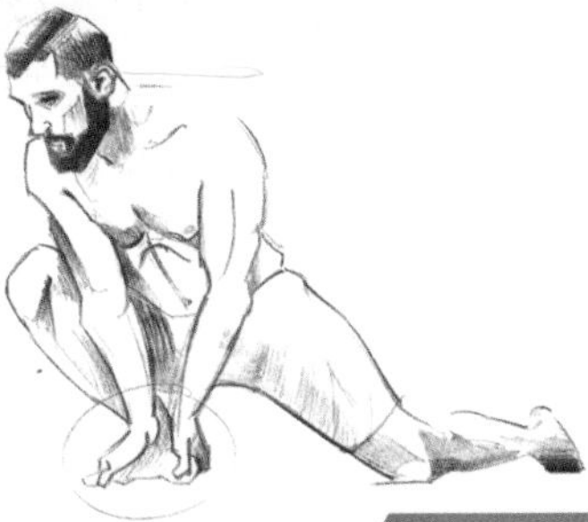

ANKLE DORSIFLEXION

1

Knighthood

Lunge toward a wall with the toes of your front foot one fist's distance away from the wall and your back knee on the floor. With your front foot flat on the floor (do not lift your heel off the floor during this test) and the instep of your back foot flat on the floor, place your hands on your hips and shift your position forward to move your front knee beyond your front foot toward the wall. If your kneecap touches the wall, you passed the test.

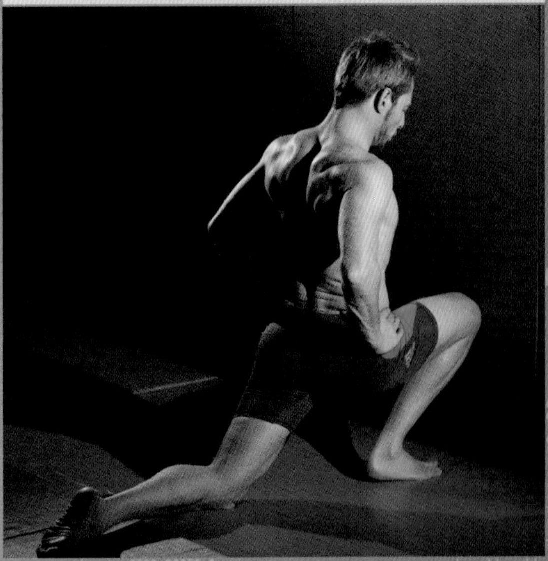

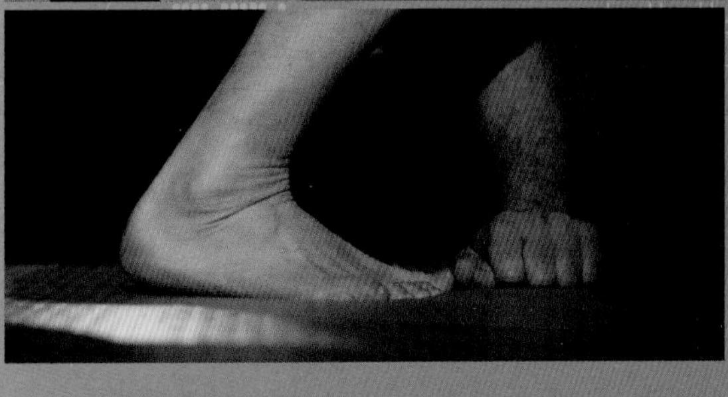

2

Pistol Test

Hang a resistance band above you and grab it with both hands. Keep one supporting foot flat on the floor (do not lift your heel off the floor) and move into a squat position on only one leg. Slow your descent using the resistance band. This test is successful if you can move into a full squat without lifting your heel.

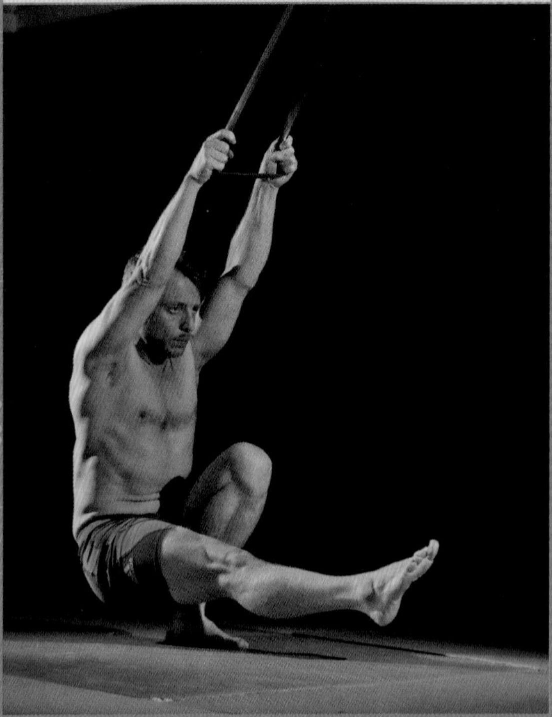

Perform one to three sets of each of the following exercises in order, alternating sides as you go along. Do not stop between exercises.

MASSAGE | STRETCHING | MOBILIZATION | WEIGHTS

solution 01

ANKLE DORSIFLEXION

01. CALF MASSAGE USING A ROLLER

Place your calf on the roller and alter the intensity of the massage by pressing your buttocks toward the floor. Intensify the massage even more, if necessary, by crossing your free leg over the one being massaged.
Perform 10 front-to-back rolls, 10 left-to-right rolls, and 10 circular ankle movements.

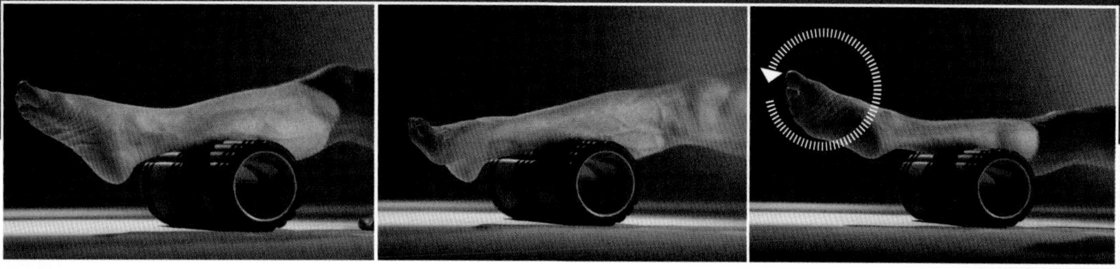

02. KNIGHTHOOD STRETCH WITH FOOT ANCHORED TO THE FLOOR

From a very low lunge position with the knee and instep of your back leg and foot on the floor, hold your front foot to anchor it to the floor. Move your front knee as far forward as you can without lifting the heel of your front foot off the floor. To increase the stretch, allow your front knee to go beyond the toes of your front foot as much as possible.
Hold the stretch for 30 seconds.

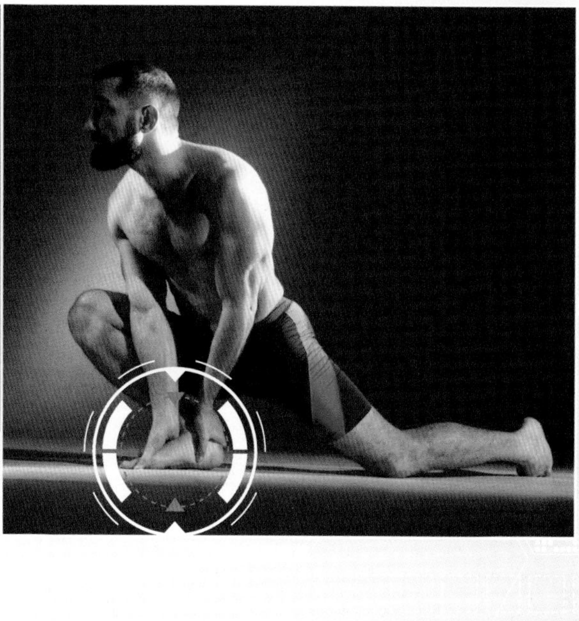

03. AIKIDO MOVES

This move is inspired by Aikido and is a powerful exercise for dynamic ankle flexibility. From a low lunge position, slowly allow the front knee to pass over the toes, delaying the moment when the heel of your front foot lifts off the floor. Once it does, place your front knee on the floor and reverse your position to work on the other ankle. (The final photo shows a stretch on both legs and feet.)

Perform by moving forward 3 times on each side.

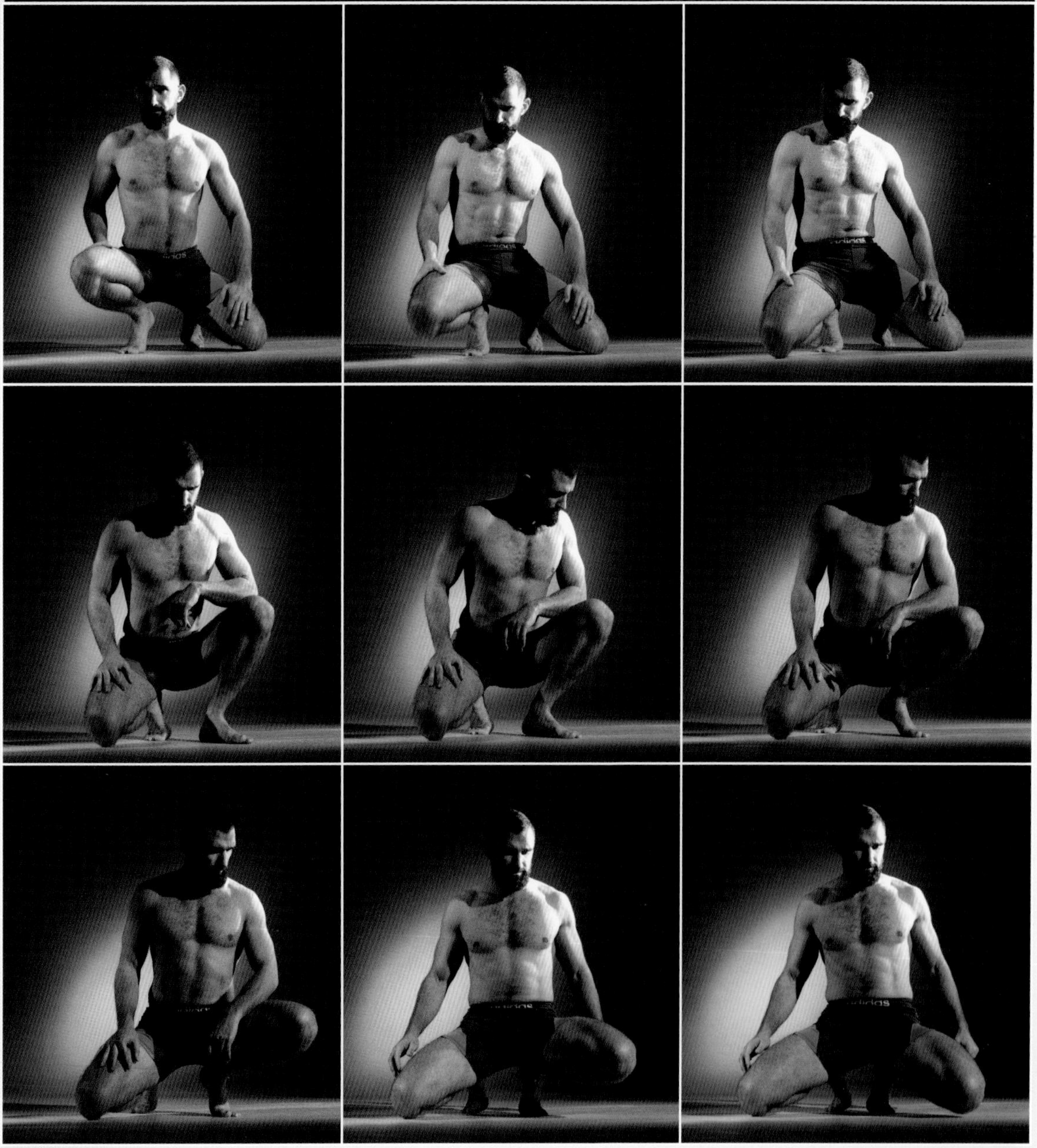

04. OPTIONAL: WALKING WITH A BAR ON THE BACK TO ACTIVATE THE CALVES

Place a weight bar on the back of your shoulders. Exaggerate a heel-to-toe walking movement by leading with the heel of your front foot and rolling through your front foot to finish on your tiptoes as you lift the other knee level to your hip. **Perform 3 steps on each side.**

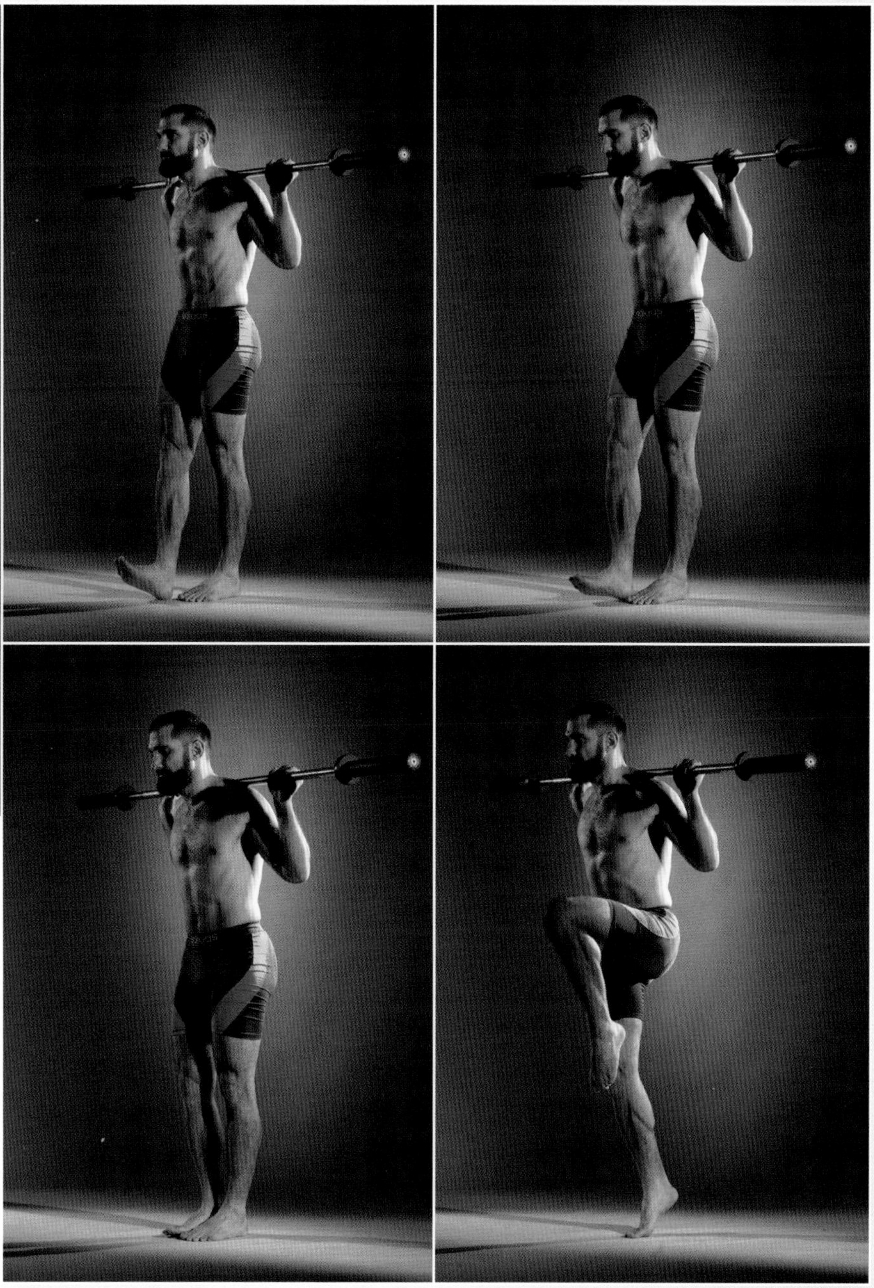

solution 02

MASSAGE | STRETCHING | MOBILIZATION | WEIGHTS

Perform one to three sets of each of the following exercises in order, alternating sides as you go along. Do not stop between exercises.

ANKLE DORSIFLEXION

01. CALF MASSAGE USING A LARGE BALL

Place your calf on a large massage ball and alter the intensity of the massage by pressing your buttocks toward the floor. Intensify the massage even more, if necessary, by crossing your free leg over the one being massaged. **Perform 10 front-to-back rolls, 10 left-to-right rolls, and 10 circular ankle movements.**

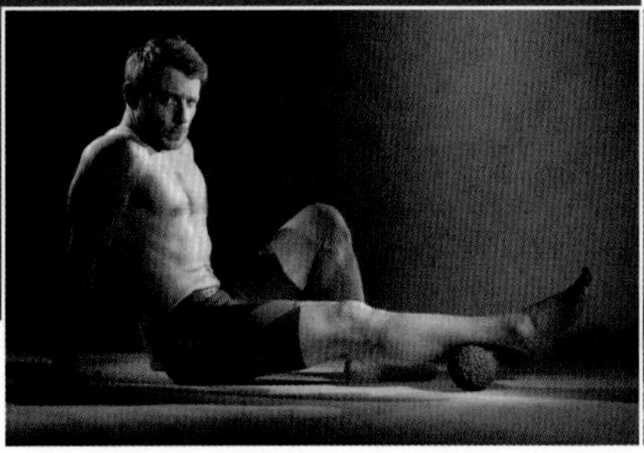

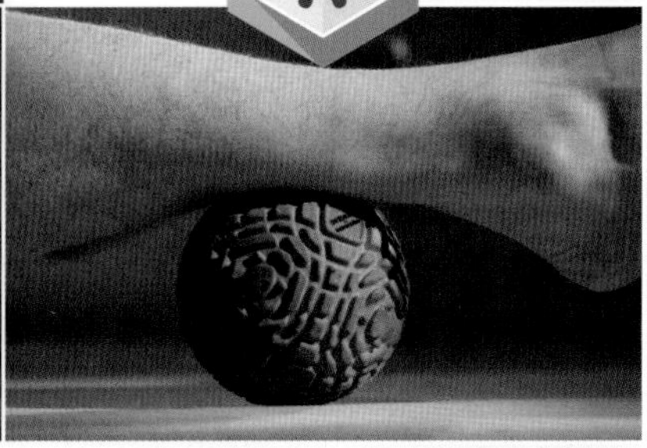

02. STRETCH AGAINST A WALL WITH KNEE EXTENDED THEN FLEXED

Lean forward to push against a wall with your arms overhead and your feet in a staggered stance. Be sure the toes of both feet point toward the wall. With the heel of your back foot flat on the floor and your back knee fully extended, shift your hips forward to create a stretch in the calf of your back leg. For an additional stretch, slightly flex your back knee. **Hold the stretch for 30 seconds.**

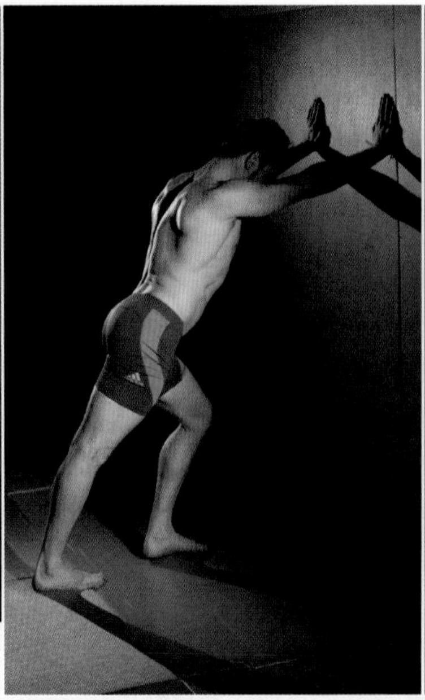

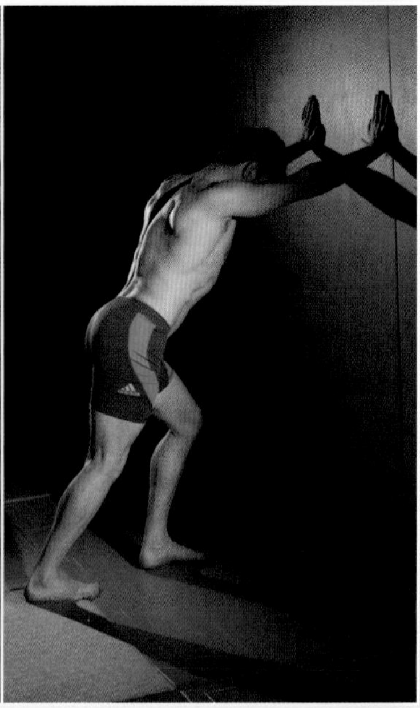

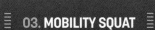

03. MOBILITY SQUAT

Make yourself as tall as possible, then move to a fully-squatted position with your heels flat on the floor and your knees pointing outward. Reach one arm overhead, then the other arm, and finally both arms. Try to keep your torso erect throughout the exercise, especially when you reach your arms overhead. If you cannot keep your heels on the floor, you can use a wedge under your heels, but work toward removing the wedge. An advanced version is to use a wedge under the balls of your feet.
Perform 5 reps of each arm, and 5 reps with both arms.

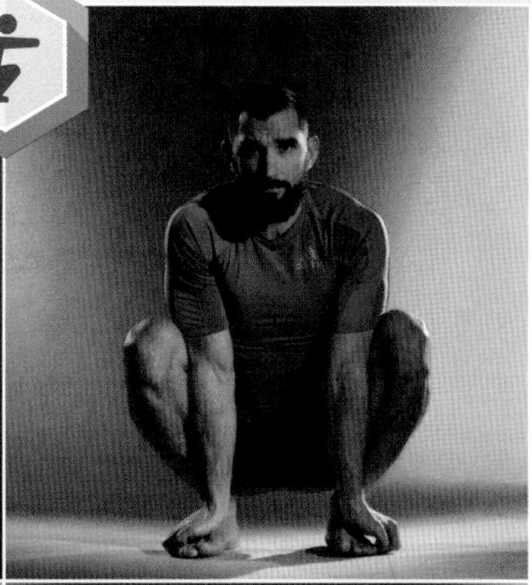

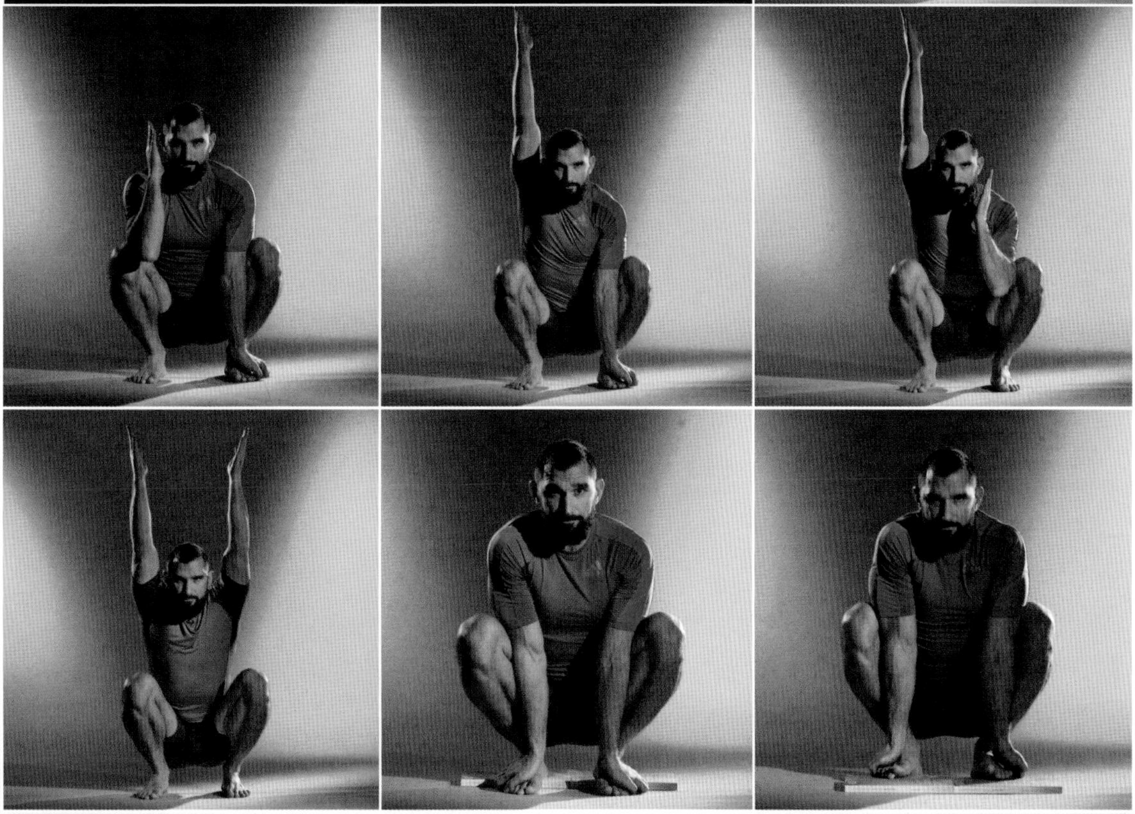

04. OPTIONAL: DEEP SQUAT USING A WEIGHT BAR

A classic squat can be used to improve mobility if you use a lighter weight and squat deeper than normal. You can also pause for several seconds in the lowest position if it is not too uncomfortable. Push your chest out, focus your eyes just above level, and keep the bar firmly anchored on the back of your shoulders using an extended wrist grip (as when accelerating on a motorcycle).
Perform 5 reps.

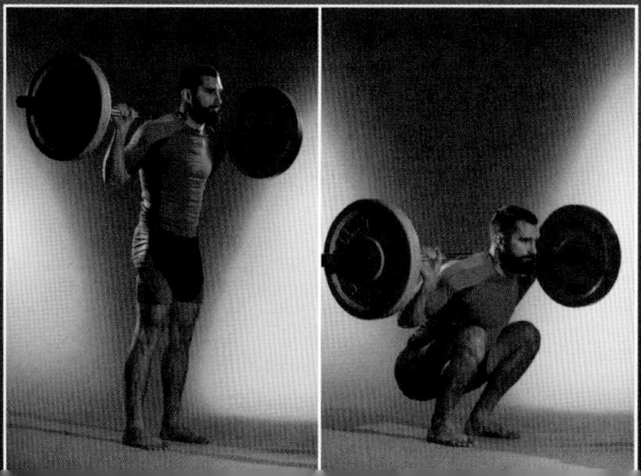

solution 03

MASSAGE | STRETCHING | MOBILIZATION | WEIGHTS

Perform one to three sets of each of the following exercises in order on the same leg. Do not stop between exercises. When they are completed, go through the series again for the other leg.

ANKLE DORSIFLEXION

01. CALF MASSAGE USING A WEIGHT BAR

Supporting your weight on your arms, place your calf on a bar (without weight plates) with your knee fully extended. Alter the intensity of the massage by extending your hip to press your calf on the bar to create the desired pressure. Intensify the massage even more, if necessary, by crossing your free leg over the one being massaged.

Perform 10 front-to-back rolls and 10 circular ankle movements (in a stationary position).

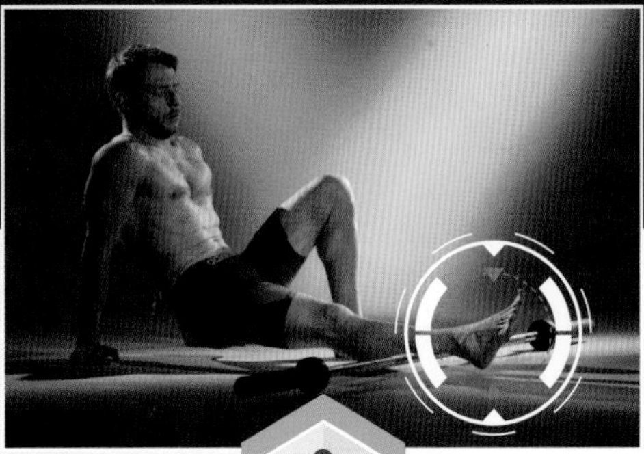

02. CALF STRETCH USING A WEIGHT PLATE AND A RESISTANCE BAND

Perform a classic calf stretch with your heel hanging off the edge of a weight plate (and touching the floor, depending on the height of the plate), then add the backward pull of a resistance band at the base of the shin

Hold the stretch for 20 to 30 seconds.

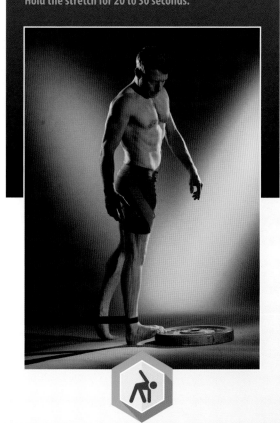

03. DORSIFLEXION AND PLANTAR FLEXION USING A BAND

Sit on the floor and place the instep of your foot in a resistance band that is anchored near the floor at a distance from you that makes the band taut. Dorsiflex your ankle to bring your toes toward you as far as possible. Relax, unattach the resistance band, loop it around the ball of your foot, and hold the taut band in your hands. Plantar flex your ankle to point your toes away from you as far as possible.

Perform 6 reps in each direction.

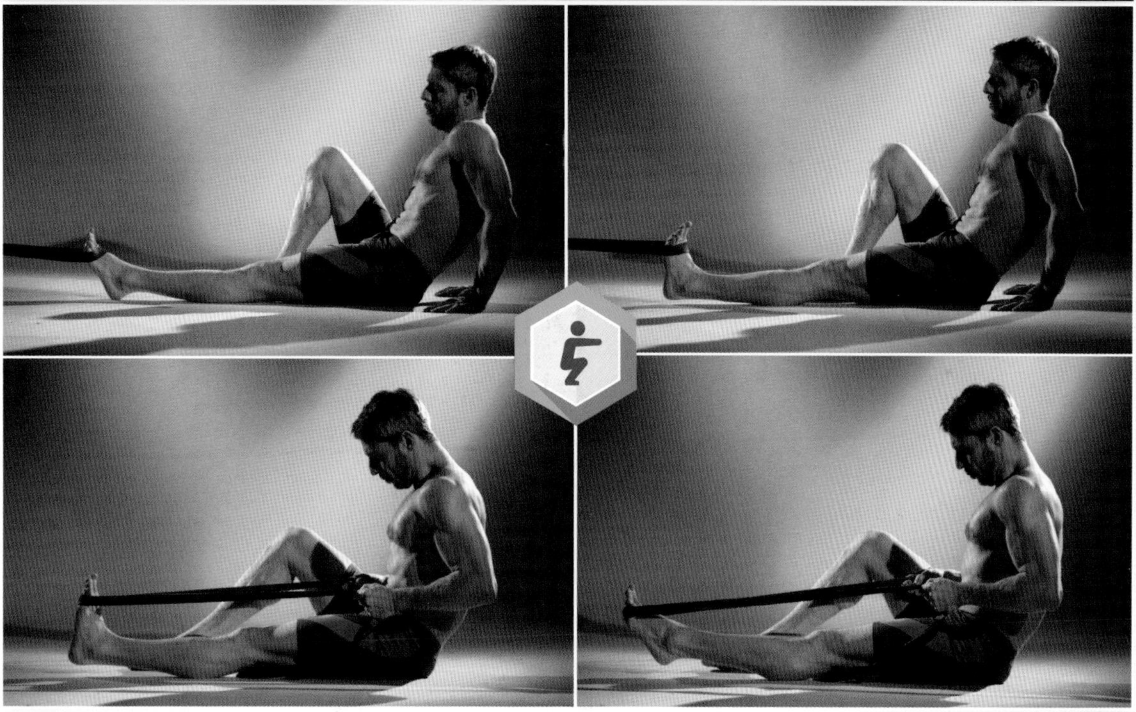

04. OPTIONAL: ROCKING CHAIR CALVES

With a weight bar on the back of your shoulders, tilt from your heels to your tiptoes in a slow, rolling movement, as if your foot were rocking a rocking chair.

Perform 10 slow reps in each direction.

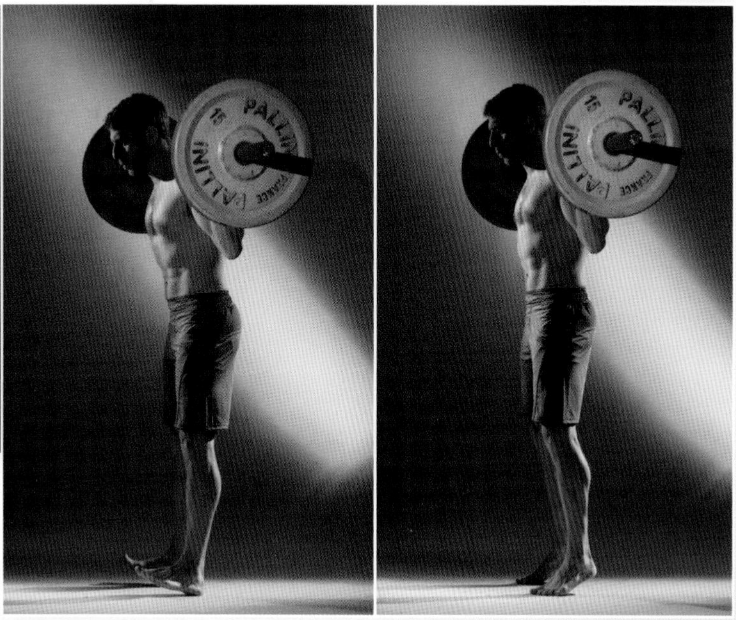

solution 04

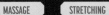

MASSAGE STRETCHING MOBILIZATION WEIGHTS

Perform one to three sets of each of the following exercises in order on the same leg. Do not stop between exercises. When they are completed, go through the series again for the other leg.

ANKLE DORSIFLEXION

01. SHIN MASSAGE USING A STICK OR SHORT BAR

With a massage stick or a short bar, roll over your shins to look for sensitive and stiff areas. Focus your work by massaging these areas.

Perform 10 up-and-down and 10 right-to-left massages.

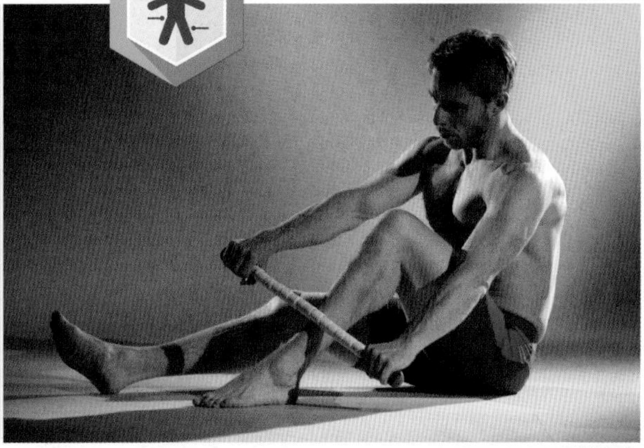

02. CALF STRETCH ON A STEP OR STACK OF BOOKS

Stand on a step or a stack of books with your heels hanging off the front edge. First, relax your calves to allow your heels to drop toward the floor. Then point your toes as far as possible, hold the contracted position, and then completely relax again.

Perform 3 to 5 reps with a 3- to 7-second hold during each rep.

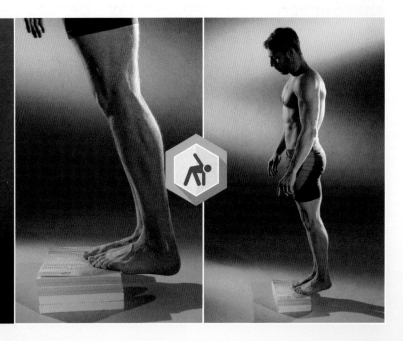

03. ALTERNATING DEEP KNIGHTHOOD LUNGE AND POSTERIOR CHAIN STRETCH

From a very low lunge position with the knee and instep of your back leg and foot on the floor, hold your front foot to anchor it to the floor. Move your front knee as far forward as you can without lifting the heel of your front foot off the floor. Then extend your front knee and flex your back knee to shift your hips to sit on top of your back leg. In the final position, the front knee should be fully extended with the toes of the front foot pointed away from you.

Perform 10 reps, holding for 3 to 5 seconds in each position.

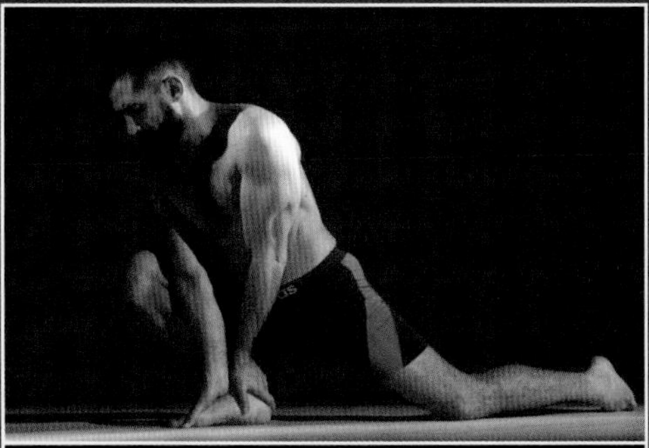

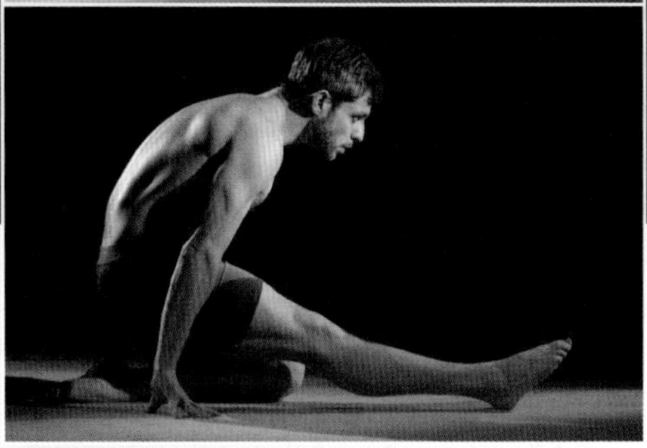

04. OPTIONAL: ONE-LEG WEIGHTED SQUAT

Place a weight bar on the back of your shoulders and the instep of your back foot solidly on a box or bench. Without any lateral compensation or rotation, flex your front hip and knee to squat toward the floor, allowing your kneecap to move over your toes. Keep the heel of your front foot in contact with the floor throughout the exercise (if it lifts up, move it a short distance farther from the box or bench). Quality technique is required for this exercise.

Perform 3 to 4 reps per leg.

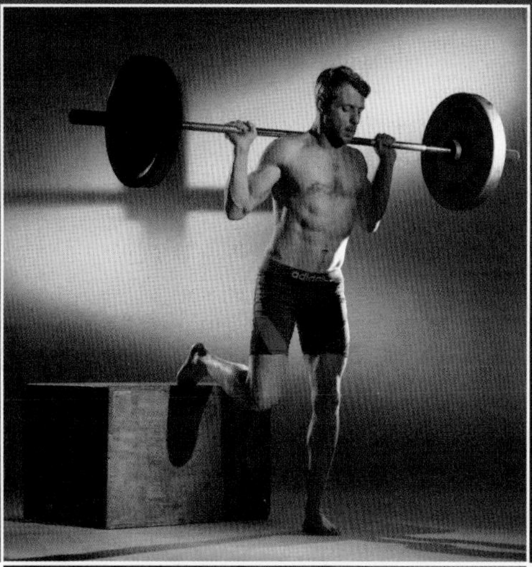

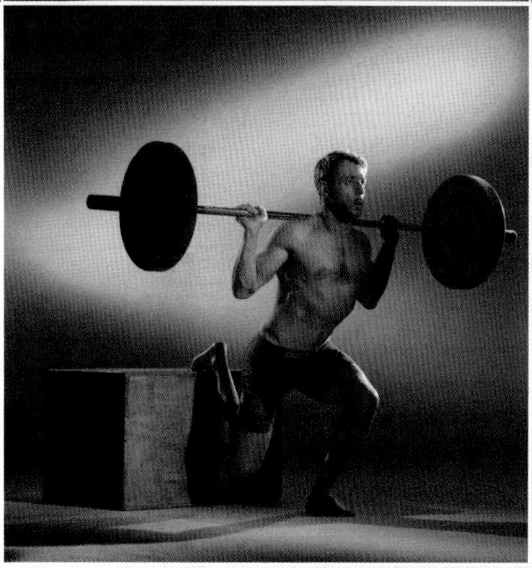

solution 05

MASSAGE | STRETCHING | MOBILIZATION | WEIGHTS

Perform one to three sets of each of the following exercises in order, alternating sides as you go along. Do not stop between exercises.

ANKLE DORSIFLEXION

01. MASSAGE USING TWO BALLS

Take a massage ball in each hand and place one on each side of your calf. Roll the balls from top to bottom and from front to back, then make circular movements. Then hold the balls tightly and slide them over the skin on each side of your calf from top to bottom. If you find a sensitive area, press the ball into the muscle and rotate or twist it to relieve the soreness.

Perform for 1 to 3 minutes on each leg. Spend more time on the most sensitive areas.

02. RAISED STRETCH ON ALL FOURS

This is a less precise version of the downward-facing dog pose. Lengthen your posterior chain, especially your calves, and place your heels on the floor. To help realign your joints, you can use a resistance band, placed at thigh level, to pull backward. If you wish to practice this move by alternating between contractions and stretches, rise onto your tiptoes to contract your calves then place your heels back on the floor to stretch them.

Perform 30 seconds of passive stretching in the downward-facing dog position. Then perform 2 sets of alternating between 10 seconds on your tiptoes and 10 seconds on your heels.

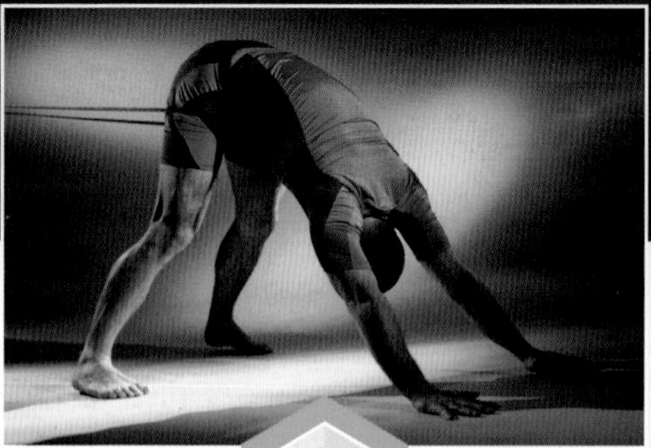

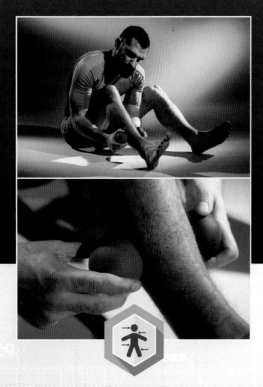

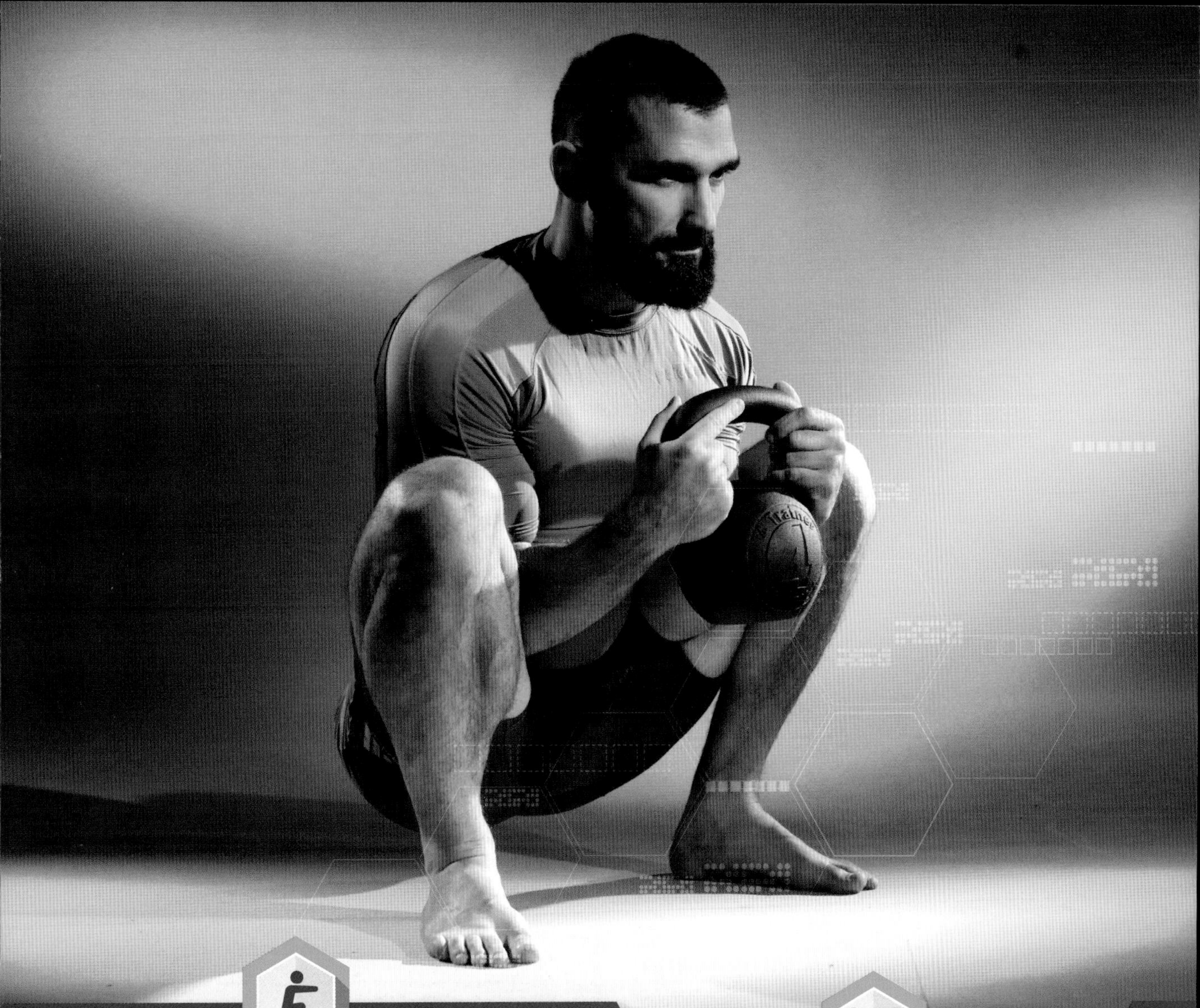

03. LOW-MOBILITY KETTLEBELL GOBLET SQUAT

From a standing position, hold a kettlebell in both hands in front of your chest. Slowly move in a controlled manner into a squat position. Do not tilt your pelvis backward. In the bottom position, press your upper arms and elbows against your inner thighs and knees to push them out (farther apart). Move the kettlebell slightly away from your torso as a counterweight, if needed. Keep your feet flat on the floor, your chest out, and your torso erect throughout the exercise. Without changing the position of your feet while in the bottom position, transfer your body weight from one foot to the other and move your knee as far forward as possible each time.

04. OPTIONAL: NORMAL-MOBILITY KETTLEBELL GOBLET SQUAT

This exercise is the same as the previous exercise except that you will control your descent as much as possible, spend at least two seconds in the bottom position, and then powerfully accelerate back up to the standing position.

Perform 6 reps.

solution
06

ANKLE DORSIFLEXION

MASSAGE

STRETCHING

MOBILIZATION

WEIGHTS

Perform one to three sets of each of the following exercises in order on the same leg. Do not stop between exercises. When they are completed, go through the series again for the other leg.

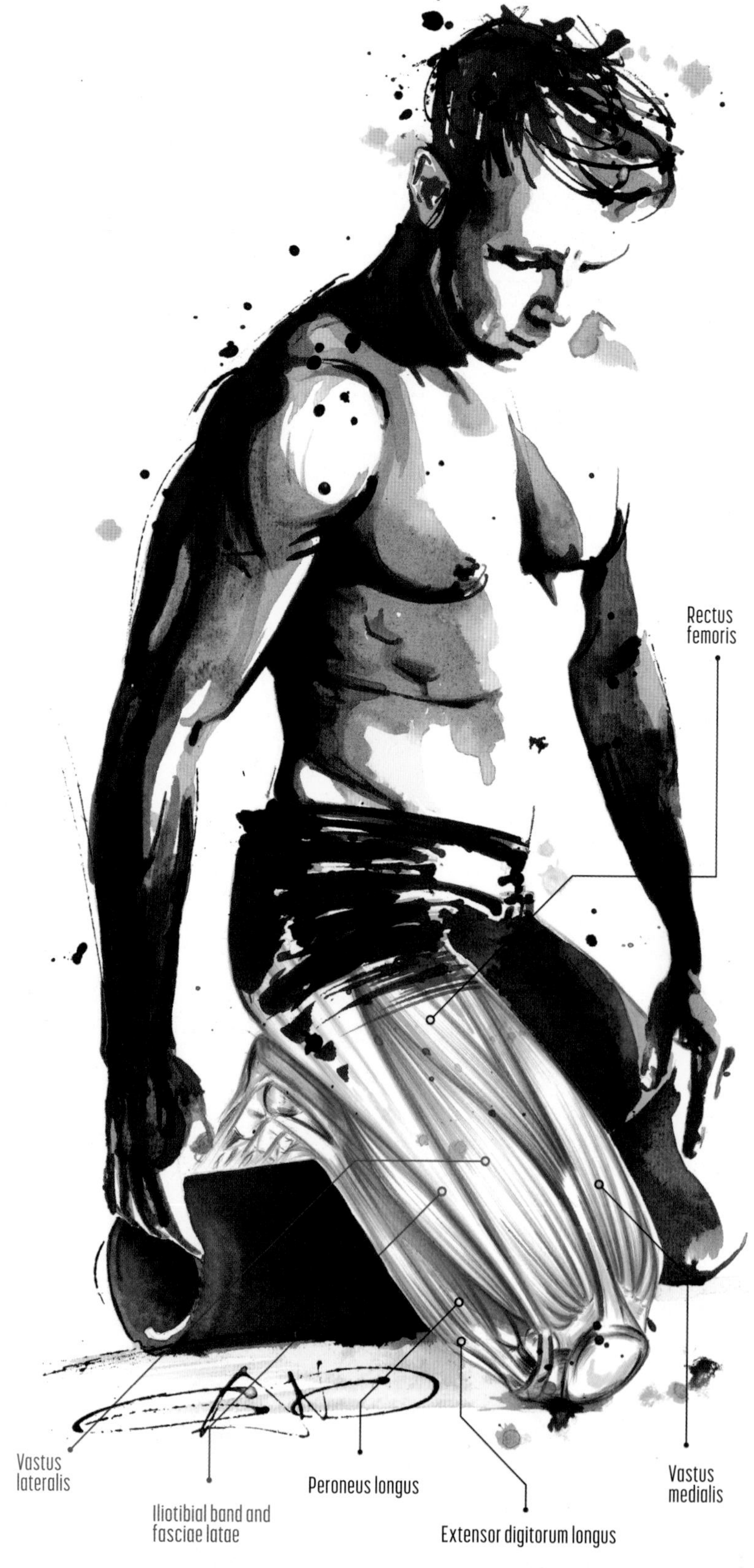

Rectus femoris
Vastus lateralis
Iliotibial band and fasciae latae
Peroneus longus
Extensor digitorum longus
Vastus medialis

01. FRONT OF THE SHIN MASSAGE USING A ROLLER

Kneel on the floor, lift one knee, place a roller under the most muscular part of the shin (the outer half), kneel back on the floor, and sit back on your heels. Initially, apply only partial pressure on the roller by shifting your weight away from the roller, then very gradually lean your weight back on that leg. Roll over a small area, looking for sensitive spots. If the pressure creates too much pain, shift away from the roller. If that is still too painful, the massage is too advanced. **Perform 10 to 15 massages from front to back over a small area.**

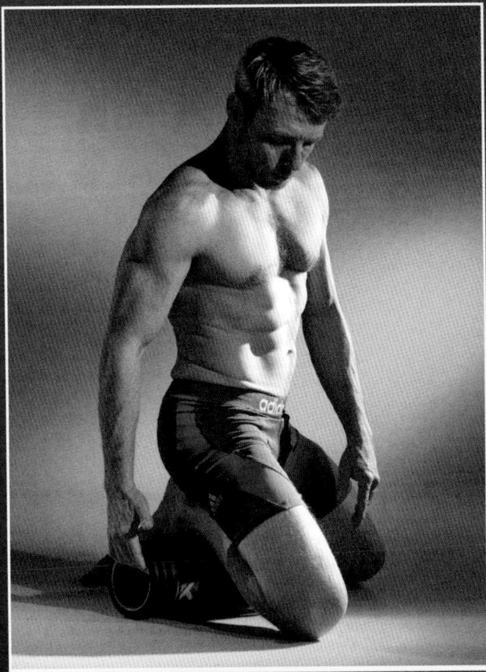

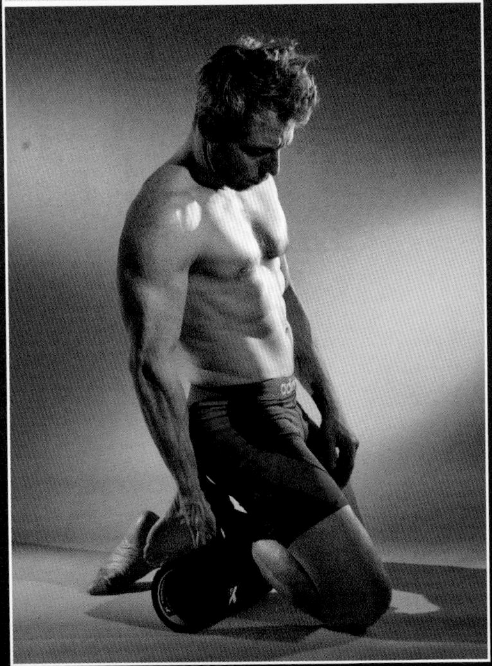

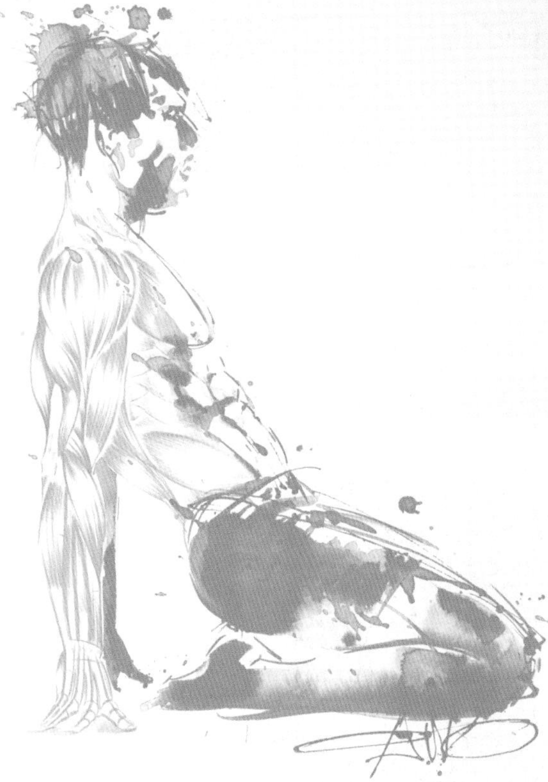

02. EXTENSION STRETCH FOR BOTH ANKLES

Kneel on the floor with your shins and insteps of both feet flat on the floor. Place your hands on the floor behind you and lean back, trying to fully sit on your heels. **Hold the final position for 20 to 30 seconds.**

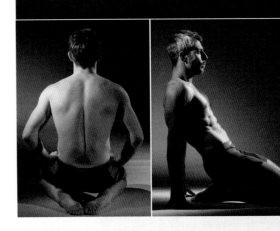

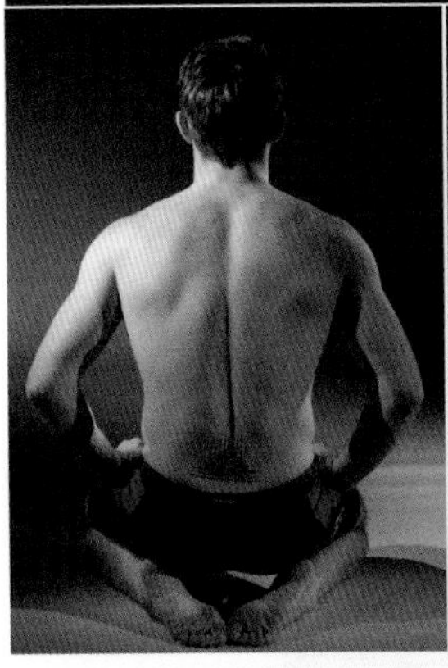

03. DOUBLE BALL MASSAGE ON A BOX WITH CIRCULAR MOVEMENTS

Kneel with your shin and instep of one foot flat on top of a box, lift the knee, and place a double massage ball between the box and your shin. Roll over a small area, looking for the most sensitive areas. Move very slightly from front to back while making circles with your ankle.

Perform at least 10 ankle circles (5 rotations in one direction then 5 in the other direction).

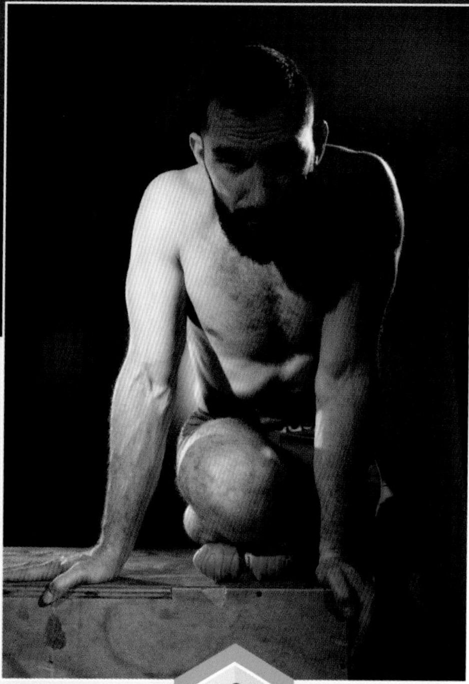

04. OPTIONAL: BONE SAW CALF SMASH

Perform the self-massage technique for the front of the shin, but this time cross your other leg or foot over the lower calf or ankle of the bottom leg. Apply pressure by gradually leaning back and toward the roller.

Perform 10 to 15 massages using short movements from front to back and 10 to 15 massages from right to left.

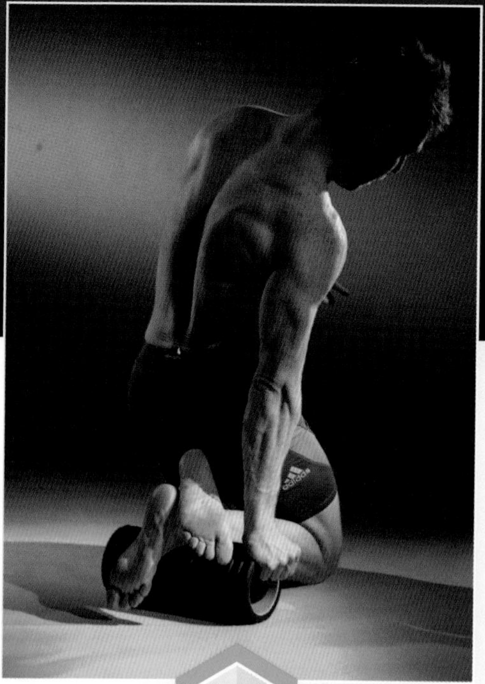

FOOT MOBILITY

1

Toe Extension

Start in the lunged knighthood position. Slowly sit back on the heel of your back foot to increase the pressure on the toes. During this test, check to see what is preventing you from doing it correctly; you should only feel pain or stiffness in the arch of your foot. Any other problems should be explored and corrected by using the other sections in this book. If you do not have any pain or stiffness in the arch of your back foot, you passed the test.

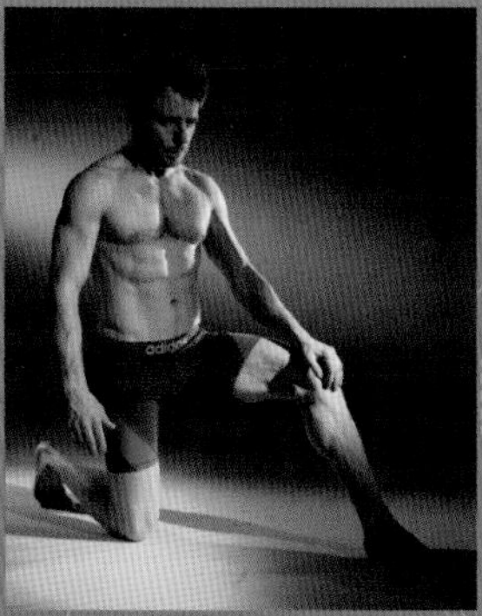

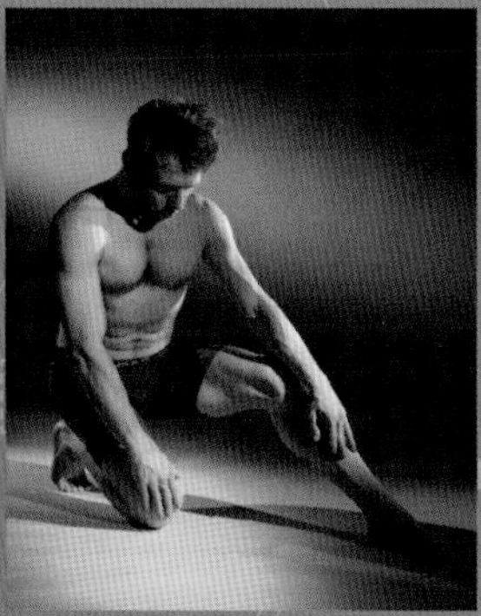

2

Toe Flexion

Sit on the floor and insert a finger knuckle (with the exception of the thumb) between each of your toes. Start with the index finger. If this exercise causes too much strain in the foot, results in a cramp, or you cannot separate the toes far enough, you have failed this test and will benefit from the corrective exercises in this section.

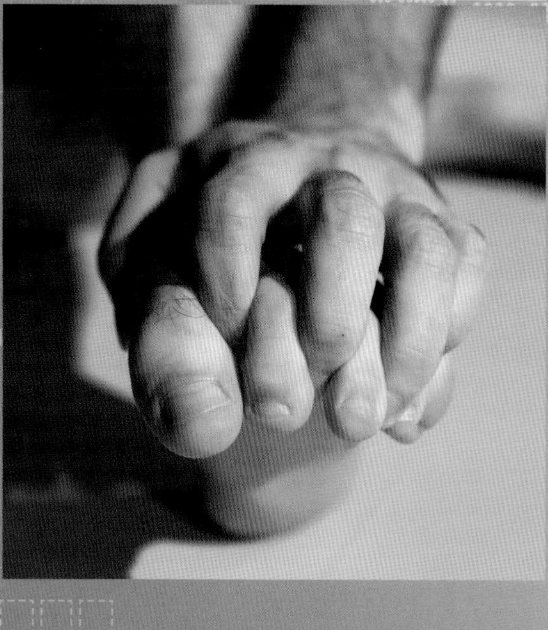

solution 01

MASSAGE | STRETCHING | MOBILIZATION | WEIGHTS

Perform one to three sets of each of the following exercises in order, alternating sides as you go along. Do not stop between exercises.

FOOT MOBILITY

01. FOOT MASSAGE USING A BALL

Stand and place a massage ball under your foot. Applying moderate pressure on the ball, follow the V-shape of your foot to roll the ball in small circles under your arch.

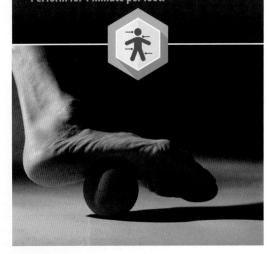

Perform for 1 minute per foot.

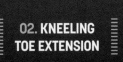

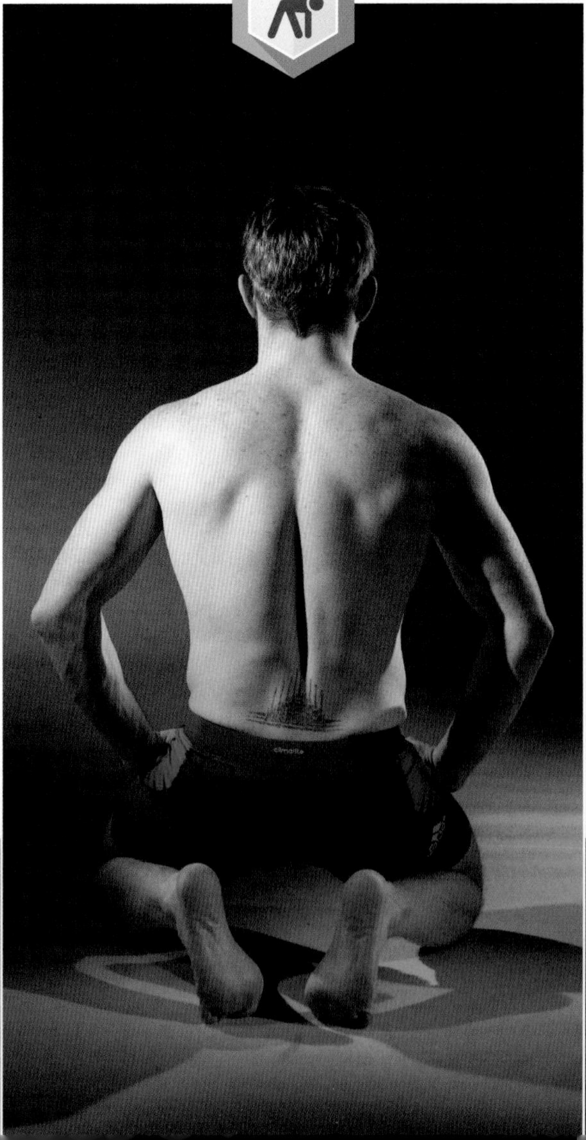

02. KNEELING TOE EXTENSION

Kneel on the floor with your toes tucked under your feet and then sit back on your heels.

Hold the stretch for 30 seconds.

03. ROLLING THROUGH THE FOOT

Walk in a straight line by placing one heel in front of the toes of your other foot and roll through your front foot (i.e., first your heel, then your full foot, then your toes) as fully and purposely as possible before taking a step with your other foot. By rolling through the foot as much as possible, you will target the mobility and proprioception of the arch of the foot.

Take 5 steps with each foot.

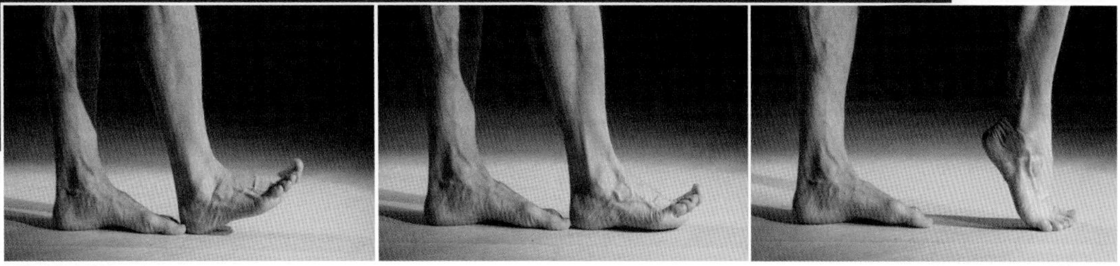

04. OPTIONAL: WEIGHTED ROLLING THROUGH THE FOOT

Hold a dumbbell in each hand and walk using the same technique as the previous exercise. This time, roll through your foot and rise onto your tiptoes at the end of each step before taking your next step.

Take 5 steps (including the extra heel raise) with each foot.

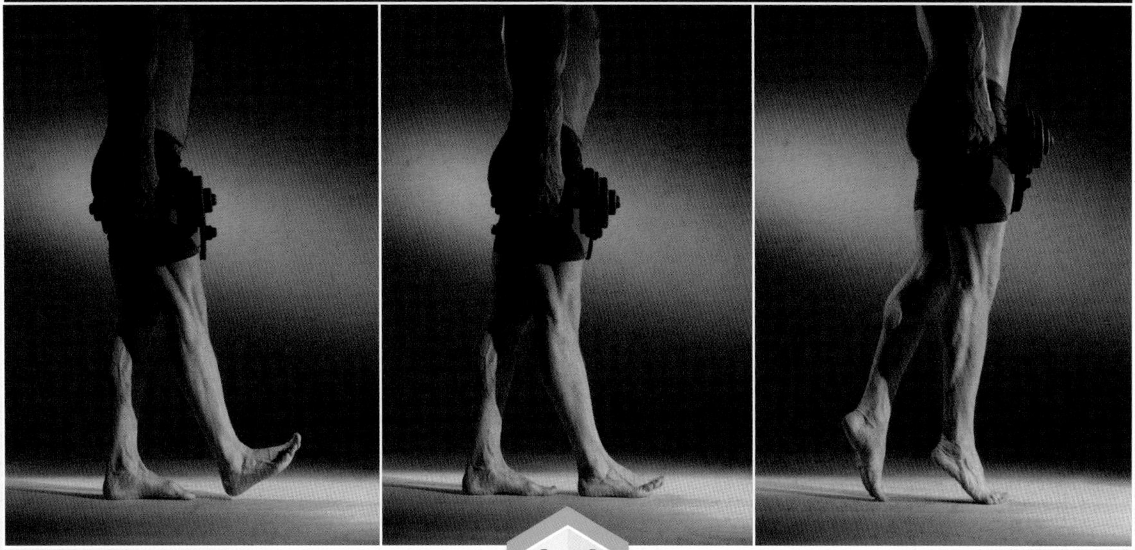

solution 02

MASSAGE | STRETCHING | MOBILIZATION | WEIGHTS

Perform one to three sets of each of the following exercises in order, alternating sides as you go along. Do not stop between exercises.

FOOT MOBILITY

01. ANKLE MASSAGE USING A BALL

Place a massage ball in the inside curve of your ankle. Pull the tissues downward to stretch your skin and then rotate or twist the ball while flexing and extending your foot.

Perform for 20 seconds on each area.

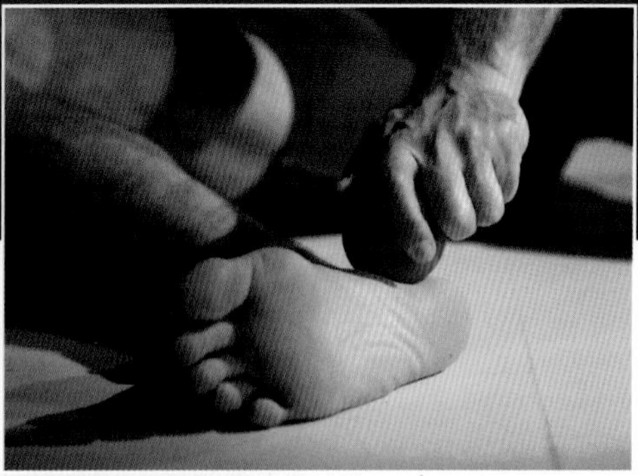

02. STRETCHING THE ACHILLES TENDON AND CALF

Place the ball of your foot against a wall, keeping your heel on the floor. Stand erect with your knee fully extended. Lean toward the wall until a stretch is felt.

Hold the position for 30 seconds.

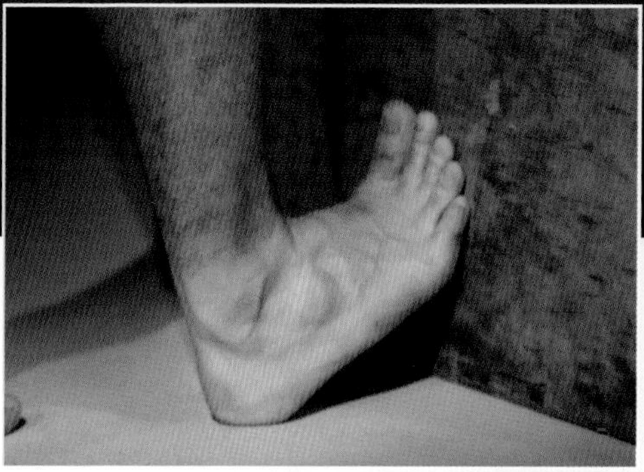

03. BENT-KNEE, RIGHT-LEFT ROTATION ON ONE FOOT

Stand on your left leg with your knee slightly flexed and with your right foot held approximately level with your left calf. Place your hands behind your head, spreading your elbows as far apart as possible. In this position, slowly and dynamically rotate your torso (not your hips) to the left. When you reach full rotation, immediately reverse direction to rotate to the right. Rotate your torso as far as possible in both directions.

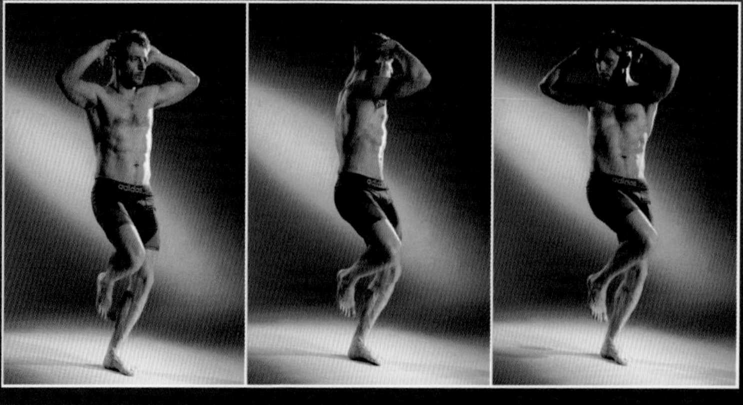

Perform 5 rotations to each direction on each ankle.

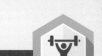

04. OPTIONAL: LUNGE USING A WEIGHT BAR

Place a weight bar on the back of your shoulders. Step with your left leg into a forward lunge position by first contacting your left heel on the floor, then roll through that foot as much as possible while exaggerating the dorsiflexed position of your right ankle. At the end of the movement, rest for a few seconds in the lunge position, allowing your left knee to move beyond the toes of your left foot (with your left heel remaining on the floor).

Perform 10 reps, alternating between the right and left legs.

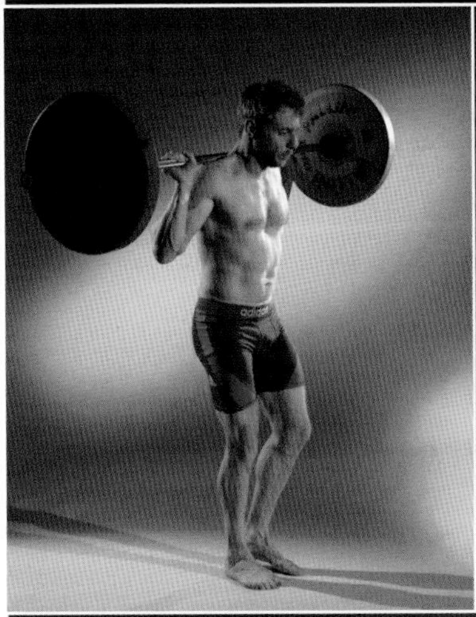

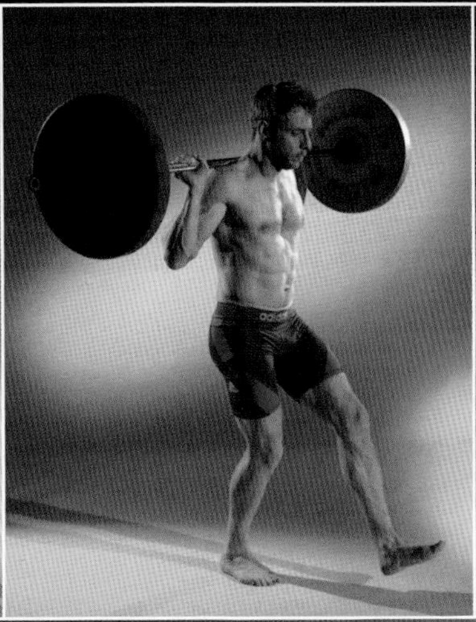

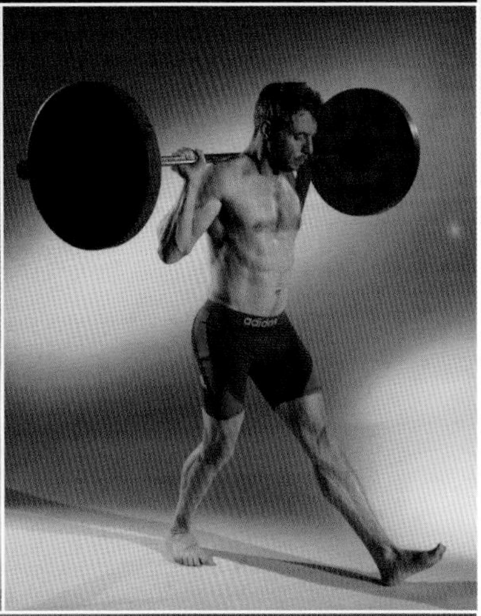

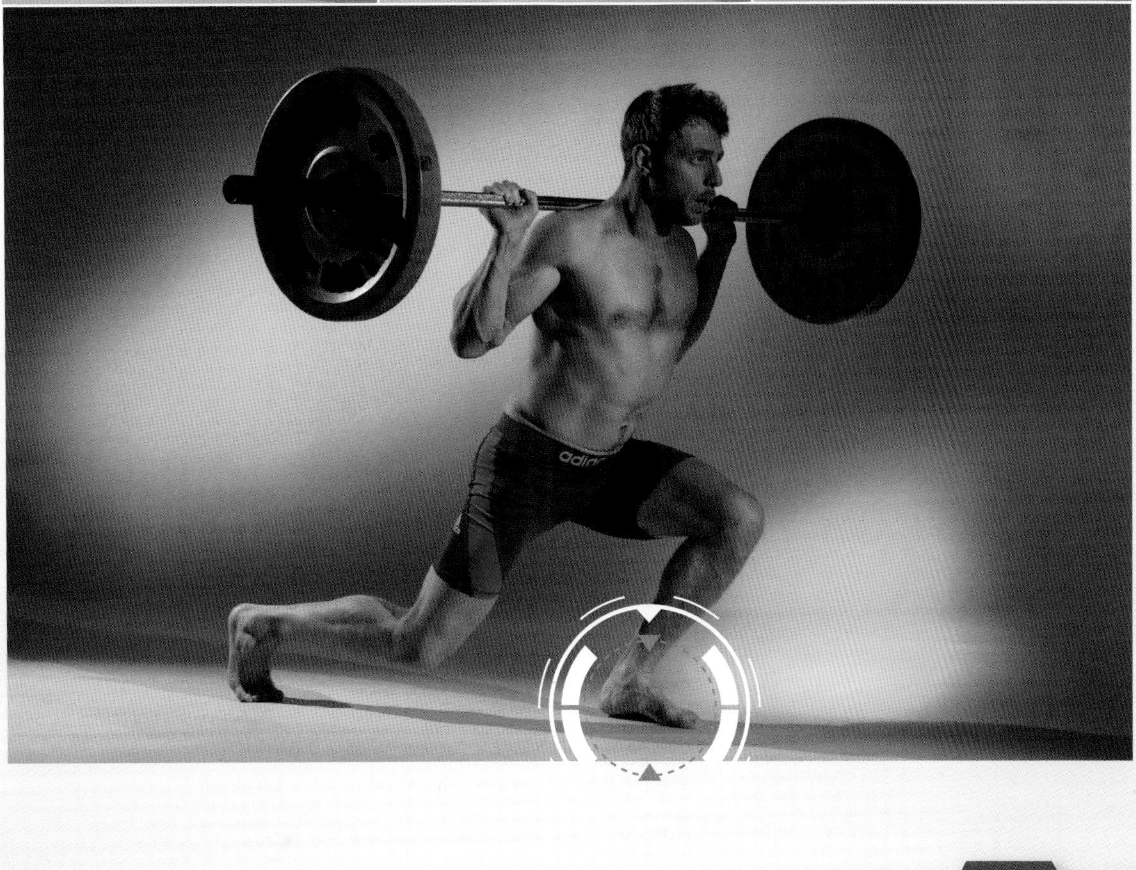

solution 03

MASSAGE | STRETCHING | MOBILIZATION | WEIGHTS

Perform one to three sets of each of the following exercises in order, alternating sides as you go along. Do not stop between exercises.

FOOT MOBILITY

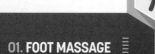

01. FOOT MASSAGE USING A BALL

Place your heel on the floor and the ball of your foot on a massage ball with moderate pressure applied to the ball. Pivoting on your heel, turn your foot from side to side to massage the full width of the ball of your foot.

Perform for 1 minute per foot.

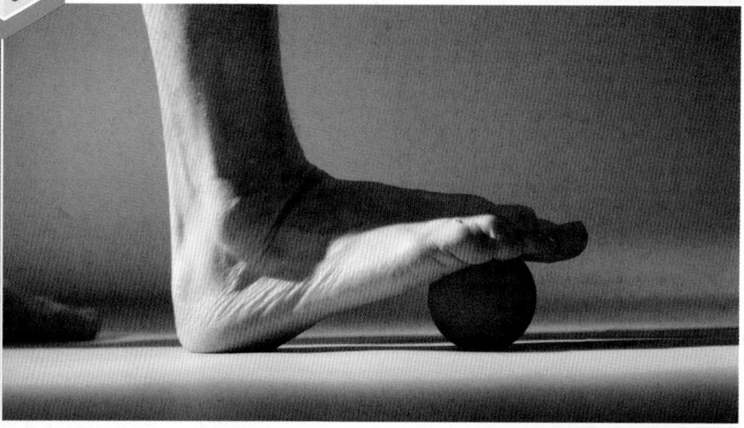

02. TOE STRETCH

Stand on your left leg with your knee slightly flexed. Lift your right knee, point your foot, flex (curl) your toes, and lower your leg to press the top side of your toes into the floor using moderate pressure.

Hold the position for 30 seconds.

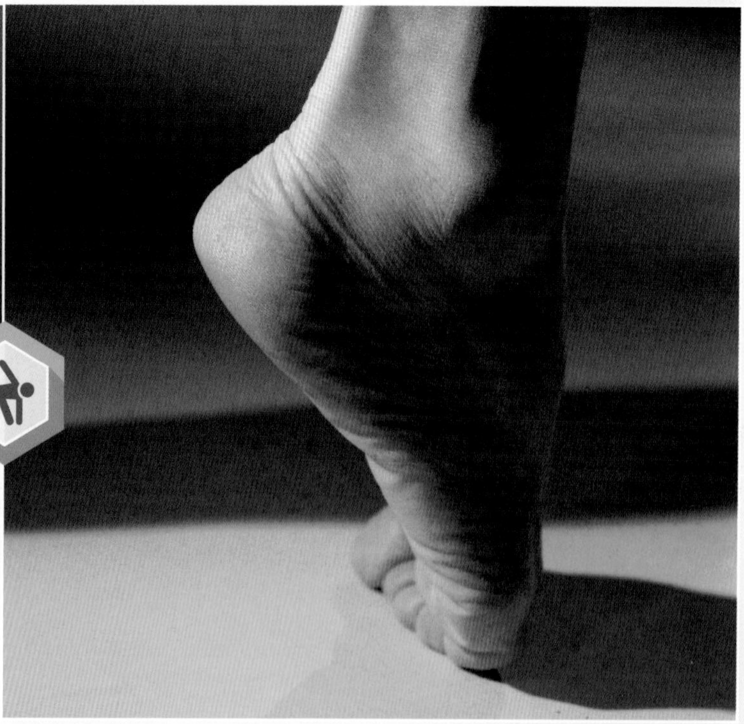

03. ROCKING CHAIR

Stand with your hands on your hips. Lean forward and shift your weight back on your heels while lifting your toes, then swing from your heels to your tiptoes as you lean backward. **Perform 5 tilts forward and 5 tilts backward.**

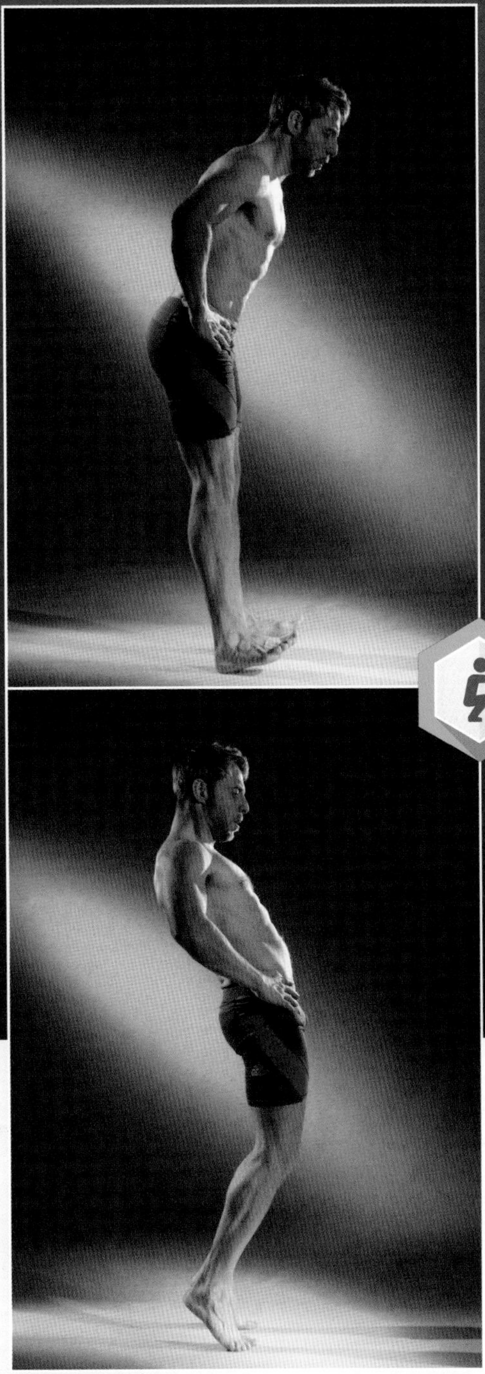

04. OPTIONAL: WEIGHTED ROCKING CHAIR

Stand with a weight bar on the back of your shoulders. Tilt from your heels to your tiptoes without flexing or extending your hips. **Perform 10 repetitions, 5 in each direction.**

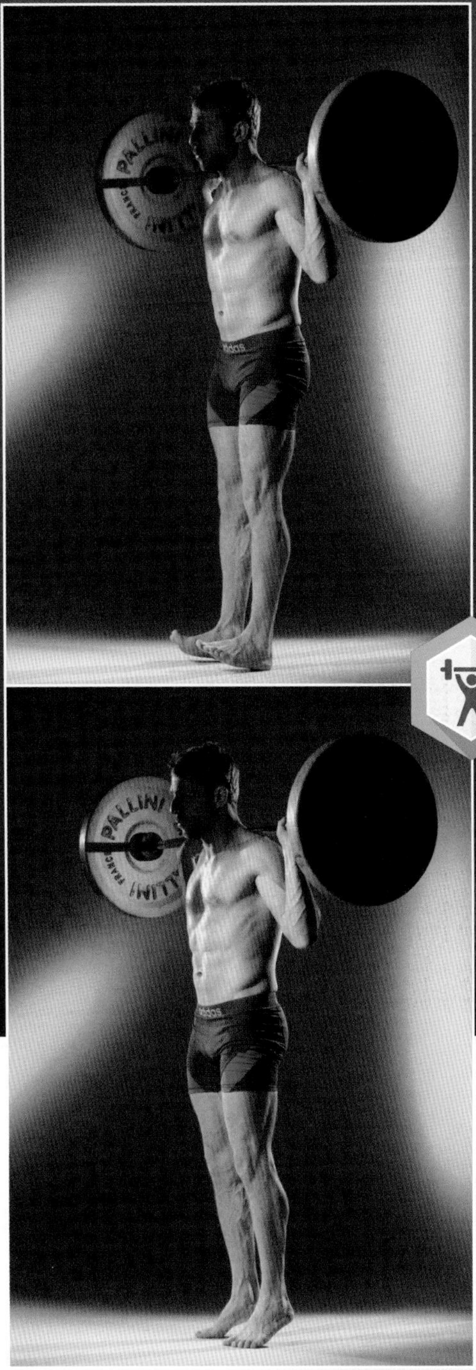

Perform one to three sets of each of the following exercises in order on the same foot. Do not stop between exercises. When they are completed, go through the series again for the other foot.

solution 04

MASSAGE · STRETCHING · MOBILIZATION · WEIGHTS

FOOT MOBILITY

01. HEEL MASSAGE USING A BALL

Place the ball of your foot on the floor and your heel on a massage ball. Roll the ball from right to left while gradually increasing pressure on the ball. **Perform for 1 minute per foot.**

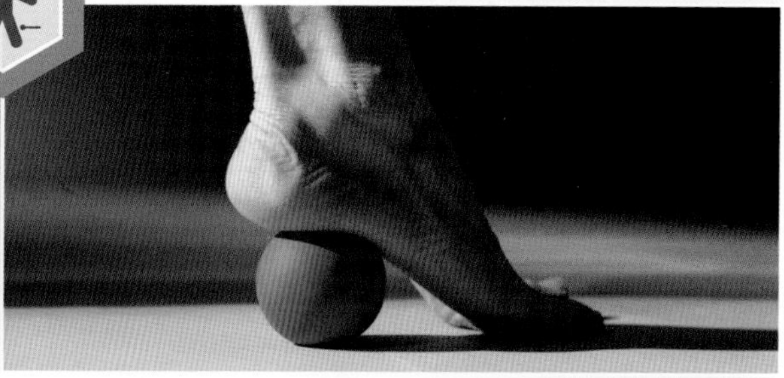

02. CALF STRETCH WITH JOINT DISTRACTION

In a staggered stance position with your right foot placed ahead of your left foot, place the ankle or lower shin of your left foot in a resistance band that is anchored near the floor behind you at a distance that makes the band taut when your left hip is in maximum extension. Slowly move the left knee forward over your second and third toes; be sure to keep your heel flat on the floor throughout the exercise. **Perform the stretch for 30 seconds.**

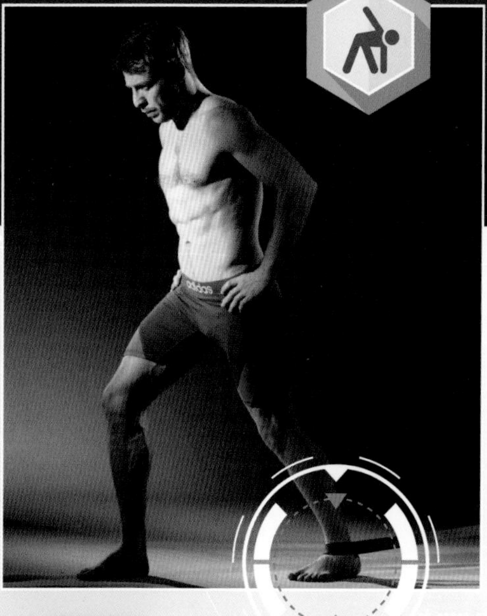

03. PROPRIOCEPTION TURN ON ONE FOOT

Stand on one leg. Gradually transfer your body weight to the front of your foot and toes, then to the outside of your foot, then to your heel, and then to the inside of the foot. Repeat the sequence in the other direction. For a more advanced version, close your eyes. **Repeat twice in each direction.**

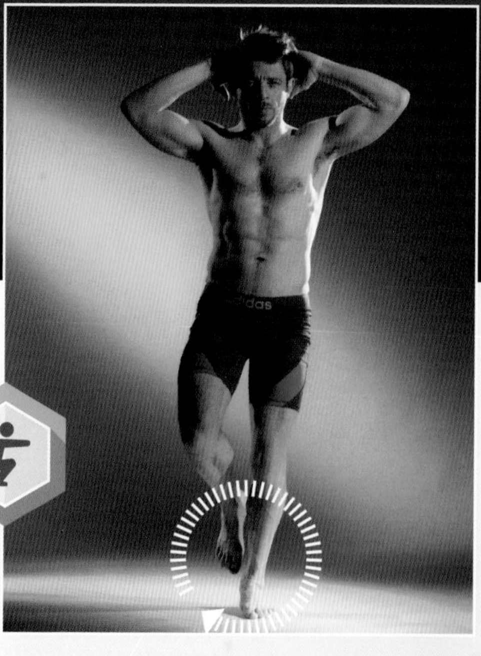

04. OPTIONAL: KETTLEBELL ROTATION ON ONE FOOT

Stand on your right leg and hold a kettlebell in your right hand. Pass the kettlebell behind your back to your left hand, bring it around in front of you, and pass it back to your right hand. As you move the kettlebell, stand tall with your chest out and your shoulders down. For a more advanced version, close your eyes. **Perform 3 rotations on each leg.**

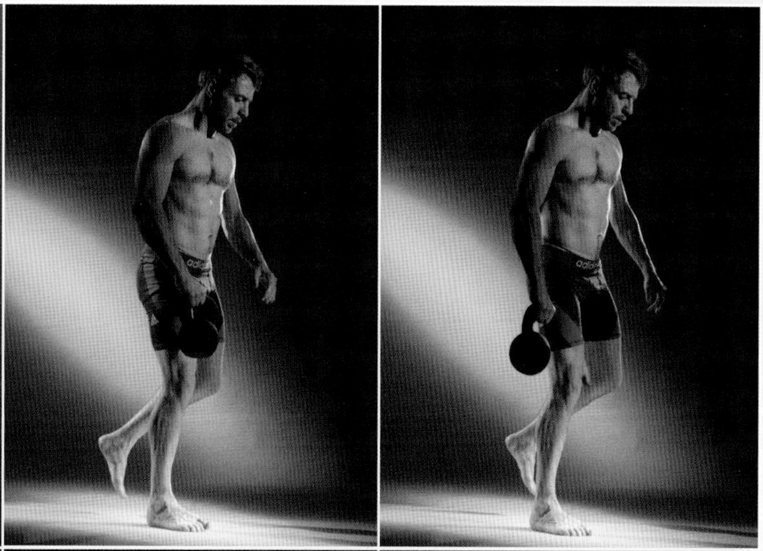

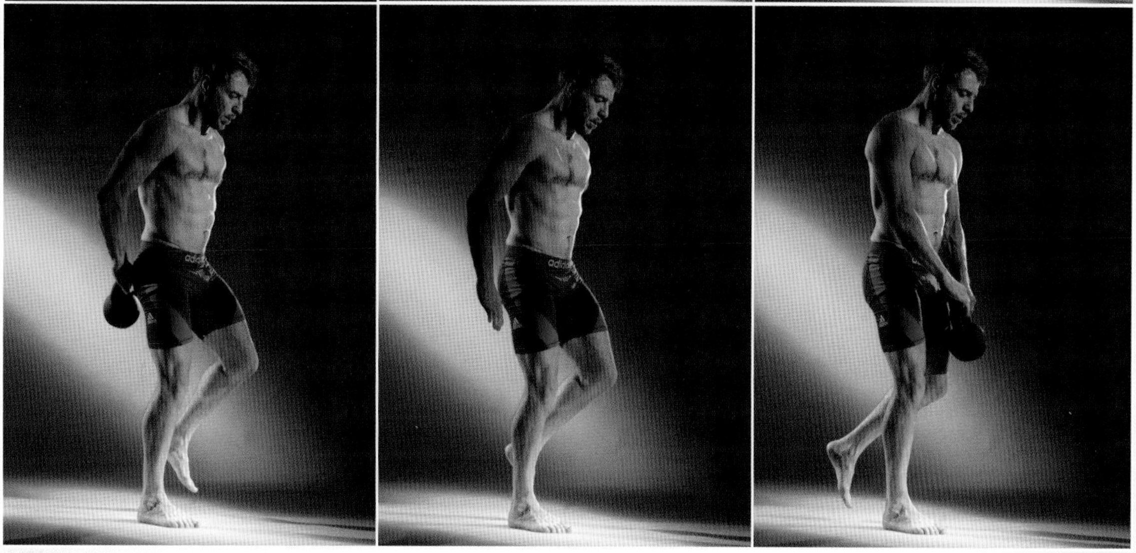

Resistance Band Position for Ankle Joint Distraction

There is debate about using a resistance band to reposition the ankle joint. Instead of looping a band around the base of the shin, it is argued that the band should be positioned over the talus bone of the ankle. This method dismisses the fact that the resistance band creates a fixed point. The decision as to where to position the band depends on the desired direction of joint distraction. If you want to realign the tibia forward, place the band over the talus or use a band anchored ahead of you at a distance from you that makes the band taut and place it around the base of the calf to pull the tibia/fibula forward. Conversely, using a band around the base of the shin to pull the tibia/fibula backward would realign them backward.

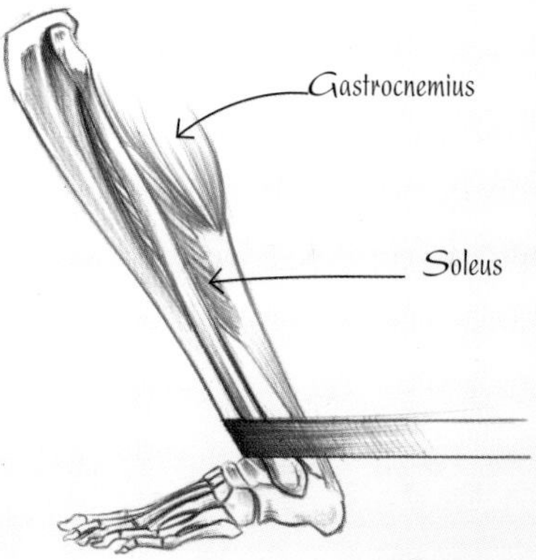

STIFFNESS IN THE PELVIS

1

Squat With Arms Extended in Front

Stand with your heels on a wedge and your arms extended out in front of you. Squat down as far as possible while keeping your back straight. If your back rounds or if you cannot keep your heels on the wedge, you will benefit from using the exercises that follow.

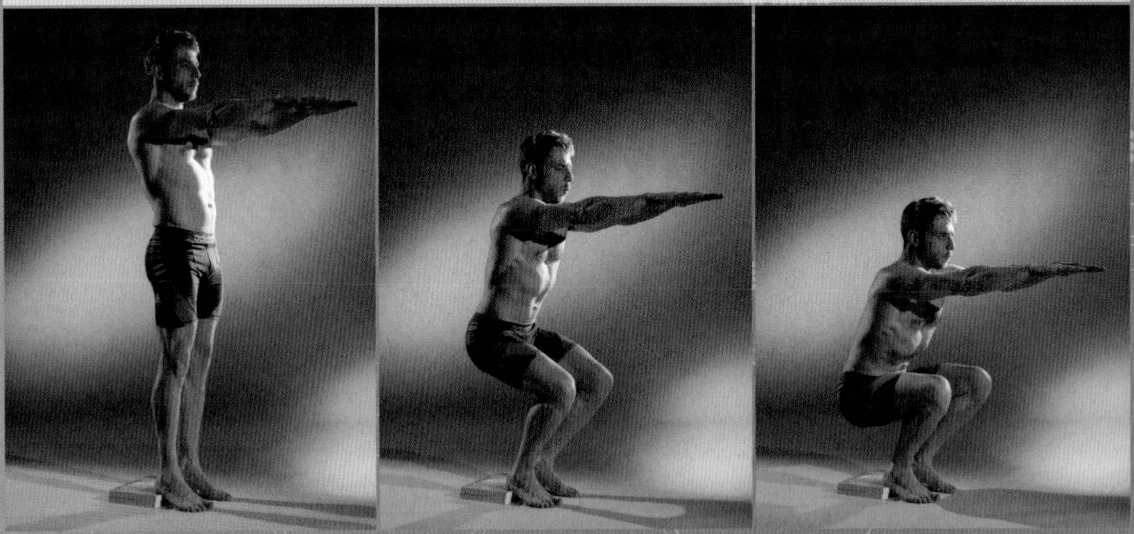

2

Kettlebell Deadlift Test

Place a 20-lb (9.1-kg) kettlebell between your feet at a short distance ahead of you. Grab it in the center with both hands. Keep your back straight, your shoulders held back, and your head in line with your back (look straight ahead through your eyebrows with your head in a neutral position). In this position, you should be able to lift the kettlebell off the floor (with only slightly flexing your knees) without compromising the position of your back and shoulders. The more you have to squat down or round your back to be able to lift the kettlebell, the more you need to perform the following exercises.

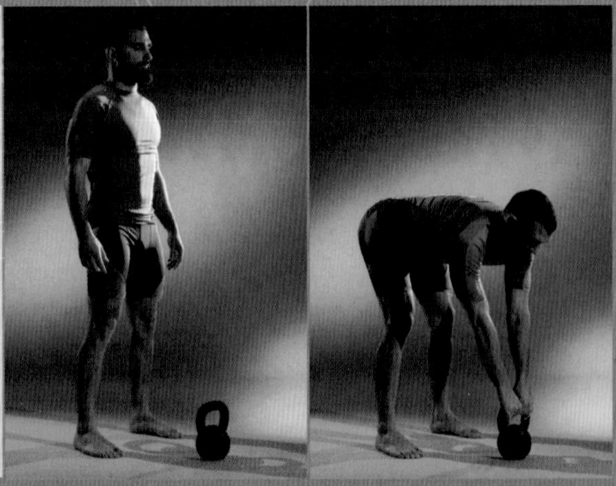

Perform one to three sets of each of the following exercises in order, alternating sides as you go along. Do not stop between exercises.

MASSAGE | STRETCHING | MOBILIZATION | WEIGHTS

solution 01

STIFFNESS IN THE PELVIS

01. GLUTEAL MASSAGE USING A ROLLER

Place a roller in line with your left thigh and position your left gluteal muscle on top of it. Cross your left ankle over your right knee and shift your hips left and right to perform the massage.

Perform 1 to 3 reps of 10 lateral massages, slightly changing the massaged area each time.

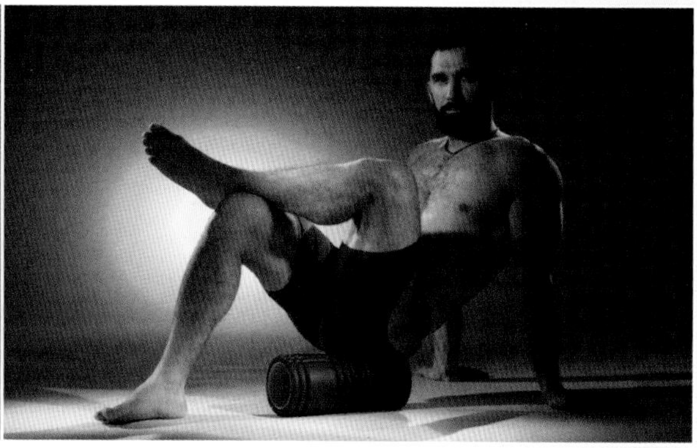

02. FIGURE FOUR SUSPENSION TRAINER STRETCH

Hold the handles of the suspension trainer, place your feet under the anchor point, and shift your hips backward. Flex your right hip and knee to a 90-degree angle and cross your left ankle over your right knee. If possible, flex your right knee farther to lower into a deep squat position.

Hold the stretch for 20 to 30 seconds.

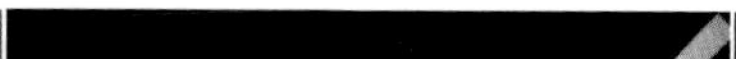

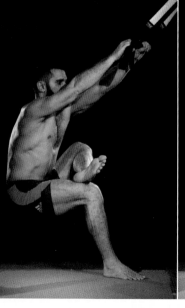

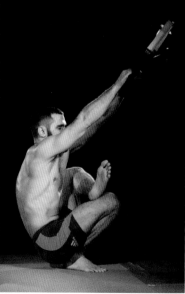

03. GET-UP

Hold the handles of the suspension trainer or a resistance band that is anchored in front of and above you at a distance that makes the band taut. Sit on the floor with your right leg flexed in front of you and your left leg flexed to the side and behind you. Using the suspension trainer or band for assistance, stand up (seen in-process in the second photo), and then sit back down with your left leg flexed in front of you and your right leg flexed to the side and behind you. **Perform 5 reps per side for a total of 10 reps.**

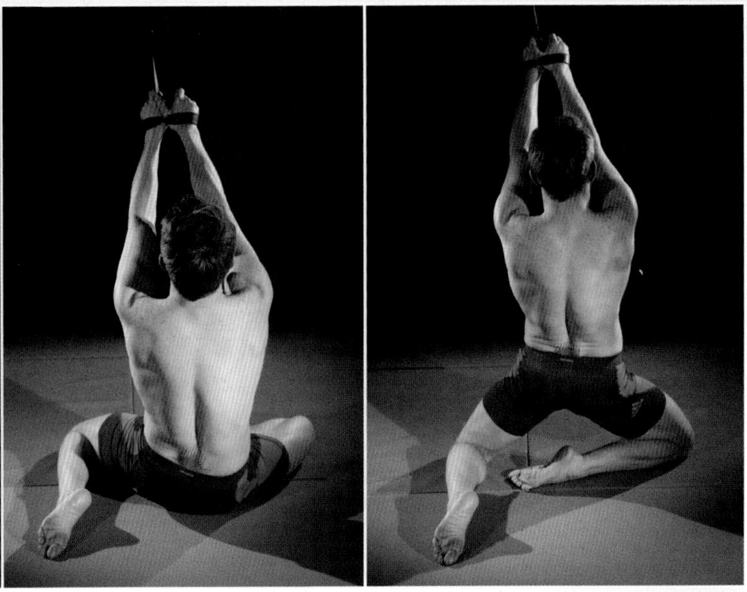

04. OPTIONAL: BARBELL BRIDGE

Sit on the floor, roll a bar over your legs, then lie down on your back. Place the bar just over your hips and hold it with a wide grip. Extend your elbows and lock them in place to keep the bar in position during the exercise. Flex your hips and knees to bring your heels toward your buttocks; in this position, your knees will be at a 90-degree angle. Inhale, quickly lift your hips as high as possible, and exhale as you lower your hips back to the floor. **Perform 4 to 7 reps.**

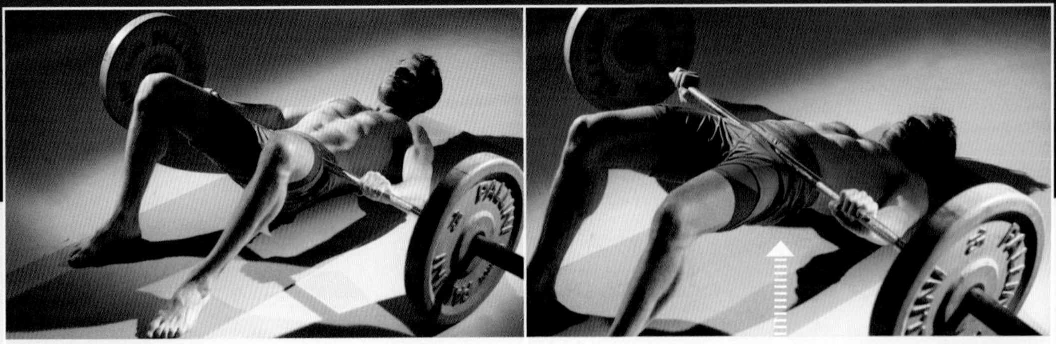

Perform one to three sets of each of the following exercises in order, alternating sides as you go along. Do not stop between exercises.

MASSAGE | STRETCHING | MOBILIZATION | WEIGHTS

solution 02

STIFFNESS IN THE PELVIS

01. GLUTEAL MASSAGE USING A BALL

Lie on your back, raise your feet, and place them on a chair or box. Slide a massage ball under your buttocks and regulate the intensity of the massage by supporting yourself with your feet, which remain on the chair or box.

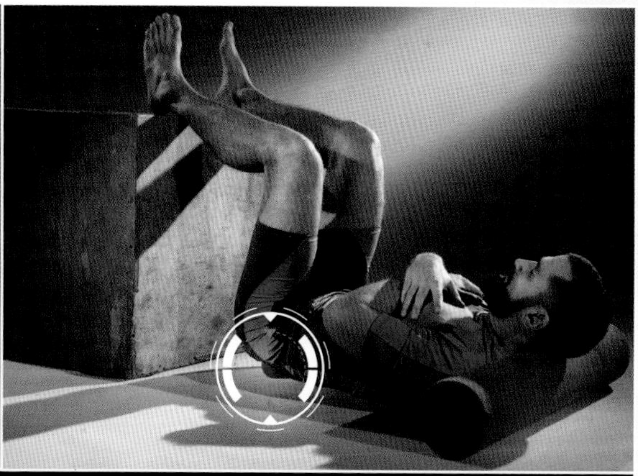

Roll 10 times from top to bottom, 10 times from left to right, and 10 times in a circular motion. Finish with 10 massages with your feet on the floor and knees apart.

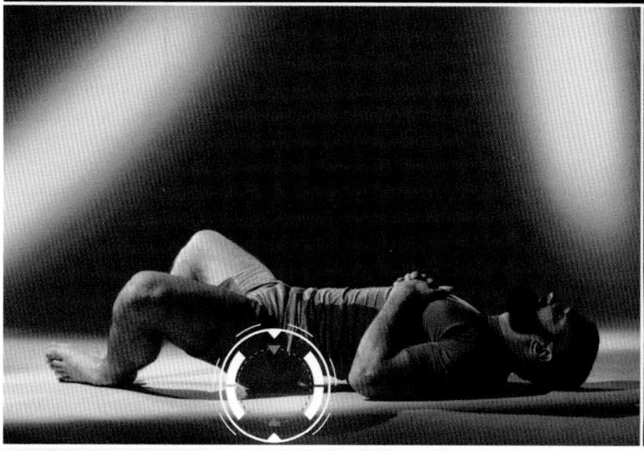

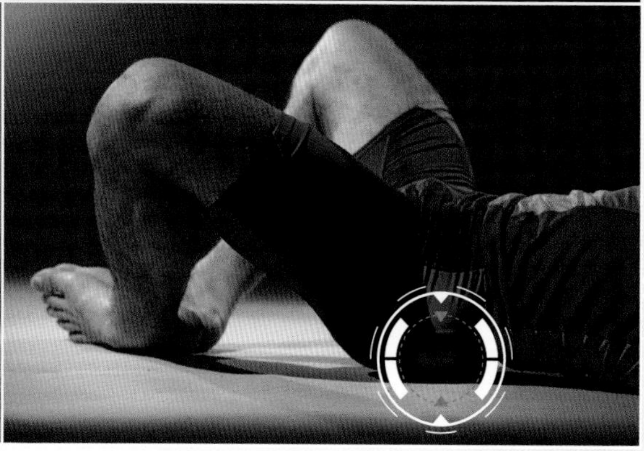

02. HIP ROTATOR WITH A BOX AND A BAND

Place one thigh and outside shin on top of a box or bench with the knee fully flexed and the sole of the foot near the hip of the other leg. Supporting your body with your hands and other leg, lean forward as far as possible. A variation is to combine this exercise with a joint realignment using a resistance band that is anchored overhead and looped around the thigh at a distance from you that makes the band taut. **Hold the stretch for 30 seconds.**

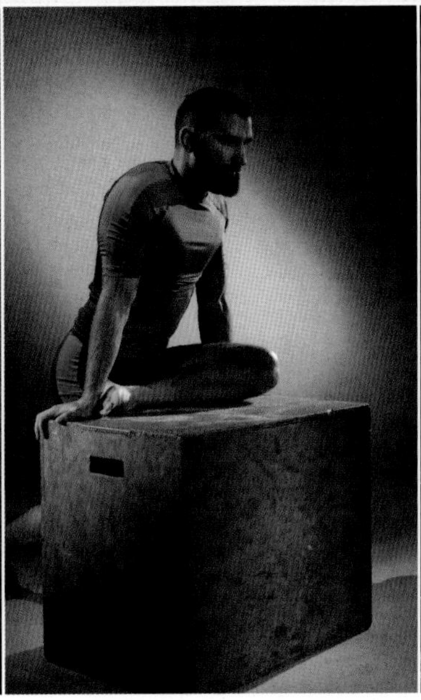

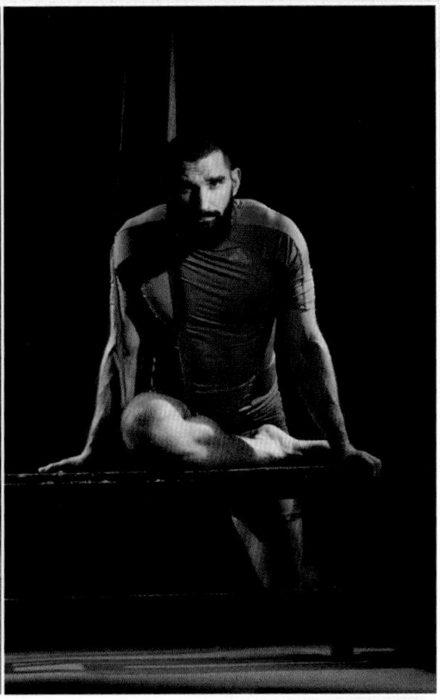

03. OPTIONAL: SIMPLE WEIGHTED GET-UP

Hold a small kettlebell (the weight is too heavy if you must change your position to be able to get up). Sit on the floor with your hips and knees flexed out in front of you and your heels on the floor. Drop the knees to one side and then extend your hips to an erect kneeling position. Sit back down on the floor, bring your legs back out in front of you in the original starting position, and repeat the same movement on the other side. **Perform 10 reps (5 on each side).**

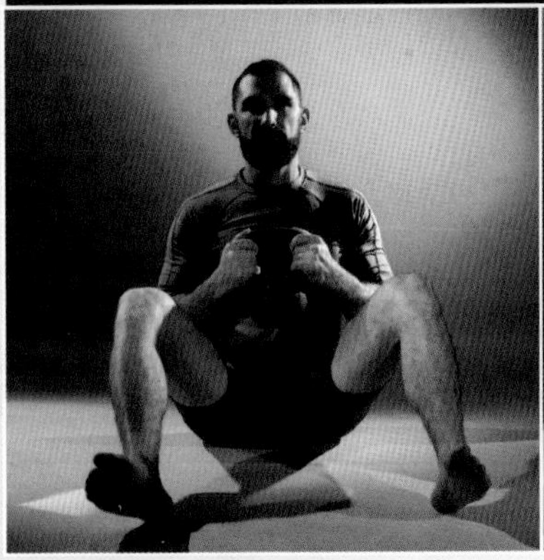

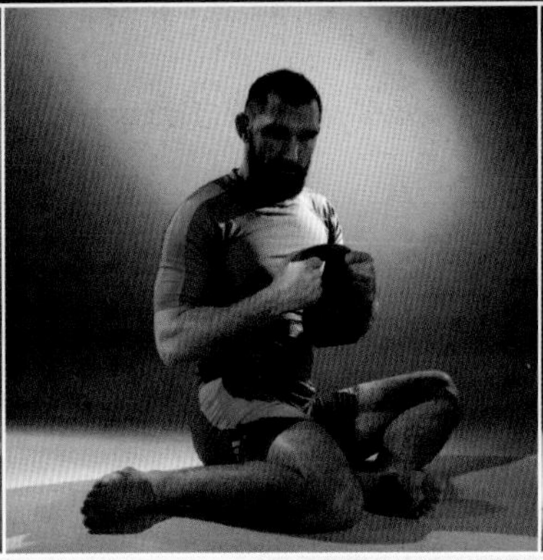

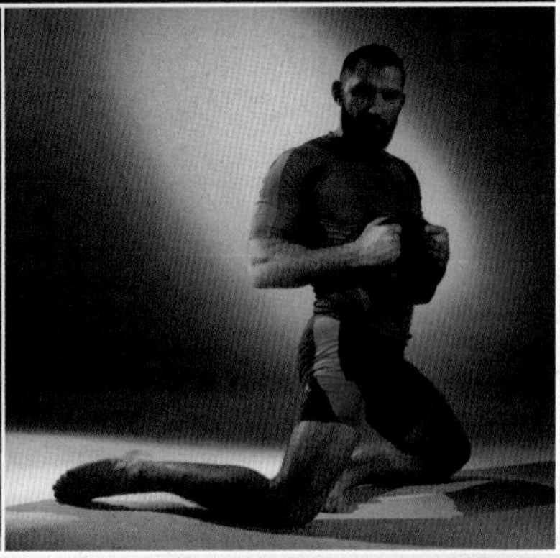

Perform one to three sets of each of the following exercises in order, alternating sides as you go along. Do not stop between exercises.

MASSAGE | STRETCHING | MOBILIZATION | WEIGHTS

solution 03

STIFFNESS IN THE PELVIS

01. LOWER BACK MASSAGE USING A DOUBLE BALL

Lie on your back, raise your feet, and place them on a box with your hips and knees flexed to 90 degrees. For comfort, you can use a foam roller under your head. Slide a double massage ball under your lower back on either side of the spine. Regulate the intensity of the massage by supporting yourself with your legs, which remain on the box. A variation is to lie on your side with the inside of the shin of your top leg on the box and a double massage ball under your torso just above your hip. Be sure to massage both sides. **Perform for 30 to 45 seconds per position.**

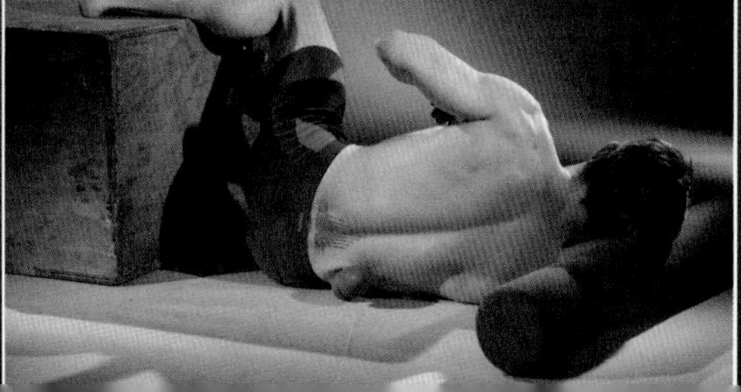

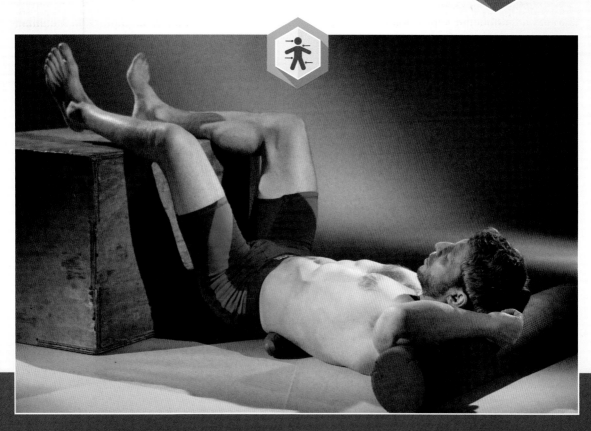

02. STRETCHING THE QUADRATUS LUMBORUM USING A BAND

Lie on your back and place your foot in a resistance band that is anchored near the floor at a distance from you that makes the band taut. Extend your arms overhead to make yourself as tall as possible and relax as much as you can. You can hold on to an anchor point (like a kettlebell or gym ladder). **Hold the stretch for 30 seconds to 1 minute.**

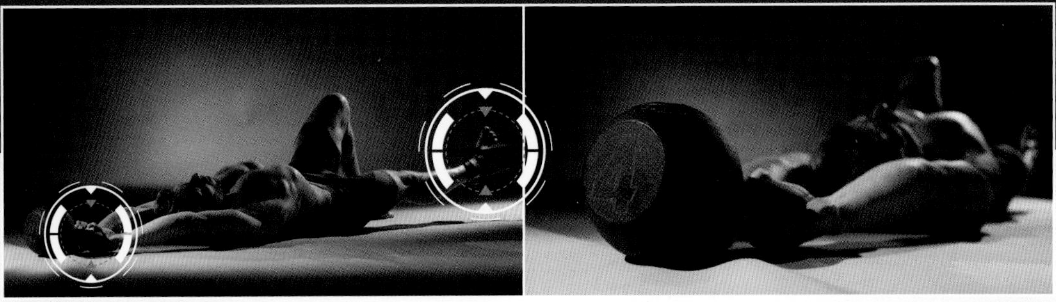

03. SCORPION

Lie face down on an exercise ball with your thighs completely on the ball and your hands on the floor in a plank torso position. Slowly rotate your hips to the side, allowing the upper leg to go as far as possible to the other side. Separate your pelvis and shoulders as much as possible and keep your shoulders parallel to the floor. As you progress, slowly increase your speed. **Perform this exercise at your own pace for 20 seconds. If you are more advanced, go faster.**

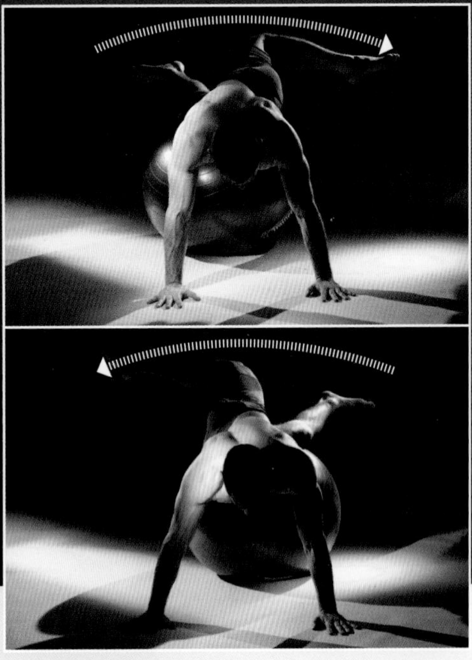

04. OPTIONAL: BACK RAISE AND ROTATION USING A BAND

With your feet held in place by a partner or a gym ladder, lie on an exercise ball with your hips on the ball and your hands holding a resistance band. Extend your torso with your chest out and your head in a neutral position until your upper body is parallel to the floor (look straight ahead through your eyebrows). As you come up, separate your hands, extend your elbows and point your thumbs up until you form a V shape. Keeping your hips on the ball, rotate your torso all the way to the right and all the way to the left, and then relax. **Perform 15 reps.**

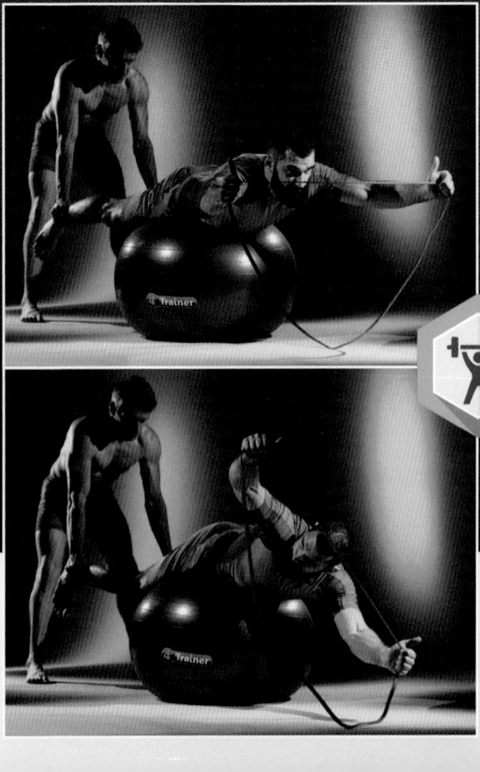

Perform one to three sets of each of the following exercises in order, alternating sides as you go along. Do not stop between exercises.

MASSAGE | STRETCHING | MOBILIZATION | WEIGHTS

solution 04

STIFFNESS IN THE PELVIS

01. ILIOPSOAS MASSAGE USING A LARGE BALL

Lie face down in a semi-plank position with your left hip and knee flexed and your right leg straight and in line with your torso. Place a large massage ball under your right hip. Roll your right hip flexors from front to back, then from left to right, and then in a circular motion. You can increase the pressure on the ball by extending your left hip, knee, or both. **Perform 10 massages of each type for 30 seconds to 1 minute on each side.**

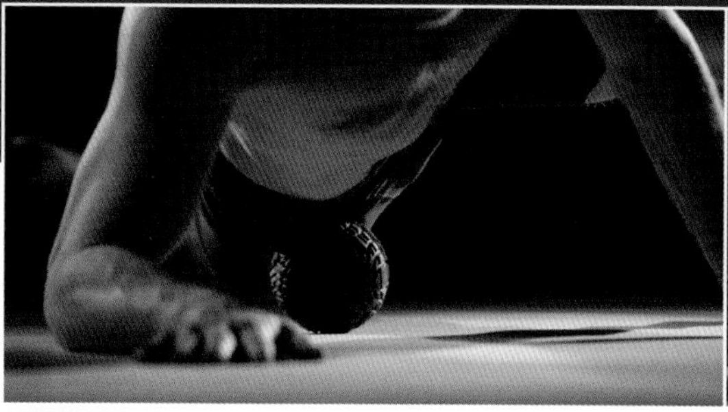

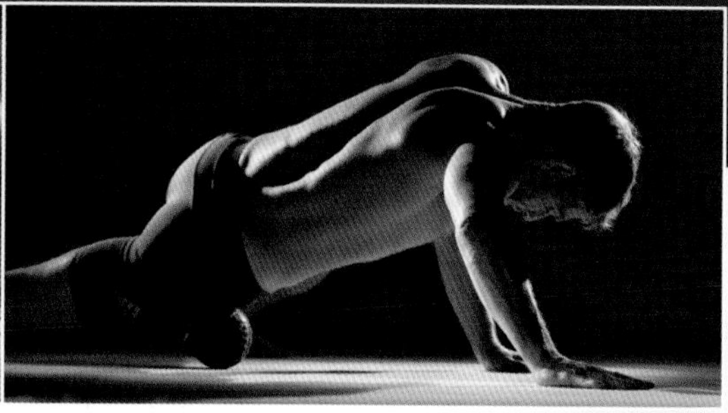

02. FORWARD LUNGE BAND STRETCH

Stand facing a box with a long resistance band that is anchored ahead of you and looped around your upper left thigh at a distance from you that makes the band taut. Place your right foot on top of the box in a deep lunge position with your left arm extended overhead and your left knee almost fully extended behind you. Tilt your torso toward your right thigh to feel the stretch. **Hold the stretch for 30 seconds.**

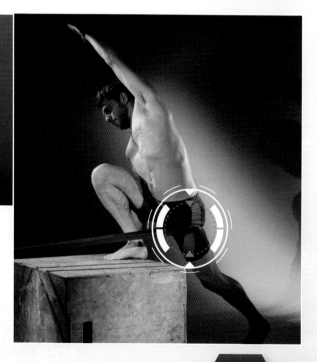

03. ALTERNATING SQUATS OR FORWARD FOLDS

Move into as low a squat as possible with your back perfectly straight and without lifting your heels (place them on a wedge if necessary). Spend three seconds moving down and three seconds in the lowest position for each repetition. Stand up and then fold your torso forward toward your legs, keeping the knees extended. Hold the forward fold position for three seconds. **Perform 4 reps of each movement.**

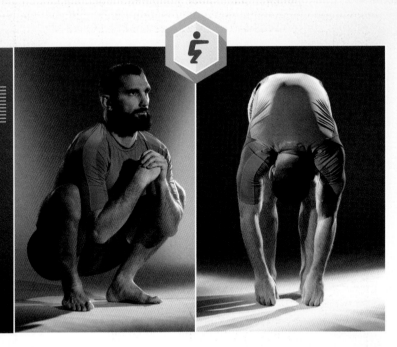

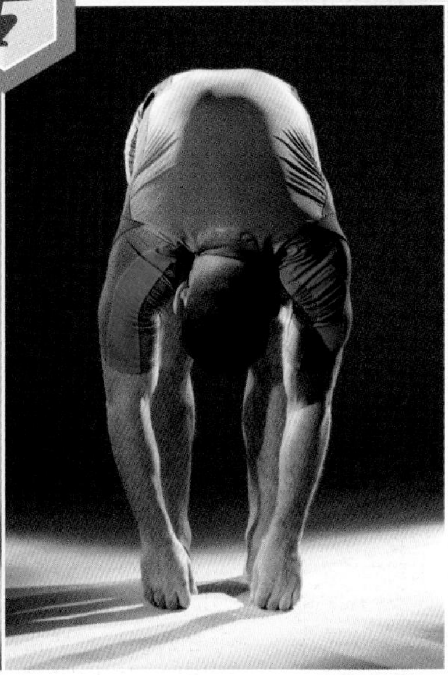

04. OPTIONAL: DEEP WEIGHTED LUNGE

Place a weight bar on the back of your shoulders. Take a step as far forward as possible, allowing the kneecap of your front knee to pass over the toes of your front foot. Open your hip as much as possible without arching your back too much. **Perform 6 reps, alternating between the right foot and the left foot.**

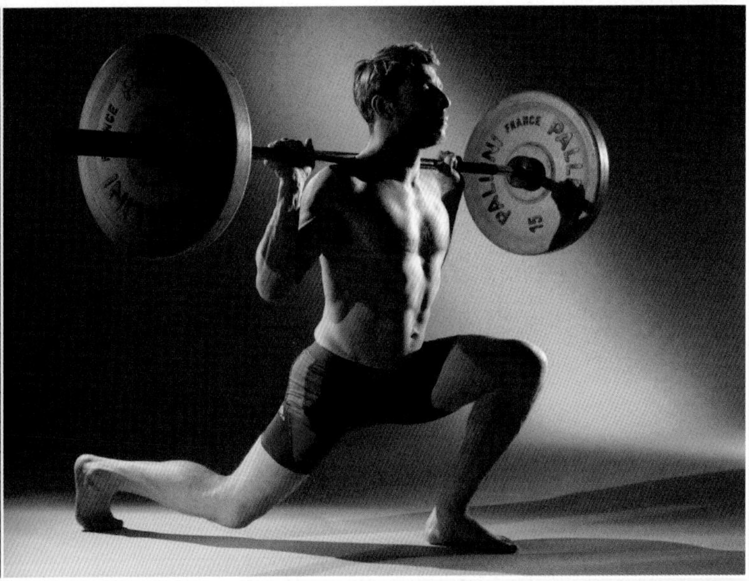

Perform one to three sets of each of the following exercises in order on the same side. Do not stop between exercises. When they are completed, go through the series again for the other side.

MASSAGE | STRETCHING | MOBILIZATION | WEIGHTS

solution 05

STIFFNESS IN THE PELVIS

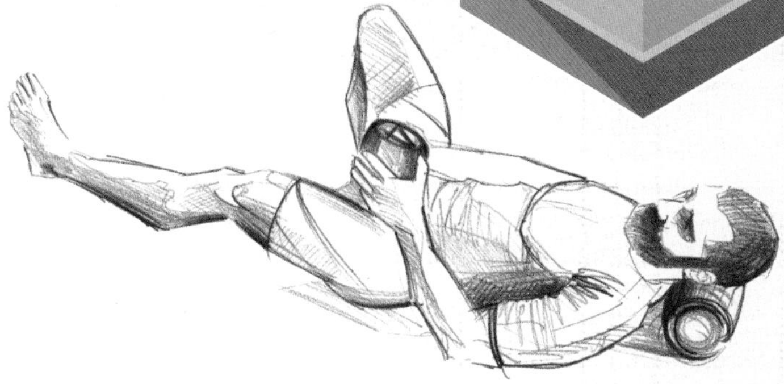

01. ILIOPSOAS MASSAGE USING A KETTLEBELL

Lie on your back and let your knees drop to one side. For comfort, you can use a foam roller under your head. Place the ball of a kettlebell on the iliopsoas of the higher hip, which is more accessible in this position. A variation for more precision is to massage the iliopsoas using your fist. **Perform by gently massaging from top to bottom and side to side for 1 minute.**

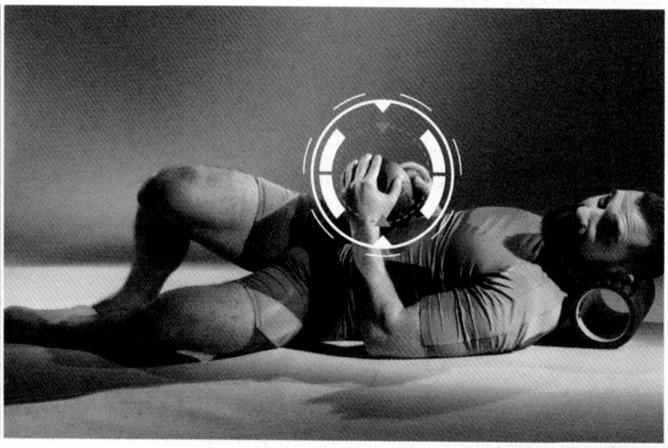

02. LUNGE STRETCH USING A BAND PULLING FORWARD

Stand in a wide split-squat lunge position with a long resistance band that is anchored ahead of you at a distance that makes the band taut when looped around your upper back thigh. Raise the arm on the same side as the back leg overhead and tilt your torso to the opposite side to feel an additional stretch. **Hold the position for 10 to 30 seconds.**

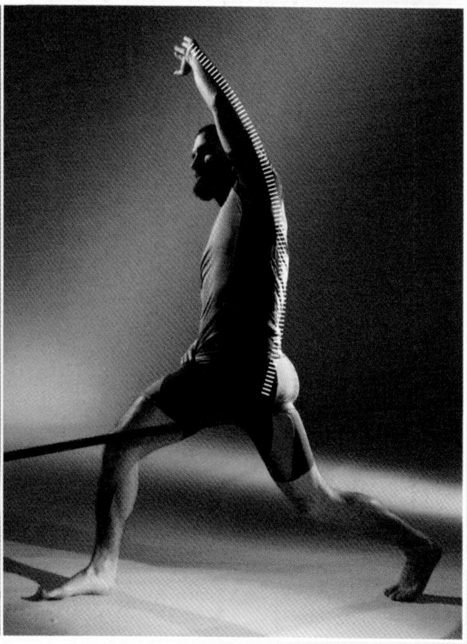

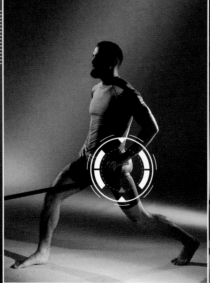

03. LUNGE WITH ARMS TOWARD THE SKY

Keeping your feet parallel to each other, lunge as deep as possible and reach your arms overhead with your palms facing each other. Look up and extend your back as much as possible. **Perform 4 reps without changing legs.**

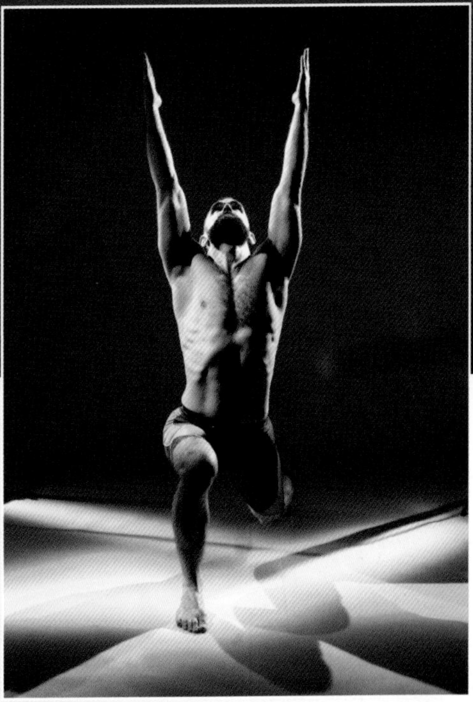

04. OPTIONAL: WEIGHTED PSOAS MOVEMENT

Lie on your back and position the handle of a kettlebell on the psoas of one hip. Fully extend your knee and raise your whole leg by flexing the hip slightly to activate the psoas. As a variation, you can flex the knee or move the leg in different directions. **Hold the position for 30 seconds to 1 minute.**

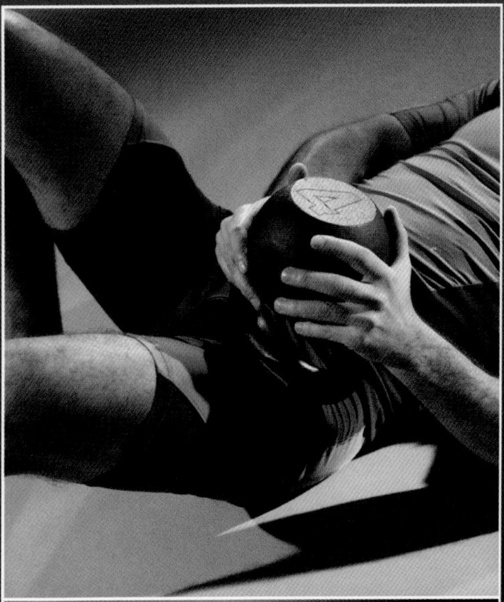

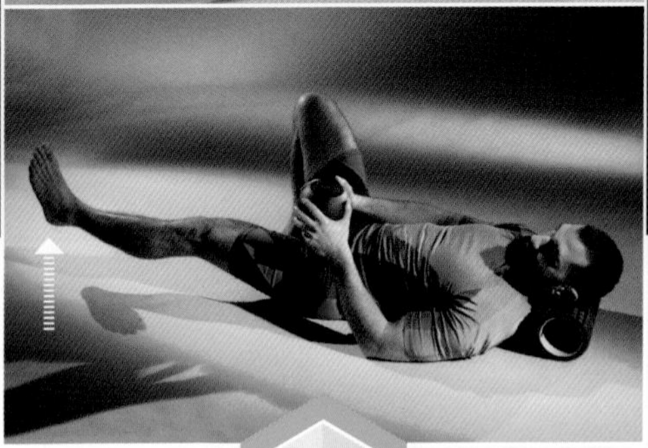

TESTS

KNEE TRAJECTORY

1

Lunge Test

Place your hands on your hips and stand with your feet together. Lunge forward then come back to the starting position. Repeat 15 times on the same leg while facing a mirror or with the help of a spotter. To pass this test, the knee must stay within the area between the small and big toes. If the knee shifts to the inside (see the second photo), you should use the following corrective exercises.

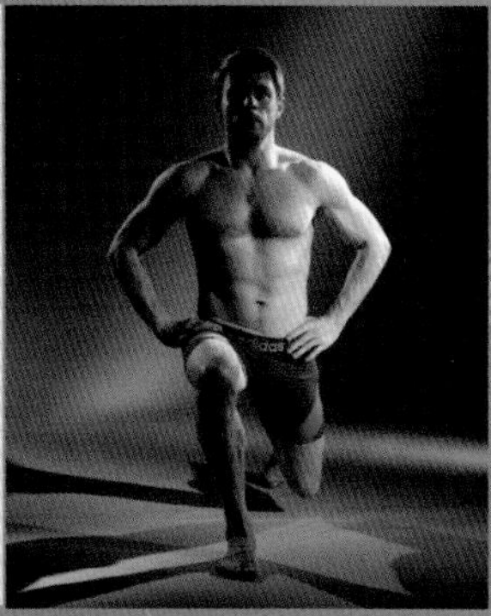

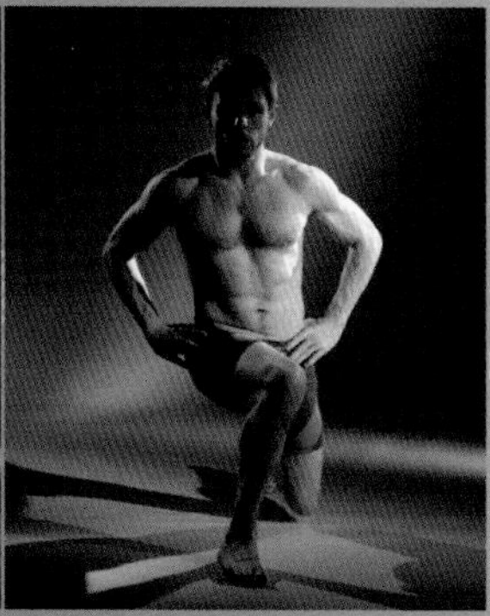

2

Wedge Test

Stand a yoga block beside you. Place your hands on your hips and squat down using one leg to touch the wedge with your other knee. You pass this test if you can touch the wedge with your knee, the movement does not cause pain, and you can maintain your balance.

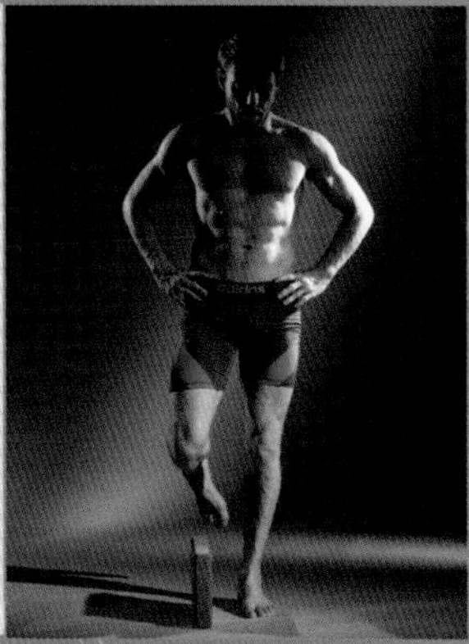

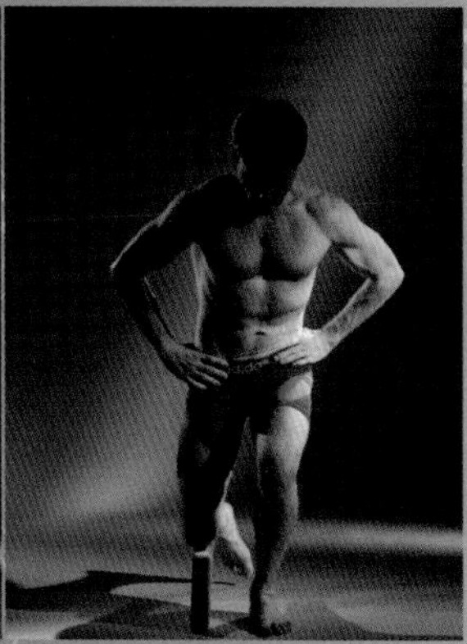

3

Monster Squat Test

Use a small band that is positioned just below your knees. Keeping your feet parallel, squat as low as possible with your hands on your hips. Keep your knees in line with your toes. If the knees shift to the inside, you should use the following corrective exercises.

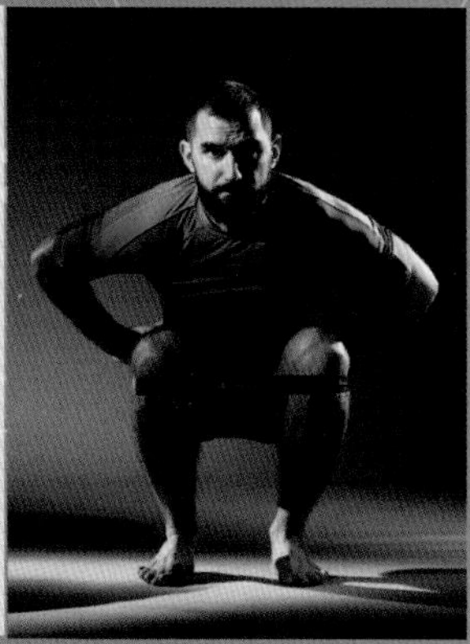

solution
01

MASSAGE | STRETCHING | MOBILIZATION | WEIGHTS

Perform one to three sets of each of the following exercises in order, alternating sides as you go along. Do not stop between exercises.

KNEE TRAJECTORY

01. ADDUCTOR MASSAGE USING A LARGE BALL

Lie face down and support yourself on your elbows. Place a large massage ball under your inner thigh and roll from front to back and then from top to bottom. Look for the stiffest and most sensitive areas and concentrate on them. **Perform 12 massages of each type.**

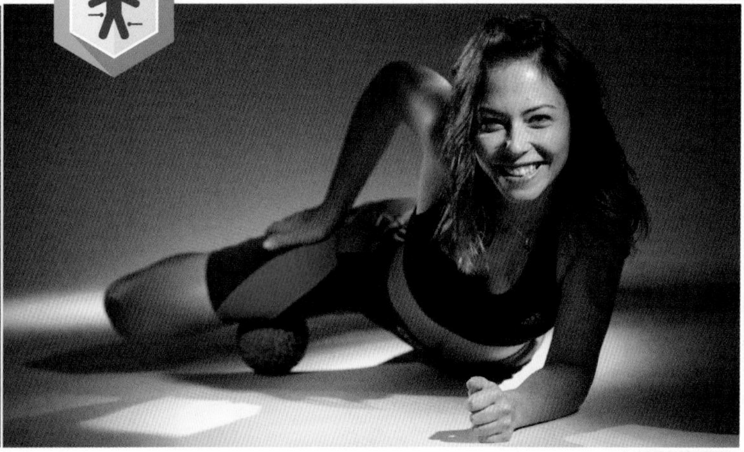

02. RESISTANCE BAND ADDUCTOR STRETCH

Lie on top of (and perpendicular to) a resistance band, bring your knees up, and place a knee into each looped end of the band. Allow the band to pull your knees as far apart as possible with your feet flat against a wall or a corner of two walls.

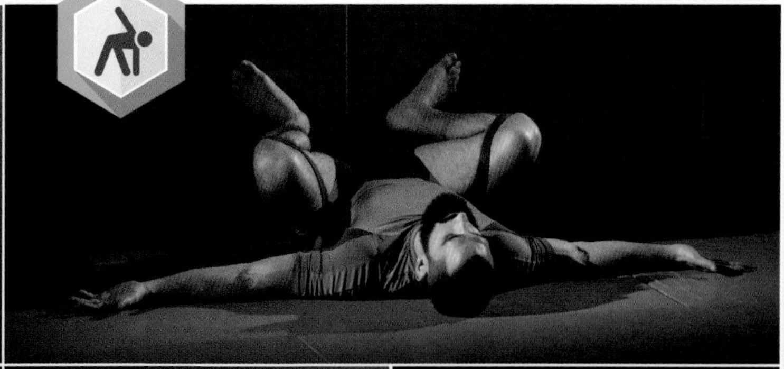

For a more advanced version, squat with your back to the wall.
Hold each position for 30 seconds to 2 minutes.

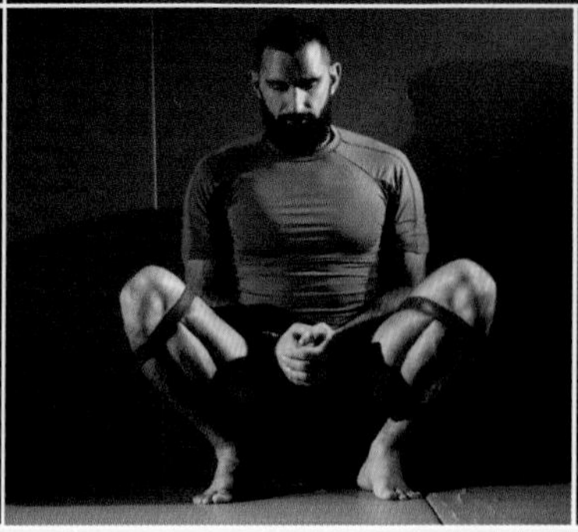

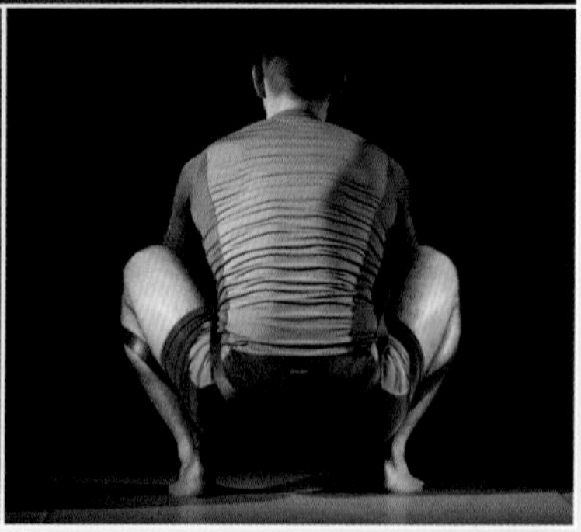

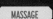

03. DEEP LATERAL SQUAT

Stand erect and, with your hands on your hips, step to the side with one leg (keep the nonstepping knee fully extended) and squat down with the support leg. Come back up and bring the extended leg back to the starting position.
Perform 4 reps to the same side before changing to the other side.

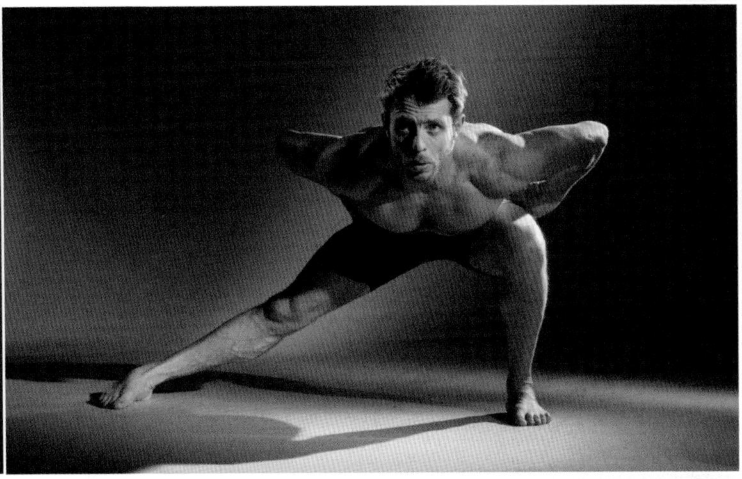

04. OPTIONAL: DEEP WEIGHTED SQUAT

Place a bar on the back of your shoulders and squat down as deeply as possible. Keep your feet flat on the floor, your chest out, and your torso erect throughout the exercise. If it hurts when you move into a deep squat, you can use a wedge under your heels, do the move without a bar, or hold on to a suspended resistance band.
Hold the bottom position for 30 seconds.

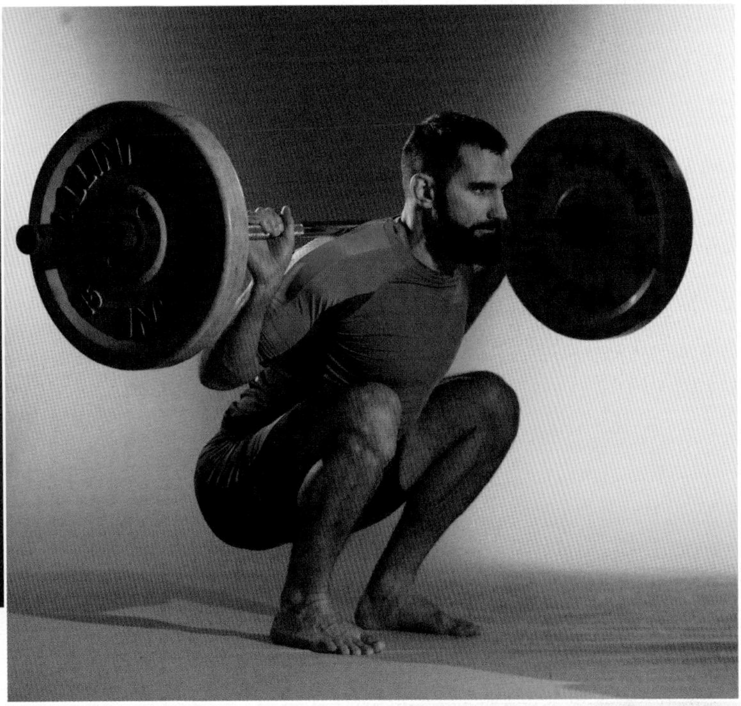

solution
02

MASSAGE | STRETCHING | MOBILIZATION | WEIGHTS

Perform one to three sets of each of the following exercises in order on the same leg. Do not stop between exercises. When they are completed, go through the series again for the other leg.

KNEE TRAJECTORY

01. ADDUCTOR MASSAGE USING A ROLLER

Lie face down and support yourself on your elbows. Place a roller under your inner thigh and roll to look for the stiffest and most sensitive areas and concentrate on them. **Perform 12 massages from left to right.**

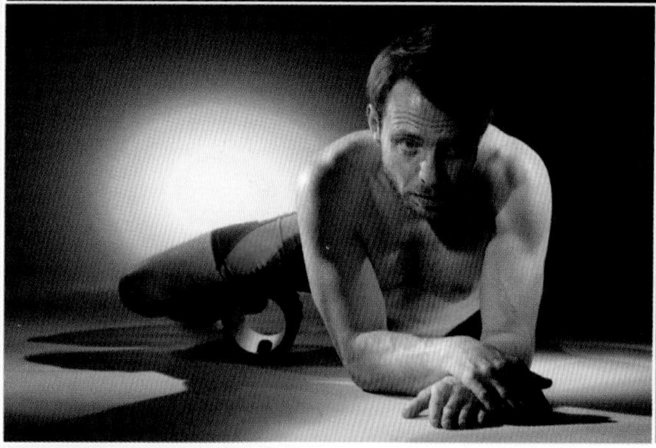

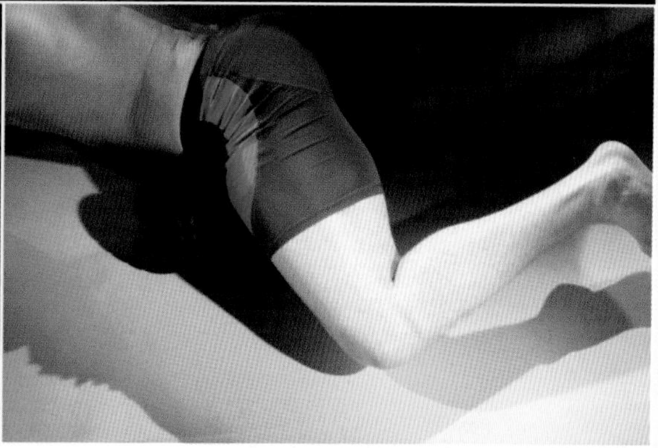

02. ADDUCTOR STRETCH ON ALL FOURS

Get into an all-fours position with your elbows on the floor, back flat, and knees flexed to about 90 degrees. Slide your knees as far apart as possible. **Hold the final position for 30 seconds to 2 minutes.**

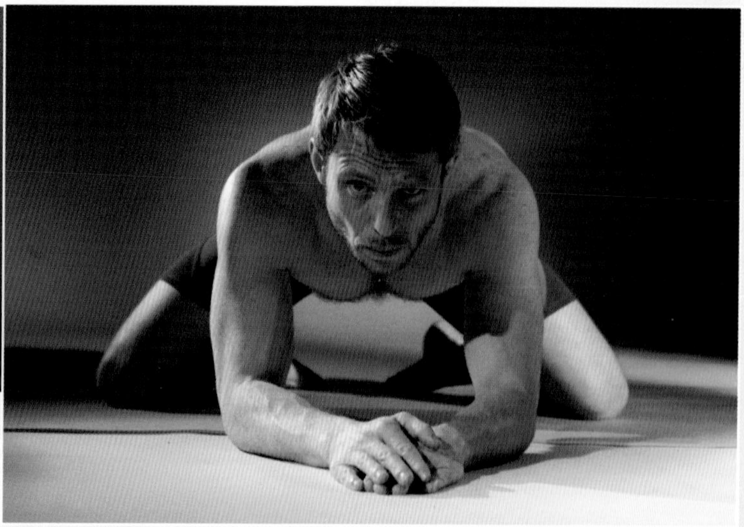

03. SUMO SQUAT

Hold on to a resistance band with both hands and extend both arms above your head. Move into a sumo squat (a squat with your feet very far apart), then lift one leg to the side by tilting your whole body to the side of your other foot. Slowly pivot on this foot to return to the same starting position, then repeat in the other direction. **Perform 3 steps in one direction and 3 steps in the other direction.**

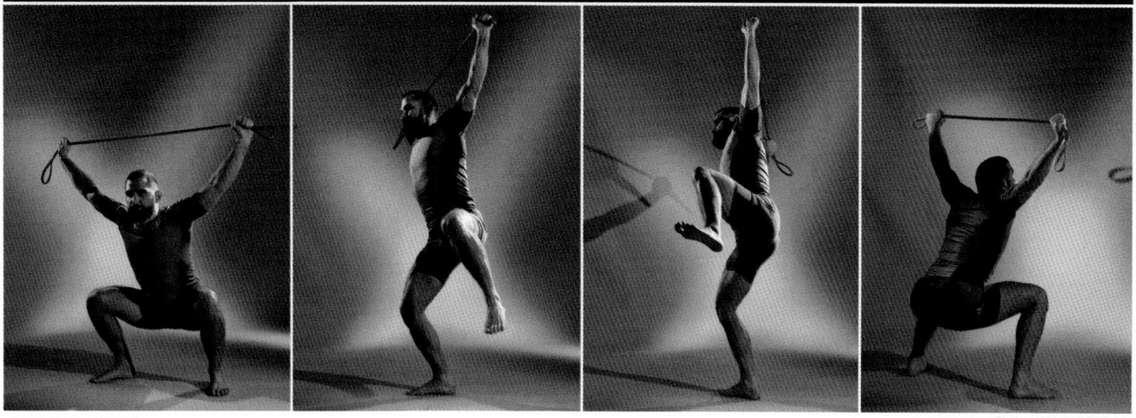

04. OPTIONAL: ONE-LEG SQUAT ON AN EXERCISE BALL

With the instep and lower shin of your back leg on top of an exercise ball, place your front foot a short distance ahead of the ball and your hands on your hips. Without any lateral compensation or rotation, flex your front hip and knee to squat toward the floor, allowing the ball to roll slightly forward and the kneecap of your front leg to follow the direction of your toes. **Perform 10 reps.**

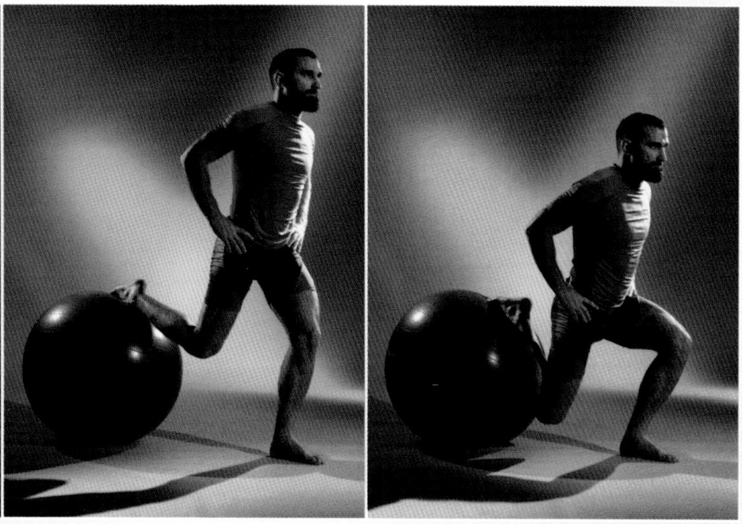

solution 03

MASSAGE STRETCHING MOBILIZATION WEIGHTS

Perform one to three sets of each of the following exercises in order, alternating sides as you go along. Do not stop between exercises.

KNEE TRAJECTORY

01. BACK OF THE KNEE MASSAGE USING A BALL

Sit down and slide a massage ball under the back of your knee. Squeeze your calf against the back of your thigh to squish the ball.

Hold the position for 20 to 30 seconds.

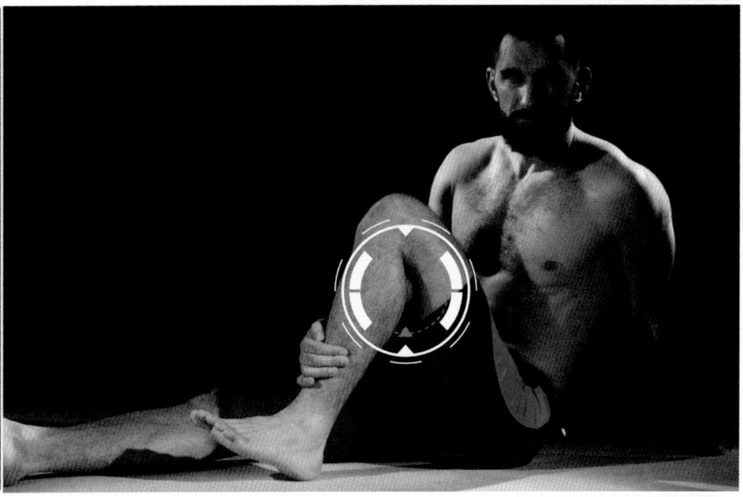

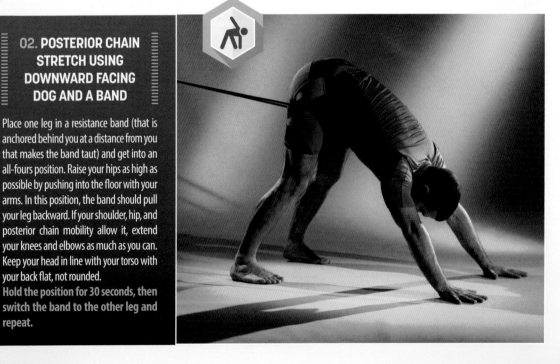

02. POSTERIOR CHAIN STRETCH USING DOWNWARD FACING DOG AND A BAND

Place one leg in a resistance band (that is anchored behind you at a distance from you that makes the band taut) and get into an all-fours position. Raise your hips as high as possible by pushing into the floor with your arms. In this position, the band should pull your leg backward. If your shoulder, hip, and posterior chain mobility allow it, extend your knees and elbows as much as you can. Keep your head in line with your torso with your back flat, not rounded.

Hold the position for 30 seconds, then switch the band to the other leg and repeat.

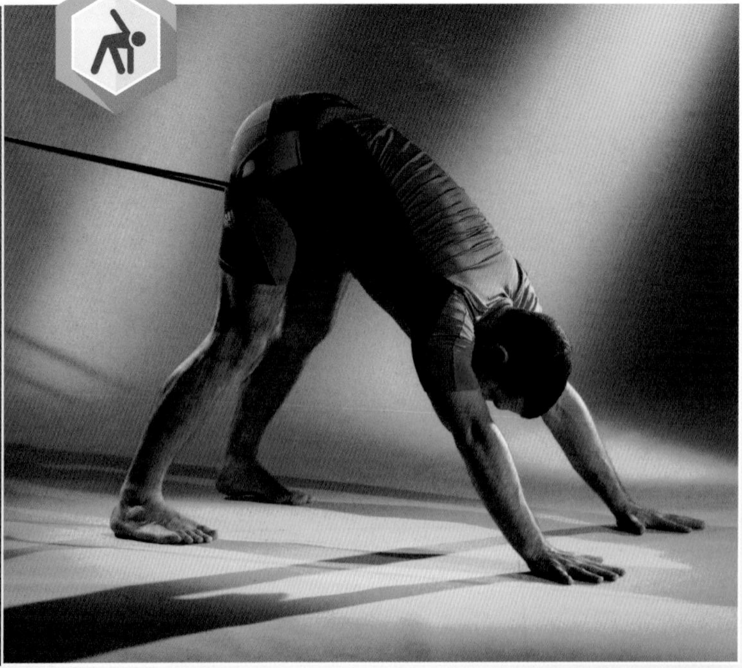

03. BALANCING ON ONE LEG USING A BAND TO DESTABILIZE THE KNEE

Wrap a resistance band around your knee that is taut enough to pull you forward. Stand on that leg (only) with your eyes closed. Ideally, ask a partner to vary the direction of the traction slightly. Try to keep your knee between your big and small toes.

Balance for 30 seconds on each leg.

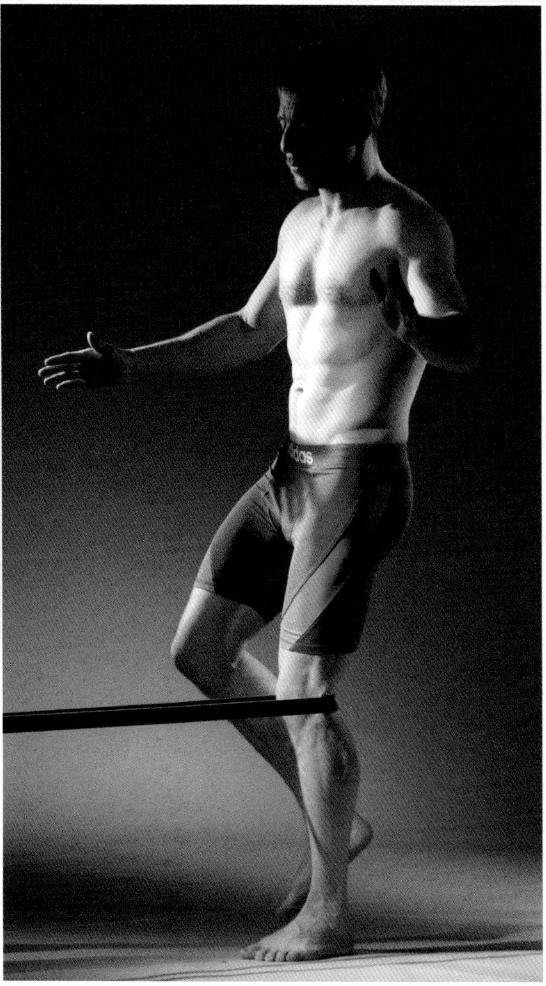

04. OPTIONAL: SQUAT USING AN EXERCISE BALL AND A WEIGHT PLATE

Place an exercise ball behind your back and stand with your feet in front of the line of your torso while holding a weight plate in front of you. While pushing back against the ball as much as possible, squat down and back up with your back perpendicular to the floor throughout the movement.

Perform 10 reps.

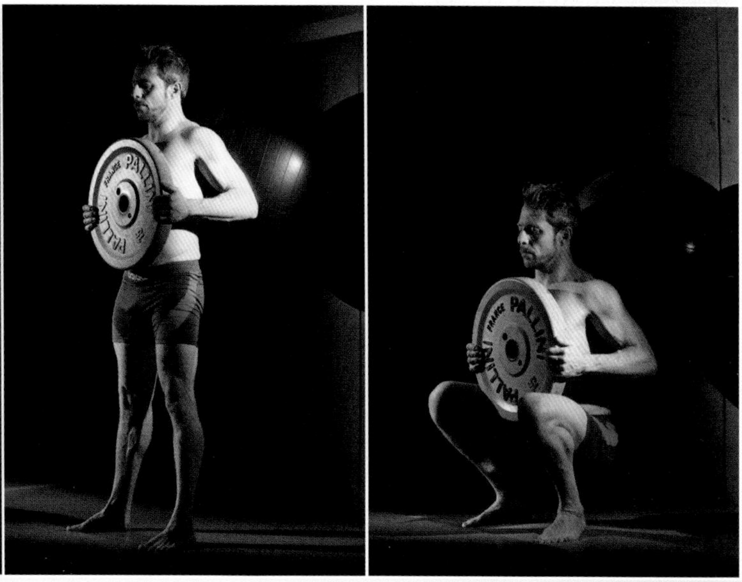

solution 04

MASSAGE | STRETCHING | MOBILIZATION | WEIGHTS

Perform one to three sets of each of the following exercises in order on the same leg. Do not stop between exercises. When they are completed, go through the series again for the other leg.

KNEE TRAJECTORY

01. PATELLAR TENDON MASSAGE USING A ROLLER

In the knighthood position, place one knee on the roller with the other leg in a lunge position. Regulate the intensity of the massage by using the front leg for support. **Roll 10 times from front to back.**

02. FORWARD LUNGE USING A BAND

Move into a forward lunge position with a resistance band anchored ahead of you and looped around your front leg at the top of your calf or shin. **Hold the position for 30 seconds.**

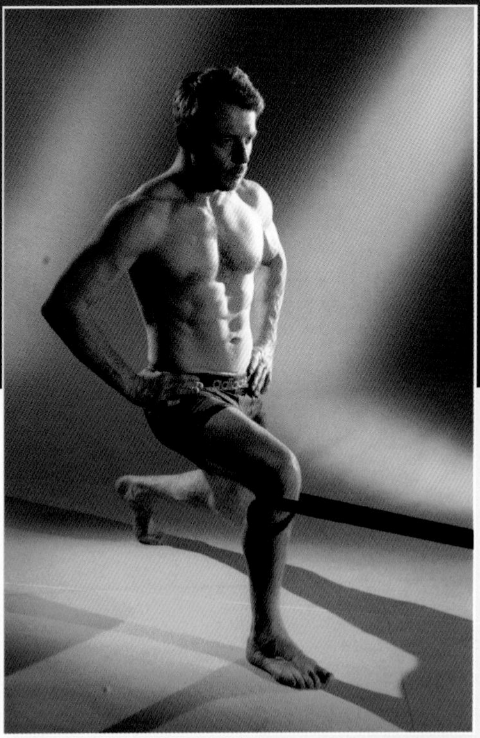

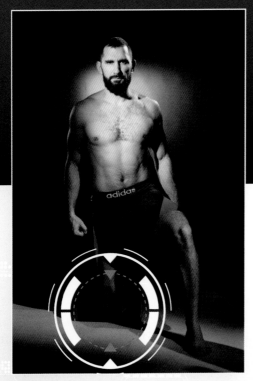

03. SUSPENSION TRAINER COSSACK SQUAT

Hold on to the suspension trainer and step to the side with one leg (keep the nonstepping knee fully extended) and squat down with the support leg. Concentrate on the trajectory of your knee, which should stay in line with your toes. **Perform 10 reps to the same side before changing to the other side.**

04. OPTIONAL: STEP-BY-STEP KNEEL USING A KETTLEBELL

Hold a kettlebell in front of you in both hands and, keeping your back as straight as possible, place one knee on the floor and then the other without flexing your hips. Sit back on your heels before shifting your legs so your shins and insteps are flat on the floor. **Perform the steps to kneel and then reverse the movement to return to a standing position. Repeat with the other leg to lead the movement.**

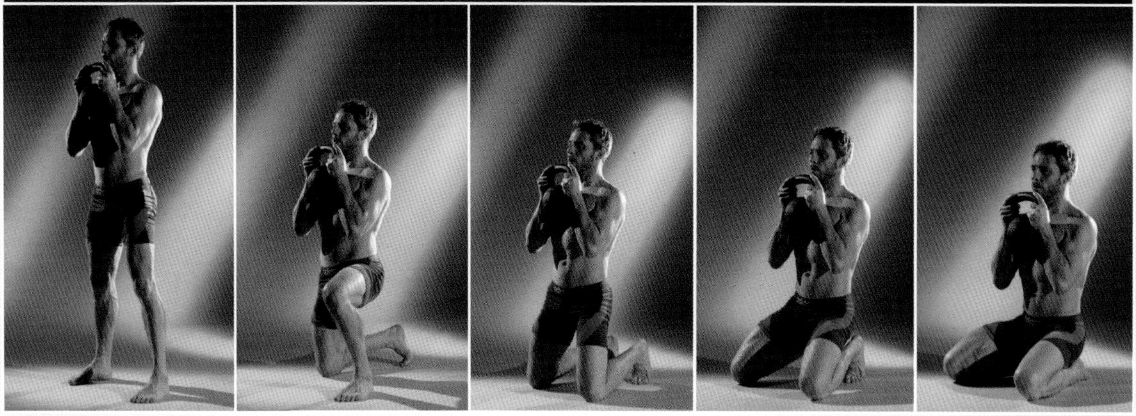

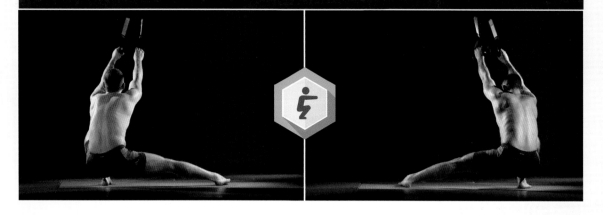

TESTS

RESTRICTIONS IN THE LOWER POSTERIOR CHAIN

1

Toe Touch

Stand and lean forward to try to touch the toes on your left foot, keeping your right knee slightly flexed. Then try to touch the toes on your right foot, keeping your left knee slightly flexed. If you cannot touch your toes on either side, it is essential that you practice the following corrective exercises. Also note the difference between the two legs; it may encourage you to focus on one side more than the other.

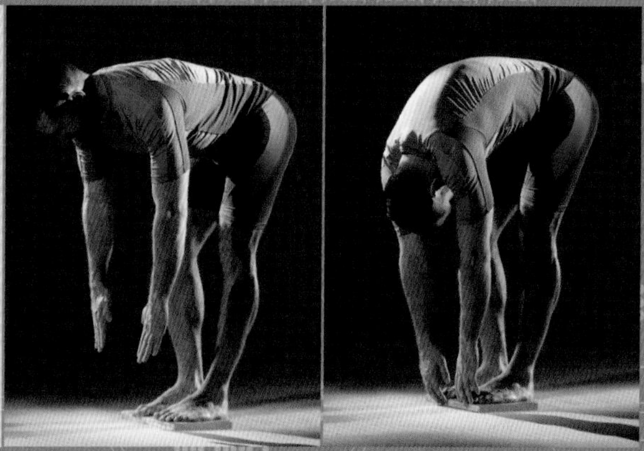

2

Kettlebell Floor Touch With a Flat Back

Holding a light kettlebell (around 10 lb [4.5 kg] for women and around 20 lb [9.1 kg] for men), push out your chest, pull your shoulders back and down, and spread your feet shoulder-width apart. With minimal knee flexion, flex your torso forward and allow the kettlebell to hang in front of you. Keep your back straight and your head neutral as you look forward. To pass this test, your torso should end up parallel to the floor (for some, the kettlebell may touch the floor).

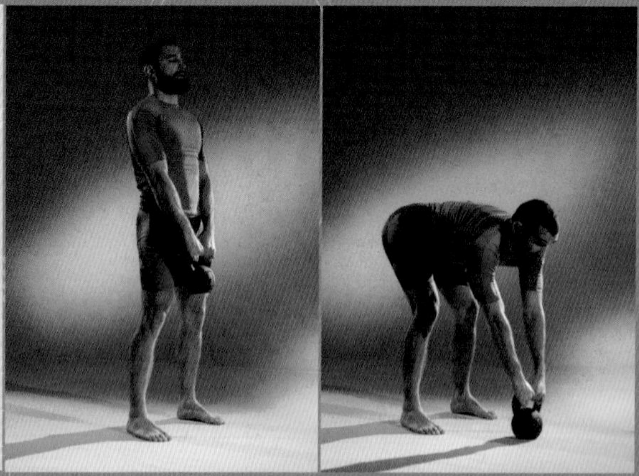

Perform one to three sets of each of the following exercises in order on the same side. Do not stop between exercises. When they are completed, go through the series again for the other side.

MASSAGE | STRETCHING | MOBILIZATION | WEIGHTS

solution 01

RESTRICTIONS IN THE LOWER POSTERIOR CHAIN

01. HAMSTRING MASSAGE USING A WEIGHT BAR

Supporting your weight on your arms and one foot, place your thigh on a bar (with added weight plates) with that knee fully extended. Alter the intensity of the massage by extending your hip to press your thigh on the bar or by flexing your elbows to lower your hips toward the floor to create the desired pressure.
Perform 10 front-to-back rolls.

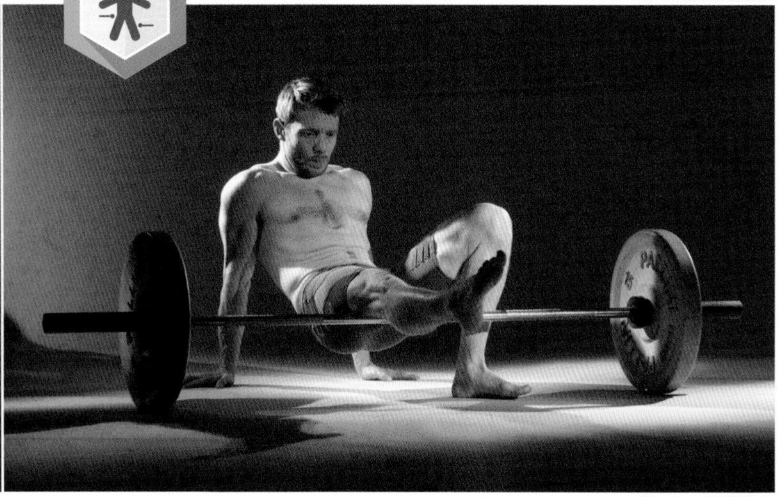

02. SINGLE-LEG STRETCH USING A BAND

Lie on your back, place your foot in the loop of a resistance band, and flex your hip to lift your leg up and toward your head, keeping your knee fully extended. With your arms anchoring the band overhead, pull on your leg. Try to not compensate by lifting your other leg off the floor or flexing either knee.
Hold the stretch for 30 seconds.

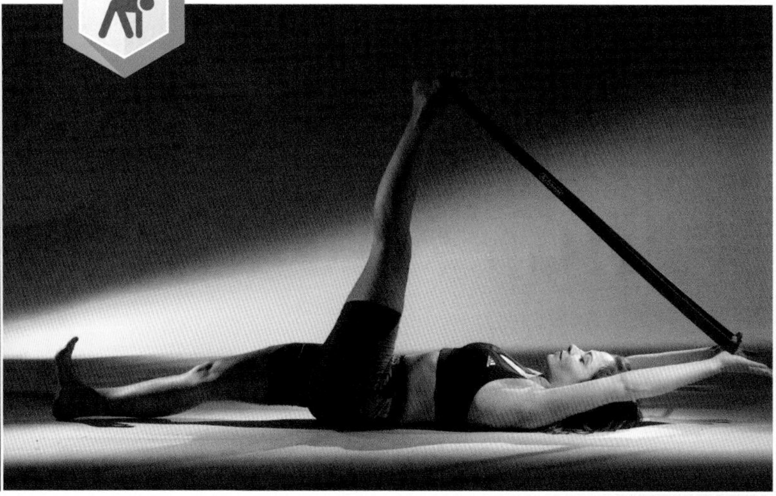

03. ASSISTED SINGLE-LEG FLEXION USING A BAND

Lie on your back, place your foot in the loop of a resistance band, and use the band to help you flex the hip with your knee fully extended. Try to not compensate by lifting your other leg off the floor or flexing either knee.
Perform 10 reps.

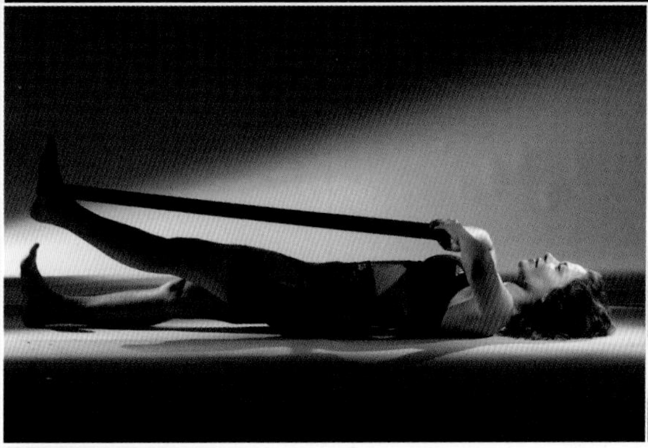

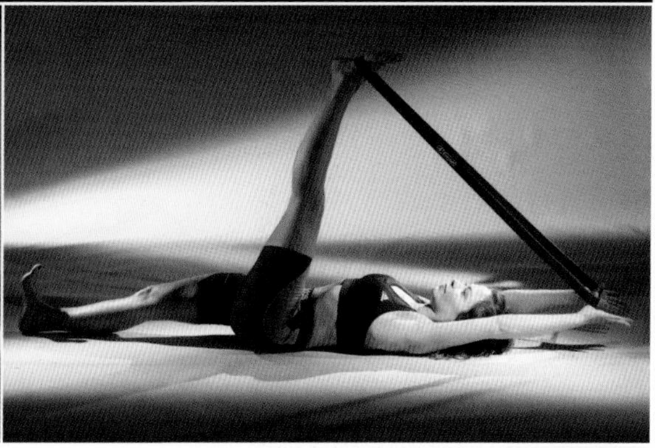

04. OPTIONAL: KETTLEBELL ARABESQUE

Stand up and hold a kettlebell in front of you with your elbows extended and feet together. Push your chest out and place your head in a neutral position. Flex your torso forward as you extend one hip to raise the leg with the knee fully extended. Your torso and lifted leg are synchronized and form a line. Do not compensate by leaning back to open your hips or flex your knees. Your torso and lifted leg should end up being parallel to the floor.
Perform 4 slow reps.

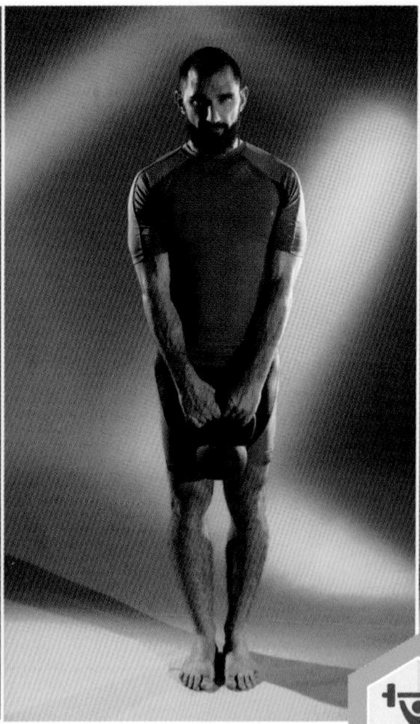

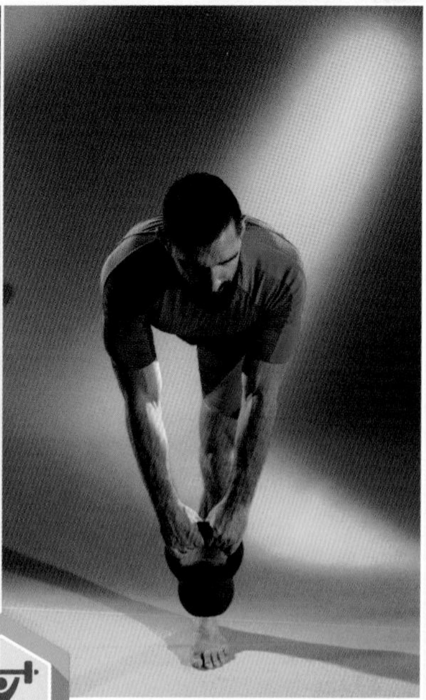

Perform one to three sets of each of the following exercises in order on the same side. Do not stop between exercises. When they are completed, go through the series again for the other side.

MASSAGE | STRETCHING | MOBILIZATION | WEIGHTS

solution 02

RESTRICTIONS IN THE LOWER POSTERIOR CHAIN

01. GLUTEAL MASSAGE USING A ROLLER

Place a roller in line with your thigh. Cross the leg of the massaged gluteal muscle over your other leg to lengthen the muscles and increase pressure.
Perform 10 to 20 left-to-right rolls.

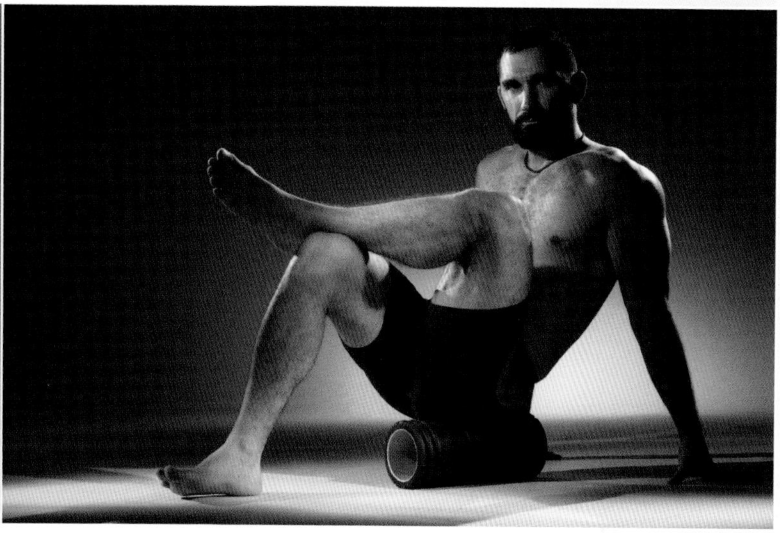

02. CROSS-LEGGED STRETCH

Sit in a cross-legged position, taking care to cross your shins, and bring your heels close to your buttocks before leaning forward. The leg on the side you just massaged should be behind the other leg.
Hold the stretch for 30 seconds.

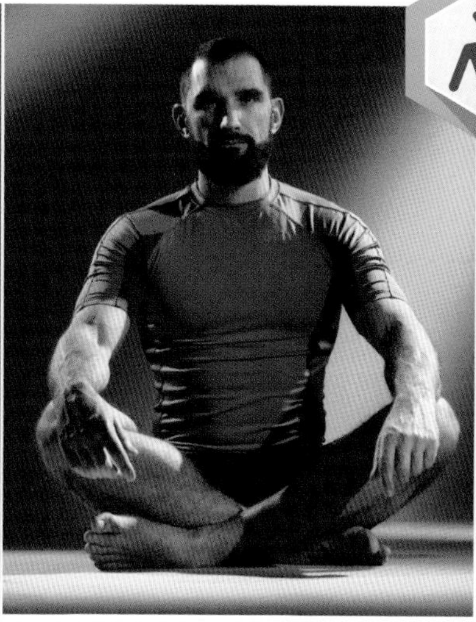

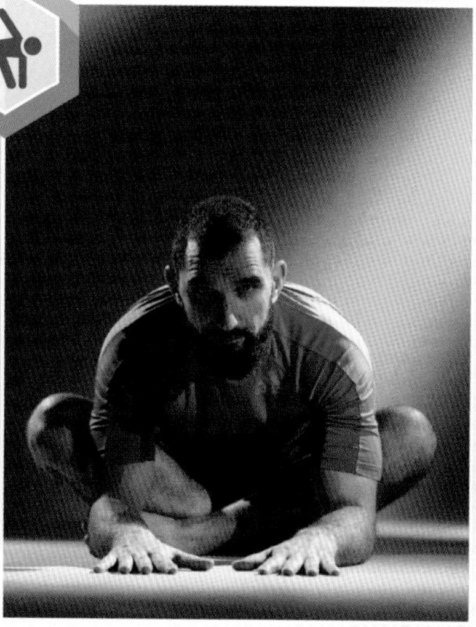

03. BALLISTIC SWEEP

Stand perpendicular to a wall. Place a hand on the wall for balance, lock your lower back, and propel your inside leg forward then backward. Do not compensate by arching or rounding your lower back. **Perform 10 sweeps per leg.**

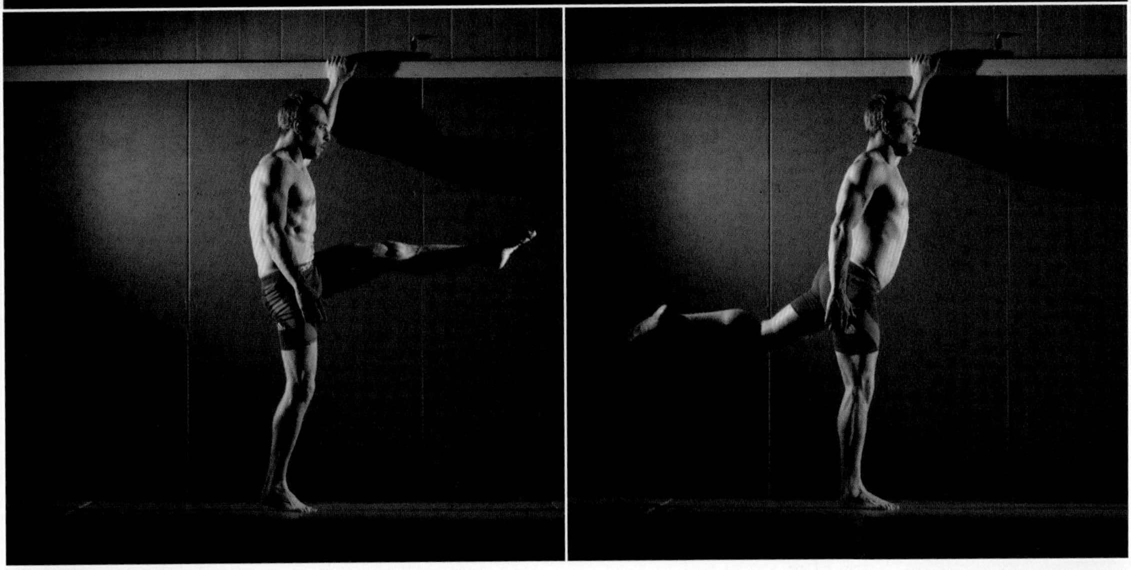

04. OPTIONAL: SHORT TRAJECTORY DEADLIFT

Place a bar on two blocks or piles of weight plates to shorten the trajectory of the movement. Stand with your feet hip-width apart and grasp the bar outside your thighs. Before starting the set of repetitions, squeeze your gluteal muscles and keep them tightened. With your back straight and chest out, stand up with the bar, pause, and lower the bar back to the starting position, taking three seconds to go down. **Perform 4 reps.**

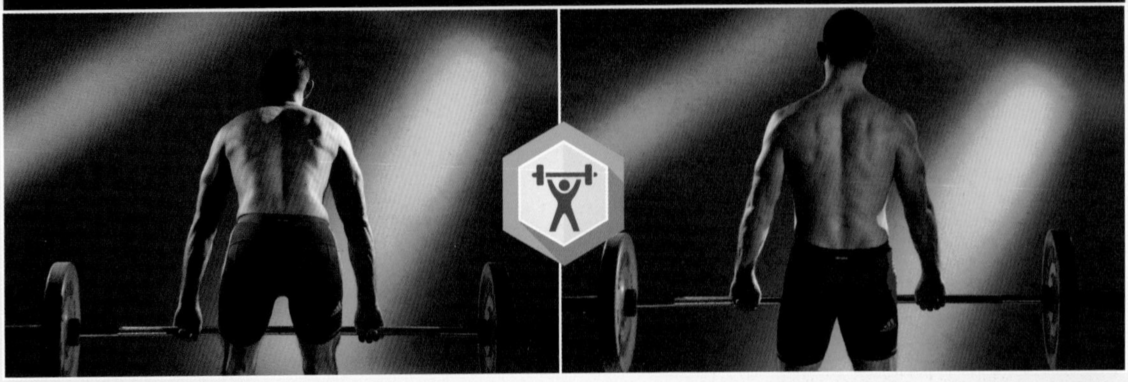

Perform one to three sets of each of the following exercises in order on the same leg. Do not stop between exercises. When they are completed, go through the series again for the other leg.

MASSAGE STRETCHING MOBILIZATION WEIGHTS

solution 03

RESTRICTIONS IN THE LOWER POSTERIOR CHAIN

01. HAMSTRING MASSAGE USING A LARGE BALL

On a table or box, sit on a large massage ball. Roll from front to back and left to right and finish with circular movements over the most sensitive and stiff areas.
Perform 10 massages of each type.

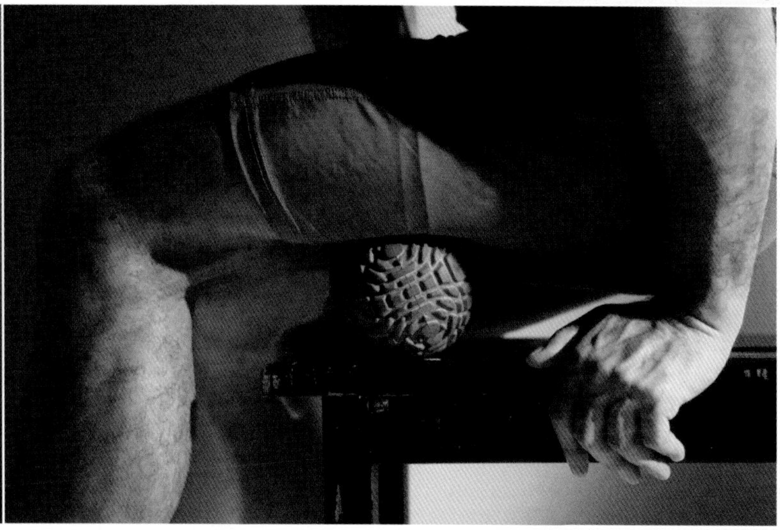

02. POSTERIOR CHAIN STRETCH ON ALL FOURS

Get into a staggered stance position with a resistance band that is anchored behind you and looped around your front leg at a distance from you that makes the band taut. Lean forward to place your hands on the floor in an all-fours position with your elbows and knees fully extended.
Hold the stretch for 30 seconds.

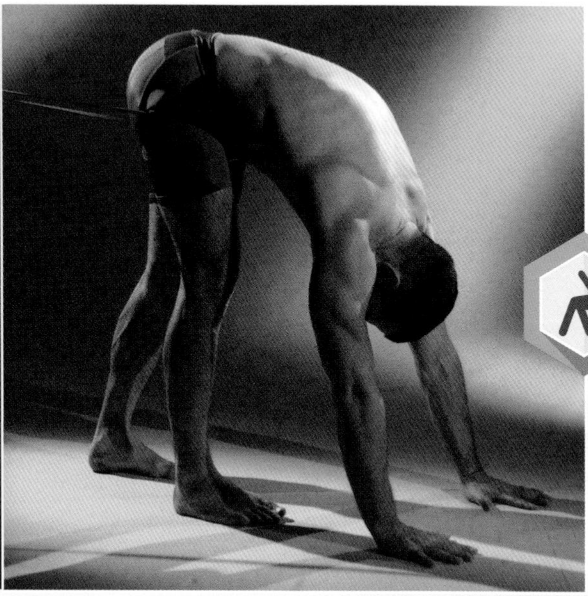

03. DYNAMIC DOWNWARD DOG

From a downward dog position, move into a push-up position by alternately moving your right and left hands forward. Do the same thing with your legs to return to the starting position. **Perform 4 reps.**

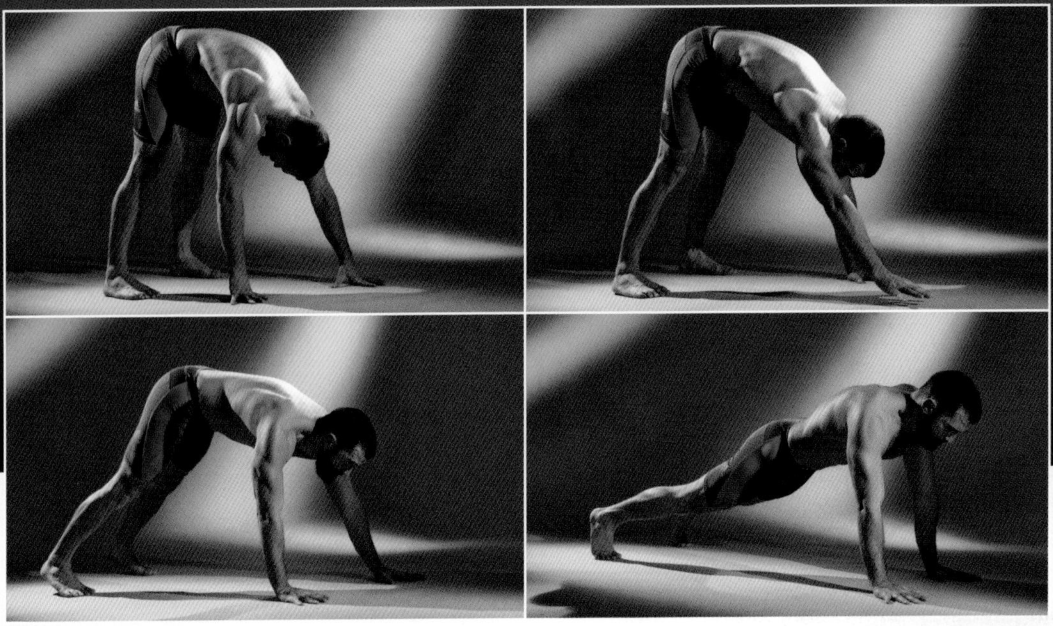

04. OPTIONAL: KETTLEBELL SWING

Place a kettlebell in front of you, forming an equilateral triangle with your legs and the kettlebell. Reach for the kettlebell and hold it in both hands without flexing your knees very far. Rotate your arms inward (as if you were turning them). Activate your gluteal muscles as much as possible and move the kettlebell backward as if you were trying to drag it on the floor. Do all of this with a minimal squatting motion. Propel the kettlebell from between your legs to simultaneously drive your kettlebell and your gluteal muscles behind you. Then reverse the movement by powerfully extending your hips to drive the kettlebell forward in the largest arc possible. Your arms do not drive the kettlebell, and your shoulders do not move up; all the movement comes from your pelvis and posterior chain muscles. The kettlebell only moves as far as the hips propel it. Inhale as the kettlebell is lowered and exhale quickly and energetically when the kettlebell is at its highest point. **Perform 6 to 8 reps.**

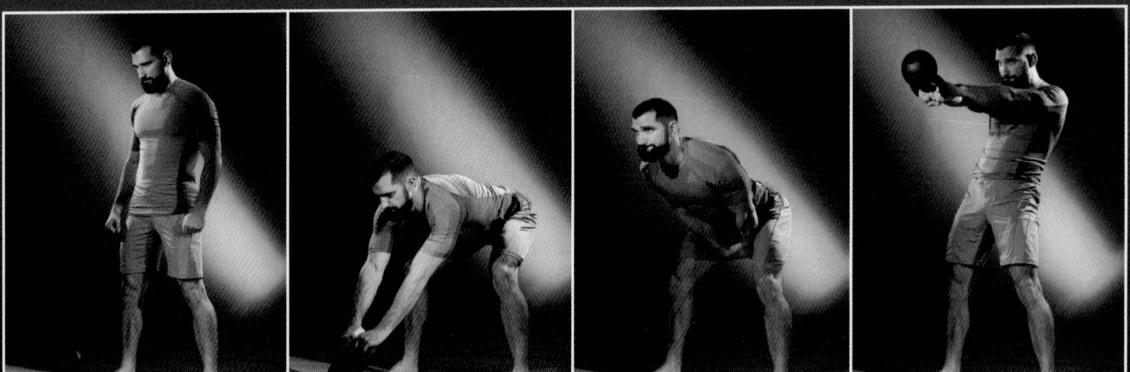

Perform one to three sets of each of the following exercises in order on the same leg. Do not stop between exercises. When they are completed, go through the series again for the other leg.

MASSAGE STRETCHING MOBILIZATION WEIGHTS

solution 04

RESTRICTIONS IN THE LOWER POSTERIOR CHAIN

01. POSTERIOR CHAIN MASSAGE USING A BALL

On a box or chair, sit on a massage ball. Roll over the most sensitive and stiff areas from front to back and left to right and finish with circular movements.

Perform 10 massages of each type.

02. POSTERIOR CHAIN STRETCH WITH HIP DISTRACTION

In a slight staggered stance position, extend your back knee and very slightly flex your front knee. Place a resistance band that is pulling backward around your back upper thigh. Lean forward, keeping your back as straight as possible.

Hold the stretch for 20 to 30 seconds.

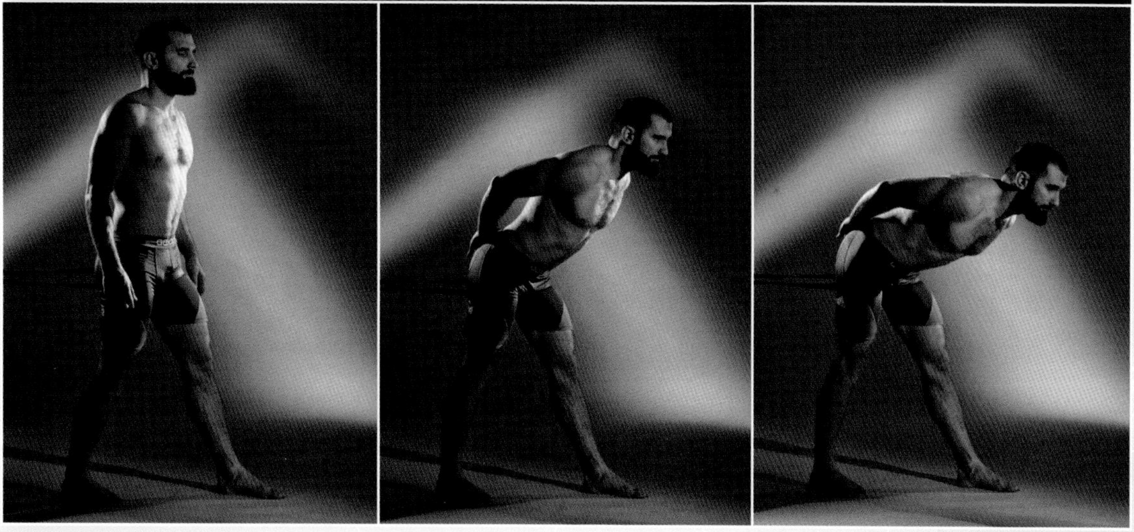

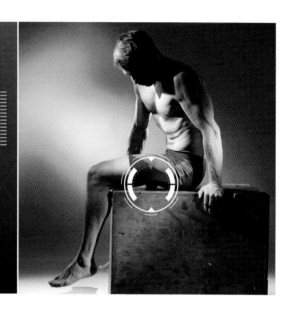

03. SUSPENSION TRAINER WINDMILLS

With your back to the suspension trainer, hold the handle in one hand and reach overhead with an extended elbow to make the strap taut. Place your feet shoulder-width apart. Lean to the side opposite of the arm holding the handle. Without letting the handle of the strap out of your sight, push the elbow of your free arm on the inside of the knee. You can flex that knee, but the goal is to keep it extended throughout the whole movement. You can use the pressure of your free arm to help extend it. Touch the floor with that hand and then come back up.

Perform 4 slow reps on each side.

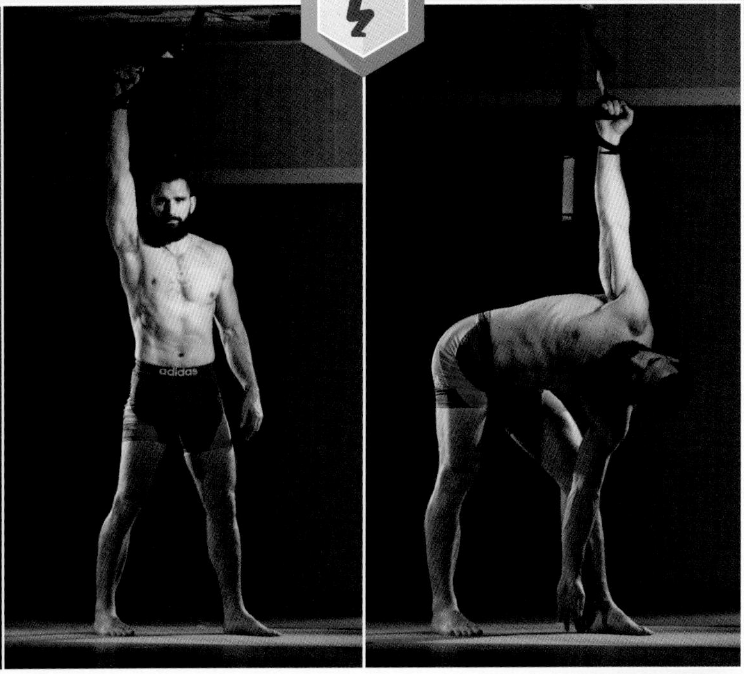

04. OPTIONAL: STIFF-LEG KETTLEBELL DEADLIFT

From a standing position holding a kettlebell in front of you, place your feet next to each other, push your chest out, and pull your shoulders back and down. Lean forward and try to place the kettlebell on the floor, keeping your knees fully extended and your back straight. As soon as your knees start to flex or your back begins to round, return to the starting position.

Perform 5 reps.

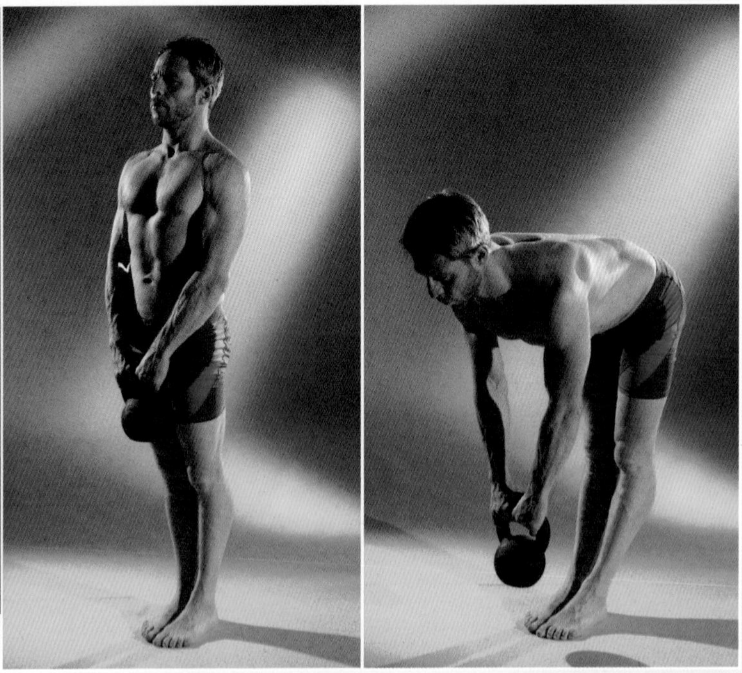

PROBLEMS IN THE UPPER BACK

1

Upper Back Extension on the Back of a Chair

Sit on a standard chair so that the top of the back of the chair is even with the middle of your upper back (the hump formed by the spine). If you are too short, sit on a pile of books. You should be able to tilt your head back to face the ceiling. If you cannot or if it hurts to do so, you need to perform the following exercises.

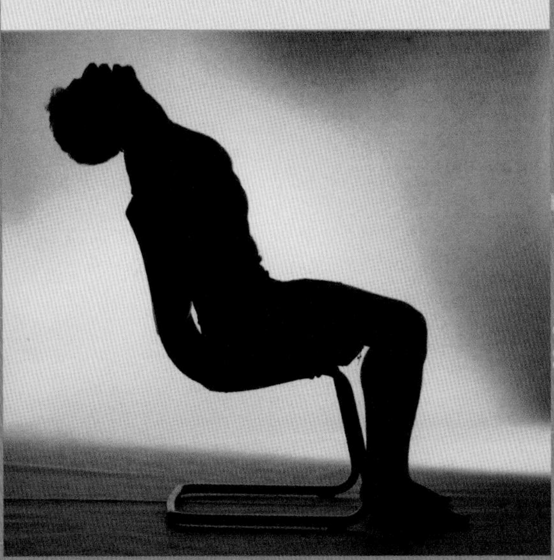

2

Upper Back Extension on an Exercise Ball Using a Kettlebell

Lie on your back on an average-sized exercise ball and hold the handle of a heavy kettlebell (at least 45 lb [20 kg]) over your head while keeping both feet on the floor. You can ask a partner to stabilize the ball if you are unbalanced. If you cannot hold the kettlebell, you cannot keep your feet on the floor, or you feel pain, incorporate these specific corrective exercises into your training.

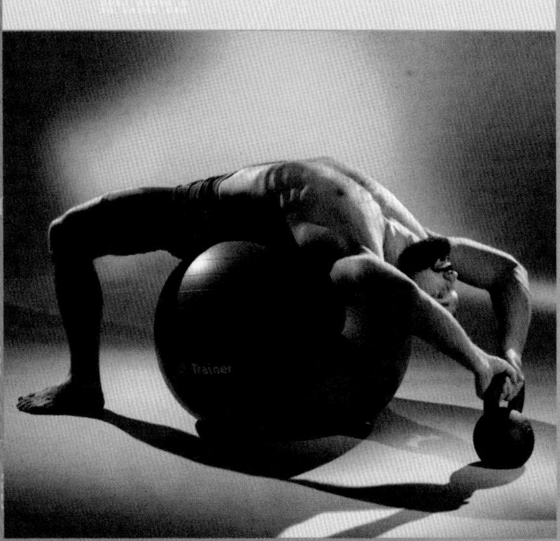

solution 01

MASSAGE STRETCHING MOBILIZATION WEIGHTS

Perform one to three sets of each of the following exercises. Do not stop between exercises.

PROBLEMS IN THE UPPER BACK

01. UPPER BACK MASSAGE USING A ROLLER

Lie on your back with your buttocks and feet flat on the floor. Place a roller under and across your upper back. Cross your arms, hold your shoulders with your hands, and slightly flex and extend your knees to move over the roller to cover your upper back. When finished, completely extend and flex your torso over the roller. **Perform for 2 minutes on all areas lacking mobility.**

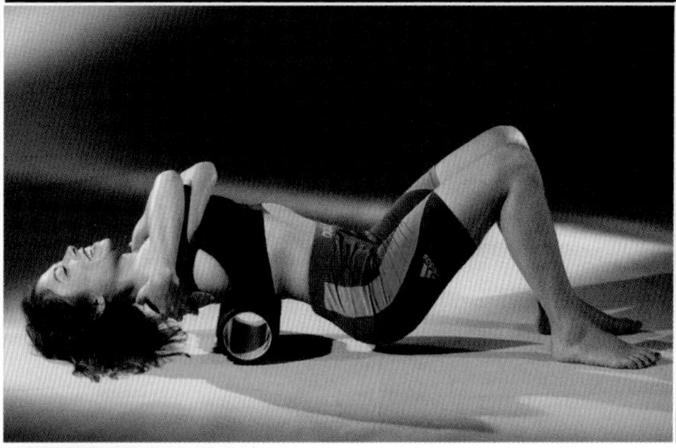

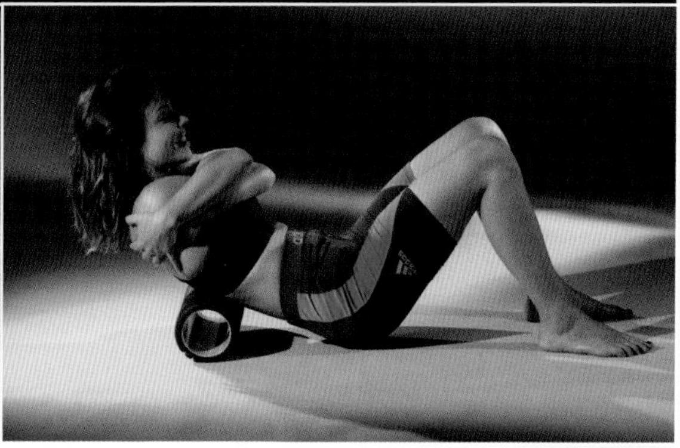

02. UPPER BACK ROLLER STRETCH USING A KETTLEBELL

Lie on your back with your legs straight and flat on the floor. Place a roller under and across your upper back. Hold the handle of a kettlebell above your head with your elbows fully extended.
Hold the position for 30 seconds to 1 minute.

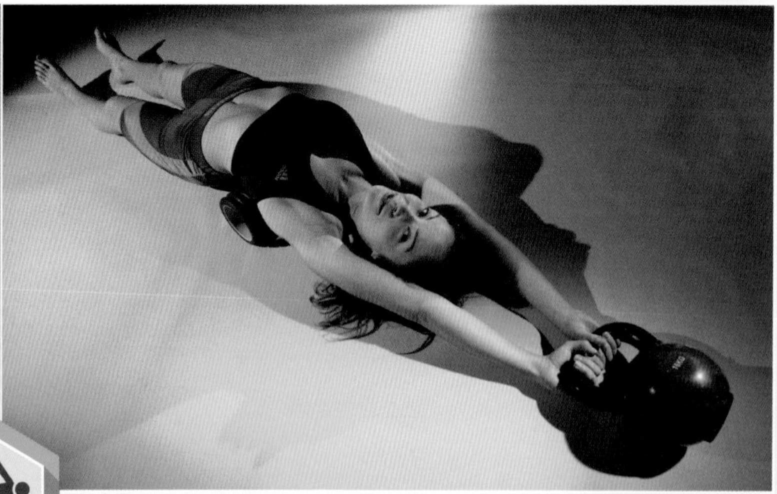

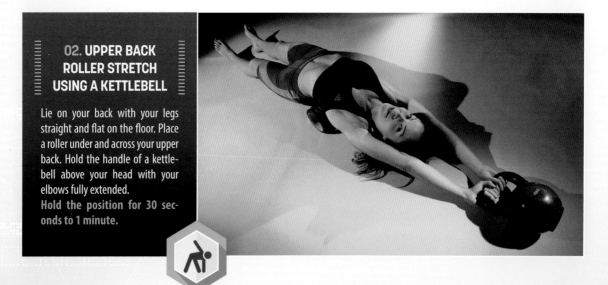

03. SWIMMING ON A ROLLER

Roll from front to back as in the Upper Back Self-Massage Using a Roller exercise and add a breaststroke movement to this exercise to add an extra dimension of mobility.

Perform 10 breaststroke movements.

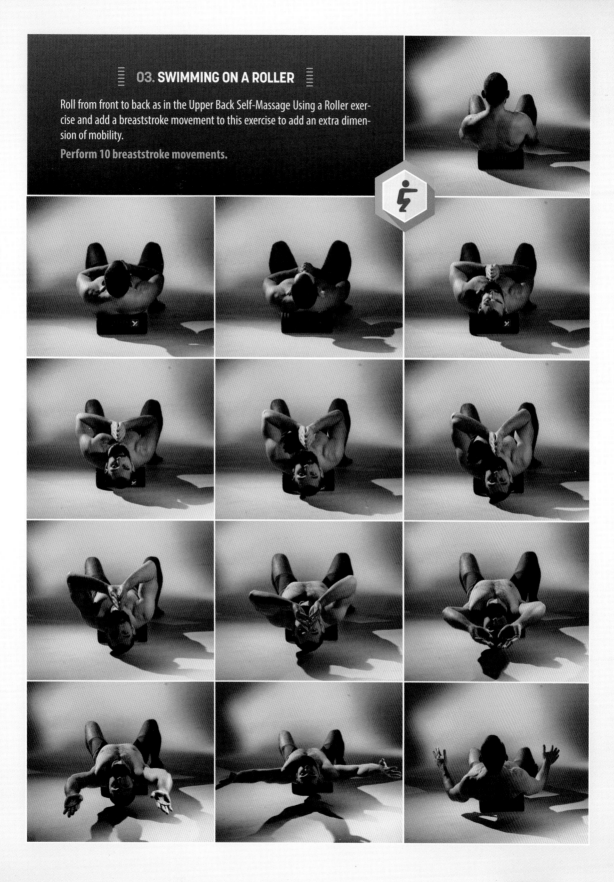

04. OPTIONAL: BACK EXTENSION ON AN EXERCISE BALL

Lie face down on an exercise ball with your thighs and hips on the ball and your feet held by a partner or a gym ladder. Place your hands at your ears and lower your torso a few degrees, then roll back on the ball until your face touches the ball. Once in the lowest position, reverse the movement by extending your back to lift your torso while lifting your head and sticking out your chest. Finish the move by returning to the starting position. Focus on rolling and unrolling your upper back for each repetition.
Perform 6 reps.

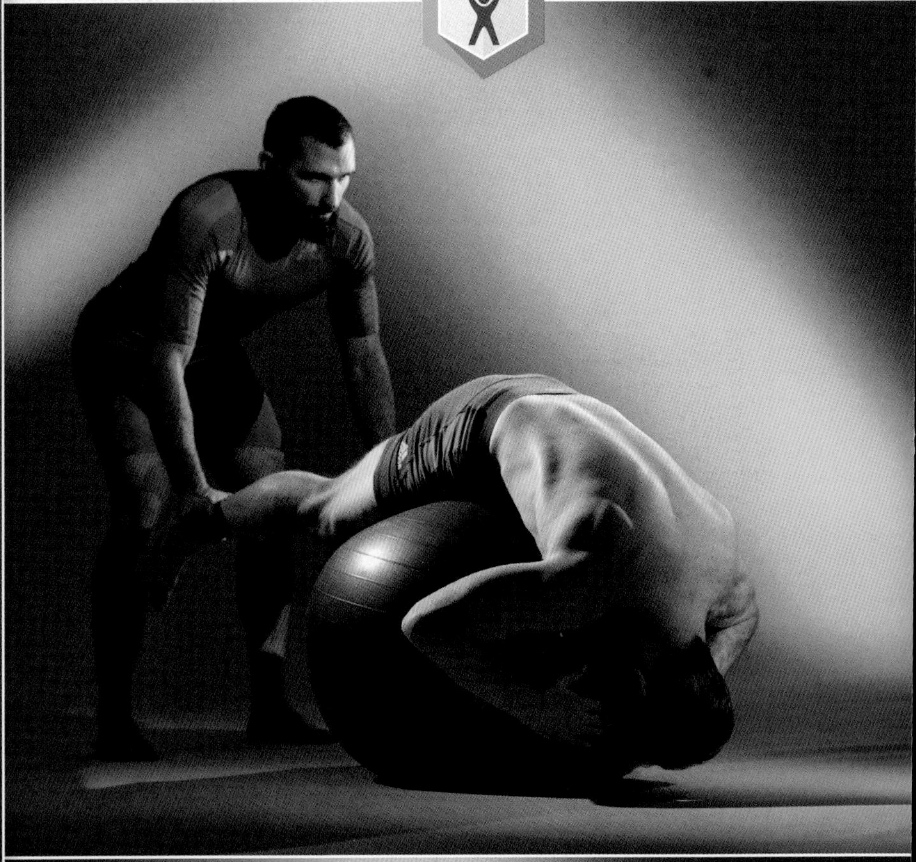

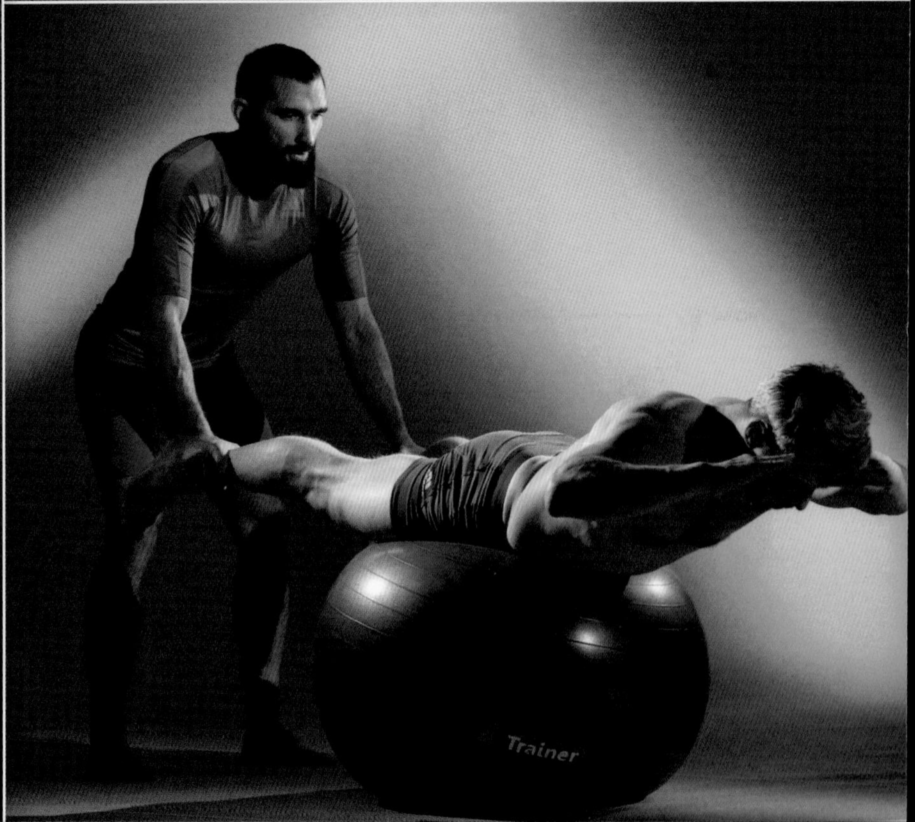

Perform one to three sets of each of the following exercises. Do not stop between exercises.

MASSAGE STRETCHING MOBILIZATION WEIGHTS

solution 02

PROBLEMS IN THE UPPER BACK

01. UPPER BACK MASSAGE USING A DOUBLE BALL AND A BAND

With two hands, grasp a resistance band that is anchored above you (at a distance from you that makes the band taut) and sit on the floor with a double massage ball under your upper back and even with your shoulder blades. Lean back on the ball to apply pressure and alter the intensity of the massage by pulling on (or relaxing) the band. **Perform 10 front-to-back rolls.**

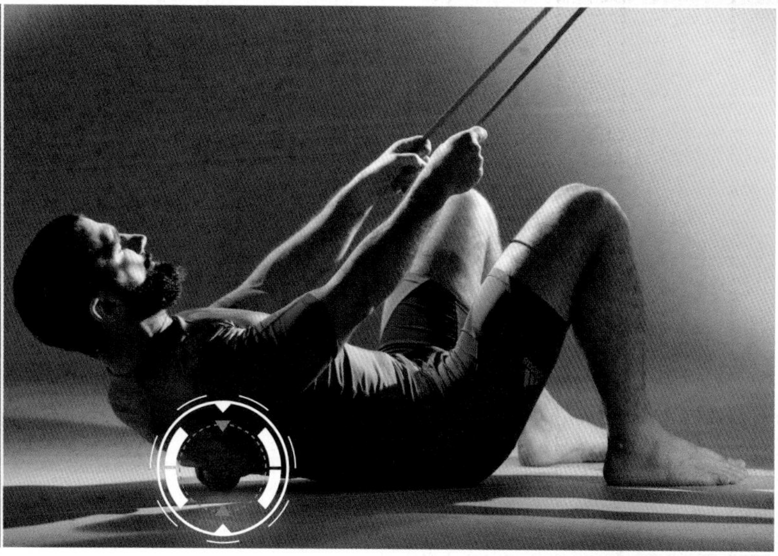

02. UPPER BACK STRETCH USING A DOUBLE BALL AND A KETTLEBELL

Lie on your back on a double massage ball placed under your upper back with your legs straight and flat on the floor. Hold the handle of a kettlebell above your head with your elbows fully extended. Move the ball to reach various pressure points. **Hold the position for 30 seconds.**

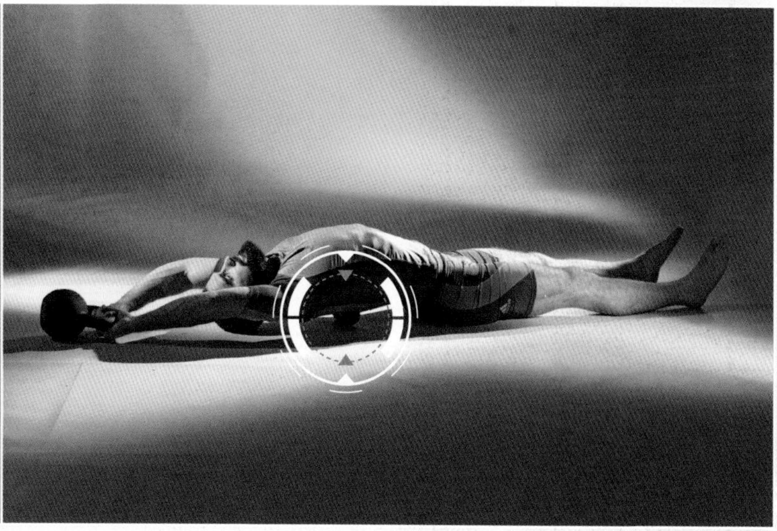

03. CAT

On all fours, lower your head and try to raise your shoulder blades as high as possible by arching your back and lowering your shoulders. Then bring your head up and arch your back and press your chest out toward the floor. **Perform 10 reps.**

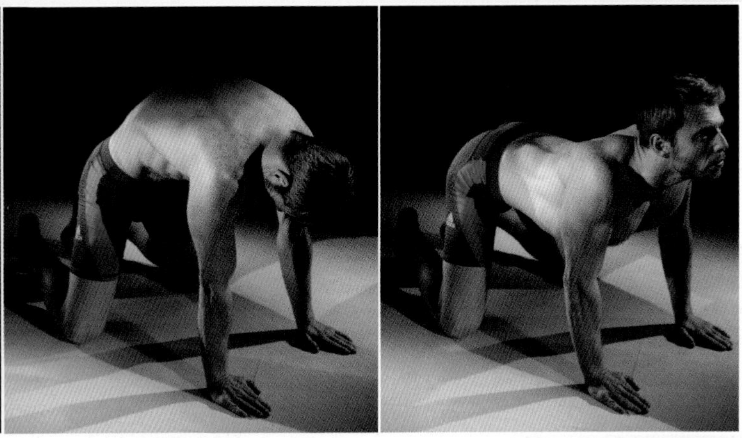

04. OPTIONAL: OVERHEAD SQUAT

Stand tall and hold a bar above your head using a very wide (snatch) grip and fully-extended elbows. Keep your head in a neutral position, hold your chest out, and focus your eyes just above level. Stand with your feet hip-width apart if you are flexible and shoulder-width apart if you are not very flexible. Slowly move down into a squat without compromising your back and head alignment. The trajectory of your knees is guided by your kneecaps, which stay in line with the toes. **Perform 4 reps.**

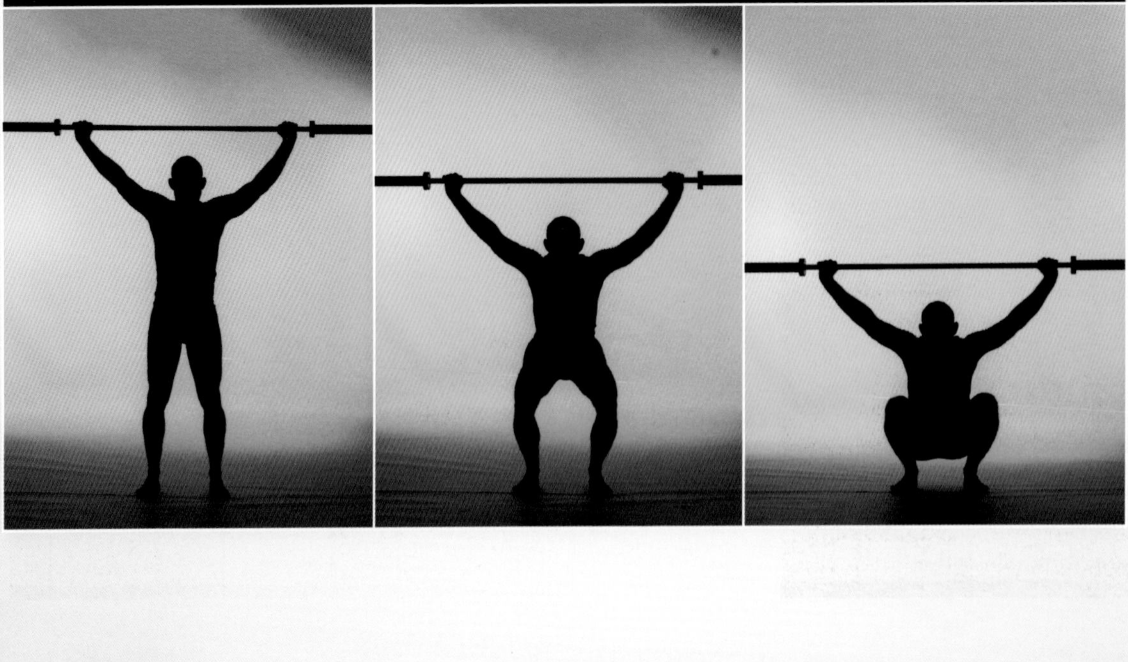

Perform one to three sets of each of the following exercises. Do not stop between exercises.

MASSAGE | STRETCHING | MOBILIZATION | WEIGHTS

solution 03

PROBLEMS IN THE UPPER BACK

01. PERPENDICULAR ROLLER MASSAGE

Lie on your back on a long foam roller aligned with your spine with your feet flat on the floor. Open your arms out to the side, relax completely, and slightly push with each leg (separately) to roll back and forth. Then cross your arms and hold your shoulders with your hands and slightly push with each leg (separately) to roll back and forth again. **Perform 10 massages of each type.**

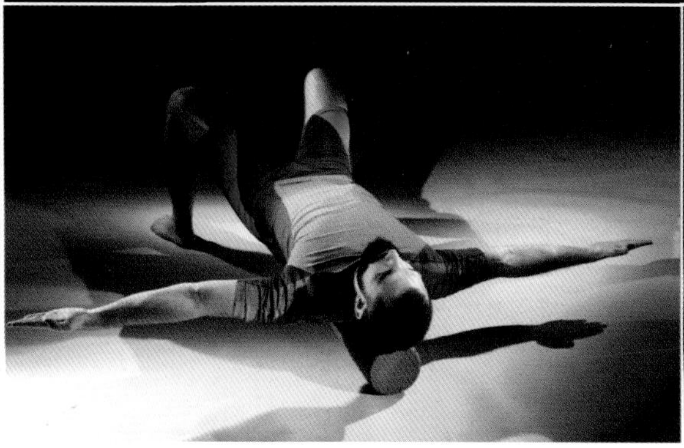

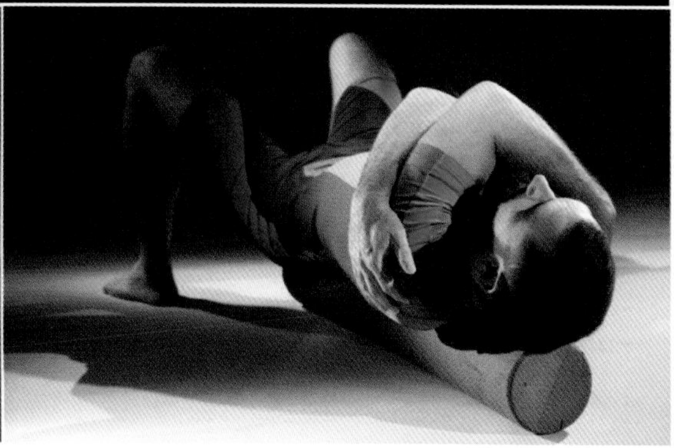

02. STRETCH ON PERPENDICULAR ROLLER WITH OPEN ARMS

Open your arms out to the side as in the last exercise and completely relax your arms so the back of your hands rest on the floor. **Hold the stretch for 30 seconds.**

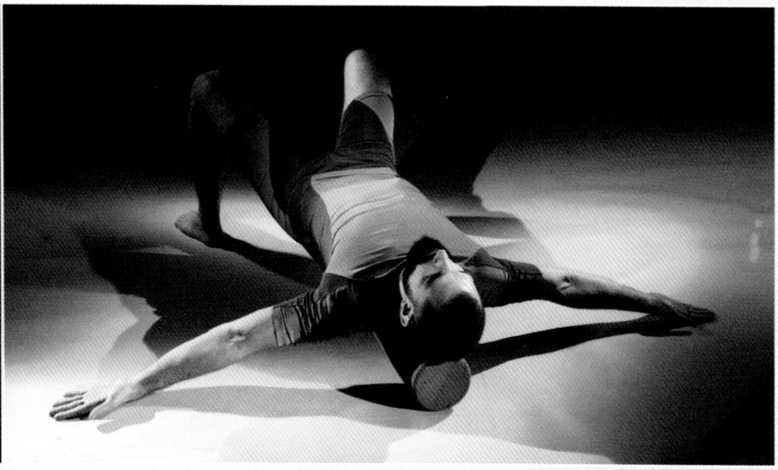

03. EXERCISE BALL PRESS

Squat with your back leaning against an exercise ball, holding a small weight plate (2.5-5 lb [1.1-2.3 kg]) in each hand. Combine a hip and knee extension with a shoulder and arm press so that you are stretched out completely over the ball. Fully lengthen your back, matching the curve of the ball. Allow the weight plates to drop your arms as low as possible while keeping your elbows extended. Reverse the move to return to the starting position. **Perform 10 reps.**

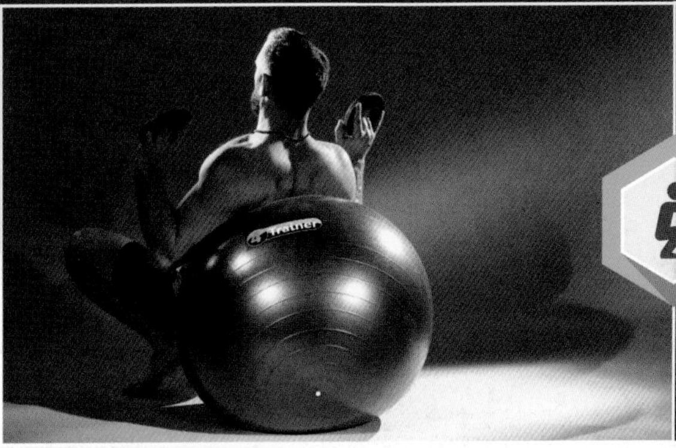

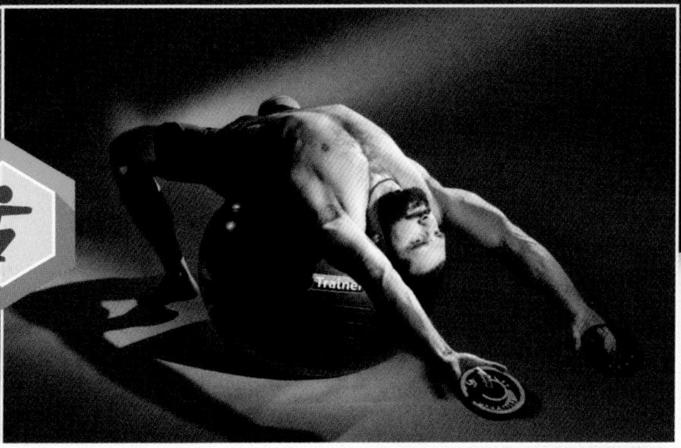

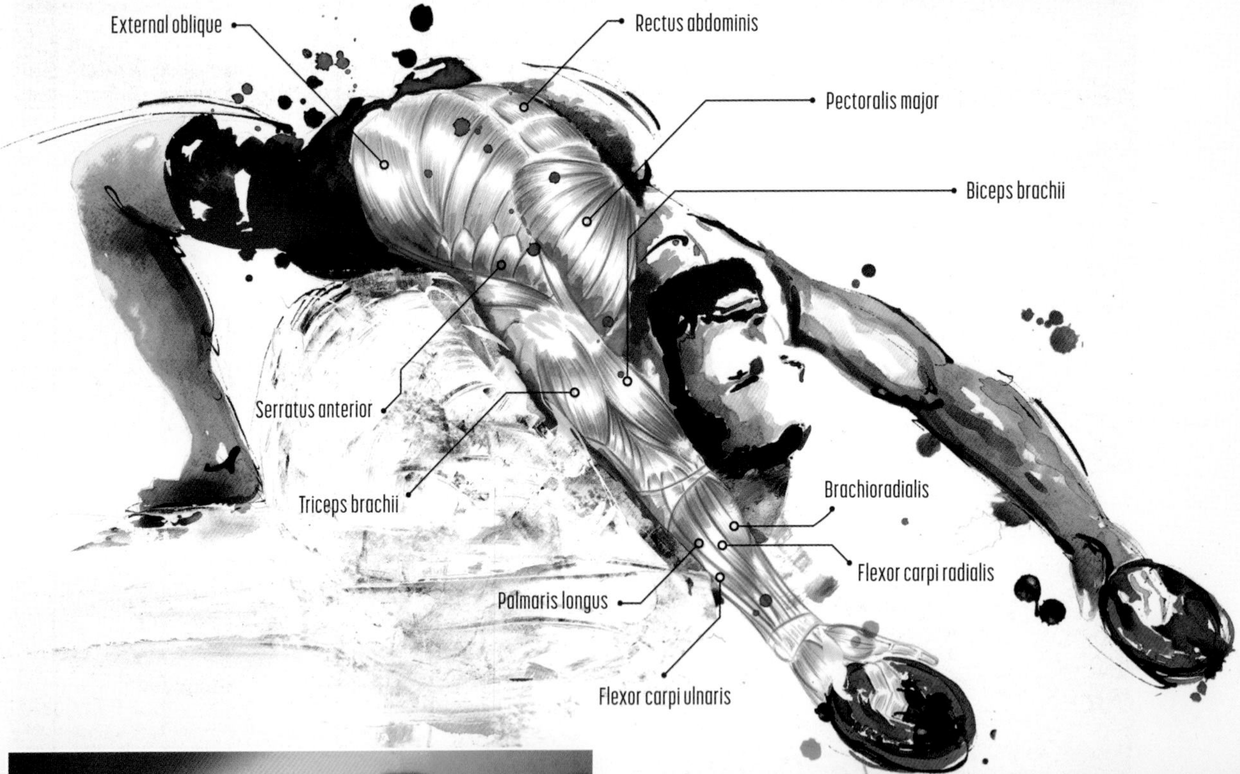

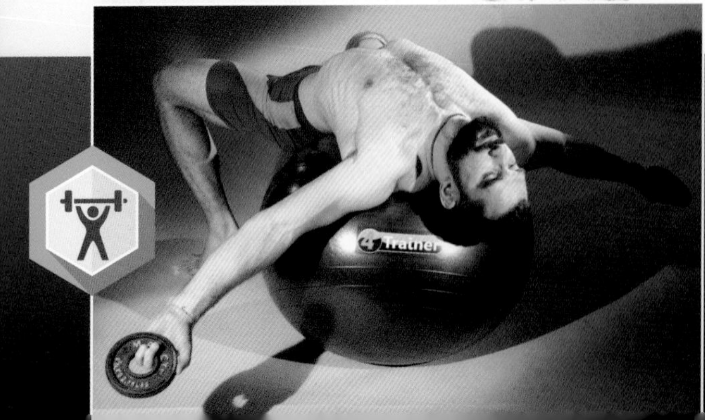

04. OPTIONAL: EXERCISE BALL FLY WITH A BOUNCE

With your back extended over an exercise ball as in the last exercise, open your arms out to the side with your palms facing up. Hold this position and make short, dynamic, bouncing movements with your arms. **Perform 10 energetic reps.**

Perform one to three sets of each of the following exercises. Do not stop between exercises.

MASSAGE | STRETCHING | MOBILIZATION | WEIGHTS

solution 04

PROBLEMS IN THE UPPER BACK

01. UPPER BACK MASSAGE USING A WEIGHT BAR AND A BAND

With two hands, grasp a resistance band that is anchored above you (at a distance from you that makes the band taut) and sit on the floor with a bar under your upper back and even with your shoulder blades. Lean back on the bar to apply pressure and alter the intensity of the massage by pulling on (or relaxing) the band. **Perform 10 front-to-back rolls.**

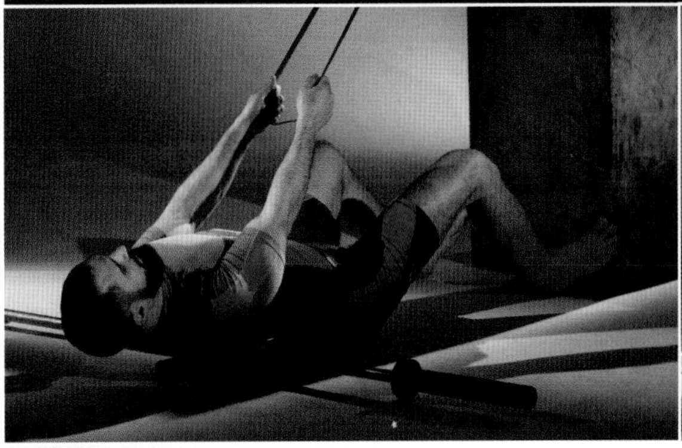

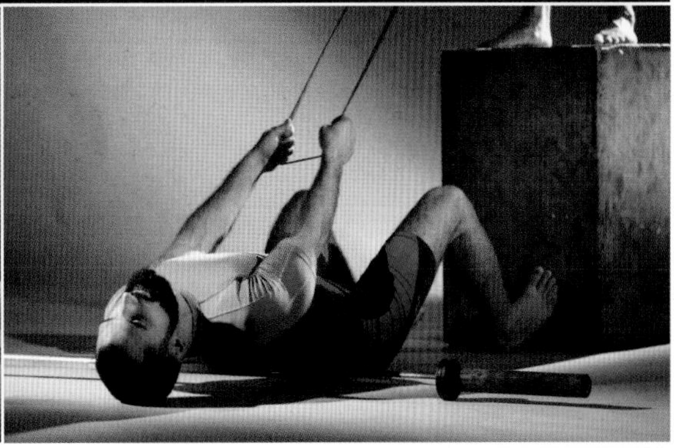

02. STRETCH ON A BAR

Sit on the floor and lean your upper back against a bar (with added weight plates) with your feet flat on the floor. Drape your elbows over the bar (to keep it from rolling) and allow the complete extension of the curve of your spine over the bar. **Hold the stretch for 30 seconds.**

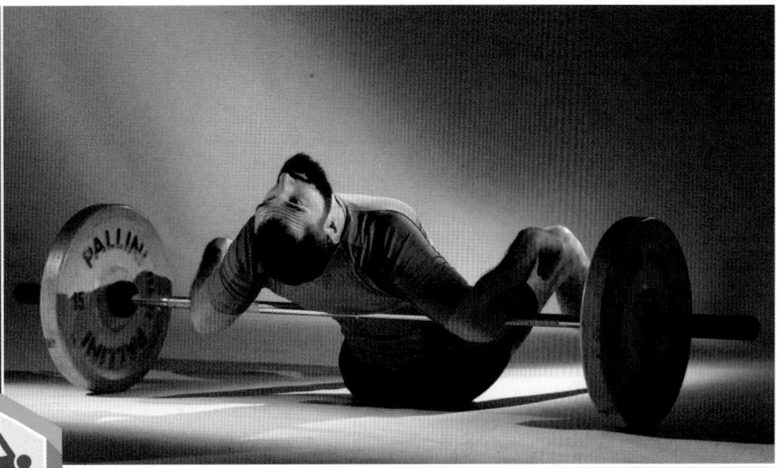

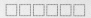

03. RHOMBOID CAT

On all fours, bring your shoulder blades together, then spread them as far apart as possible by rounding your back.
Perform 10 reps.

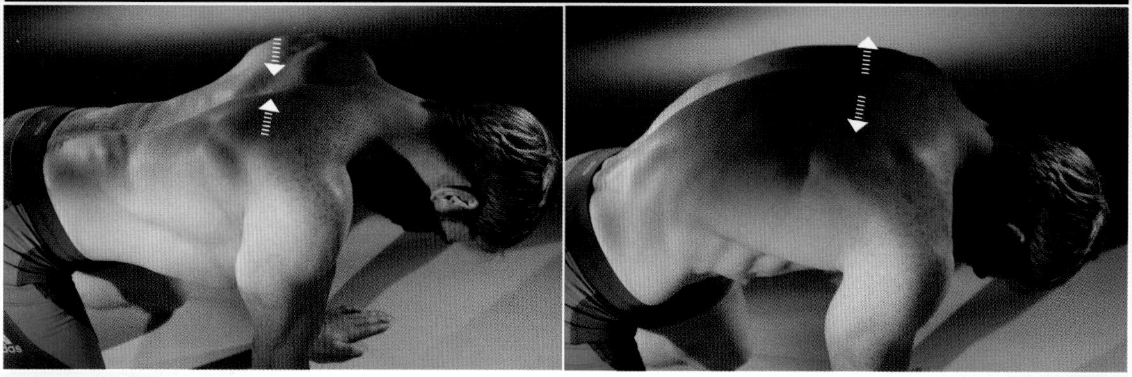

04. OPTIONAL: WEIGHTED CROSS-UNCROSS ON AN EXERCISE BALL

Hold a small weight plate (2.5-5 lb [1.1-2.3 kg]) in each hand and lie on your back over an exercise ball. Alternate between opening your arms out to the side with your palms facing up and crossing them over your chest. Bounce your weight on the ball after each time you change your arm position. Pause for a moment when your arms are completely open.
Perform 10 dynamic reps.

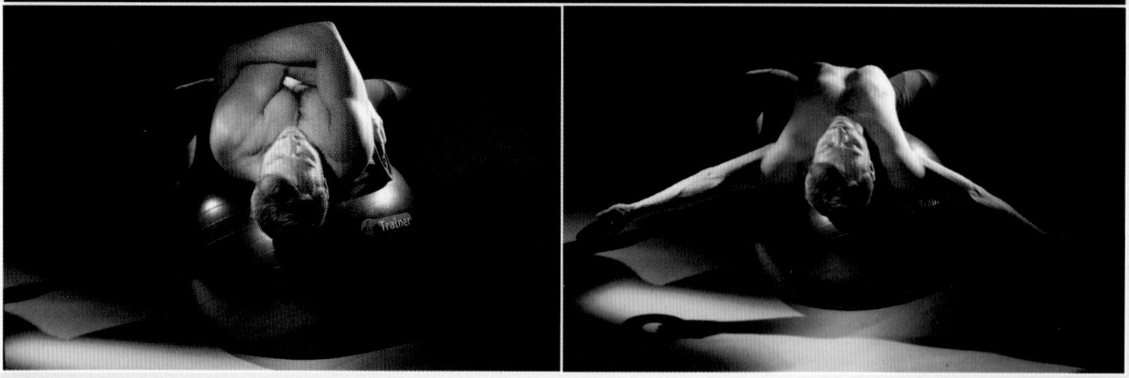

TESTS

TENSION IN THE LUMBAR AREA

1

Sphinx

Lie on your abdomen with your legs and insteps of your feet flat on the floor. Place the palm of your hands flat on the floor at the sides of your body at rib height. Push up with your arms to a fully-extended elbow position to completely extend your spine. If you have pain in your lower back, you should visit a health care professional. Any range of motion limitations should prompt you to develop your mobility through a corrective exercise program.

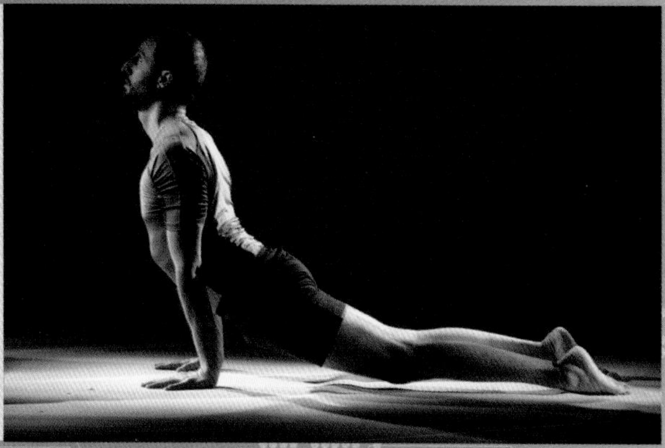

2

Back Hyperextension

Lie face down on the floor with your hands at your ears and your feet fixed in a gym ladder at floor level or held by a partner. Fully extend your back until you are looking upward. If you cannot look at the ceiling for several seconds in a row, you lack mobility.

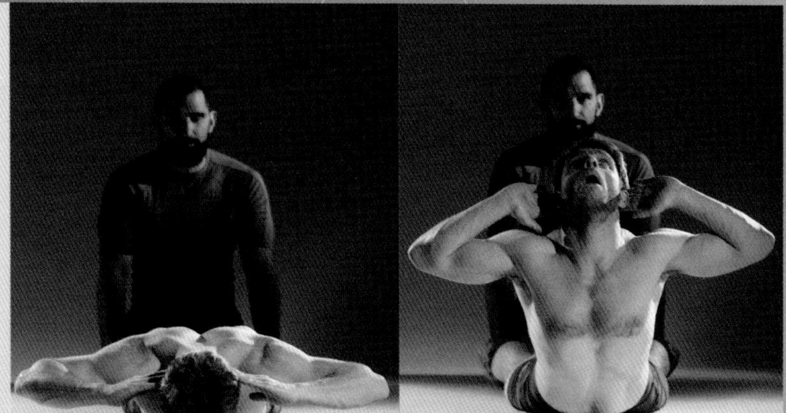

MASSAGE STRETCHING MOBILIZATION WEIGHTS

Perform one to three sets of each of the following exercises. Do not stop between exercises.

solution 01

TENSION IN THE LUMBAR AREA

01. LUMBAR CURVE MASSAGE USING A ROLLER

Lie on your back with your buttocks and feet flat on the floor. Place a roller under and across your lumbar region (the curve of your lower back). Cross your arms, hold your shoulders with your hands, and slightly flex and extend your knees to move over the roller to cover your lower back. When finished, completely extend and flex your torso over the roller.
Perform for 2 minutes, focusing on the sensitive areas by applying pressure.

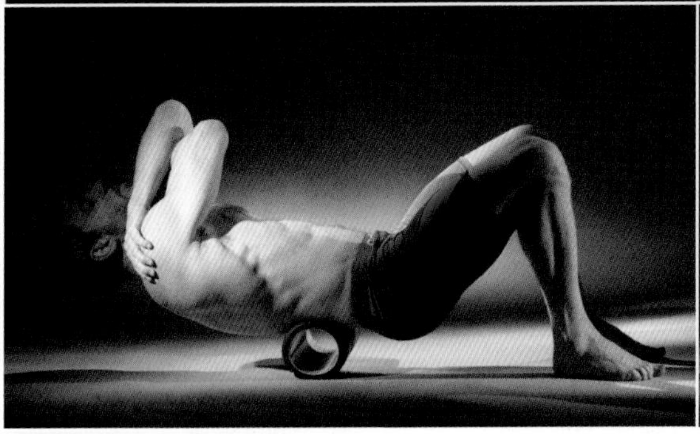

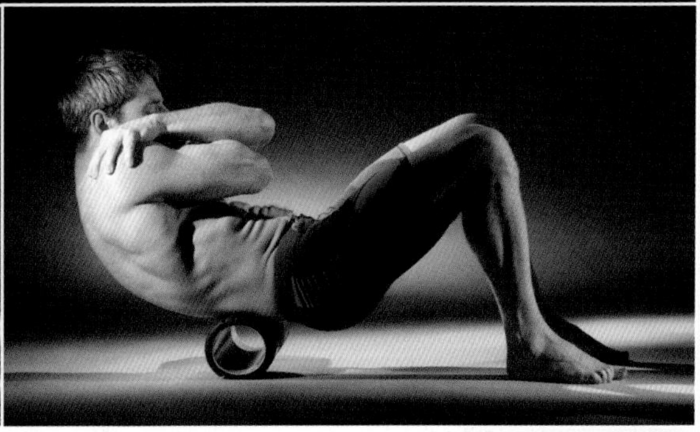

02. LUMBAR CURVE ROLLER STRETCH USING A BAND

Lie on your back with your legs straight and flat on the floor. Place a roller under the curve of your lower back. With two hands, grasp a resistance band that is anchored behind your head at a distance from you that makes the band taut. Hold the band above your head with your elbows fully extended and relax. **Hold the stretch for 30 seconds.**

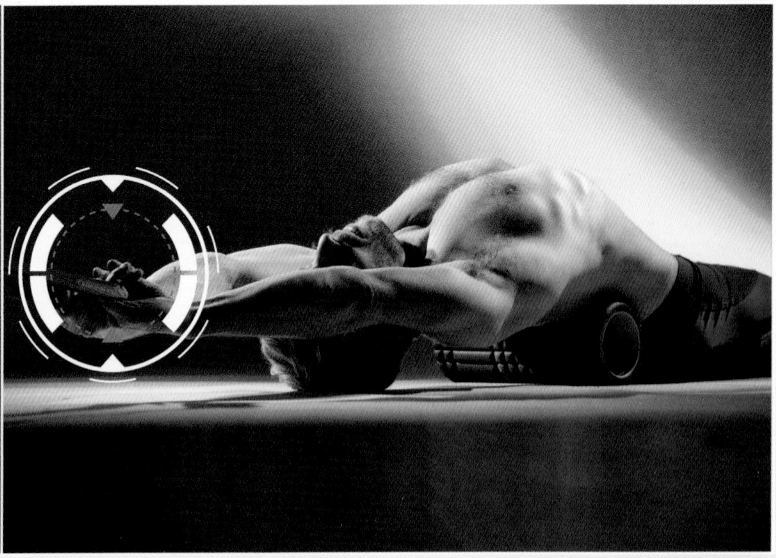

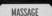

03. TUCKS ON AN EXERCISE BALL

Place your hips and the top of your thighs on an exercise ball and lean on your hands in a plank or push-up position. Flex your hips and knees to tuck your legs to bring the ball to the side as far as possible, then tuck your knees into your chest in alignment with your torso (see center photo). Continue the movement on the other side and then untuck your legs to return to the starting position. You are working to increase mobility by trying to make circles on the floor with the ball. Aim for relaxation, fluidity, and speed of execution. As your mobility improves, increase your speed while maintaining a perfectly relaxed movement. **Perform 10 reps (5 rotations to the right and 5 rotations to the left).**

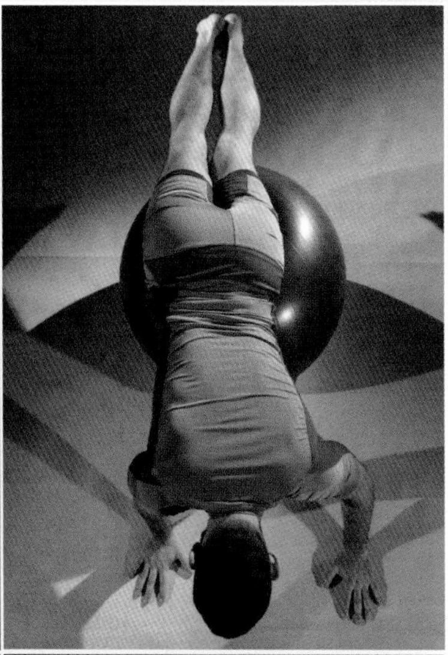

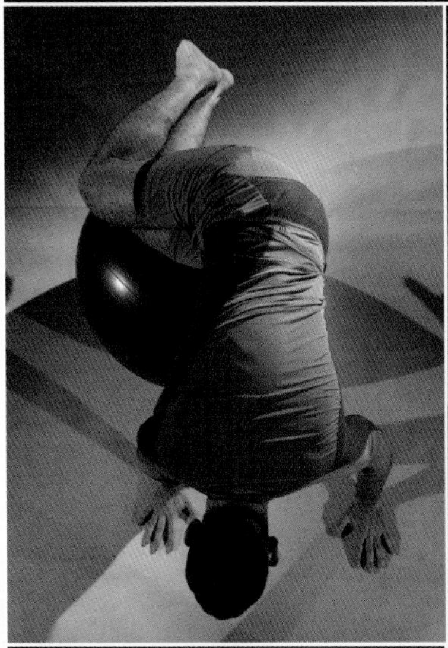

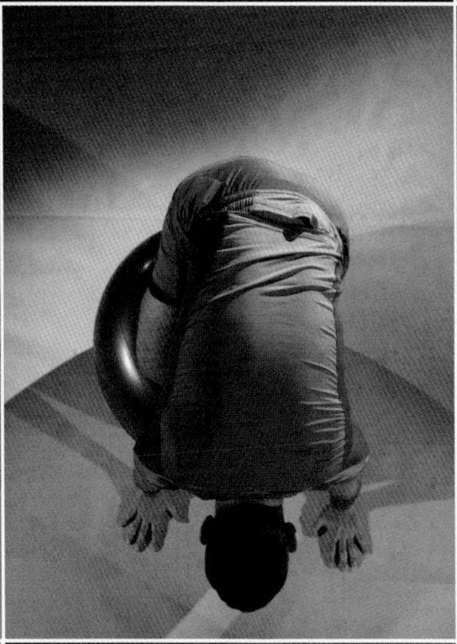

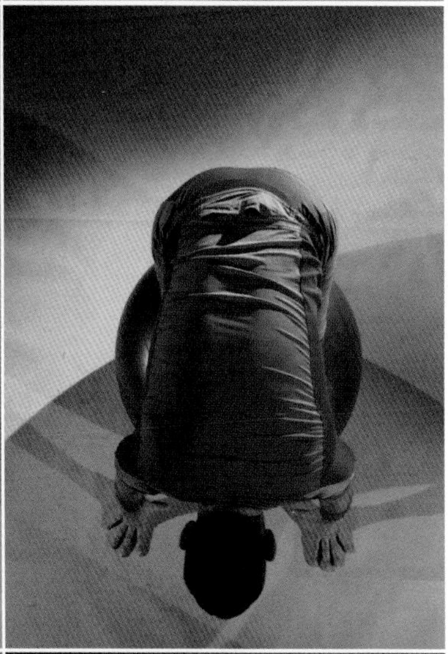

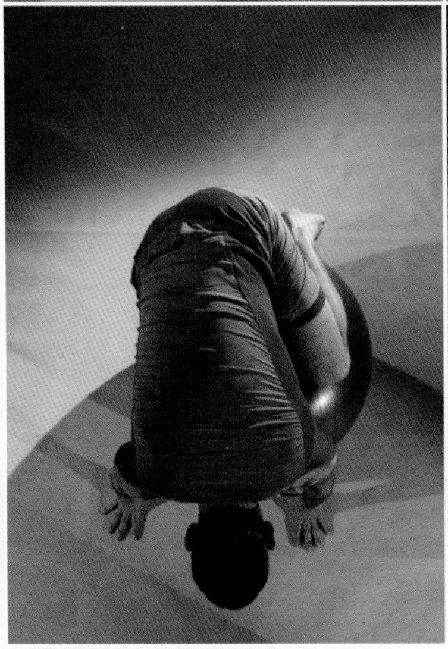

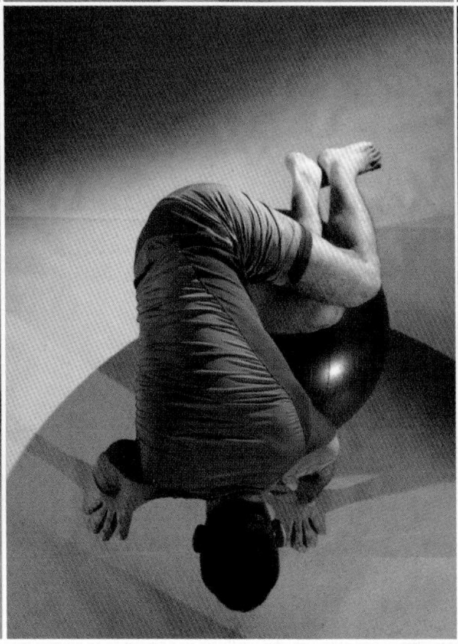

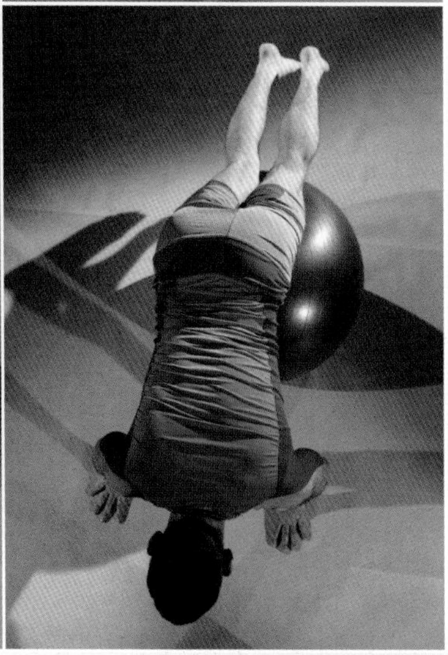

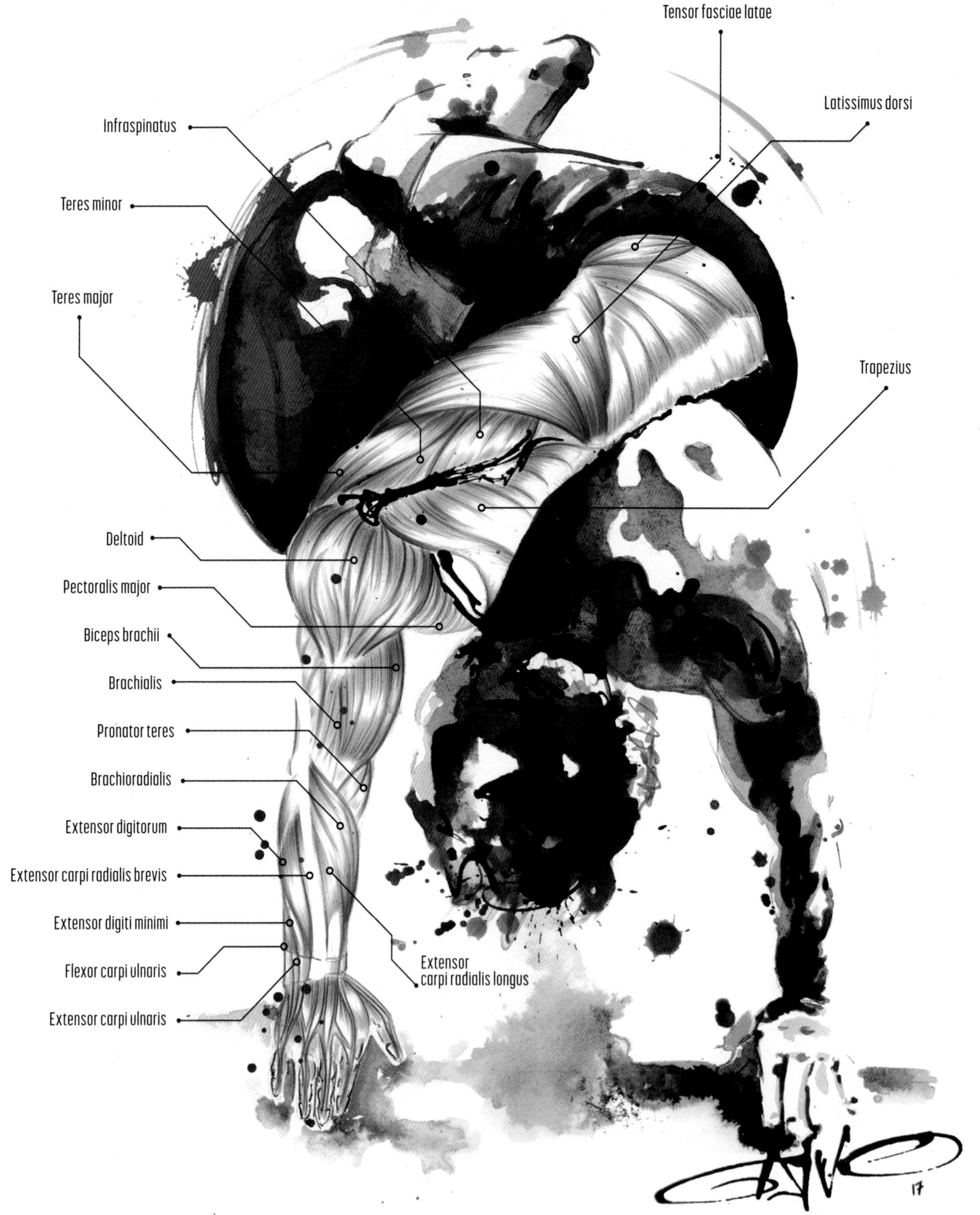
Tensor fasciae latae
Latissimus dorsi
Infraspinatus
Teres minor
Teres major
Trapezius
Deltoid
Pectoralis major
Biceps brachii
Brachialis
Pronator teres
Brachioradialis
Extensor digitorum
Extensor carpi radialis brevis
Extensor digiti minimi
Flexor carpi ulnaris
Extensor carpi ulnaris
Extensor carpi radialis longus

04. OPTIONAL: EXTENSION ON A BOX

Lie face down on top of a box with your hips pressed against the front edge. Grasp the sides of the box with your hands and use your arms to squeeze the box (if possible). Allow your hips to flex until your thighs are against the front side of the box. Flex your knees to 90 degrees to lift your feet off the floor. Once in a stable position, kick your heels back to fully extend your hips and knees and then relax back to the starting position. Keep your head in a neutral position and control your speed throughout the exercise. **Perform 10 reps.**

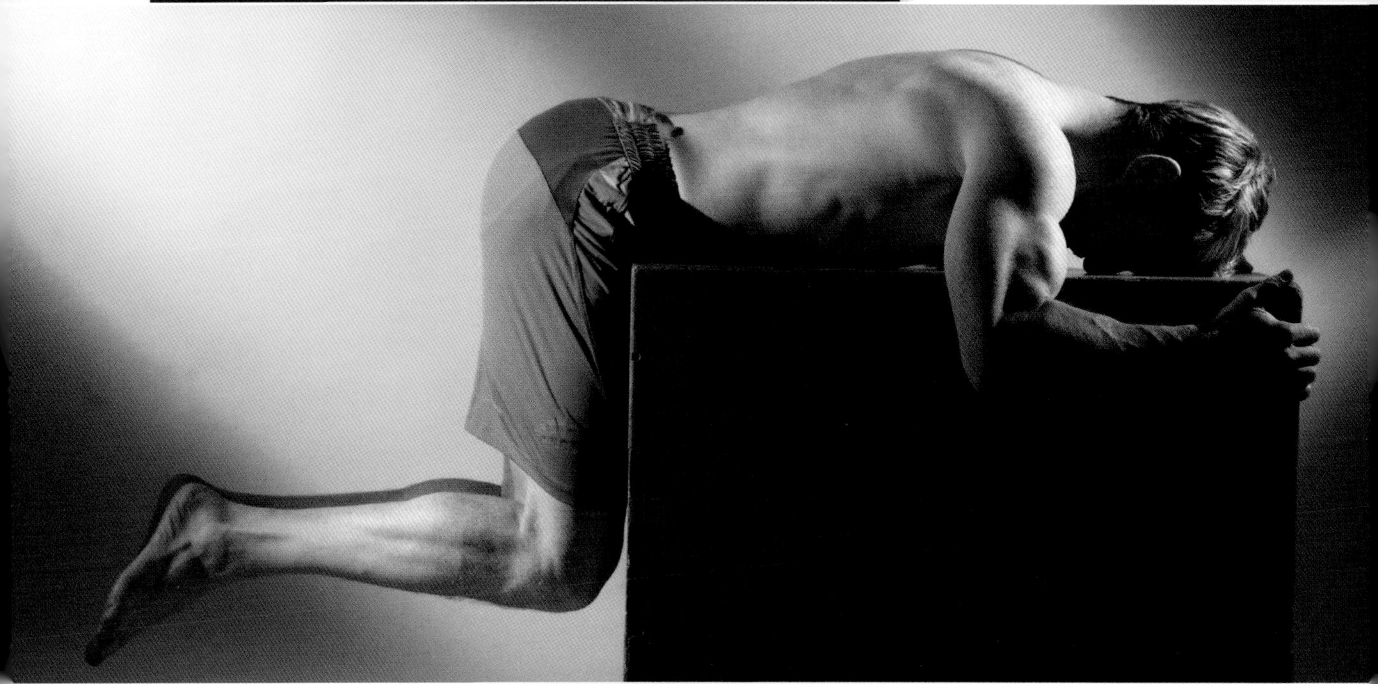

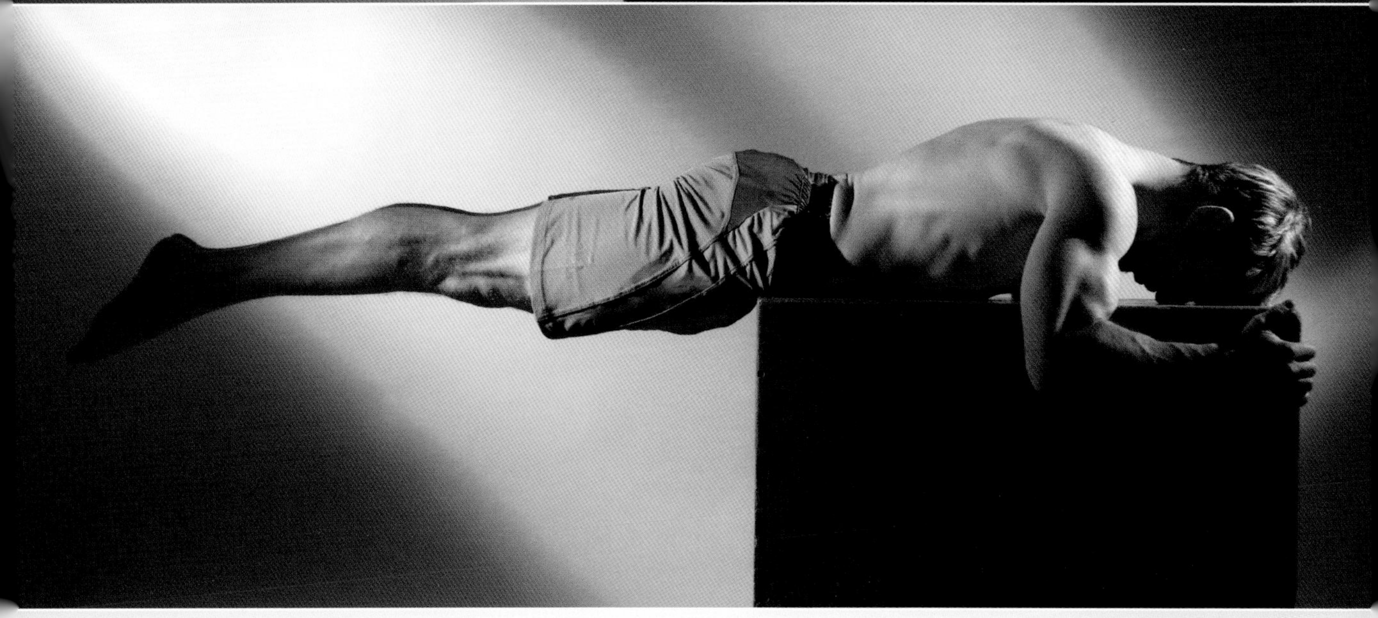

solution 02

MASSAGE | STRETCHING | MOBILIZATION | WEIGHTS

Perform one to three sets of each of the following exercises. Do not stop between exercises.

TENSION IN THE LUMBAR AREA

01. LUMBAR CURVE MASSAGE USING A LARGE BALL

Lie on your back, raise your feet, and place them on a box. Slide a large massage ball on one side of your spine in the curve of your lower back. Cross your arms across your chest and regulate the intensity of the massage by supporting yourself with your feet, which remain on the box. **Perform 10 right-to-left massages, 10 top-to-bottom massages, and 10 massages in a circular movement.**

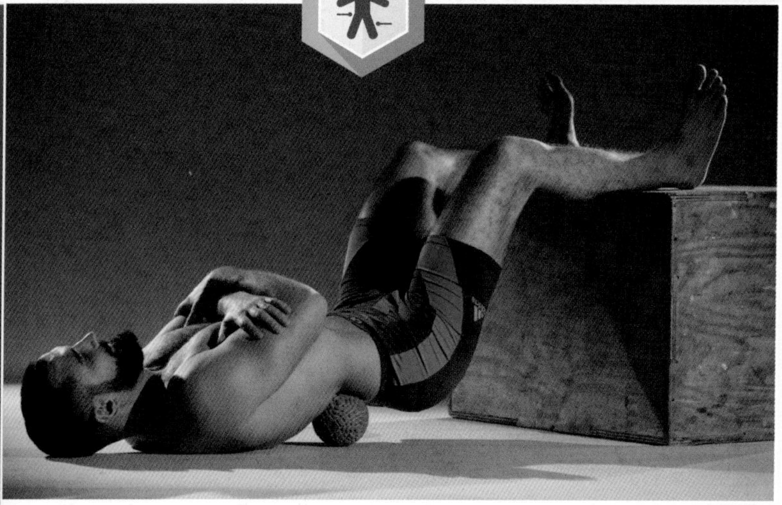

02. STRETCH ON A LARGE BALL

Keeping the large massage ball in the same place as the previous exercise, place your feet on the floor and allow your knees to fall to the same side as the ball.

Hold the position for 30 seconds.

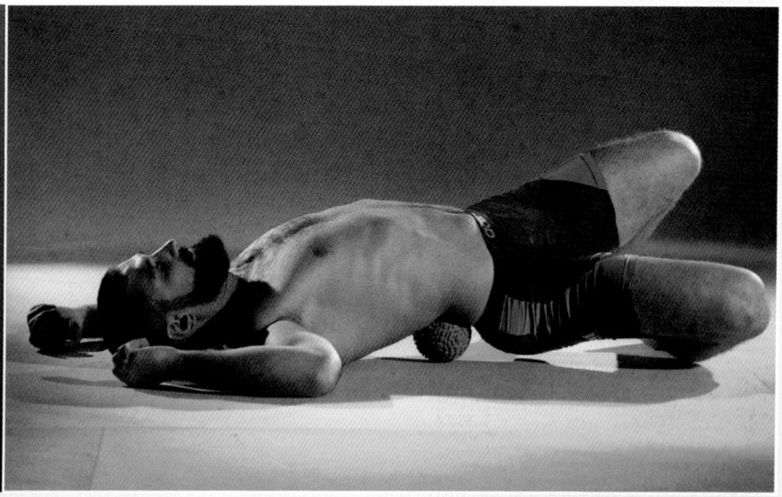

03. SUSPENSION TRAINER SCISSORS

In the plank or push-up position, place one foot in each handle, then pivot your hips to reverse the position of your legs. **Perform 5 pivots to the right and 5 pivots to the left.**

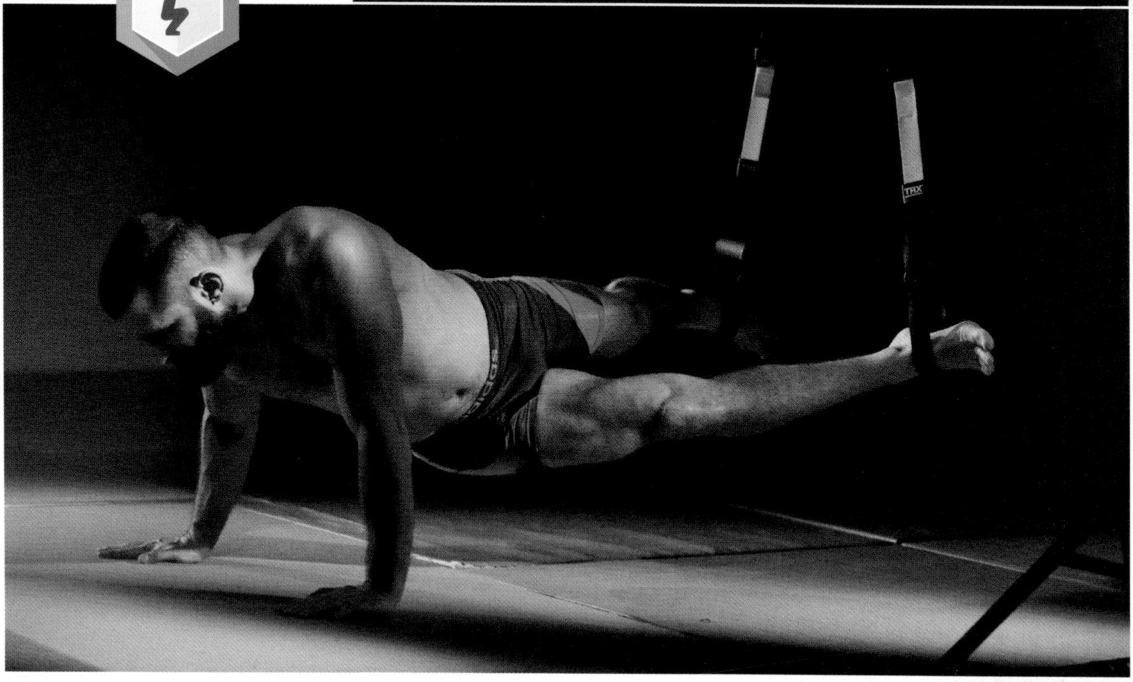

04. OPTIONAL: EXTENSION ON AN EXERCISE BALL

Lie flat on your abdomen on an exercise ball. Allow your hips to flex until your thighs are against the ball. Flex your knees to lift your feet off the floor. Have a partner hold your hands to help you keep your balance. Kick your heels back to fully extend your hips and knees and then relax back to the starting position. Keep your head in a neutral position and control your speed throughout the exercise. **Perform 10 reps.**

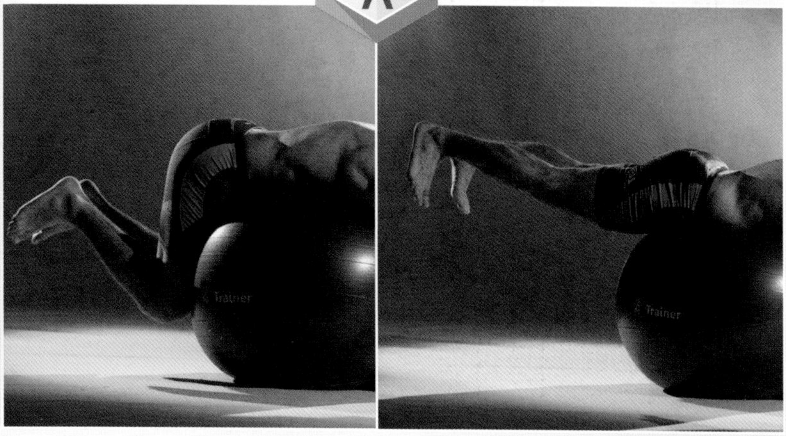

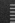

solution 03

MASSAGE STRETCHING MOBILIZATION WEIGHTS

Perform one to three sets of each of the following exercises. Do not stop between exercises.

TENSION IN THE LUMBAR AREA

01. LUMBAR CURVE MASSAGE USING A DOUBLE BALL

Lie on your back with your buttocks and feet flat on the floor. Place a double massage ball under and across your lumbar region. Cross your arms, hold your shoulders with your hands, and rotate your torso to move over the ball to cover your lower back. When finished, completely extend and flex your torso over the ball. **Perform for 2 minutes, focusing on the sensitive areas by applying pressure.**

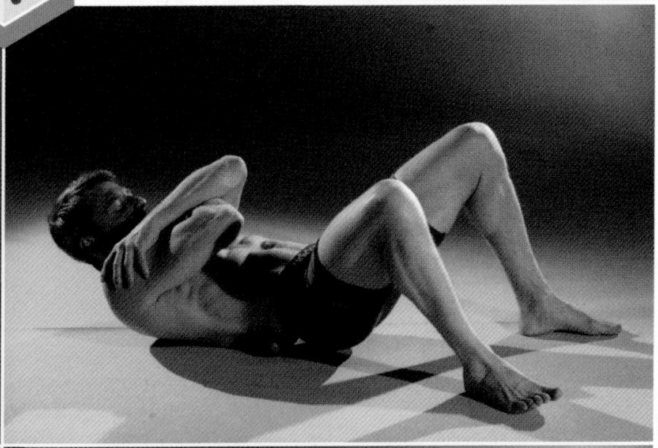

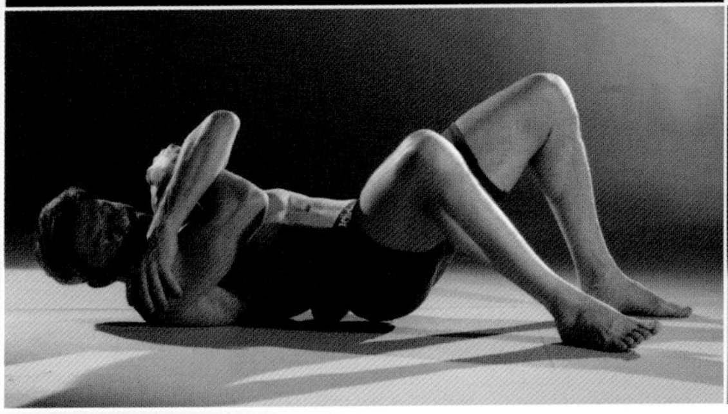

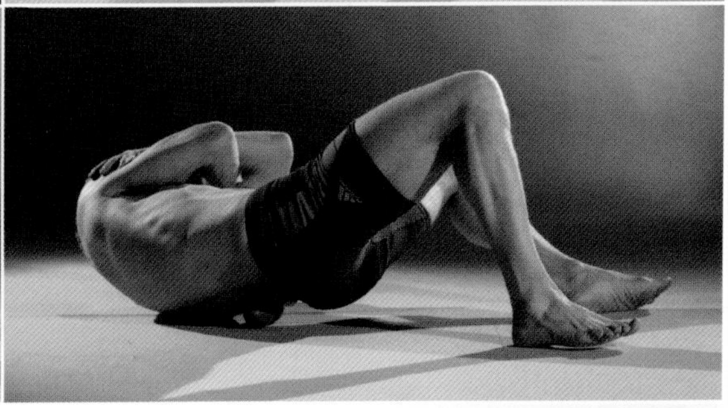

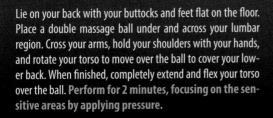

02. LOWER BACK STRETCH USING A DOUBLE BALL AND A BAND

Wrap a resistance band (anchored near the floor beyond your feet at a distance from you that makes the band taut) around one ankle. Lie on your back with your legs straight and flat on the floor. Place a double massage ball under the curve of your lower back. Cross your arms, hold your shoulders with your hands, and allow the band to lengthen your body as much as possible. **Hold the stretch for 30 seconds, switch the band to the other ankle, and repeat.**

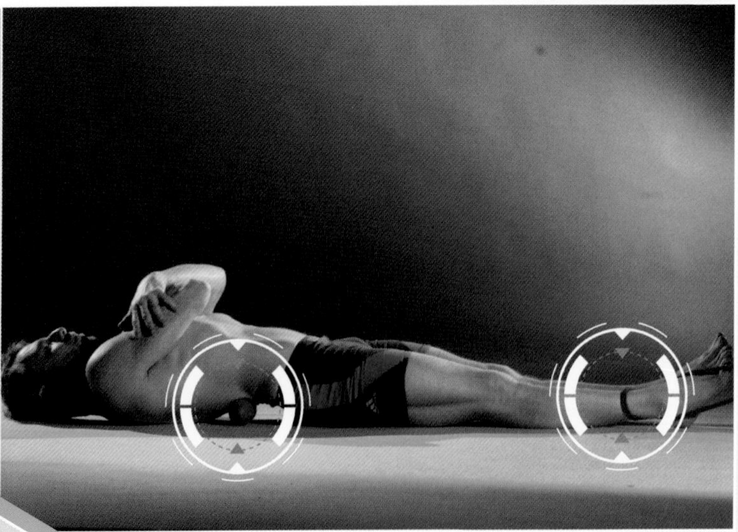

03. PELVIC MOBILITY WHILE SITTING ON AN EXERCISE BALL

Sit erect on an exercise ball with your feet flat on the floor and hands on your knees. Without changing the position of your back, move your pelvis. **Tilt from front to back and then from back to front, 5 times each.**

Tilt to from right to left and then from left to right, 5 times each.

Put your hands on your hips and circle to the right and then to the left, 5 times each.

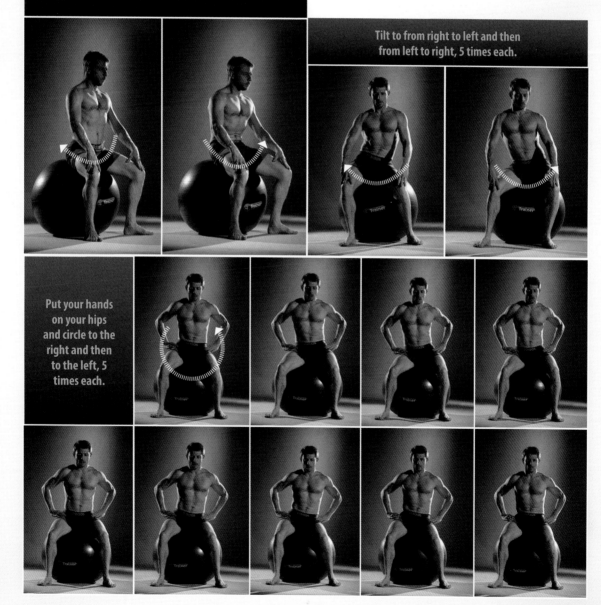

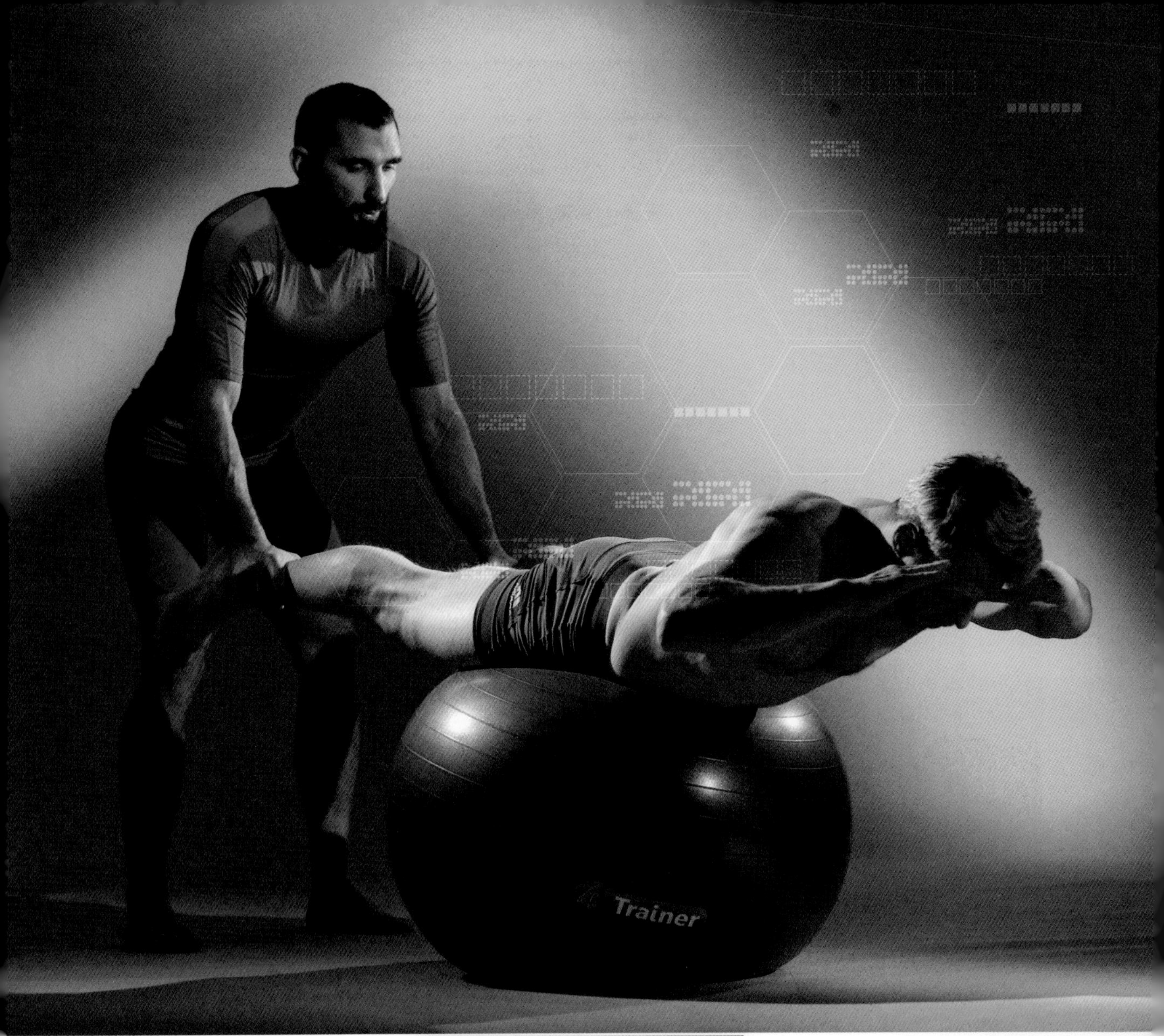

04. OPTIONAL: BACK EXTENSION ON AN EXERCISE BALL

Lie face down on an exercise ball with your thighs and hips on the ball and your feet held by a partner or a gym ladder. Place your hands at your ears (or, ideally, hold a weight in front of your chest) and lower your torso until your face touches the ball. Once in the lowest position, reverse the movement by extending your back to lift your torso while lifting your head and sticking out your chest. **Perform 6 reps.**

Perform one to three sets of each of the following exercises. Do not stop between exercises.

MASSAGE STRETCHING MOBILIZATION WEIGHTS

solution 04

TENSION IN THE LUMBAR AREA

01. LOWER BACK MASSAGE USING TWO BALLS OR A DOUBLE BALL

Lie on your back, raise your feet, and place them on a chair or box with your hips and knees flexed to 90 degrees. Slide two massage balls—one on each side of the spine (see the second photo in the top row)—or one double massage ball under your lower back. Regulate the intensity of the massage by supporting yourself with your legs, which remain on the box. A variation is to lie on your side with the inside of the shin of your top leg on the box and a double massage ball under your torso just above your hip. Be sure to massage both sides. **Perform 10 massages in each position.**

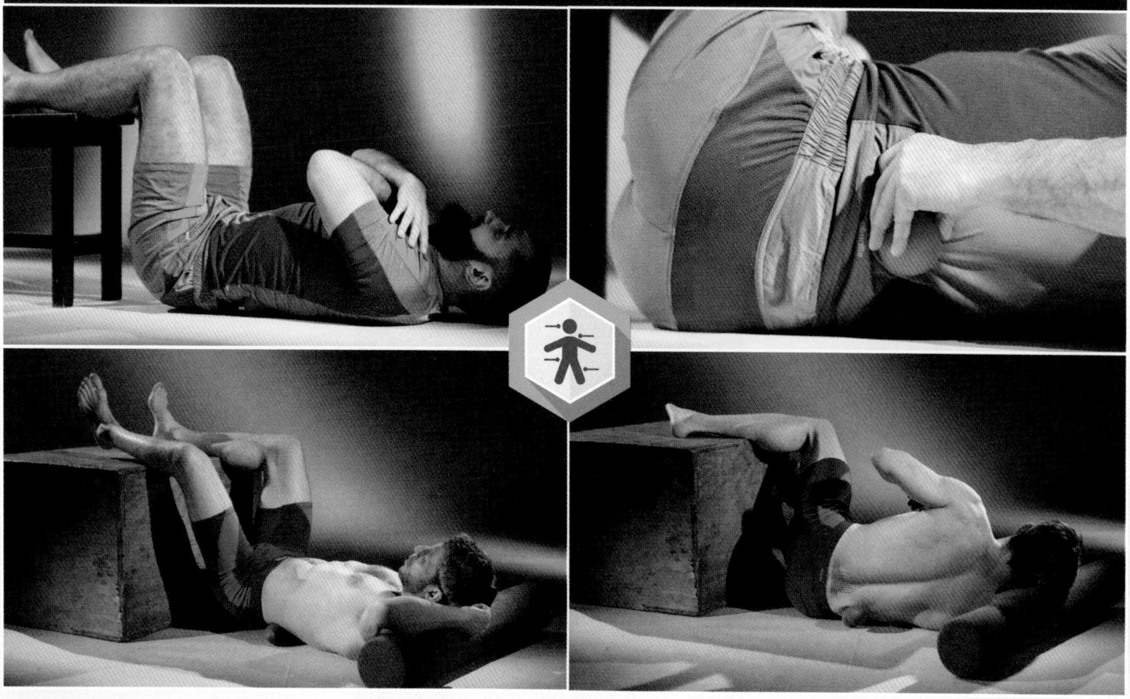

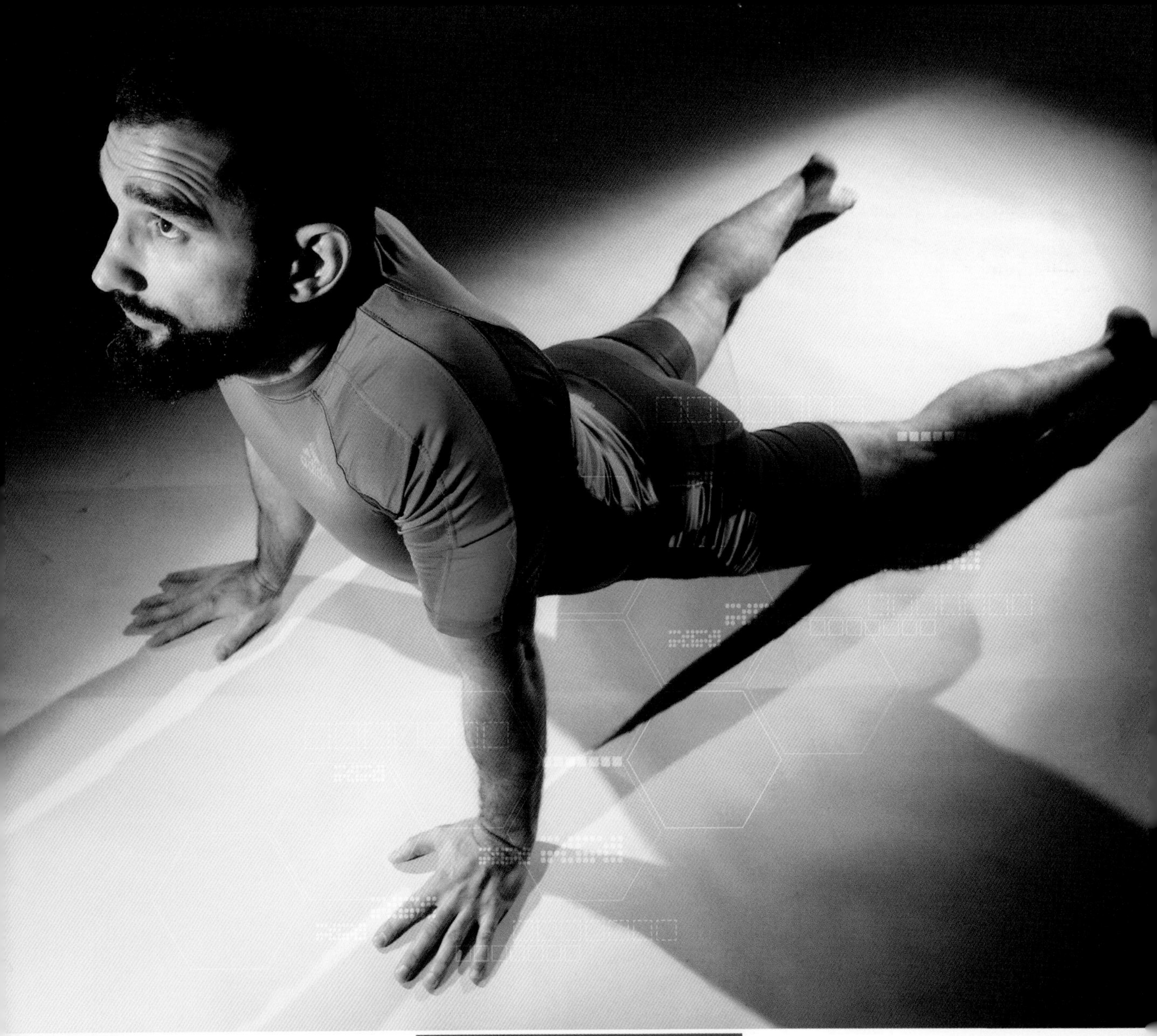

02. SPHINX STRETCH (WITH OR WITHOUT A BAND)

Lie on your abdomen with your legs and the insteps of your feet flat on the floor. Place the palm of your hands flat on the floor at the sides of your body at rib height. Push up with your arms to a fully-extended elbow position to completely extend your spine. You can wrap an exercise band around your upper back and anchor the ends under each hand to increase the effect of this exercise. **Hold the stretch for 30 seconds.**

03. BACKWARD-FORWARD QUADRUPED VARIATIONS

On all fours, shift your hips back until your elbows are extended and you are sitting on your heels (the first photo does not show the final position). Then push your hips forward, flatten the palm of your hands on the floor at the sides of your body at rib height, and push up to a fully-extended elbow position. Completely extend your spine and look up at the ceiling. **Hold each position for 5 to 10 seconds and perform 6 reps of each.**

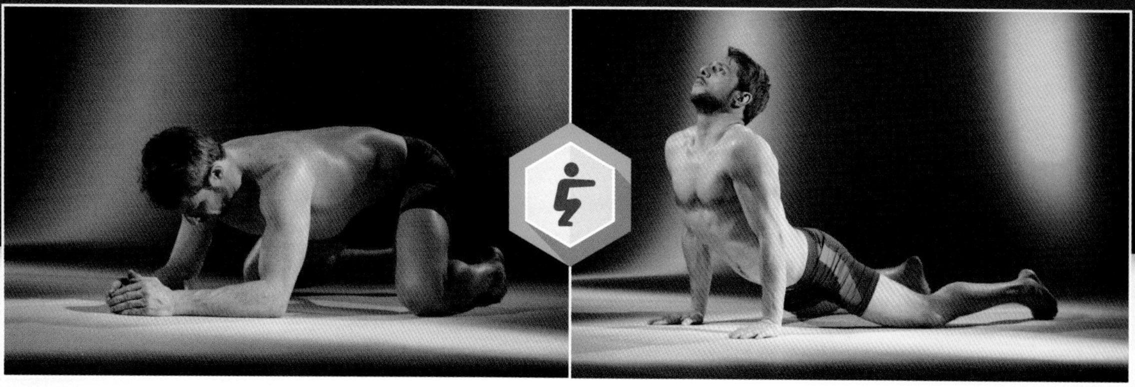

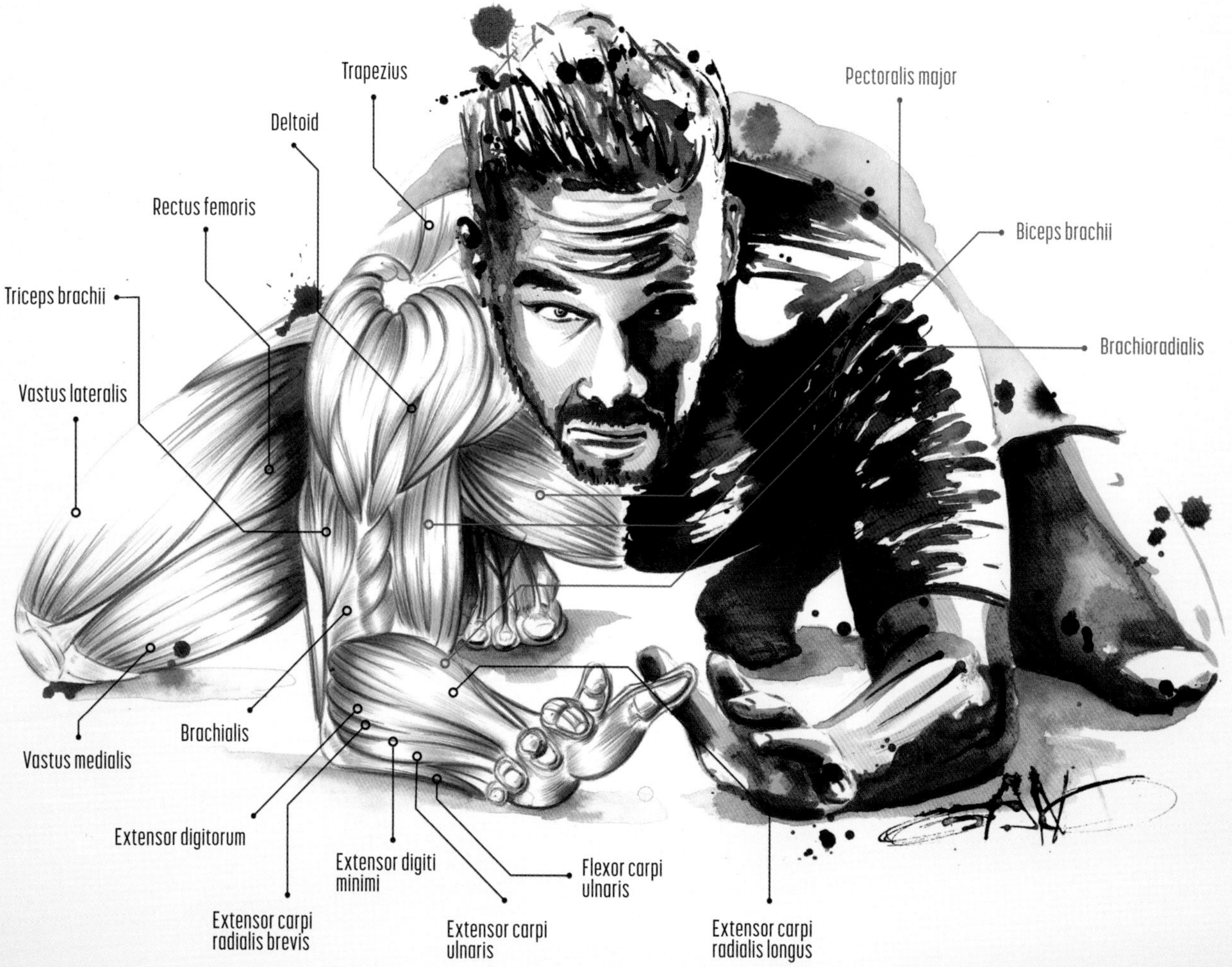

04. OPTIONAL: MEDICINE BALL BACK EXTENSION ON AN EXERCISE BALL WITH ROTATION

Lie face down on an exercise ball with your thighs and hips on the ball and your feet held by a partner or a gym ladder. Hold a medicine ball in front of your chest and lower your torso until the medicine ball touches the ground. Once in the lowest position, reverse the movement by extending your back to lift your torso while lifting your head and sticking out your chest. At the end of each raise, rotate your torso to one side and extend your elbows. Rotate back to the neutral position, perform another back extension repetition, and then rotate your torso to the other side. Do not change the alignment of your back during the exercise.

Perform 6 reps, alternating sides with each repetition.

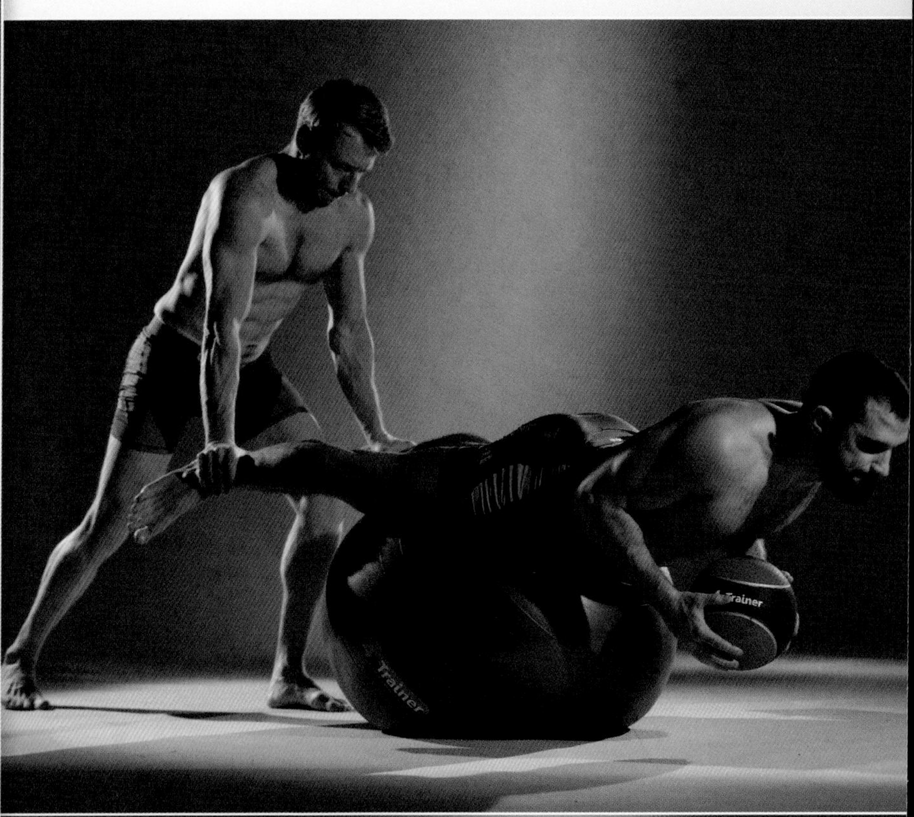

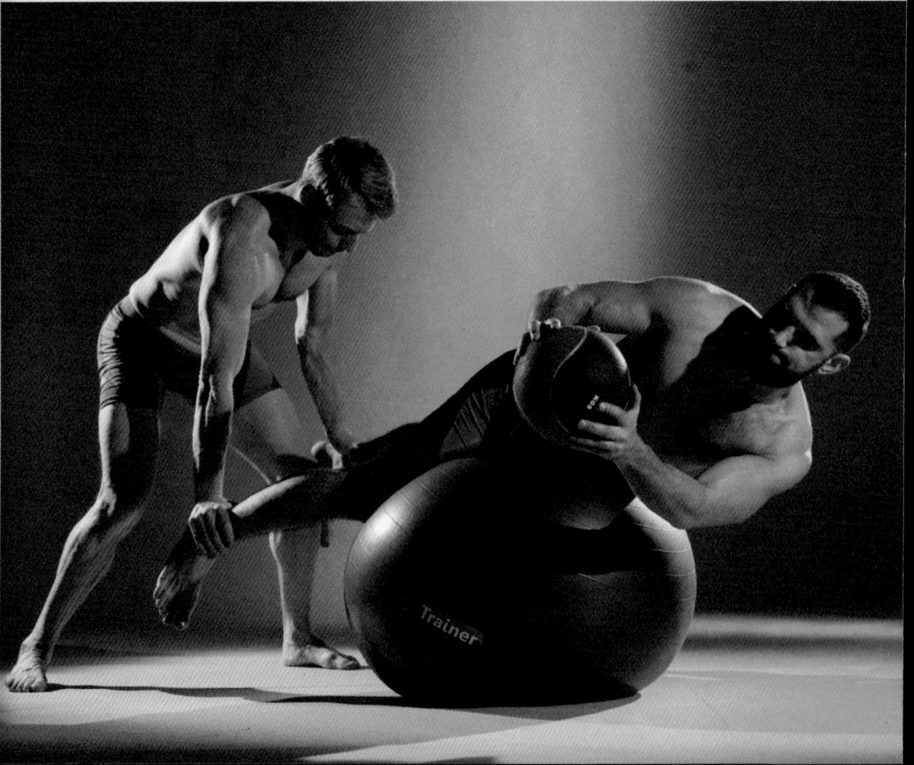

FUNCTIONAL TRAINING 01

A functional approach to movement that relies on mobility is at the heart of the training programs inspired by the sports of track and field, gymnastics, and weightlifting.

Human movement can be specific to a particular sport, but it is also a part of everyday life. Simply said, ***movement that is functional allows us to live life.*** A basic approach to maintain and develop mobility is the key to training because it does the following:

- Uses the three dimensions of space
- Encourages an awareness of breathing
- Promotes eccentric and concentric muscle actions
- Includes exercises with and without weights
- Involves a balance between agonist and antagonist muscles
- Creates a perception of the position and movement of the body
- Improves the strength and tone of muscle tissue

Training is no longer only about prioritizing strength or building endurance. Instead, we add a component that improves basic mobility for any physical activity, then we keep it consistent throughout all workouts and phases of training. This allows us to transfer different physical qualities to movement and to combat the harmful effects of certain training practices (or of everyday life) on motor function.

NOTE

A large part of mechanical restrictions in movement, and even pathological restrictions, stems from a loss of motor control (Comerford and Mottram 2012).

TAKE BACK CONTROL

Breathing, emotional, and physical disorders (injuries, overtraining, poor form, etc.) can cause serious muscle compensations and various imbalances in the short or long term. In part, the body loses control over its movement, becoming a nonfunctioning machine drowning under the weight of restrictions and problems.

You must take back control

Mastering optimal movement—guided by good feedback from the nervous system; proper coordination of movement in all directions; and limited stiffness, adhesions, and muscle imbalances—are the keys to a life free of pain and restrictions in movement, whatever your daily level of physical activity.

Modern literature has studied unstructured movement a great deal, and this, unless it is caused by an injury, often results from poorly controlled movement.

Compensatory movements, muscle imbalances, and the overuse of powerful motor muscles are objectively addressed by many sources in the scientific community (Comerford and Mottram 2001; Sahrmann 2002; Richardson et al. 2004; Jull et al. 2000).

MUSCLE FIBER TYPES AND MOVEMENT

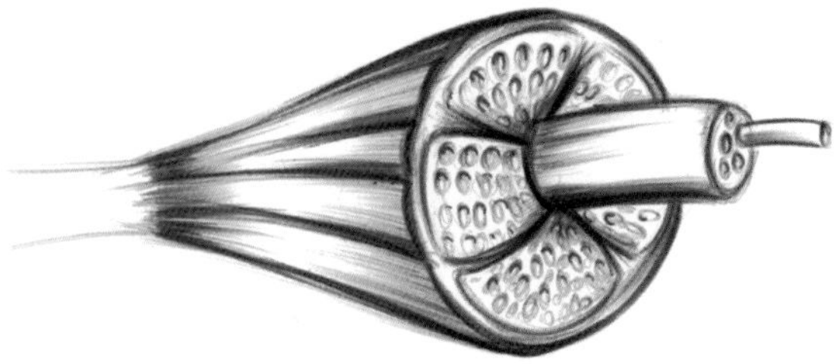

Muscle is comprised of fast-twitch fibers and slow-twitch fibers, and their relative proportion has a large influence on training. Fast-twitch muscle fibers are designed to generate quick, explosive movements that produce contractions of high intensity, but they tire easily. Conversely, slow-twitch muscle fibers, which are less easily fatigued, control movement and posture.

As a result, there are two different dimensions in the physical training of the human body: speed and strength on one hand and endurance and motor control on the other hand. For optimal performance, both are involved. It is a bit like a computer: There is the machine, and there is the software. To be as powerful as possible, you need to upgrade to the best hardware and the best software. Over the years, we have been trying to improve the human machine as if it were a computer: We add a better graphics card, a better processor, or faster memory without improving the operating system. For a maximum function, these things must go hand in hand: Use the best motor functions, link them with optimized muscles, and promote balance (antigravity and postural control) and mobility (weighted or quick movements).

Throughout your training sessions, always remember to combine mobility and balance. One does not work without the other. In your training, you must always keep a dimension of quality, fluidity, and speed and use the whole range of practice time and the number of recommended sets and repetitions.

Take the example of the scorpion exercise (see page 208). As described, the exercise is done using quick movements, but it can also be done slowly, with pauses at the different points of maximum range, ensuring alignment of the body and engaging the deep abdominal muscles. You can do 3 sets of 10 controlled repetitions with 40 seconds of recovery. This means you are following a program that is clearly focused on balance.

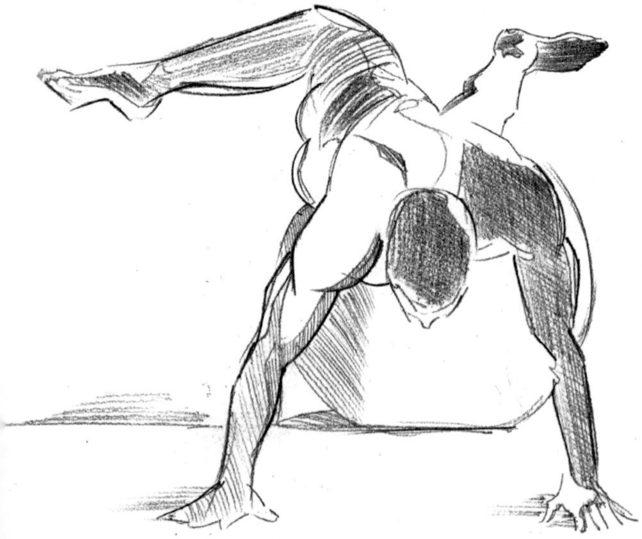

Conversely, you can also practice the scorpion exercise by relaxing. In this case, you are not measuring a number of reps or elapsed time but rather fluidity of movement or speed of execution. In this example, the idea is not to go faster just to go faster but to perform the moves in full range with control. Speed is built on the base of fluid movement.

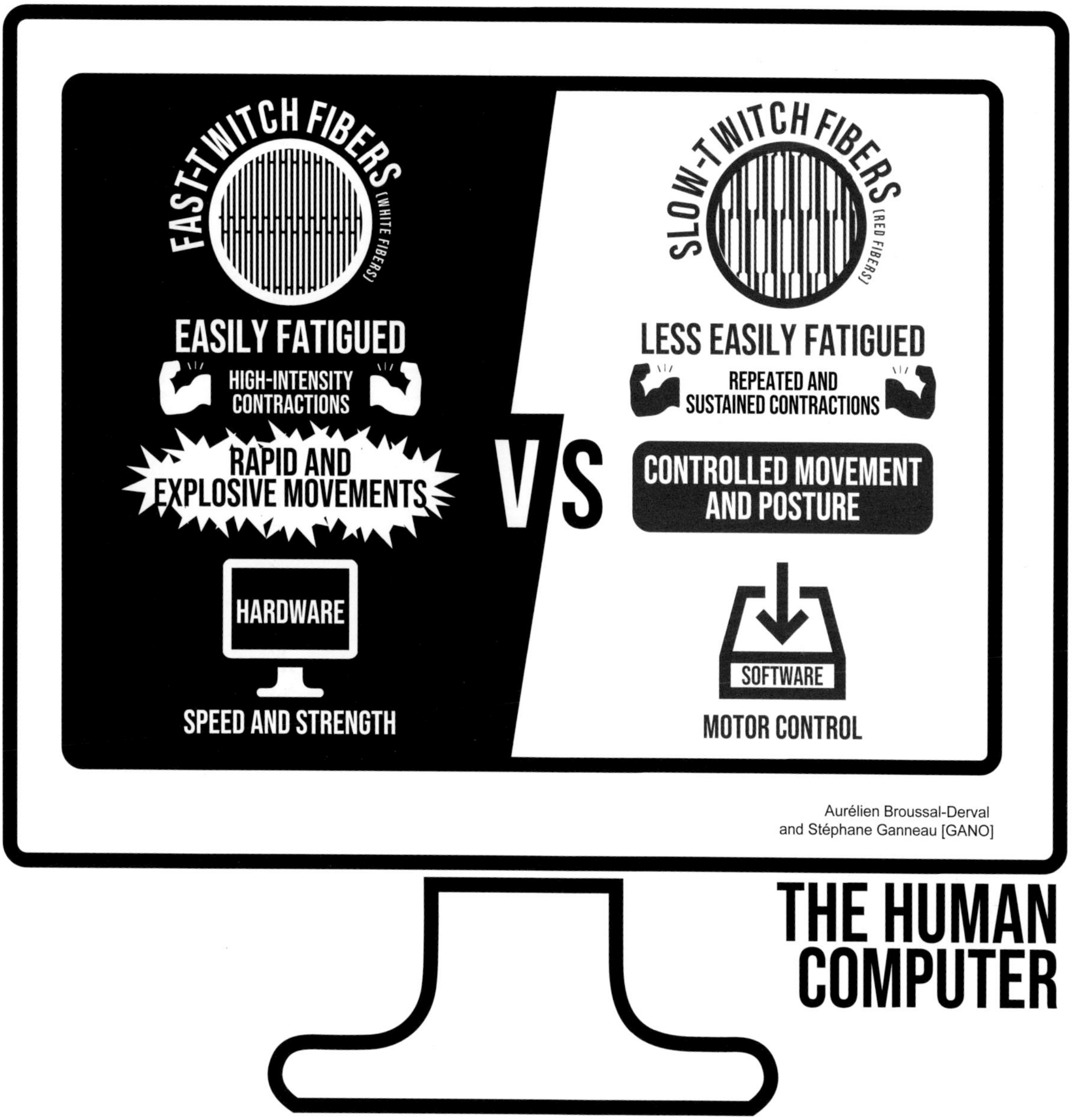

THE HUMAN COMPUTER

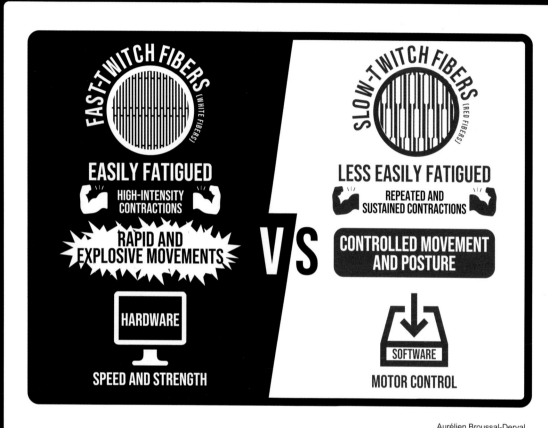

Exercise Series

The variations of these exercises are presented in order of difficulty. As you advance, work through the variations. In all cases, be sure not to bypass the first several exercises; over time, they will become warm-up exercises as you progress.

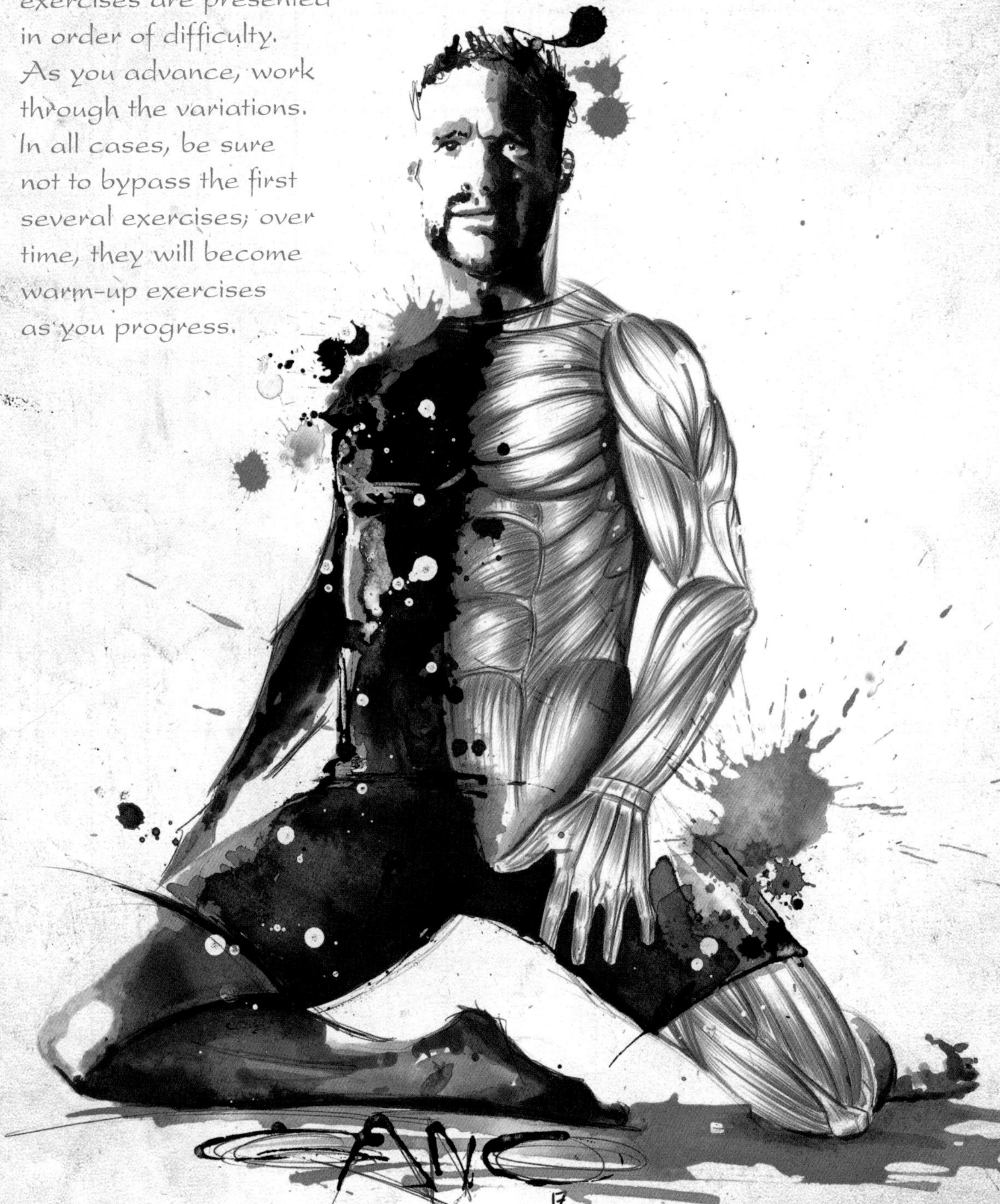

SHOULDER-OPENING
SERIES

The goal of these exercises is to optimize shoulder mobility and control. They are also a powerful combination of dynamic core training and motor control using the spiral chains. The movements should be done as slowly as possible, and all the principles of core stability apply (i.e., position of the back, activation of the transversus, and control over the pelvic floor). It is also essential to have total control over your breathing (see the section on breathing starting on page 78).

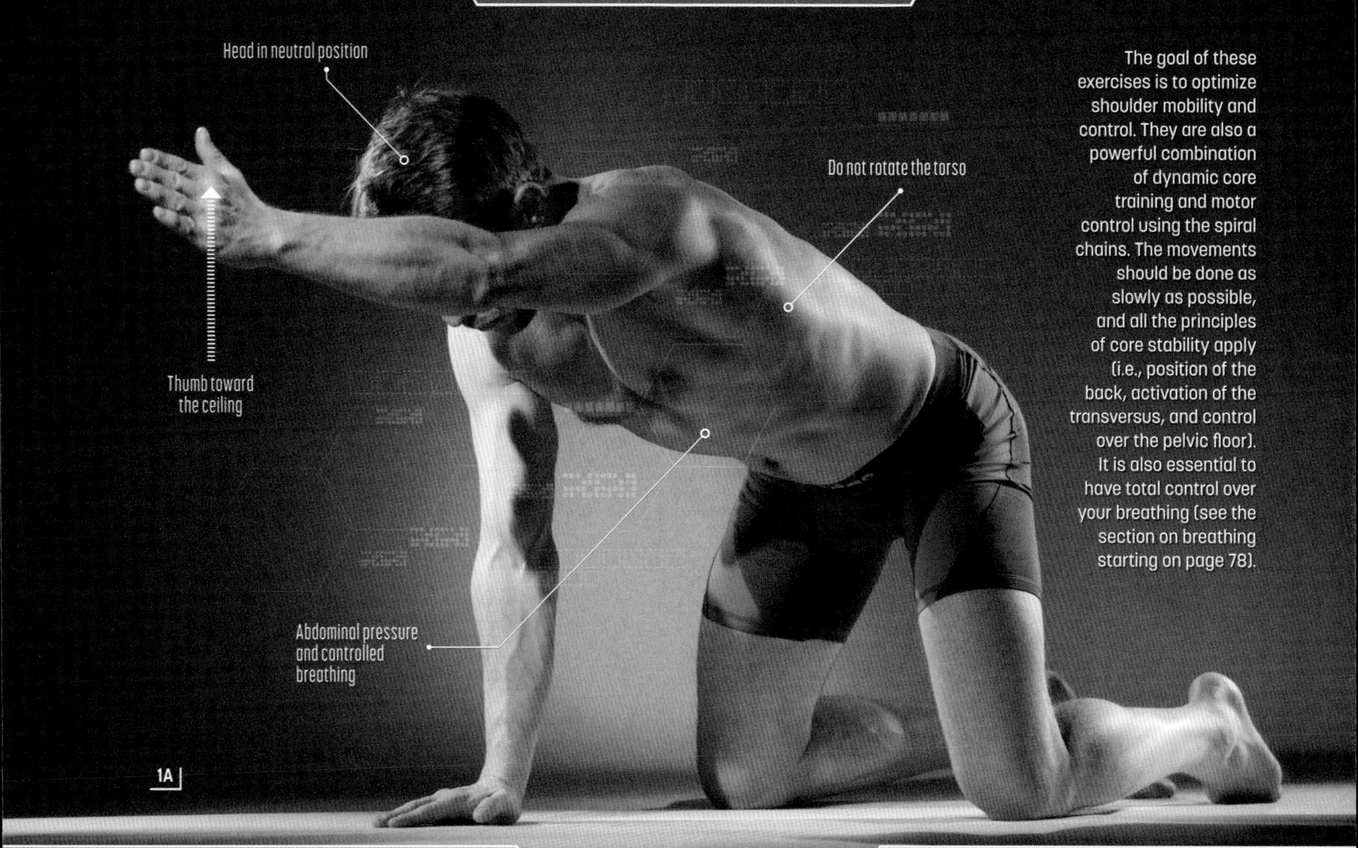

Head in neutral position
Do not rotate the torso
Thumb toward the ceiling
Abdominal pressure and controlled breathing
1A

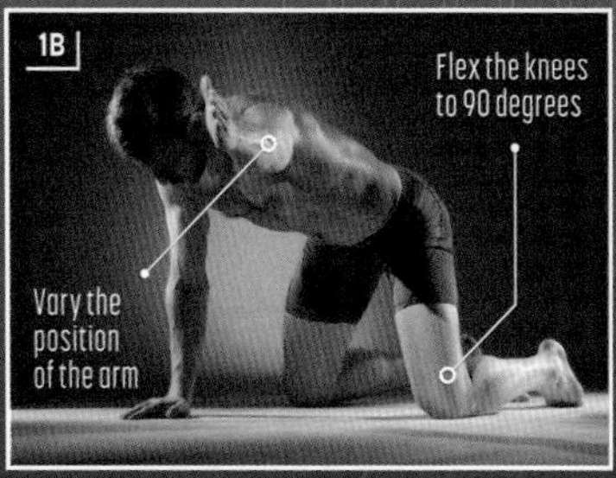

1B
Flex the knees to 90 degrees
Vary the position of the arm

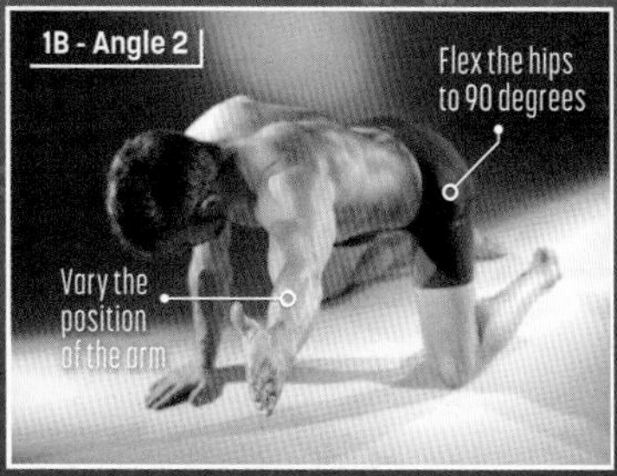

1B - Angle 2
Flex the hips to 90 degrees
Vary the position of the arm

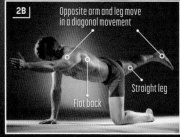

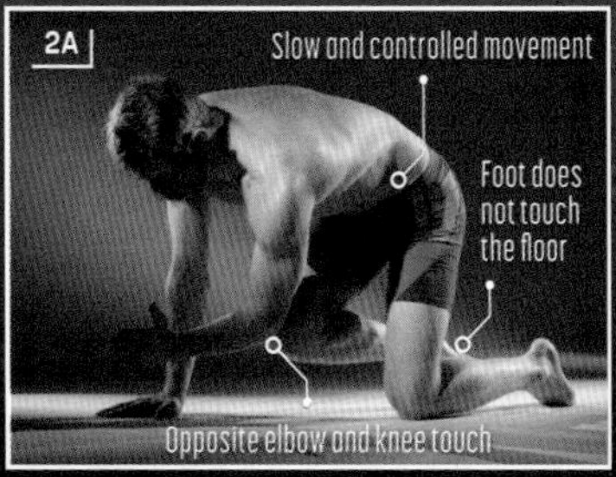

2A
Slow and controlled movement
Foot does not touch the floor
Opposite elbow and knee touch

2B
Opposite arm and leg move in a diagonal movement
Straight leg
Flat back

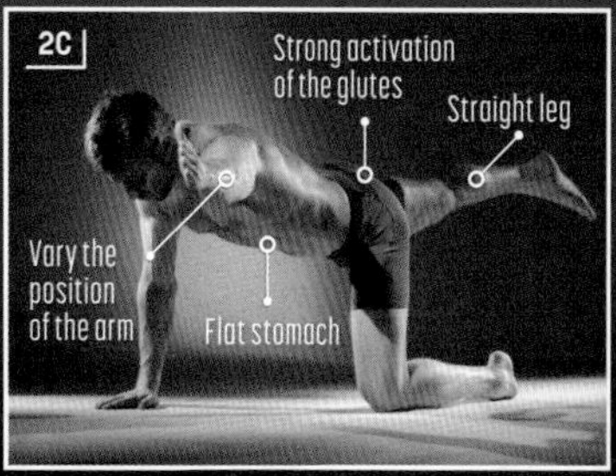

2C
Strong activation of the glutes
Straight leg
Vary the position of the arm
Flat stomach

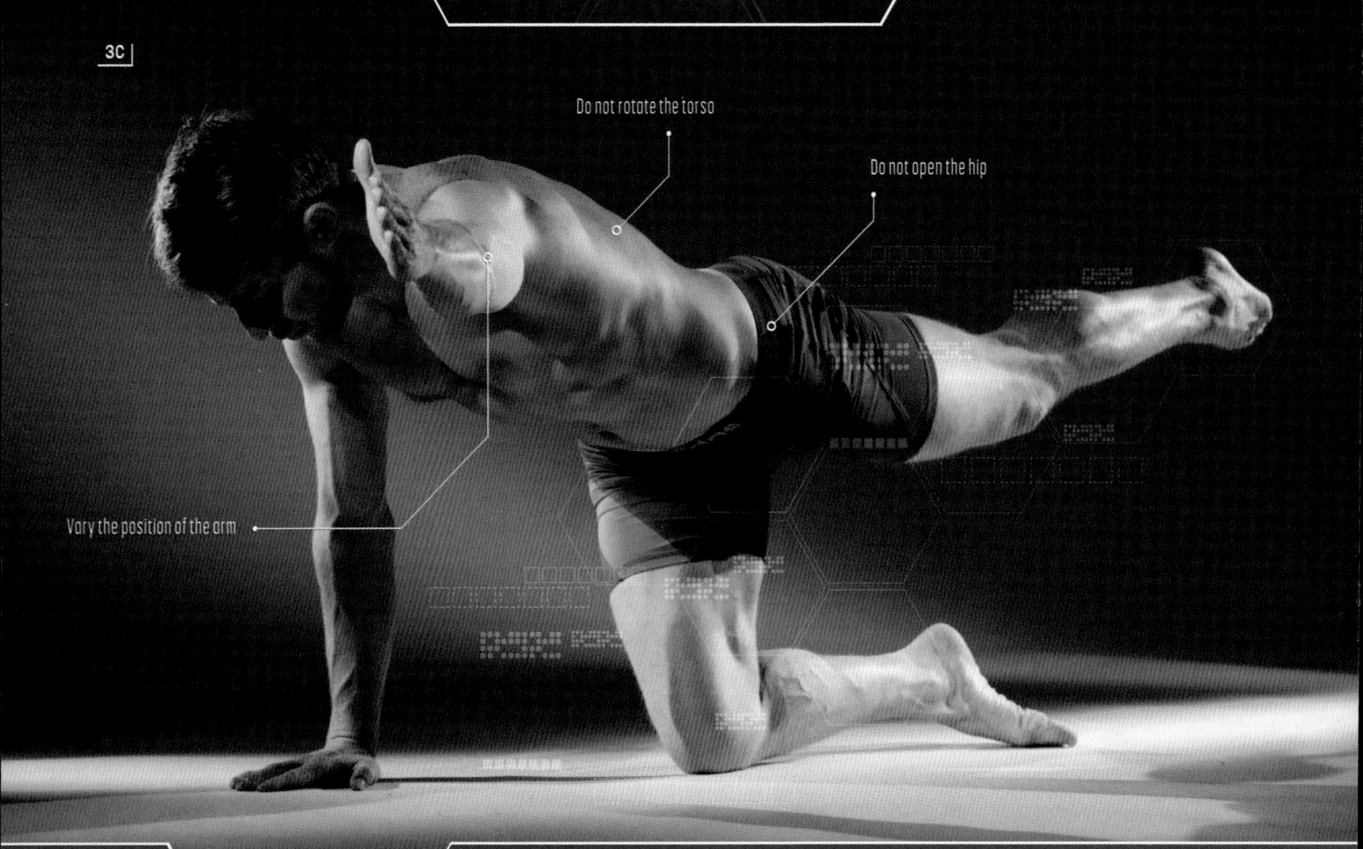
3C
Do not rotate the torso
Do not open the hip
Vary the position of the arm

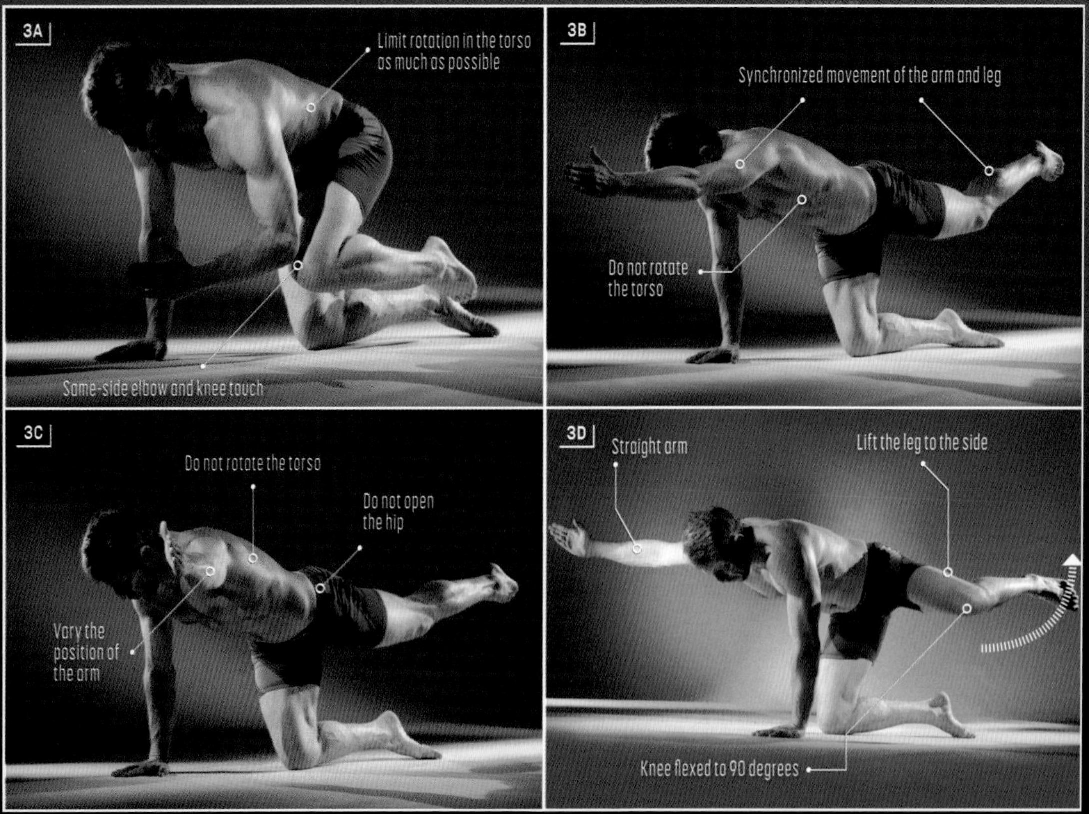
3A
Limit rotation in the torso as much as possible
Same-side elbow and knee touch
3B
Synchronized movement of the arm and leg
Do not rotate the torso
3C
Do not rotate the torso
Do not open the hip
Vary the position of the arm
3D
Straight arm
Lift the leg to the side
Knee flexed to 90 degrees

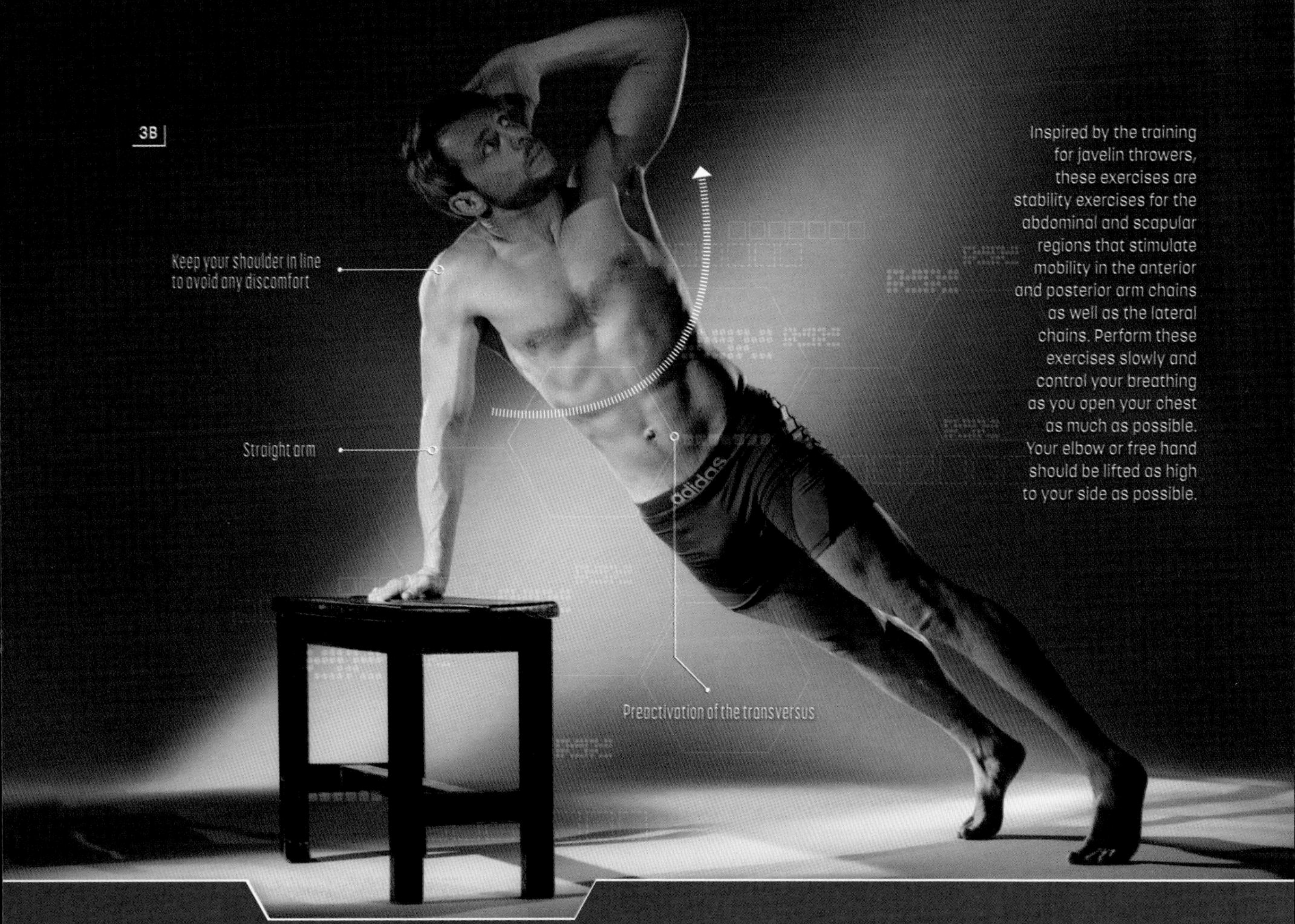
3B
Keep your shoulder in line to avoid any discomfort
Straight arm
Preactivation of the transversus

Inspired by the training for javelin throwers, these exercises are stability exercises for the abdominal and scapular regions that stimulate mobility in the anterior and posterior arm chains as well as the lateral chains. Perform these exercises slowly and control your breathing as you open your chest as much as possible. Your elbow or free hand should be lifted as high to your side as possible.

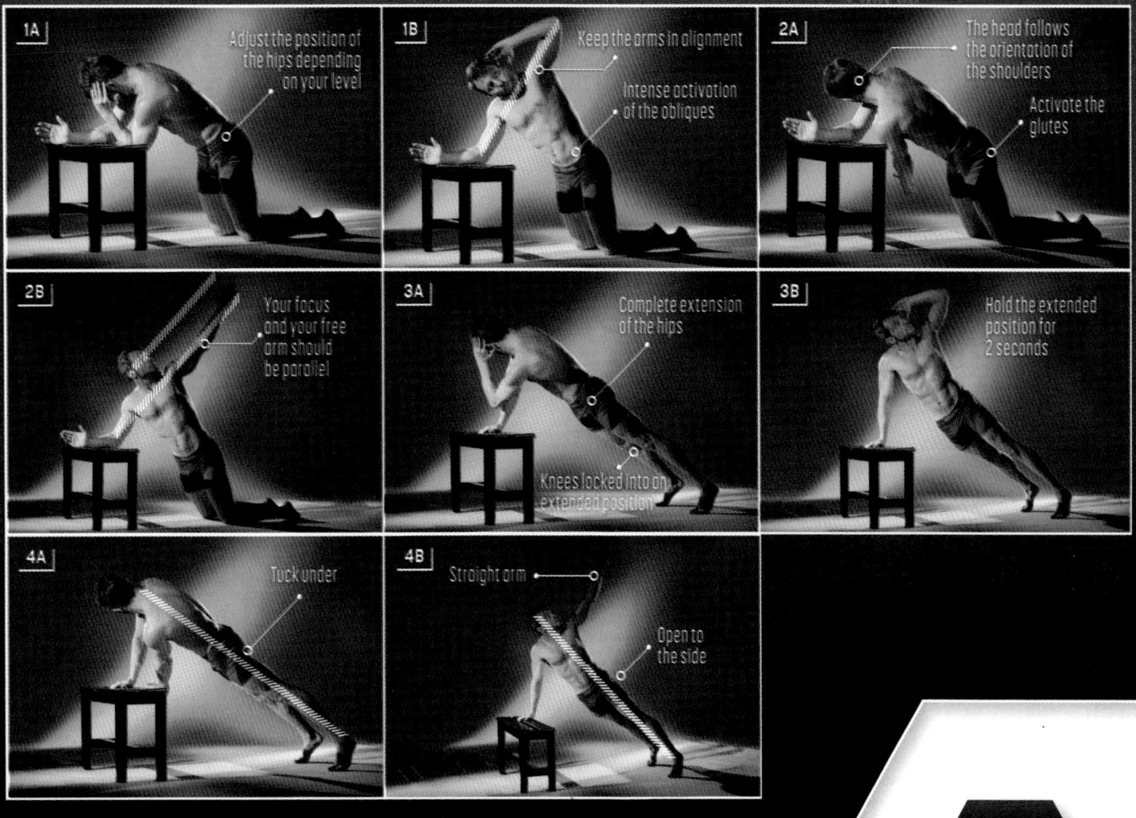
1A
Adjust the position of the hips depending on your level
1B
Keep the arms in alignment
Intense activation of the obliques
2A
The head follows the orientation of the shoulders
Activate the glutes
2B
Your focus and your free arm should be parallel
3A
Complete extension of the hips
Knees locked into an extended position
3B
Hold the extended position for 2 seconds
4A
Tuck under
4B
Straight arm
Open to the side

SPHINX
SERIES

The extension of the back is an essential prerequisite for functional human movement. Since it is often not the focus of training, its mobility can gradually deteriorate over time. Progressively performing variations of the sphinx is an effective tool to maintain and improve back extension. Be prudent to move through the steps slowly; do not try to do the most advanced levels right away. For each variation, try to reach and maintain the fullest back extension position that is possible based on your level of mobility. For all of the movements, press your hips into the floor, open your chest, and (when applicable) focus your eyes on the ceiling.

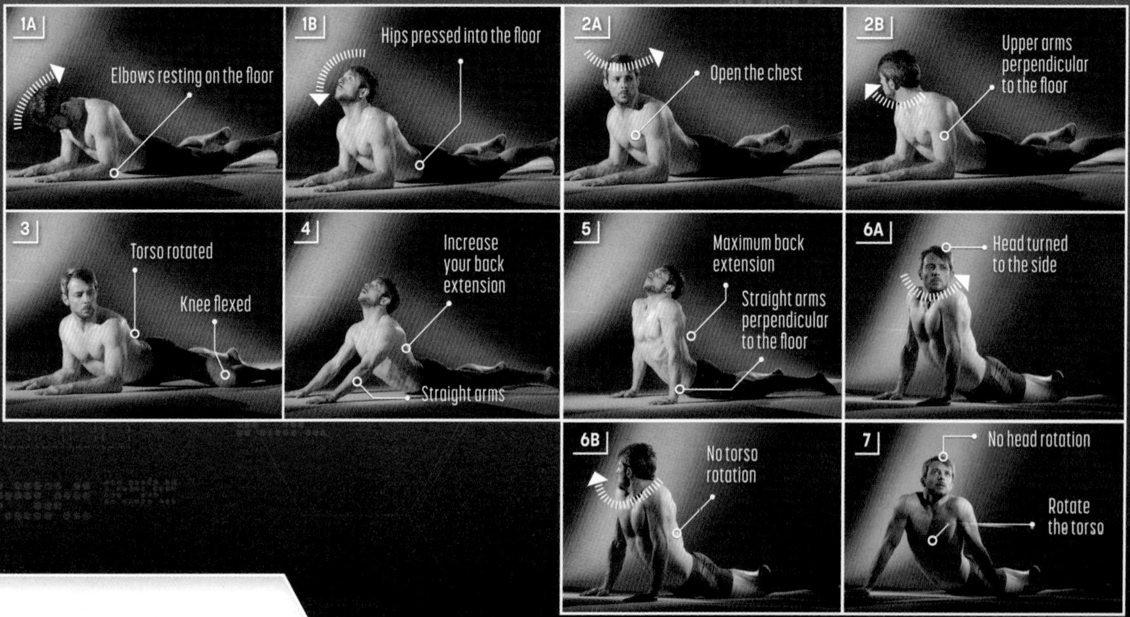

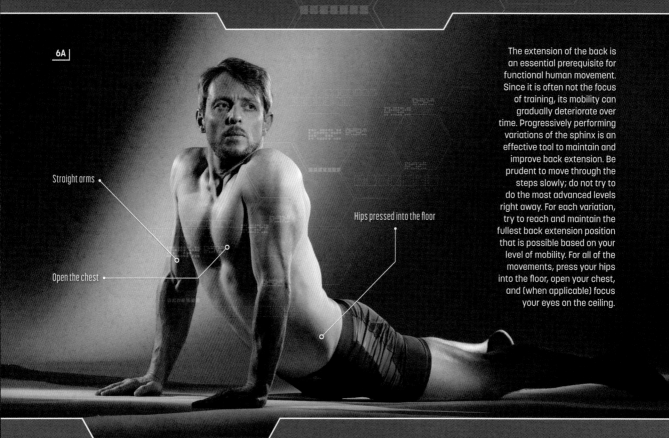

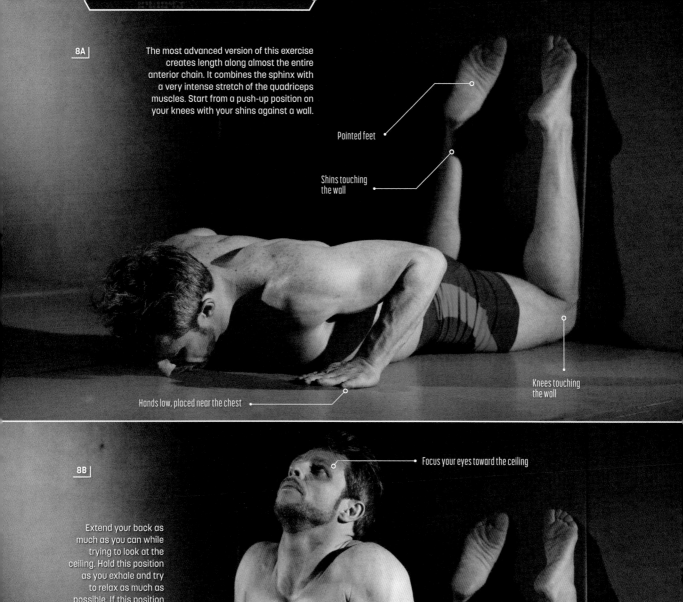

8A

The most advanced version of this exercise creates length along almost the entire anterior chain. It combines the sphinx with a very intense stretch of the quadriceps muscles. Start from a push-up position on your knees with your shins against a wall.

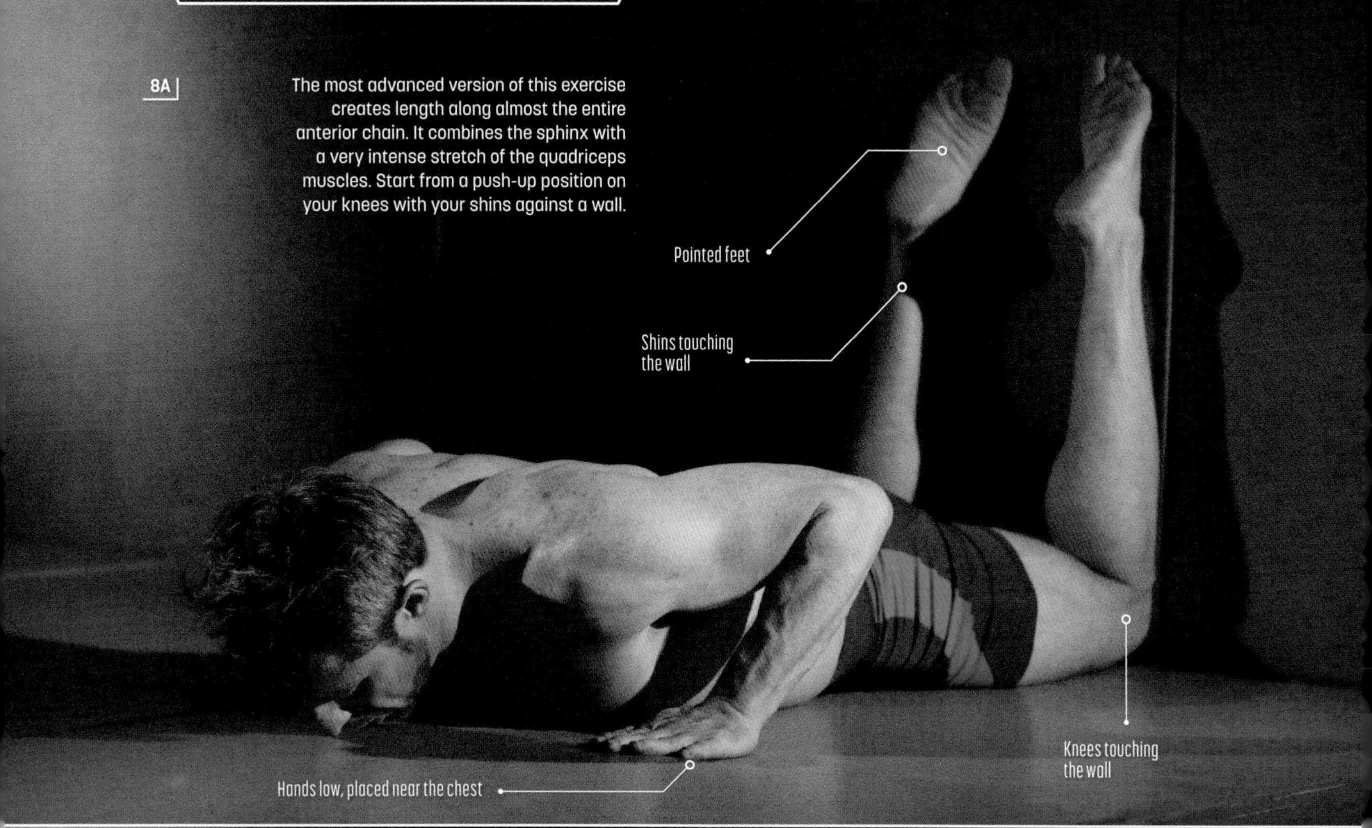
Pointed feet
Shins touching the wall
Knees touching the wall
Hands low, placed near the chest

8B

Extend your back as much as you can while trying to look at the ceiling. Hold this position as you exhale and try to relax as much as possible. If this position is easy or becomes easy for you, then you can increase the range of motion by looking at the ceiling until you can see the wall behind you. You can also press your hips into the floor as much as possible.

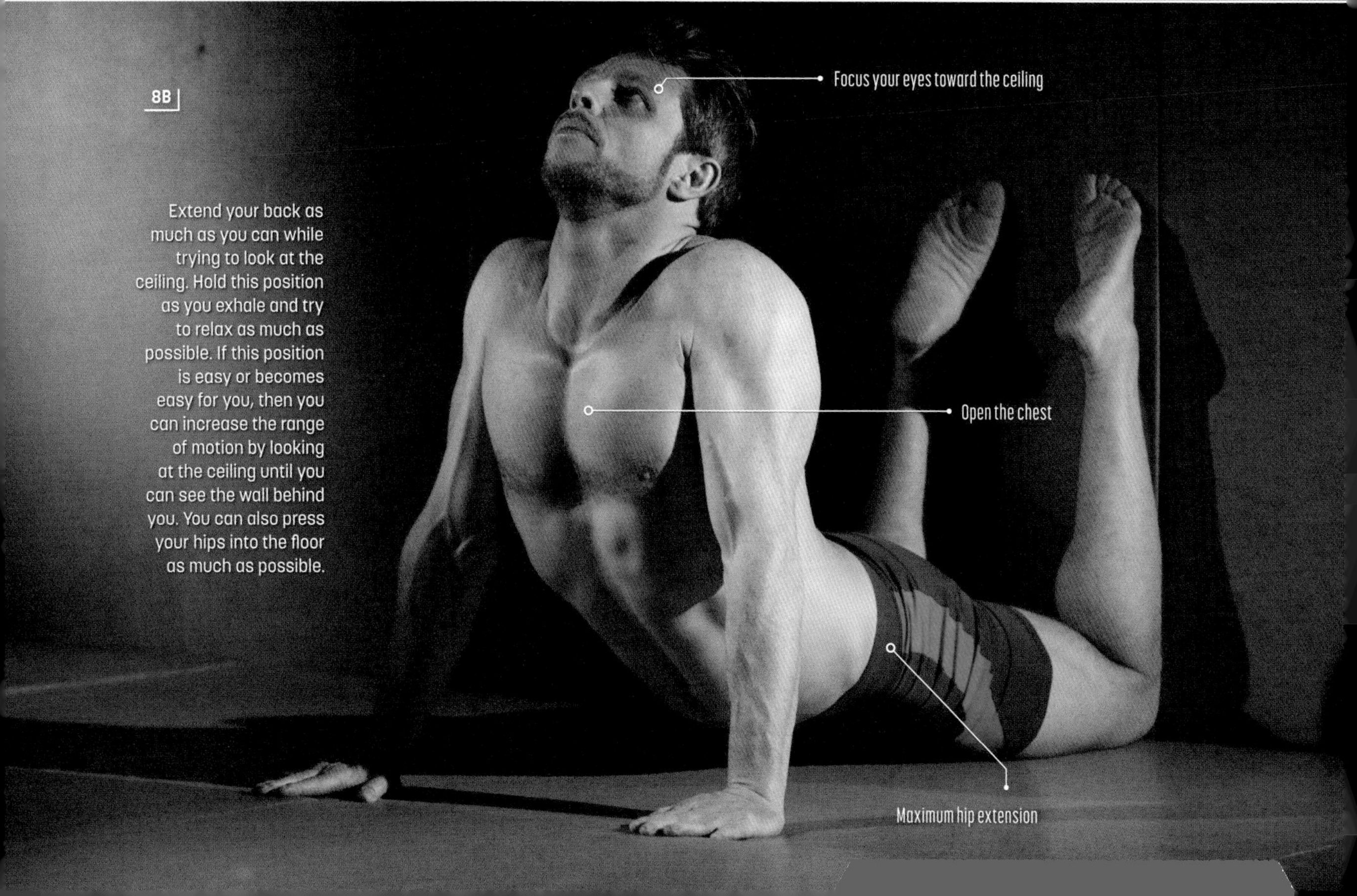
Focus your eyes toward the ceiling
Open the chest
Maximum hip extension

These exercises aim to (re)take control over the pelvis to the point that you can specifically focus on that part of your body. Over time, you can learn to mobilize the hips in different planes without equipment or, as seen in several of the photos, using a medium-sized medicine ball or an exercise ball.

1A

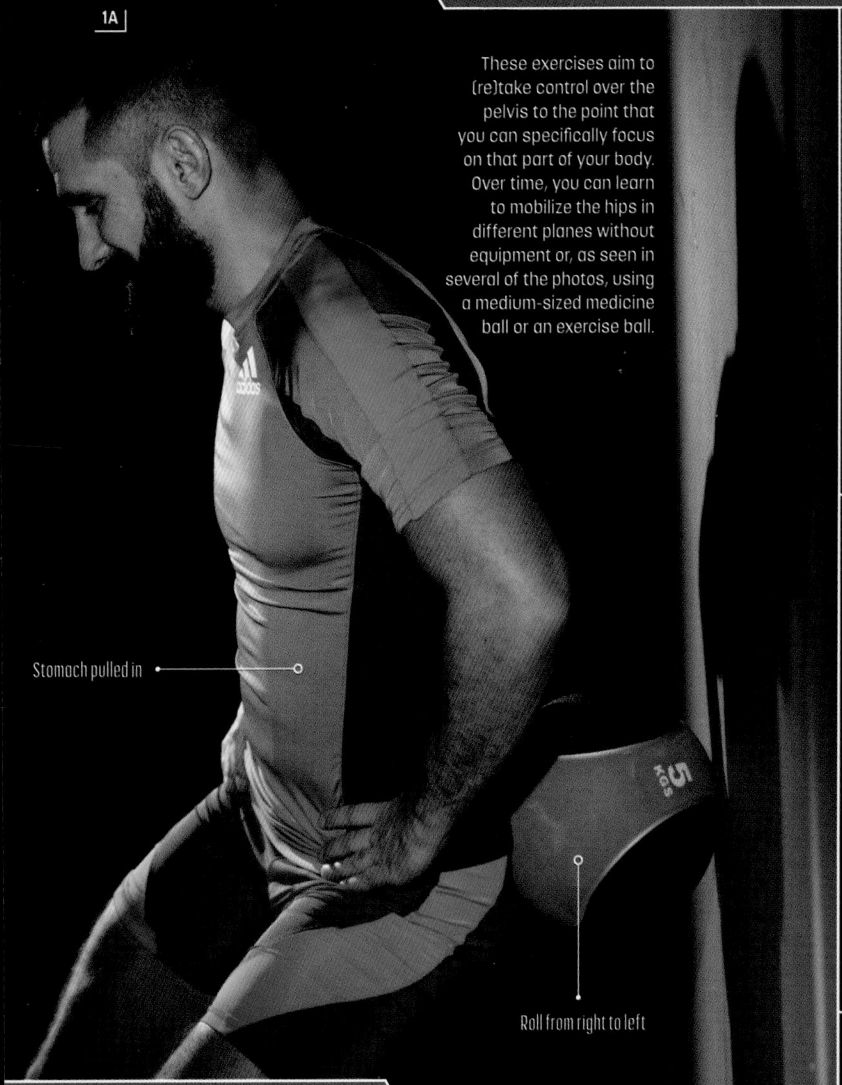

Stomach pulled in
5 KGS
Roll from right to left

1B

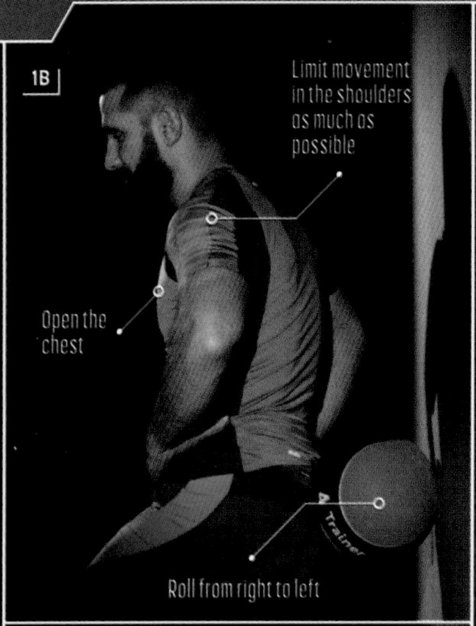

Limit movement in the shoulders as much as possible
Open the chest
Roll from right to left

2A

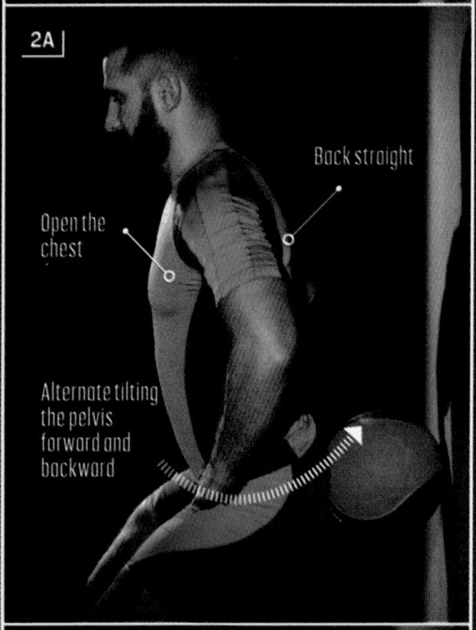

Back straight
Open the chest
Alternate tilting the pelvis forward and backward

2B

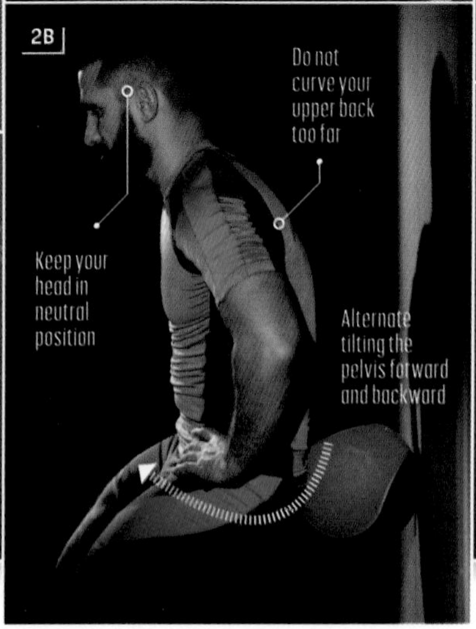

Do not curve your upper back too far
Keep your head in neutral position
Alternate tilting the pelvis forward and backward

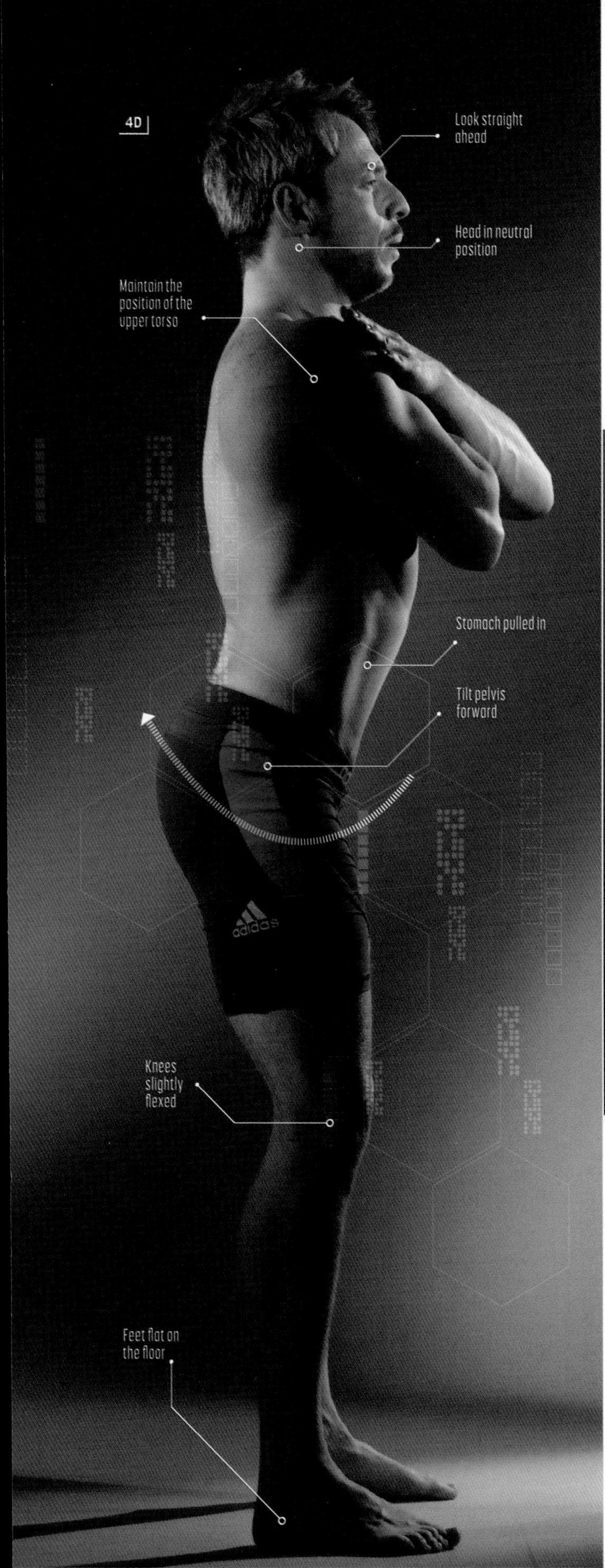
4D
Look straight ahead
Head in neutral position
Maintain the position of the upper torso
Stomach pulled in
Tilt pelvis forward
Knees slightly flexed
Feet flat on the floor

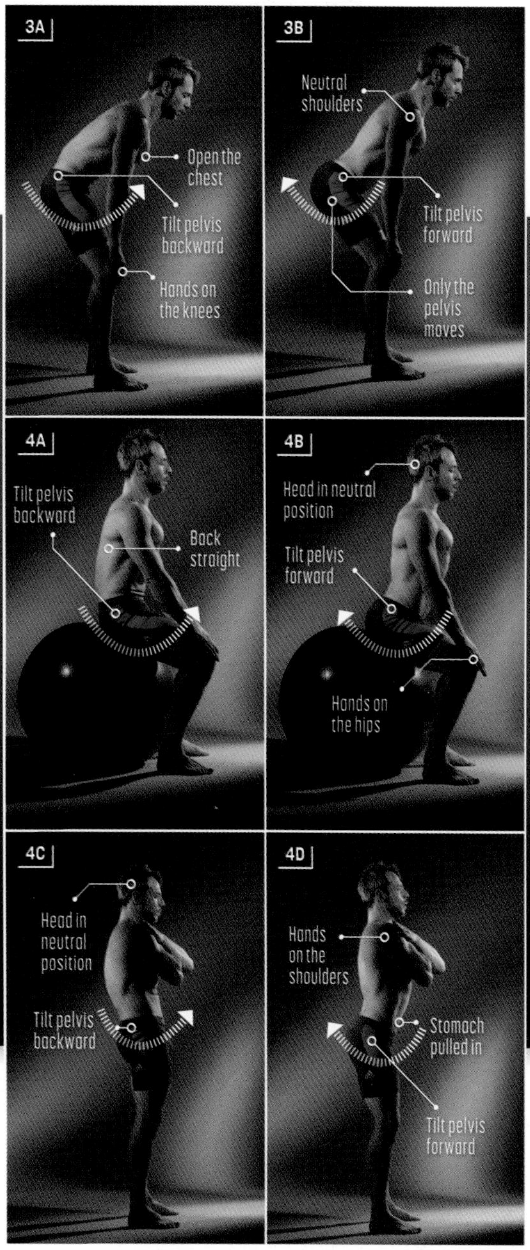
3A
Open the chest
Tilt pelvis backward
Hands on the knees
3B
Neutral shoulders
Tilt pelvis forward
Only the pelvis moves
4A
Tilt pelvis backward
Back straight
4B
Head in neutral position
Tilt pelvis forward
Hands on the hips
4C
Head in neutral position
Tilt pelvis backward
4D
Hands on the shoulders
Stomach pulled in
Tilt pelvis forward

OMOPLATA
SERIES

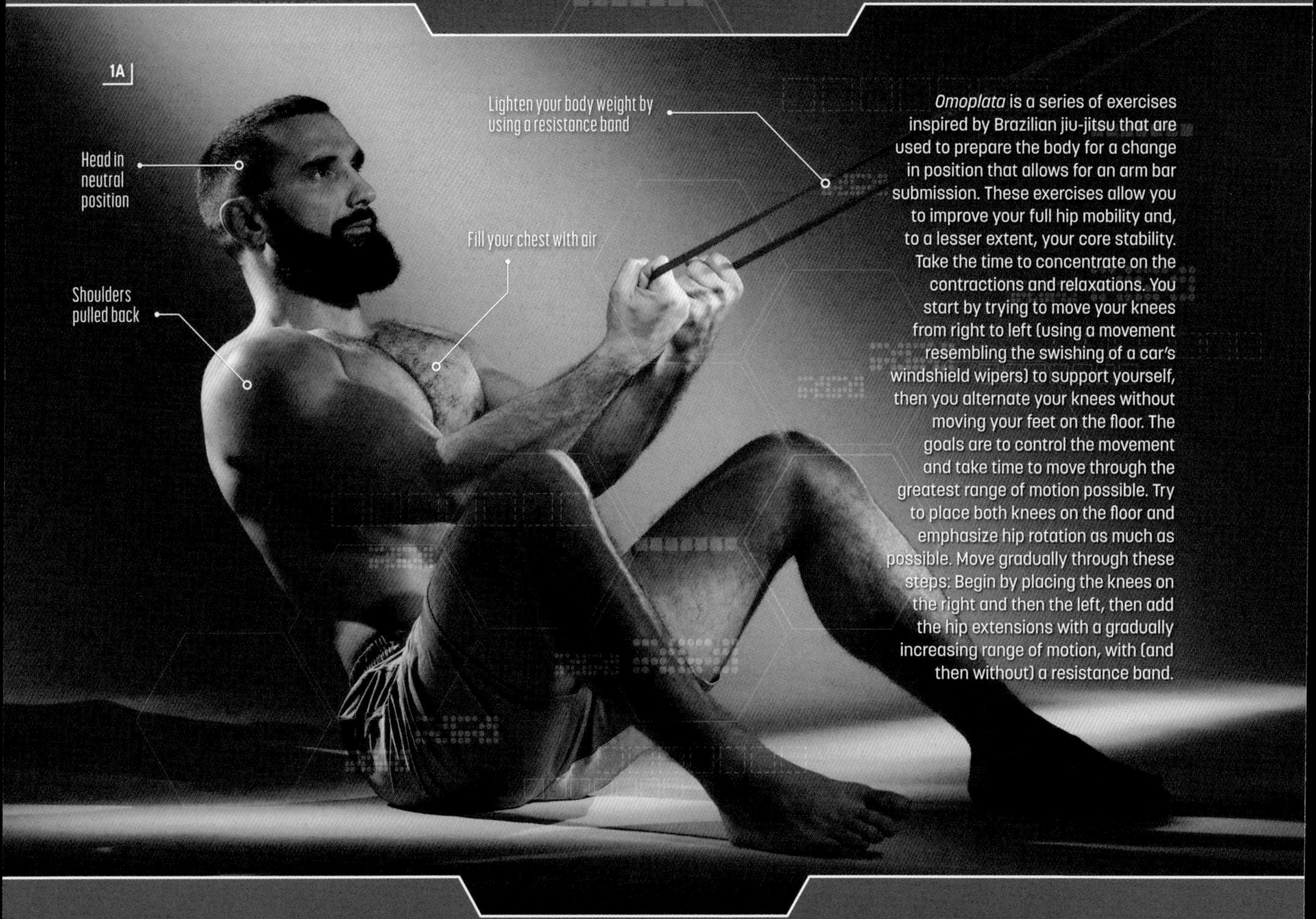
1A
Head in neutral position
Lighten your body weight by using a resistance band
Fill your chest with air
Shoulders pulled back

Omoplata is a series of exercises inspired by Brazilian jiu-jitsu that are used to prepare the body for a change in position that allows for an arm bar submission. These exercises allow you to improve your full hip mobility and, to a lesser extent, your core stability. Take the time to concentrate on the contractions and relaxations. You start by trying to move your knees from right to left (using a movement resembling the swishing of a car's windshield wipers) to support yourself, then you alternate your knees without moving your feet on the floor. The goals are to control the movement and take time to move through the greatest range of motion possible. Try to place both knees on the floor and emphasize hip rotation as much as possible. Move gradually through these steps: Begin by placing the knees on the right and then the left, then add the hip extensions with a gradually increasing range of motion, with (and then without) a resistance band.

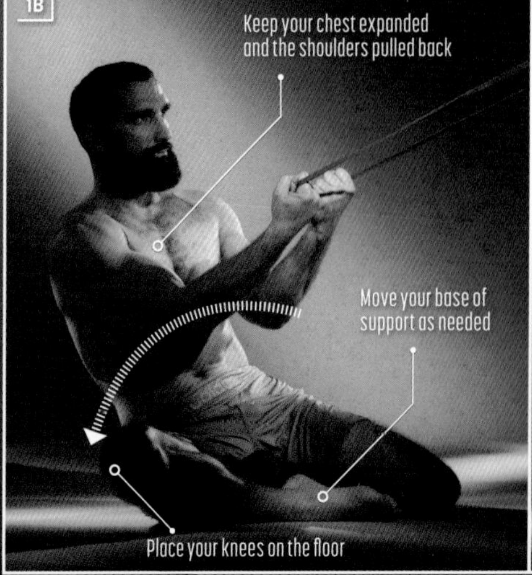
1B
Keep your chest expanded and the shoulders pulled back
Move your base of support as needed
Place your knees on the floor

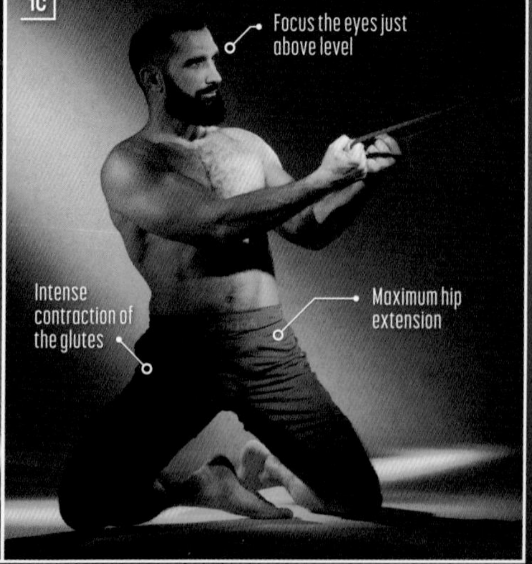
1C
Focus the eyes just above level
Intense contraction of the glutes
Maximum hip extension

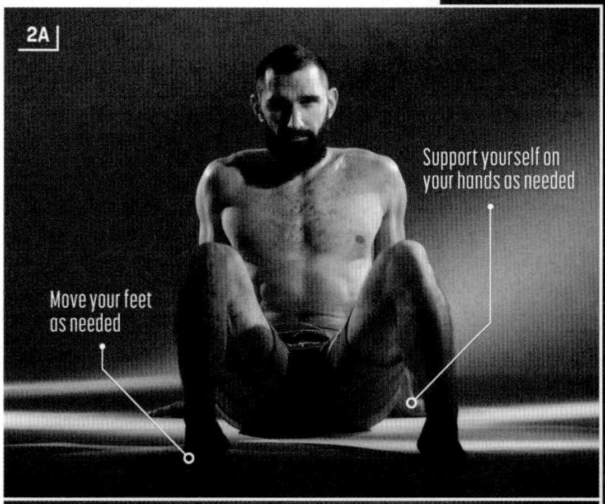
2A
Support yourself on your hands as needed
Move your feet as needed

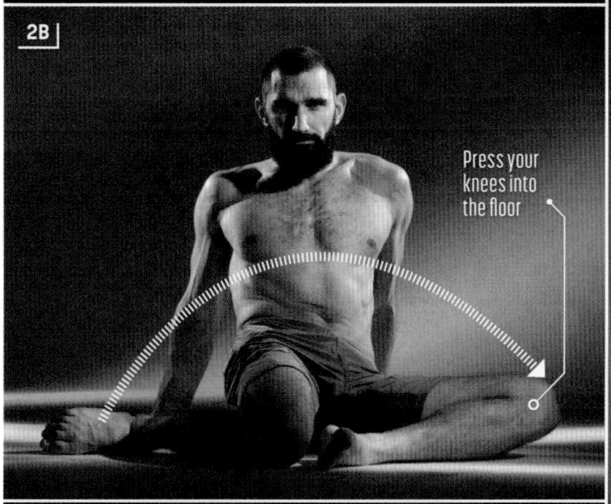
2B
Press your knees into the floor

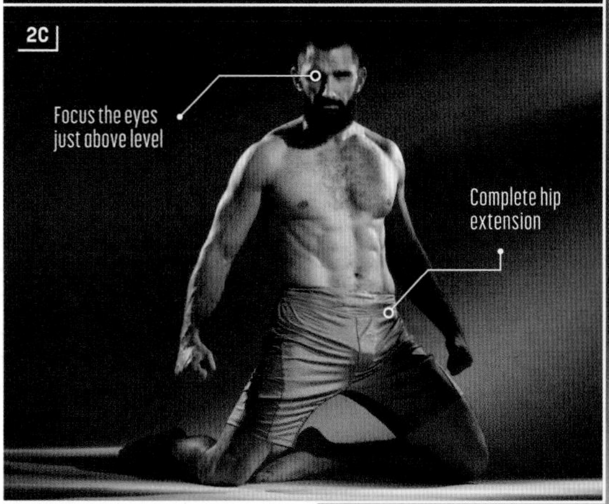
2C
Focus the eyes just above level
Complete hip extension

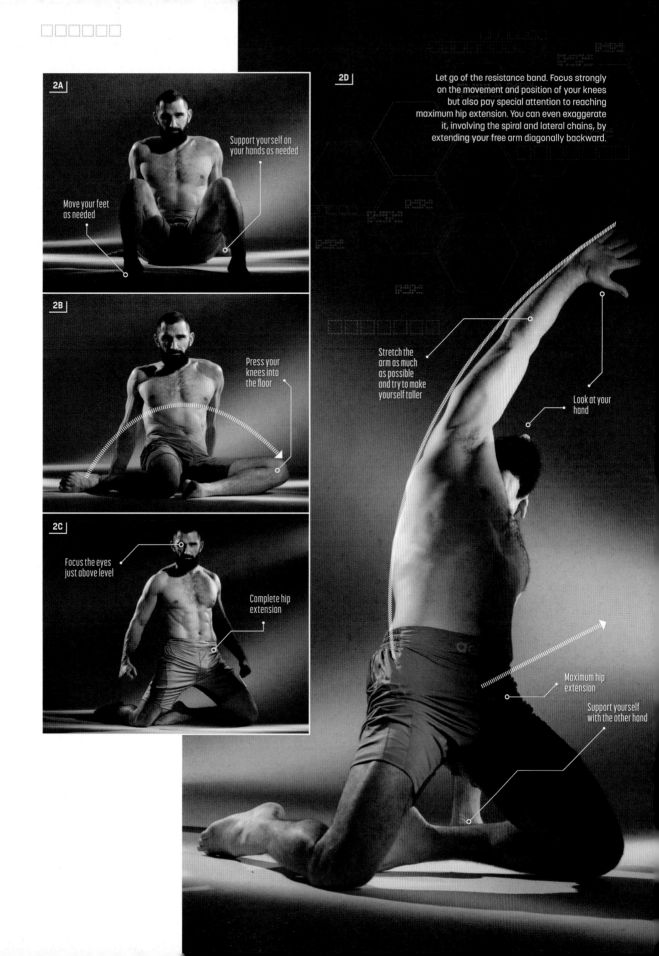

2D Let go of the resistance band. Focus strongly on the movement and position of your knees but also pay special attention to reaching maximum hip extension. You can even exaggerate it, involving the spiral and lateral chains, by extending your free arm diagonally backward.

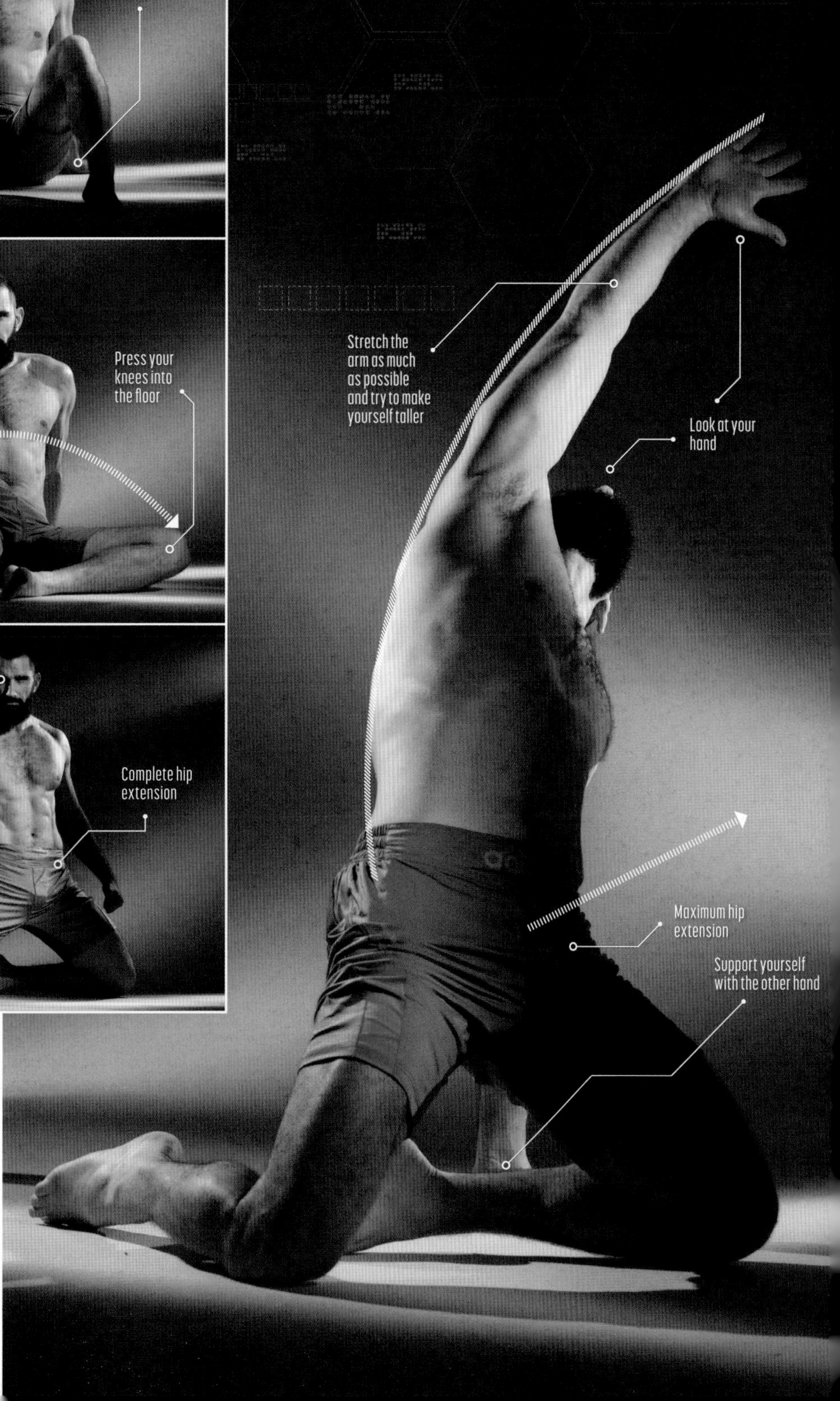
Stretch the arm as much as possible and try to make yourself taller
Look at your hand
Maximum hip extension
Support yourself with the other hand

3C

For this exercise, you will not use your hands or move your feet on the floor. The support of your feet at the beginning of the exercise is your only support. Place both knees on the floor and extend your hips. Once you are up, reverse the position of your lower legs (shins) through a sweeping movement from left to right. Control the descent to return to the starting position and begin again (do not let yourself fall back into a sitting position).

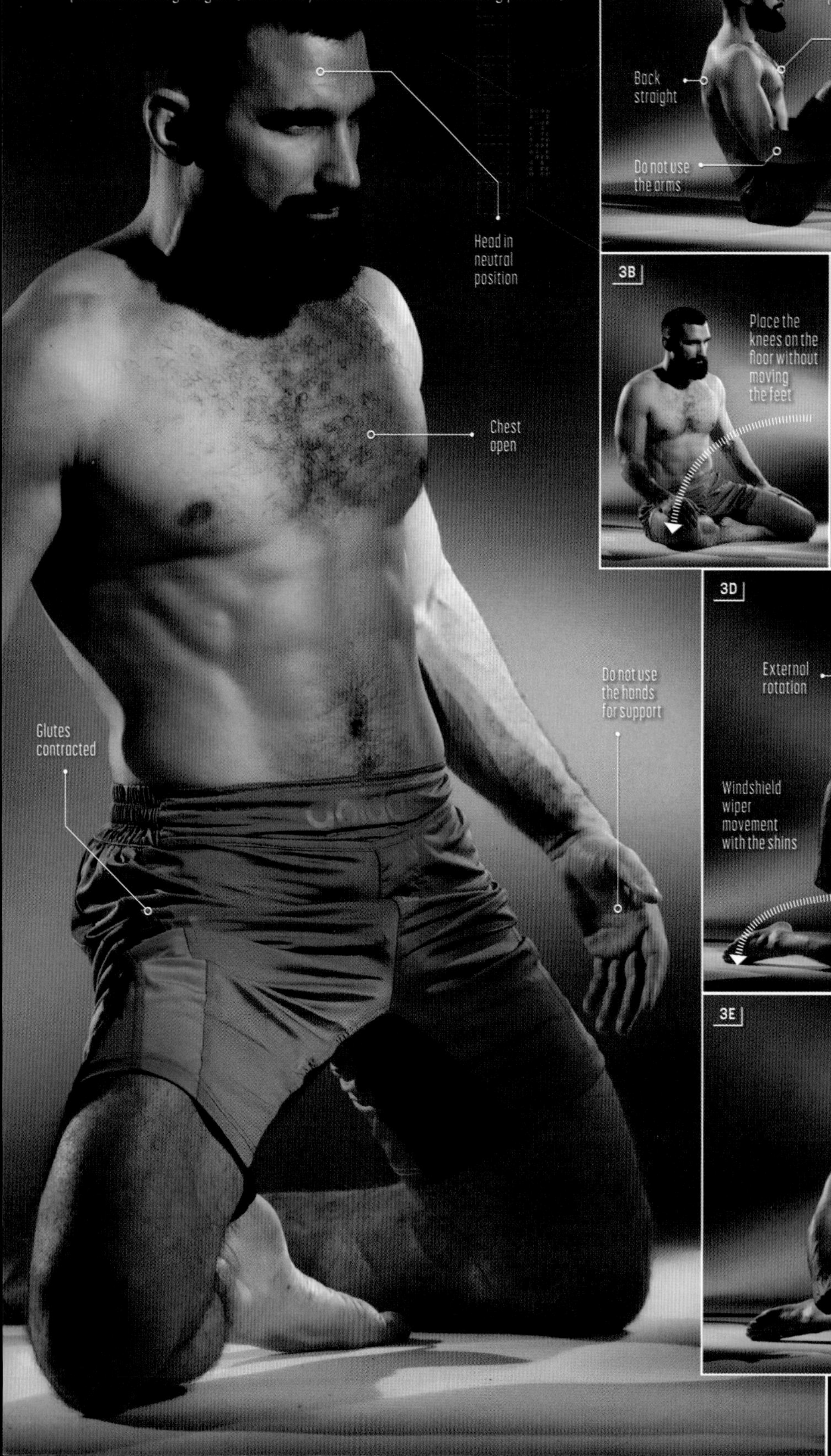
Head in neutral position
Chest open
Glutes contracted
Do not use the hands for support

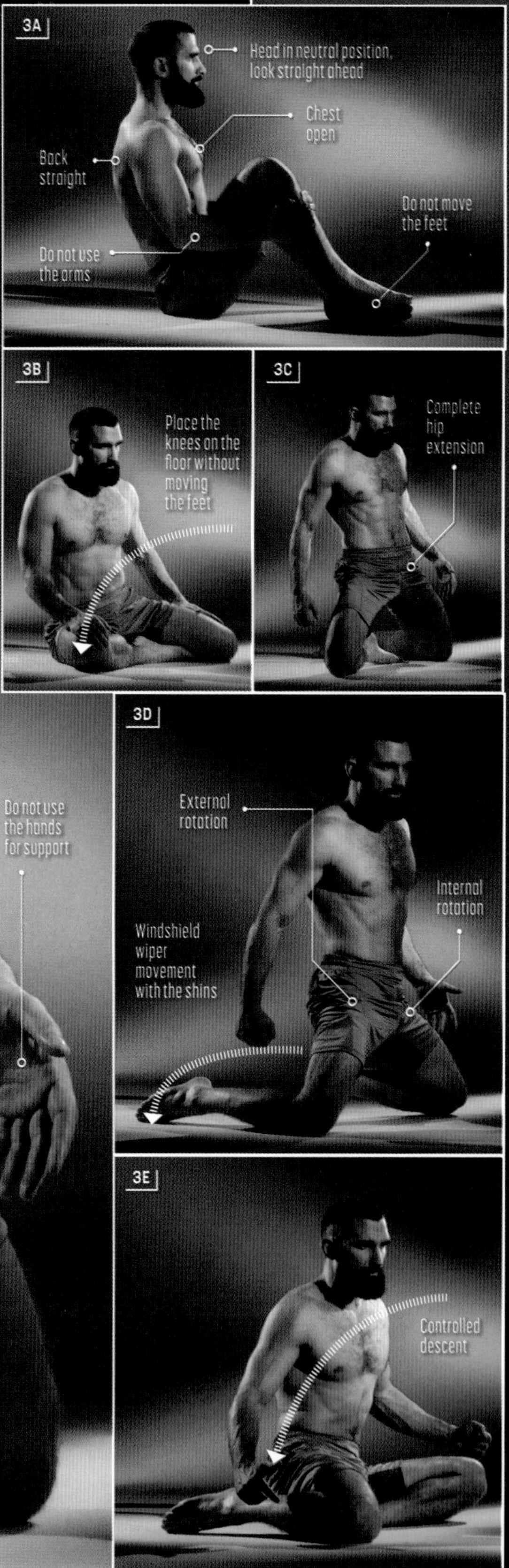
3A
Head in neutral position, look straight ahead
Chest open
Back straight
Do not move the feet
Do not use the arms
3B
Place the knees on the floor without moving the feet
3C
Complete hip extension
3D
External rotation
Internal rotation
Windshield wiper movement with the shins
3E
Controlled descent

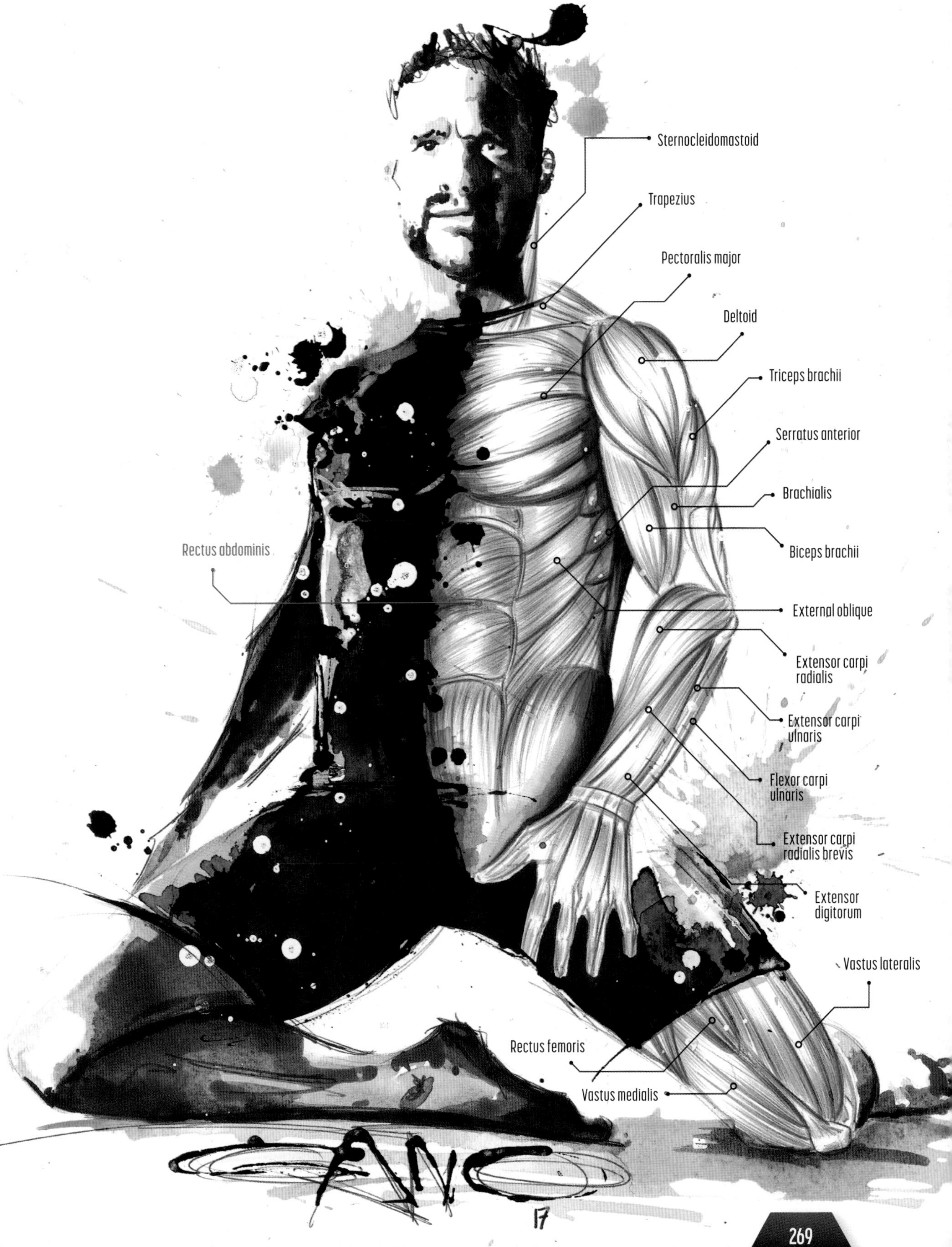
Sternocleidomastoid
Trapezius
Pectoralis major
Deltoid
Triceps brachii
Serratus anterior
Brachialis
Biceps brachii
Rectus abdominis
External oblique
Extensor carpi radialis
Extensor carpi ulnaris
Flexor carpi ulnaris
Extensor carpi radialis brevis
Extensor digitorum
Vastus lateralis
Rectus femoris
Vastus medialis

4C

This final step in the omoplata series combines torso rotations with an initial windshield wiper move. Once you have mastered this entire combination, it is a powerful warm-up tool before any type of athletic activity. When you place your knees on the floor, pivot your torso as far as possible and look behind you. When you do the full hip extension, extend your arm to the back and diagonally and try to sit up taller.

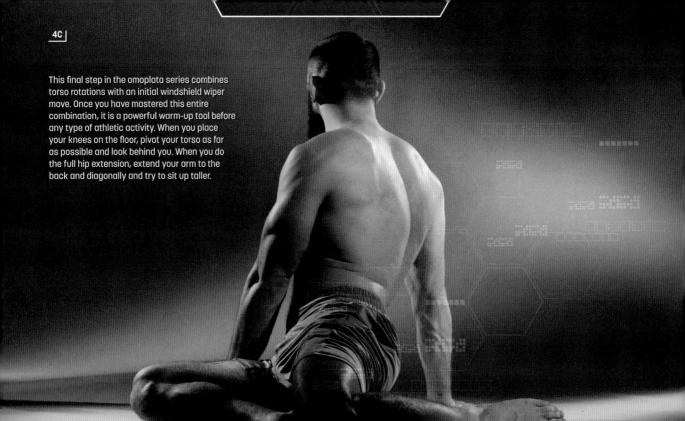

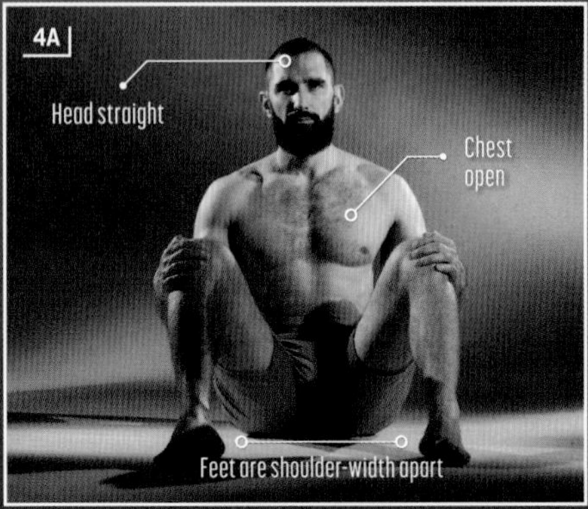

4A
Head straight
Chest open
Feet are shoulder-width apart

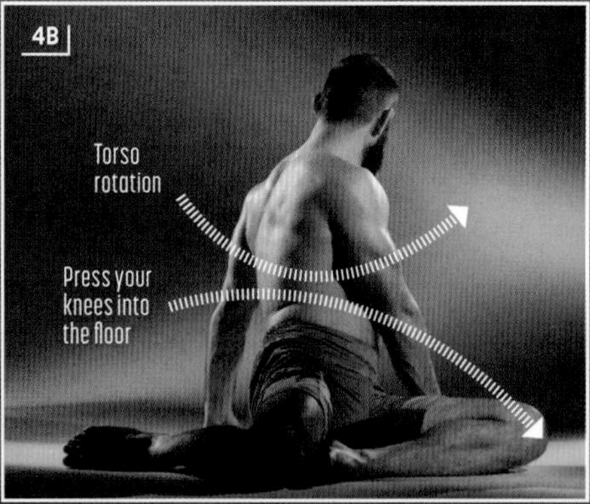

4B
Torso rotation
Press your knees into the floor

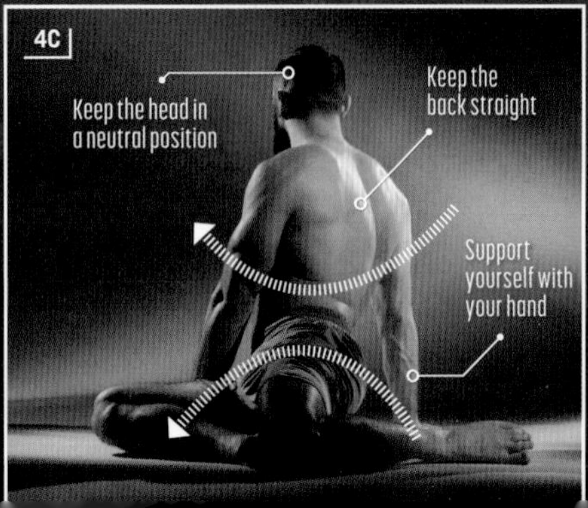

4C
Keep the head in a neutral position
Keep the back straight
Support yourself with your hand

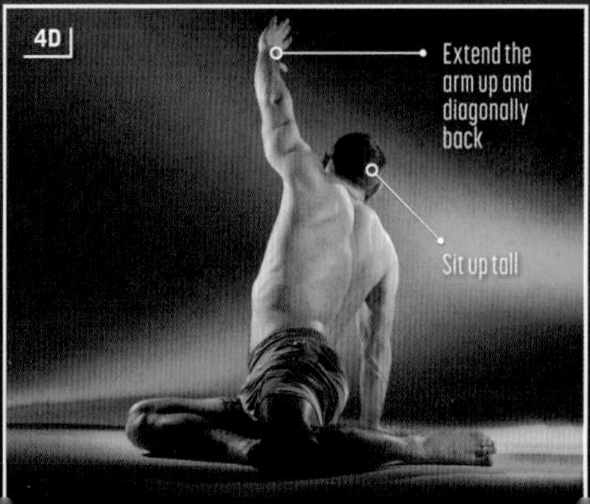

4D
Extend the arm up and diagonally back
Sit up tall

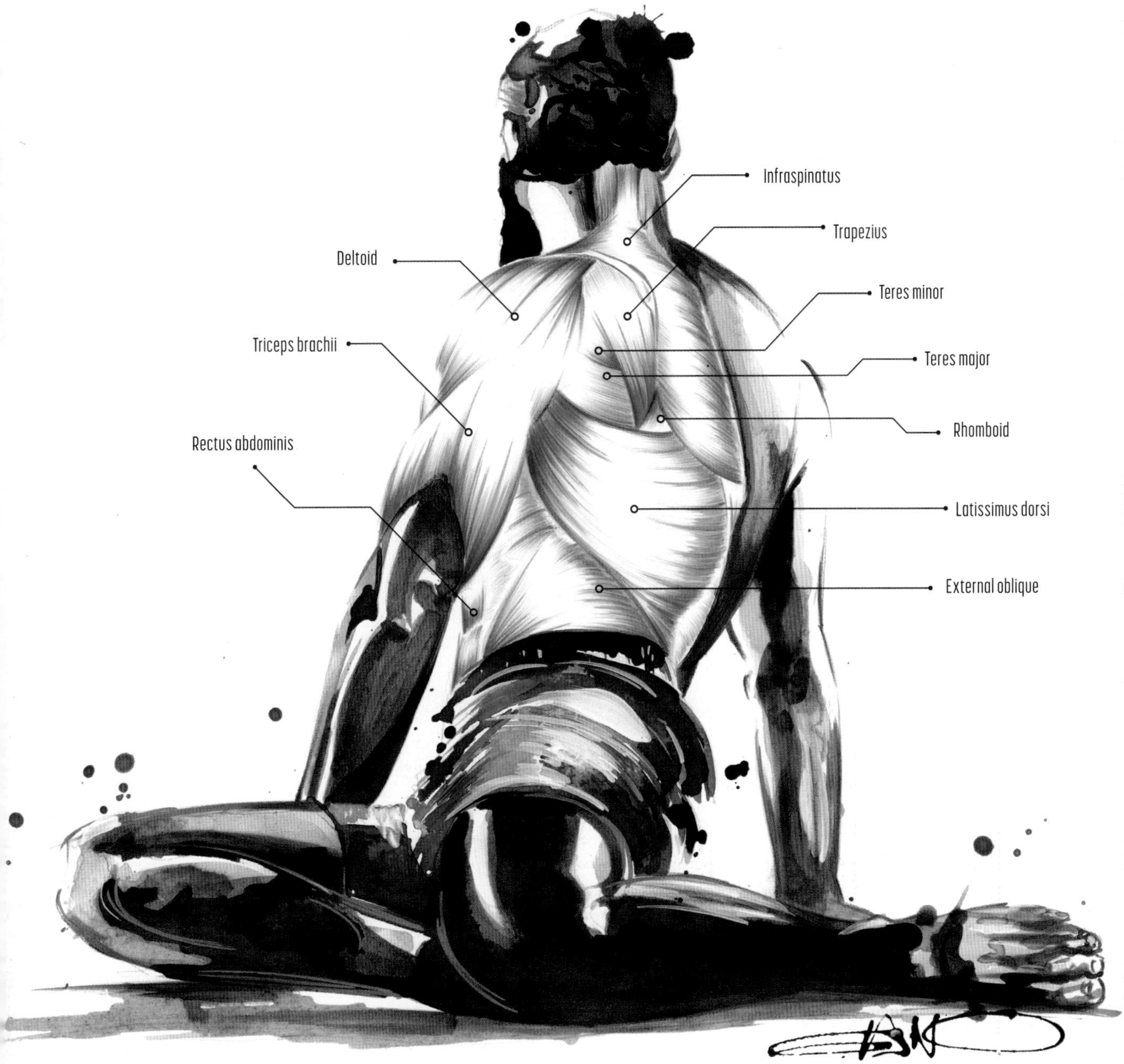
Infraspinatus
Trapezius
Deltoid
Teres minor
Triceps brachii
Teres major
Rhomboid
Rectus abdominis
Latissimus dorsi
External oblique

BASIC GET-UP 1
SERIES

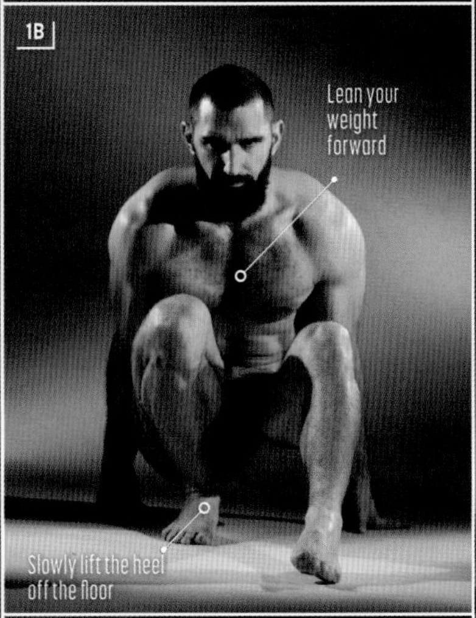

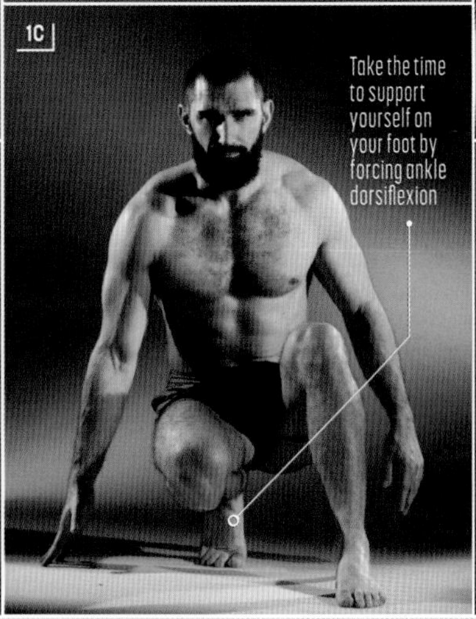

Lean your weight forward

This series improves ankle mobility, but it is not about simply getting up from a crouching position. It is also about forcing dorsiflexion of the ankle in a front and backward movement using the entire body. From a seated position, bring one heel as close as possible to (and under) your buttocks so that the leg becomes your base of support. Then slowly, using your hands and the other leg (that was placed on the floor ahead of your body) for balance, stand up and allow the heel of your support leg to slowly lift off of the floor.

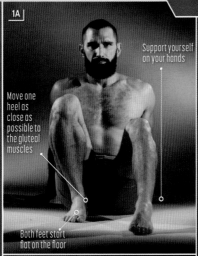

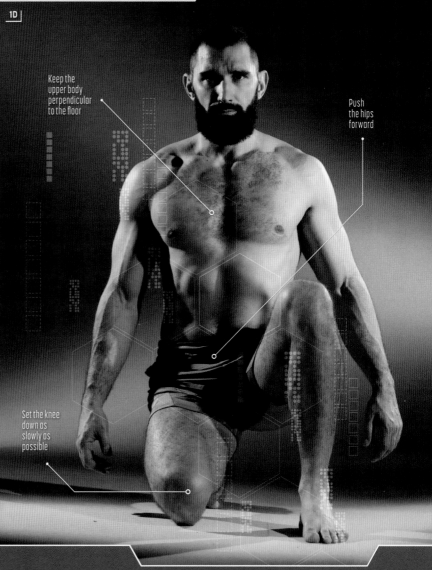

2E

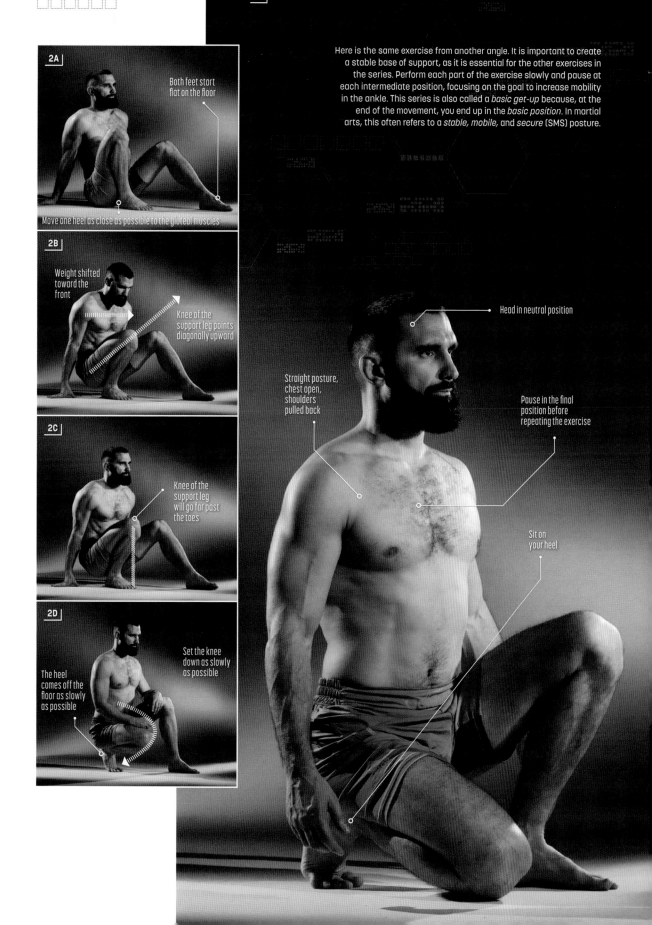

Here is the same exercise from another angle. It is important to create a stable base of support, as it is essential for the other exercises in the series. Perform each part of the exercise slowly and pause at each intermediate position, focusing on the goal to increase mobility in the ankle. This series is also called a *basic get-up* because, at the end of the movement, you end up in the *basic position*. In martial arts, this often refers to a *stable, mobile,* and *secure* (SMS) posture.

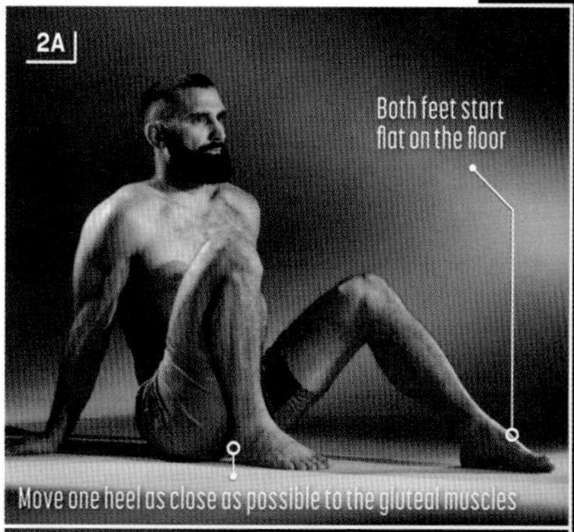
2A
Both feet start flat on the floor
Move one heel as close as possible to the gluteal muscles

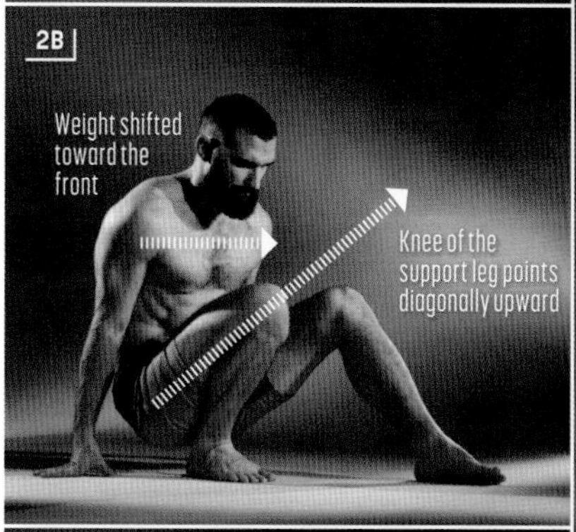
2B
Weight shifted toward the front
Knee of the support leg points diagonally upward

2C
Knee of the support leg will go far past the toes

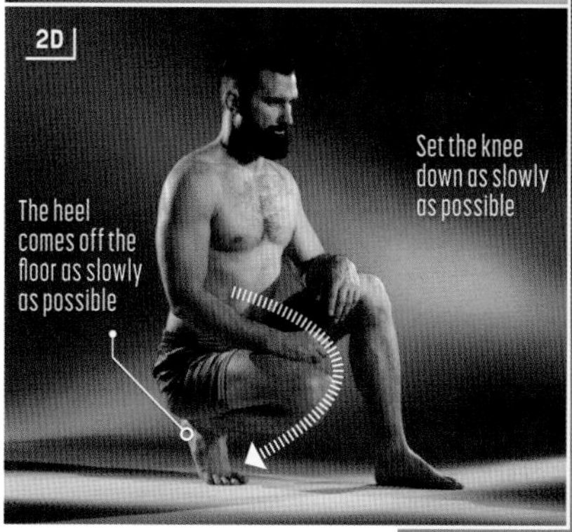
2D
Set the knee down as slowly as possible
The heel comes off the floor as slowly as possible

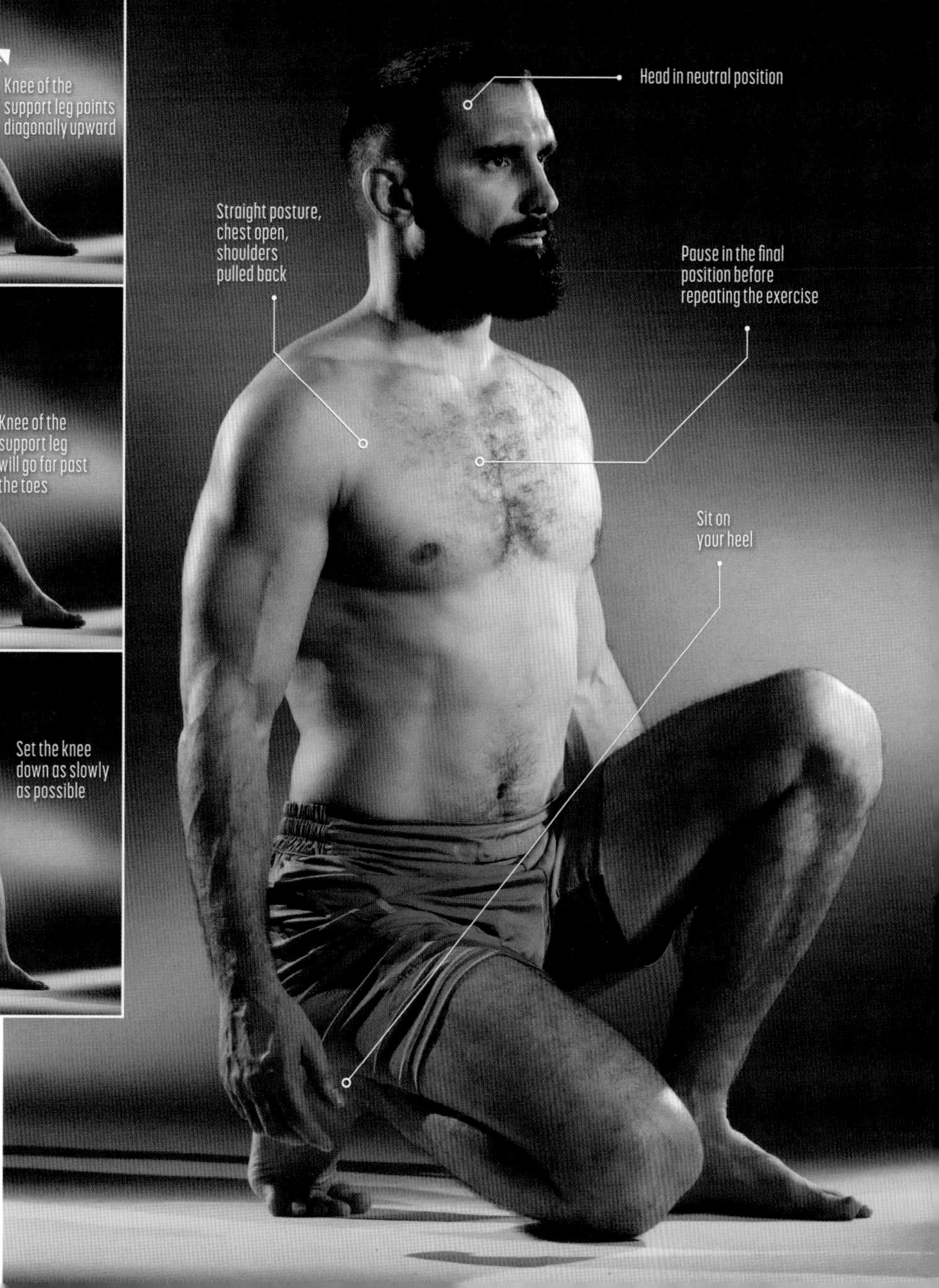
Head in neutral position
Straight posture, chest open, shoulders pulled back
Pause in the final position before repeating the exercise
Sit on your heel

These two exercises add movement and speed to the ankle dorsiflexion portion of the previous exercise. The number of repetitions does not matter, nor does the time it takes to perform the exercise. You are aiming for fluidity in the movement, relaxation, and combining the moves without stopping. You should be especially interested in balance and in trying to maximize ankle dorsiflexion. Do a roll before you do the basic get-up. In the first case, you will stay in line, as in the previous step. In the second case, combine the roll with a rotation in the hips so that you stand up with one knee on the floor and one knee lifted.

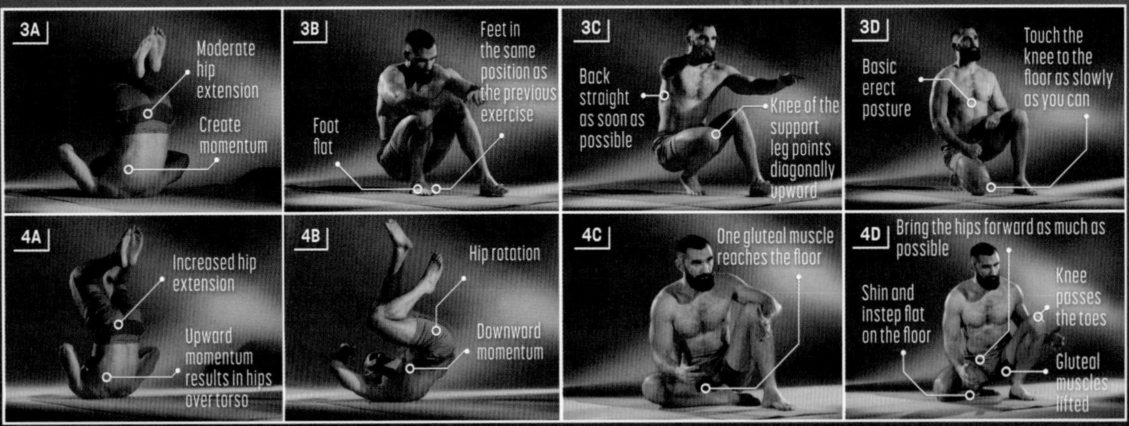

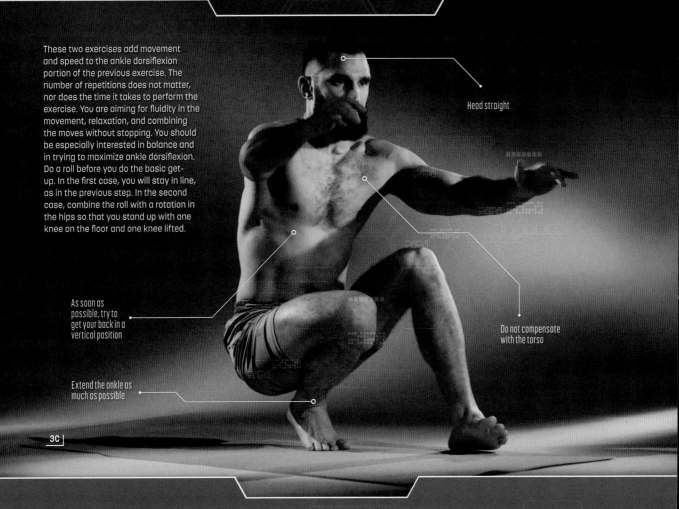

As soon as possible, try to get your back in a vertical position

Extend the ankle as much as possible

Create momentum

Basic erect posture

Upward momentum results in hips over torso

Downward momentum

Knee passes the toes

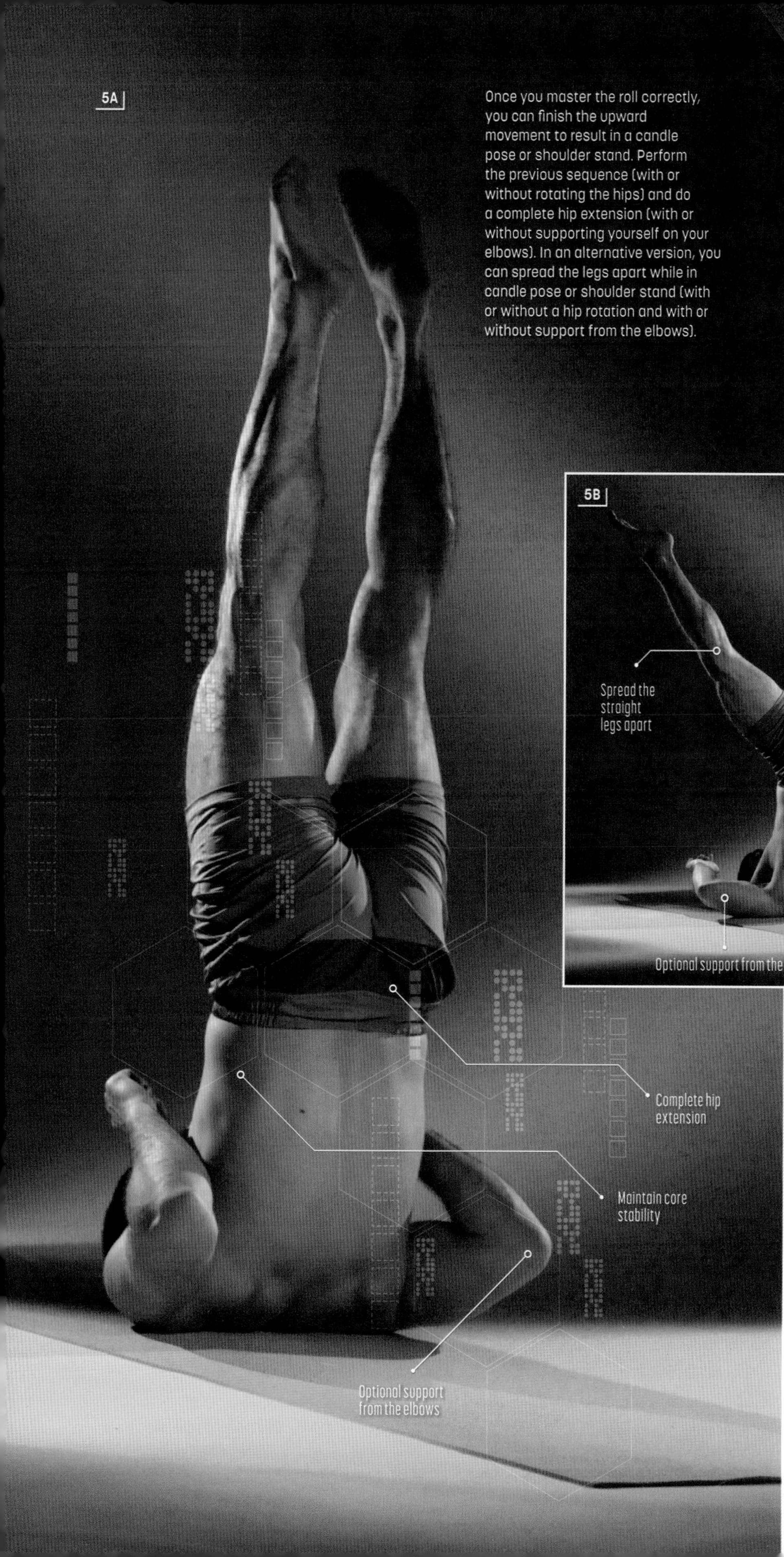
5A
Complete hip extension
Maintain core stability
Optional support from the elbows

Once you master the roll correctly, you can finish the upward movement to result in a candle pose or shoulder stand. Perform the previous sequence (with or without rotating the hips) and do a complete hip extension (with or without supporting yourself on your elbows). In an alternative version, you can spread the legs apart while in candle pose or shoulder stand (with or without a hip rotation and with or without support from the elbows).

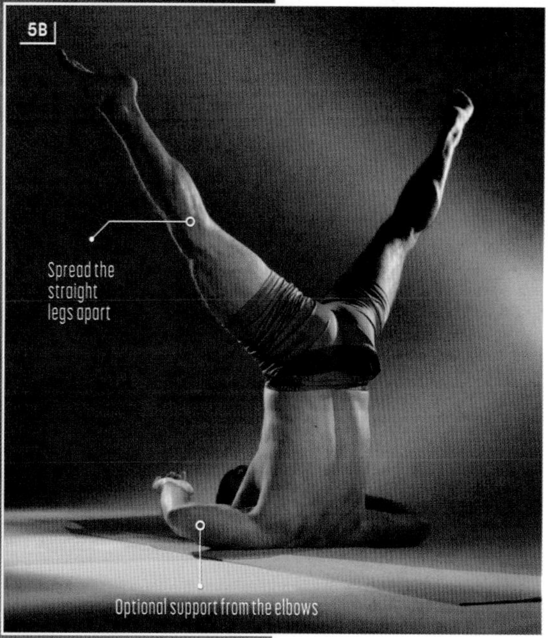
5B
Spread the straight legs apart
Optional support from the elbows

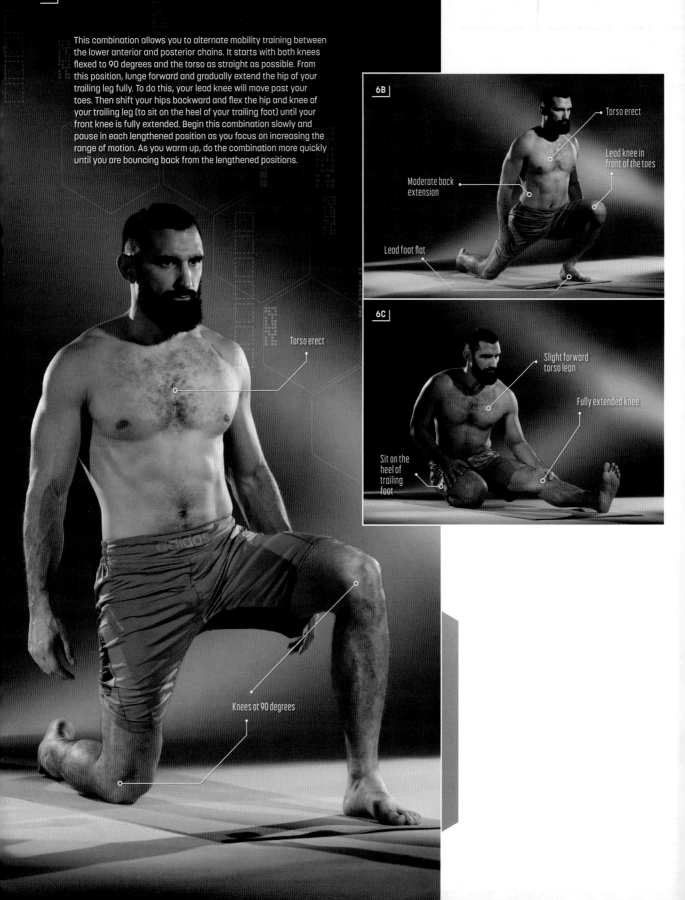

6A

This combination allows you to alternate mobility training between the lower anterior and posterior chains. It starts with both knees flexed to 90 degrees and the torso as straight as possible. From this position, lunge forward and gradually extend the hip of your trailing leg fully. To do this, your lead knee will move past your toes. Then shift your hips backward and flex the hip and knee of your trailing leg (to sit on the heel of your trailing foot) until your front knee is fully extended. Begin this combination slowly and pause in each lengthened position as you focus on increasing the range of motion. As you warm up, do the combination more quickly until you are bouncing back from the lengthened positions.

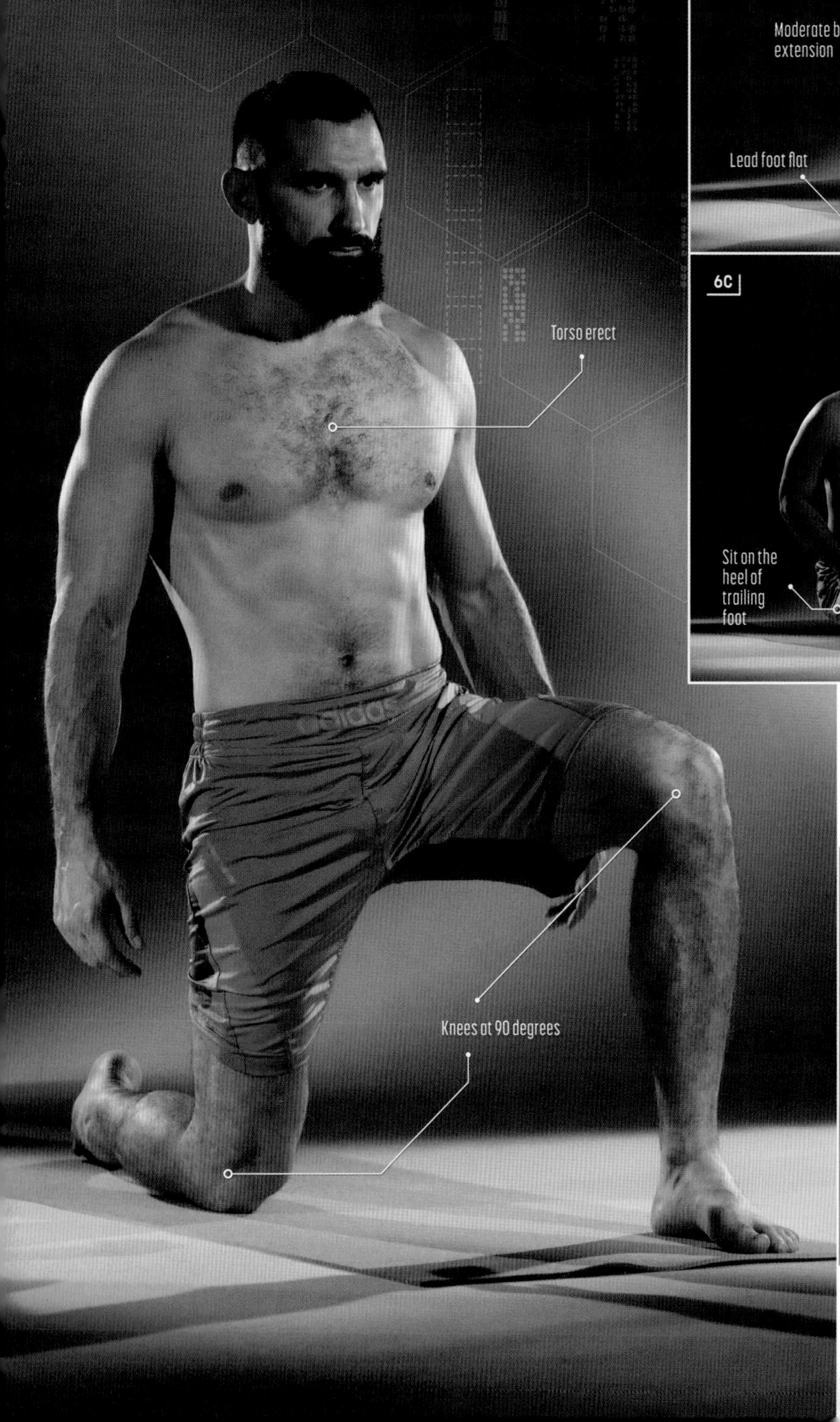

6B

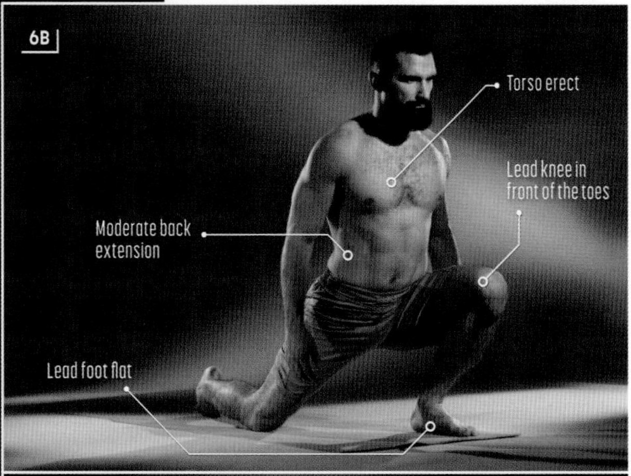

6C

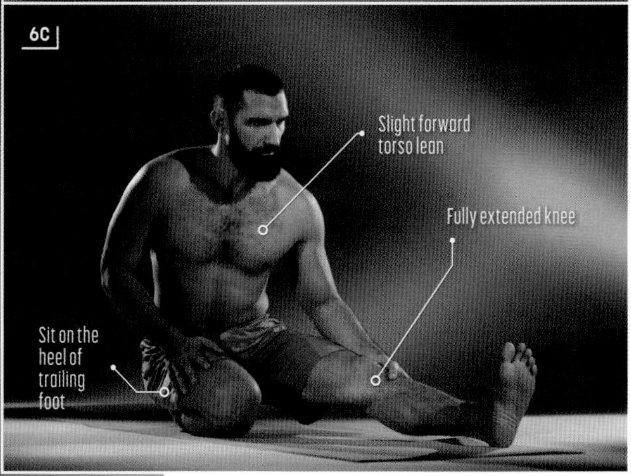

BASIC GET-UP 2
SERIES

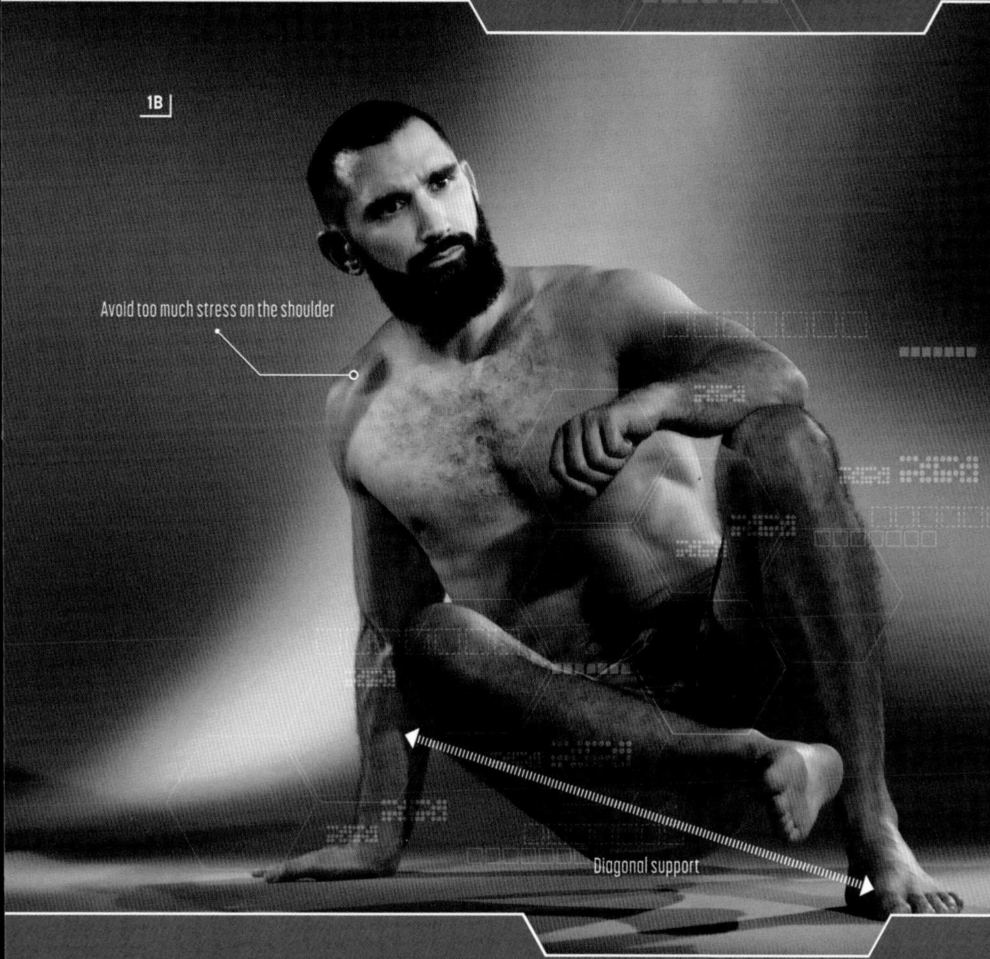

1B
Avoid too much stress on the shoulder
Diagonal support

This series also provides an exceptional warm-up. Returning to the basic position (see the concept of SMS on page 273) takes you from sitting to a standing position through different steps that mobilize every muscle chain. Inspired by martial arts, this series introduces the essential concept of diagonal support, which is particularly effective for moving from one muscle chain to another through the functional and spiral chains. Sit on one buttock and support yourself using one of your feet and the hand on the opposite side. Using just these two supports allows you to lighten your pelvis and lift it to move from front to back. You can then evolve on your diagonal to extend the leg to the front or place your knee (or your foot, in the second version of this exercise) directly beyond the hand. The exercise ends with a classic lunge with the knee on the floor or in a squat followed by a standing extension, depending on the version.

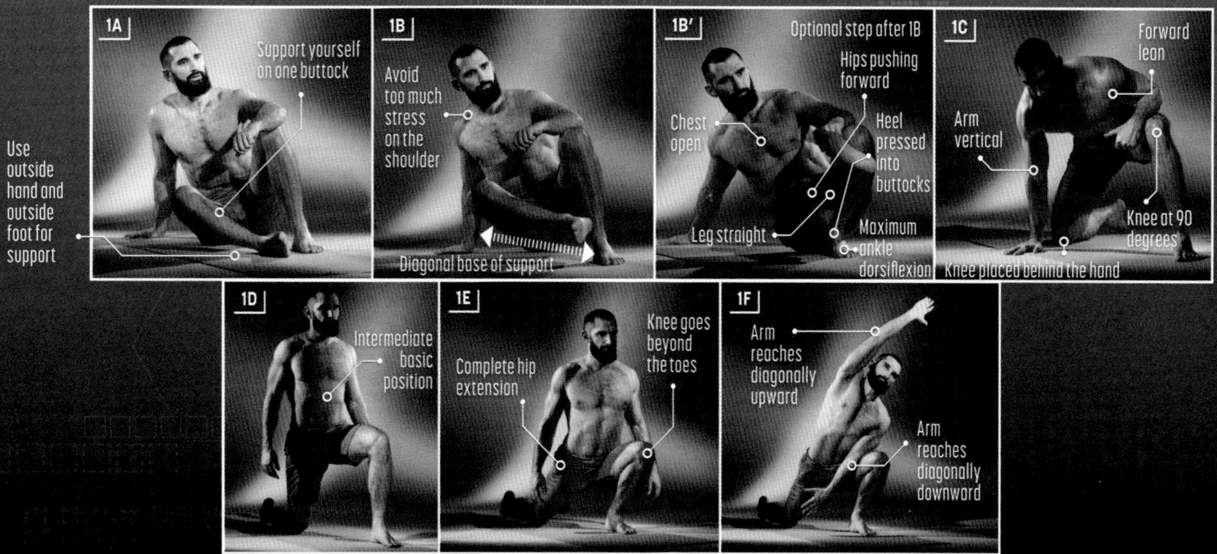

1A
Support yourself on one buttock
Use outside hand and outside foot for support
1B
Avoid too much stress on the shoulder
Diagonal base of support
1B′
Optional step after 1B
Hips pushing forward
Chest open
Heel pressed into buttocks
Leg straight
Maximum ankle dorsiflexion
1C
Forward lean
Arm vertical
Knee at 90 degrees
Knee placed behind the hand
1D
Intermediate basic position
1E
Complete hip extension
Knee goes beyond the toes
1F
Arm reaches diagonally upward
Arm reaches diagonally downward

2A

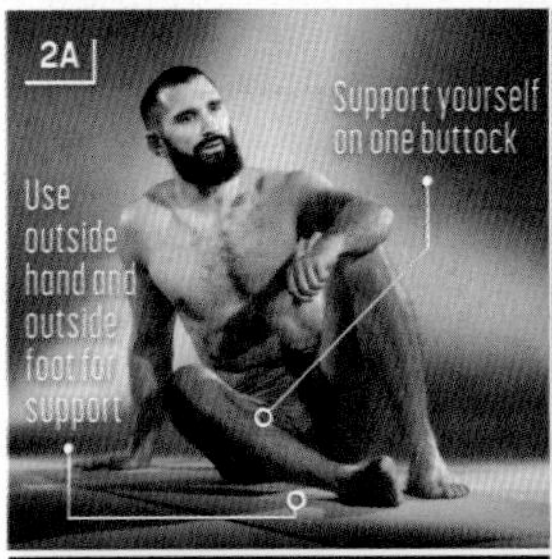
Support yourself on one buttock
Use outside hand and outside foot for support

2B

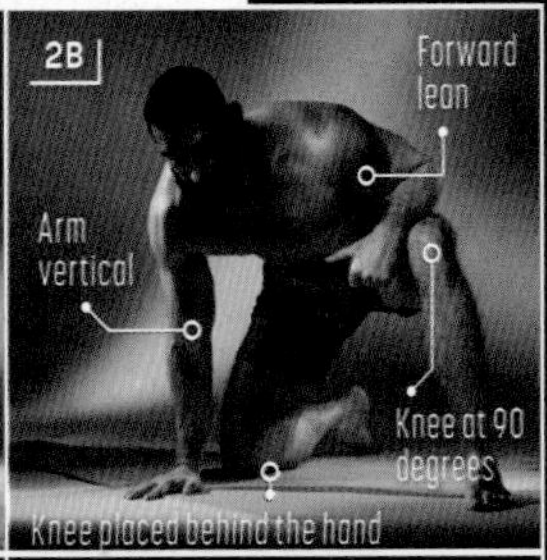
Forward lean
Arm vertical
Knee at 90 degrees
Knee placed behind the hand

2C

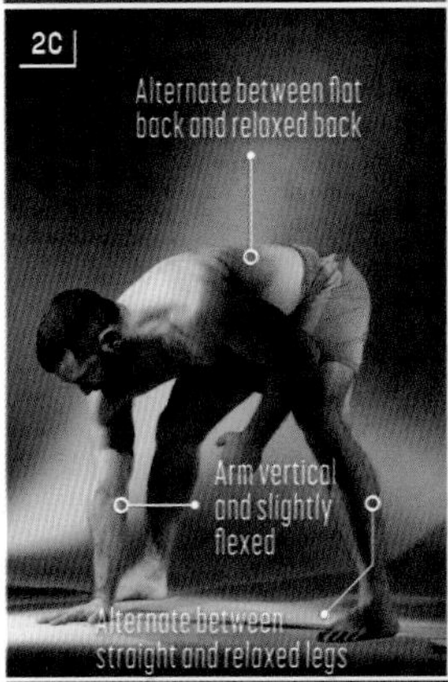
Alternate between flat back and relaxed back
Arm vertical and slightly flexed
Alternate between straight and relaxed legs

2D

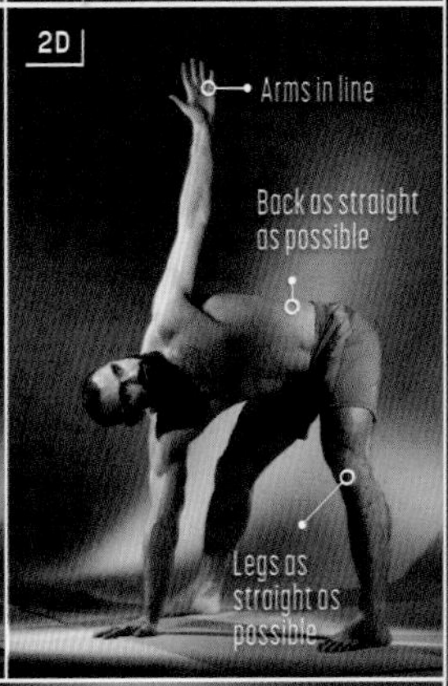
Arms in line
Back as straight as possible
Legs as straight as possible

2D'

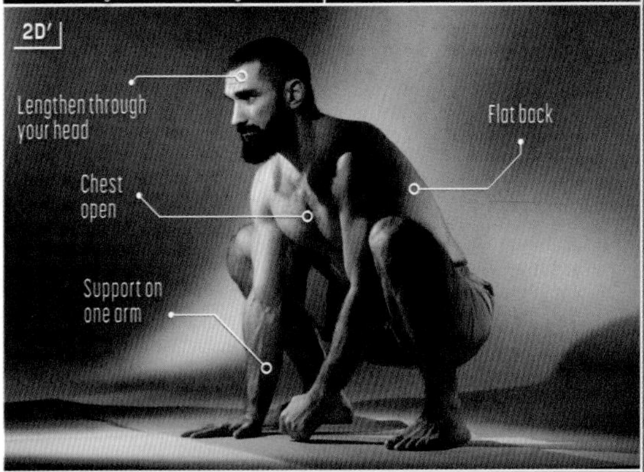
Lengthen through your head
Flat back
Chest open
Support on one arm

2D''

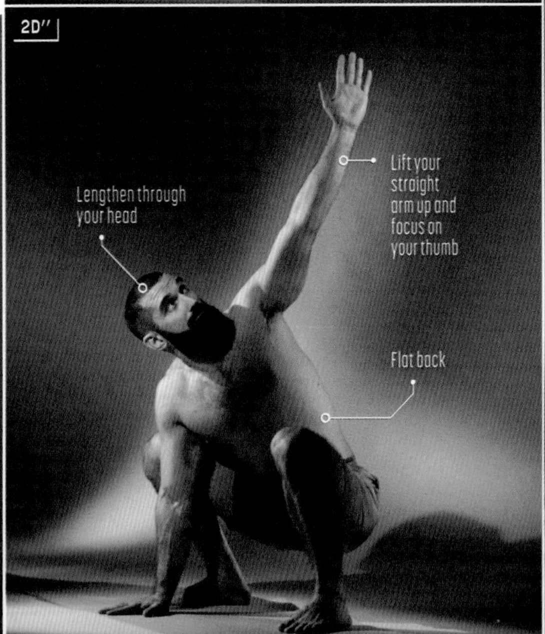
Lift your straight arm up and focus on your thumb
Lengthen through your head
Flat back

2E

This second version in the series allows you to stand up with various optional steps: torso rotation, a squat, or a squat with rotation. In all cases, it ends with a complete extension of the spine. The starting point is the same as the previous exercise, but this version involves placing the foot (instead of the knee) directly on the floor in step 2C. Take the time to focus on each step separately or repeat each step multiple times.

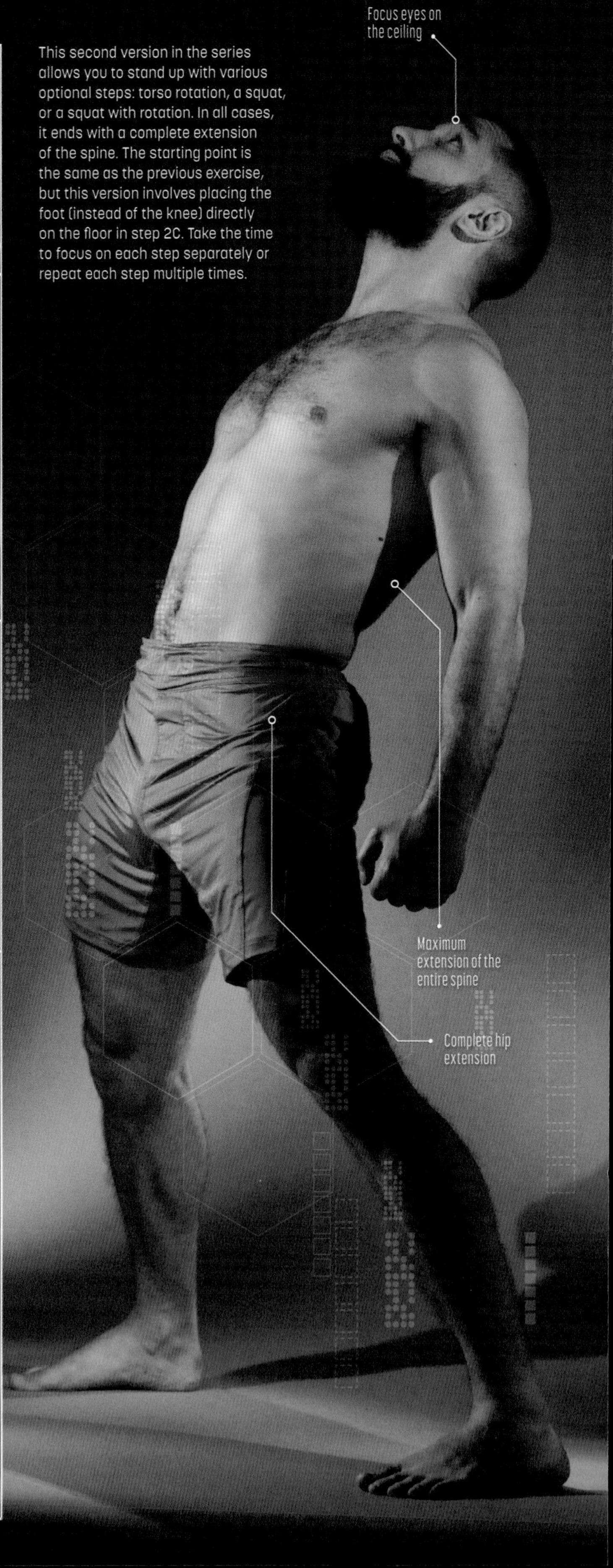
Focus eyes on the ceiling
Maximum extension of the entire spine
Complete hip extension

BRIDGE SERIES

1C

This series has two goals: mobility and stability of the pelvis through support from the posterior chain and gradual tension in the joints, especially the scapula. No matter what level of this series you are doing (steps A, B, and C of level 1 or 2), focus on the extension of the hips for a certain period of time or for a certain number of repetitions. Core stability remains the primary objective, but mobility in the hips is also important.

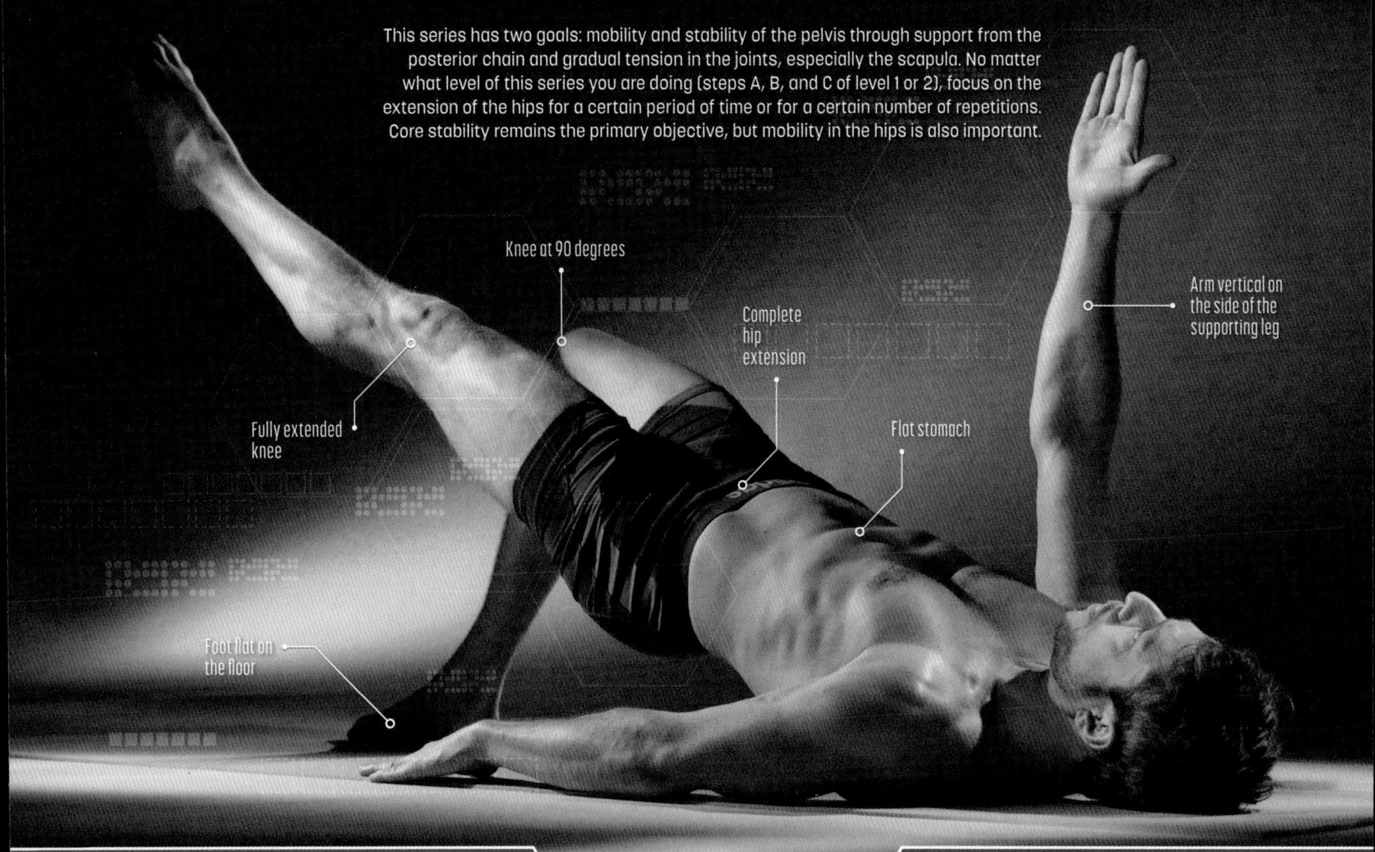

Knee at 90 degrees
Complete hip extension
Arm vertical on the side of the supporting leg
Fully extended knee
Flat stomach
Foot flat on the floor

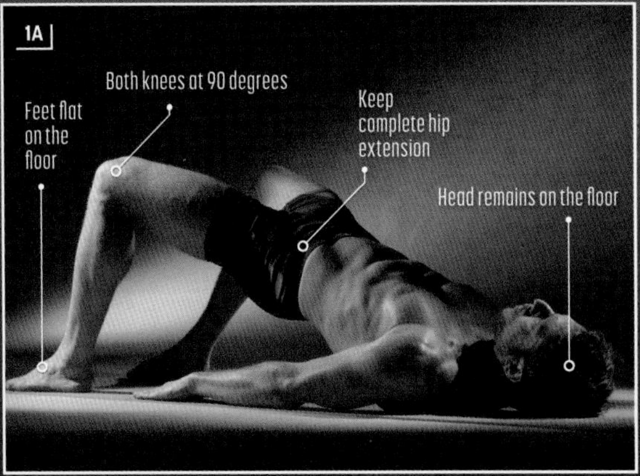

1A
Both knees at 90 degrees
Feet flat on the floor
Keep complete hip extension
Head remains on the floor

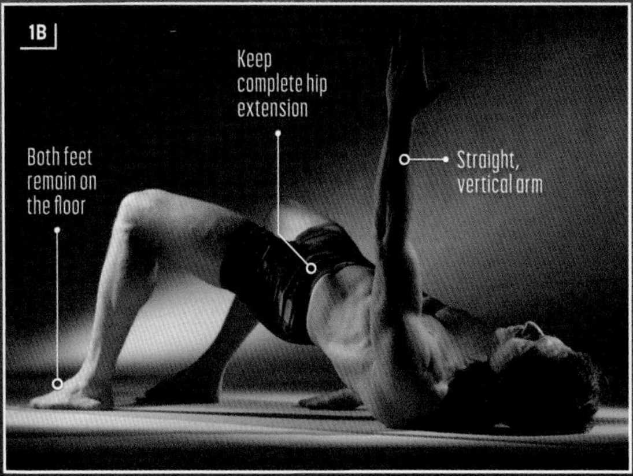

1B
Keep complete hip extension
Both feet remain on the floor
Straight, vertical arm

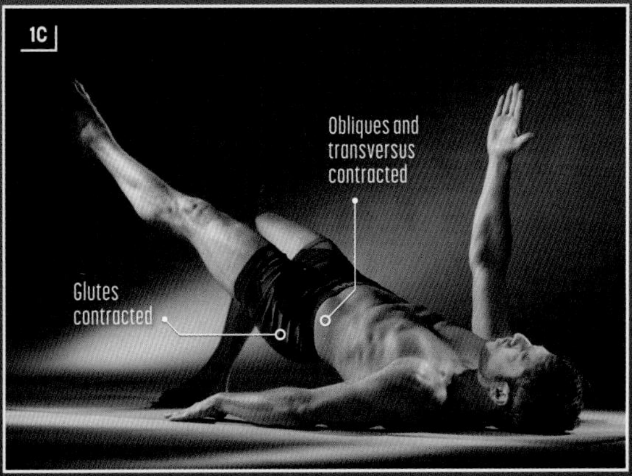
1C
Obliques and transversus contracted
Glutes contracted

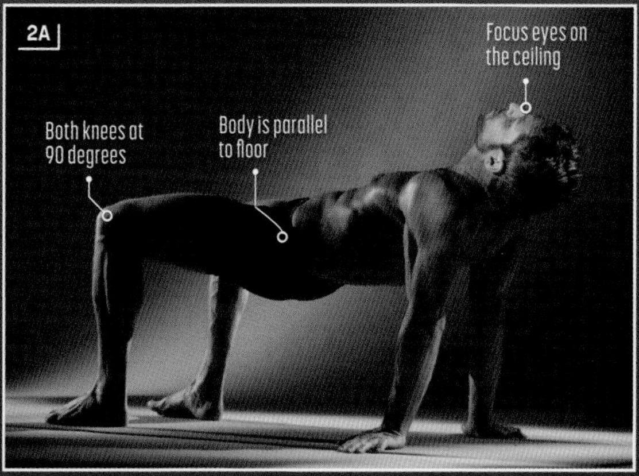
2A
Focus eyes on the ceiling
Both knees at 90 degrees
Body is parallel to floor

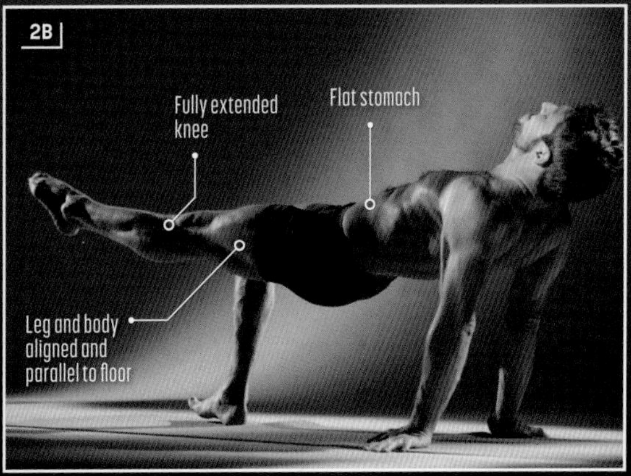
2B
Fully extended knee
Flat stomach
Leg and body aligned and parallel to floor

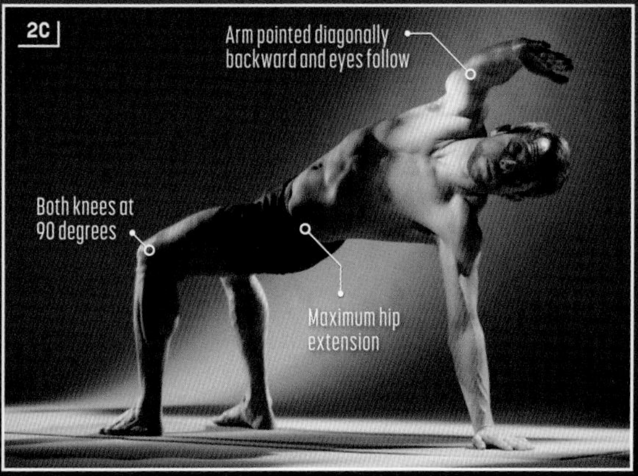
2C
Arm pointed diagonally backward and eyes follow
Both knees at 90 degrees
Maximum hip extension

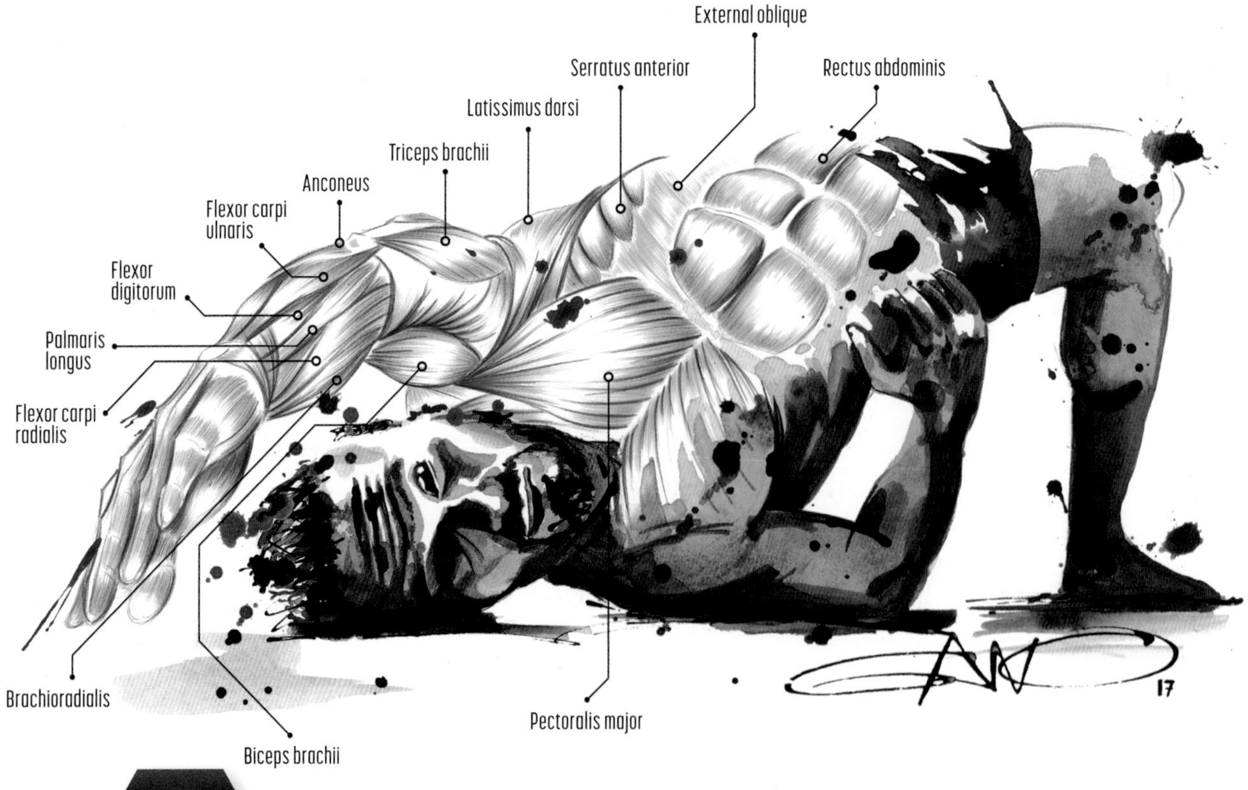
External oblique
Serratus anterior
Rectus abdominis
Latissimus dorsi
Triceps brachii
Anconeus
Flexor carpi ulnaris
Flexor digitorum
Palmaris longus
Flexor carpi radialis
Brachioradialis
Biceps brachii
Pectoralis major

LEG DROP SERIES

This six-exercise series was inspired by the flips done in martial arts during ground fighting, such as in judo or Brazilian jiu-jitsu. For these exercises, active core stability, dissociation between the pelvis and the shoulders, and mobility of the pelvis are essential. For these three reasons, the leg drop series is an extremely effective warm-up strategy. This series initially involves gaining control over the pelvis through core stability and opening and closing the hips to move from a lying position to a seated position without using your back to compensate. Next, side-to-side leg movements are used to control the rotation of the pelvis. The third step also targets pelvic rotation but by dissociating the legs. Once you have mastered each of these three steps, you will learn to combine them. In all versions, do not extend your back to compensate and stop opening the torso and legs the moment you have to arch your back to continue lowering your legs.

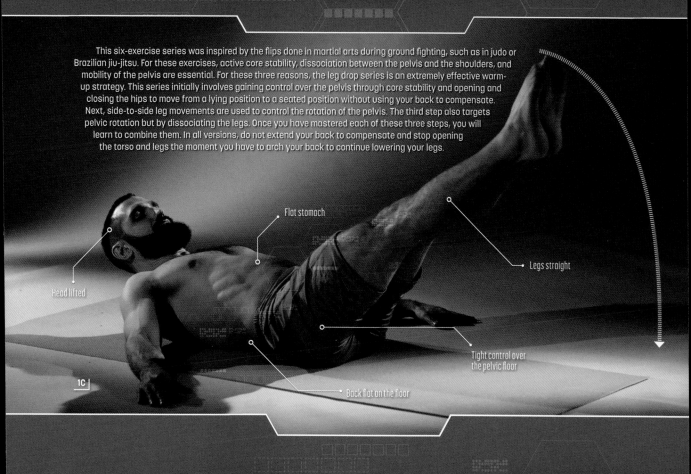

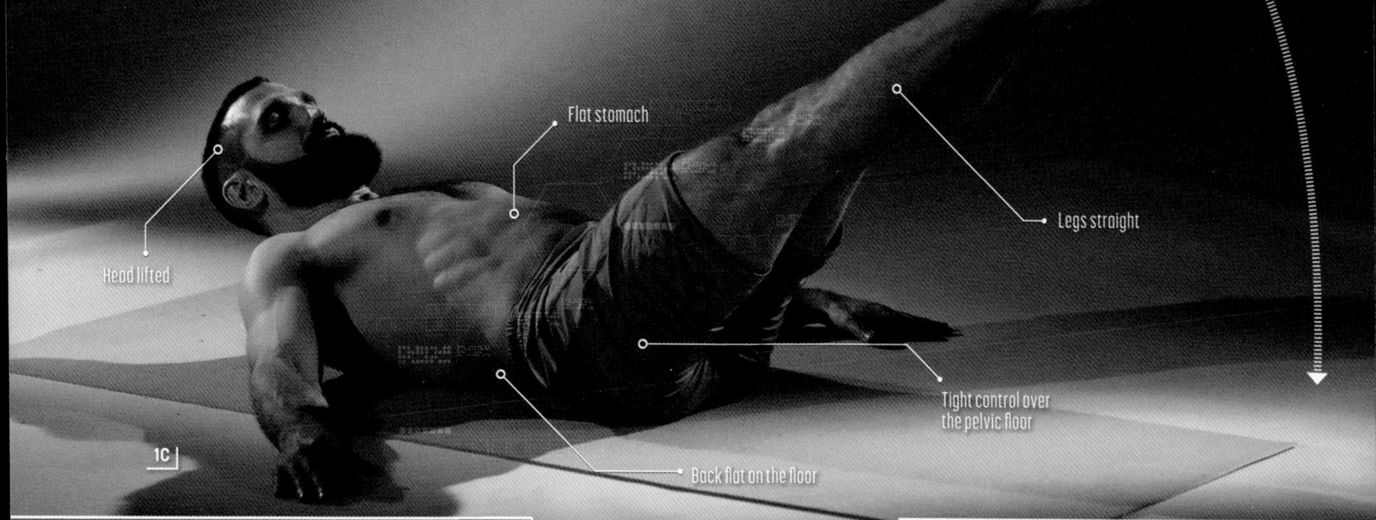

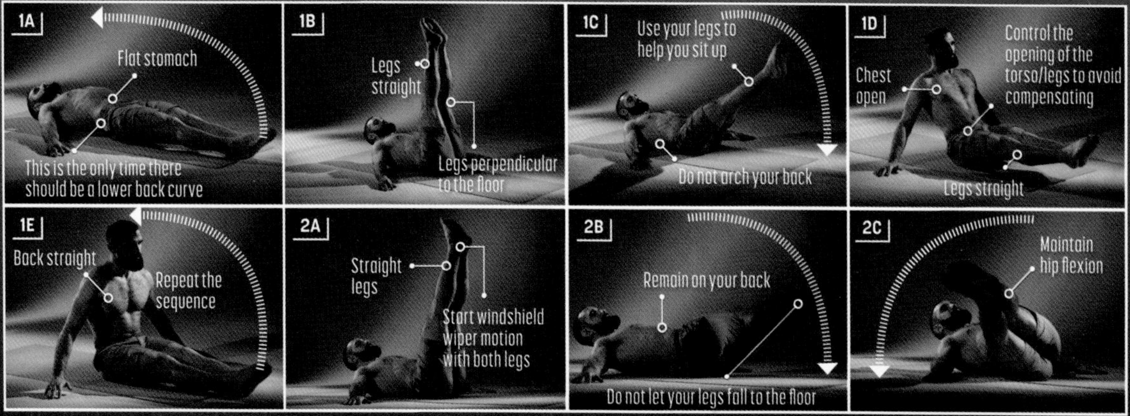

These exercises can be performed in one of two ways: slowly and in control or quickly and relaxed. In either case, the focus is not on the number of repetitions or the total time spent in the exercise. Instead, you should focus on relaxation and fluidity or on control and precision. For the latter version, simply move one leg to the side then move the other leg. Be sure to keep the knees of both legs completely extended throughout the exercise.

3A

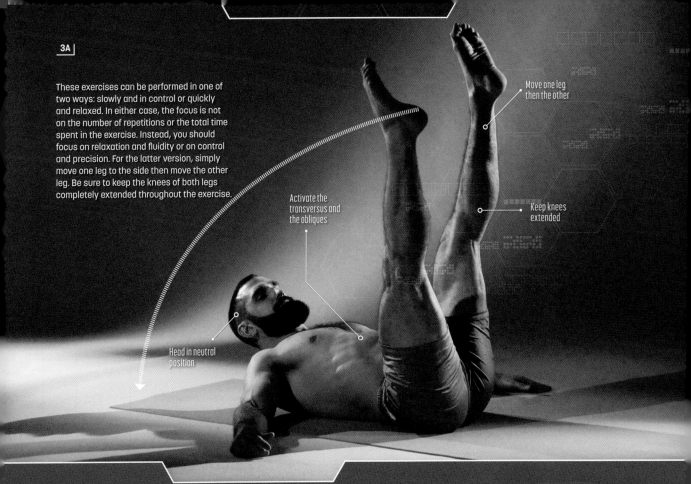

Move one leg then the other
Activate the transversus and the obliques
Keep knees extended
Head in neutral position

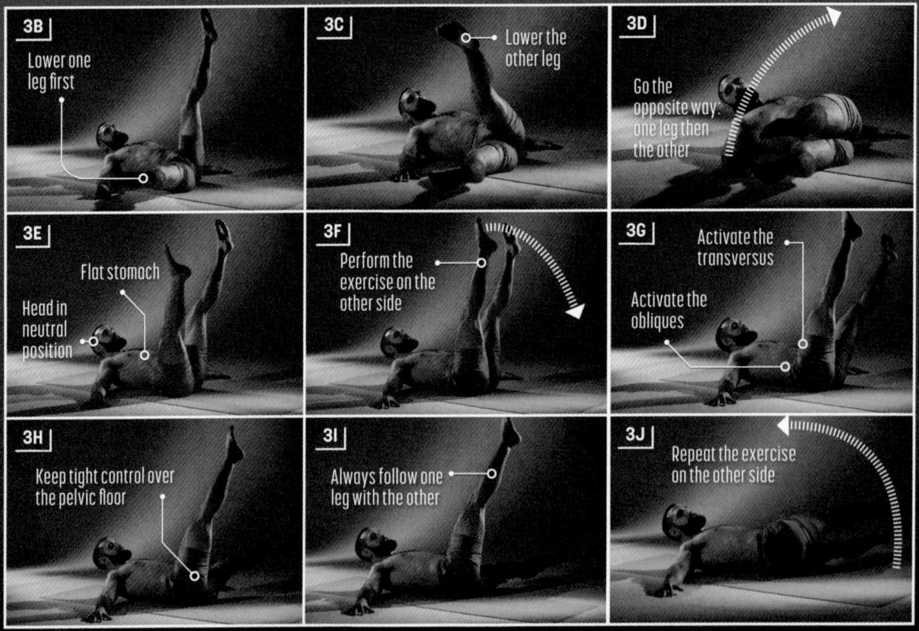

3B
Lower one leg first
3C
Lower the other leg
3D
Go the opposite way: one leg then the other
3E
Flat stomach
Head in neutral position
3F
Perform the exercise on the other side
3G
Activate the transversus
Activate the obliques
3H
Keep tight control over the pelvic floor
3I
Always follow one leg with the other
3J
Repeat the exercise on the other side

4B

This time, you will use your hips through all of the planes of motion. As before, keep your legs straight but this time squeeze them together. The rocking movement that you use to sit up will be enhanced by pivoting your hips to the side—without changing the position of the torso—to end up sitting on your side.

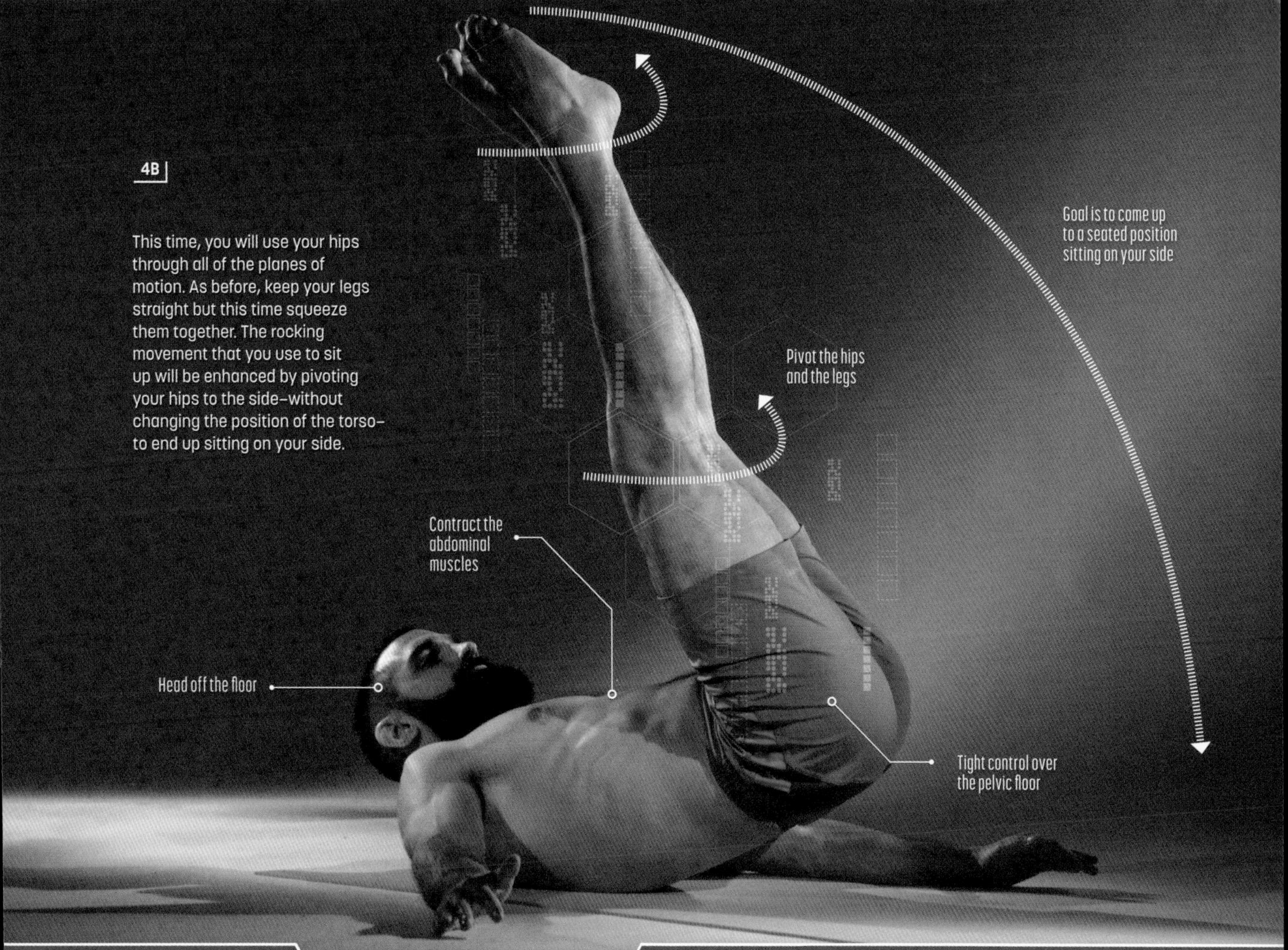

Goal is to come up to a seated position sitting on your side
Pivot the hips and the legs
Contract the abdominal muscles
Head off the floor
Tight control over the pelvic floor

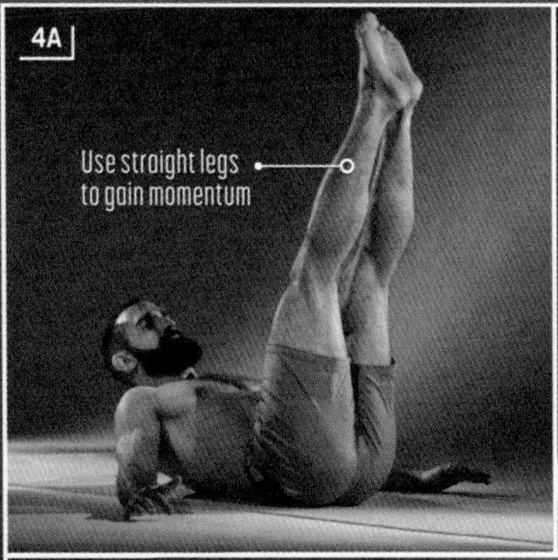

4A
Use straight legs to gain momentum

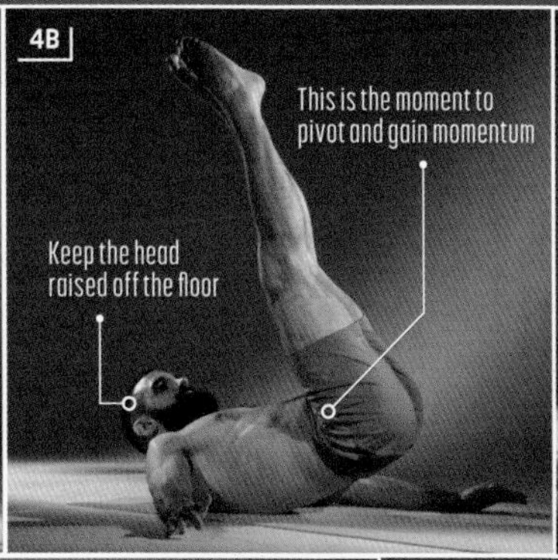

4B
This is the moment to pivot and gain momentum
Keep the head raised off the floor

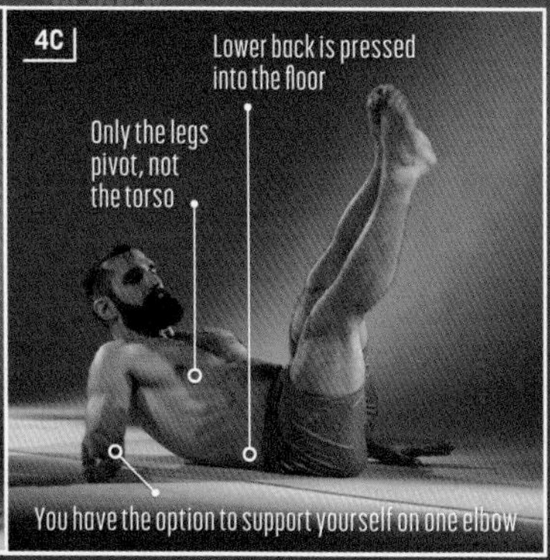

4C
Lower back is pressed into the floor
Only the legs pivot, not the torso
You have the option to support yourself on one elbow

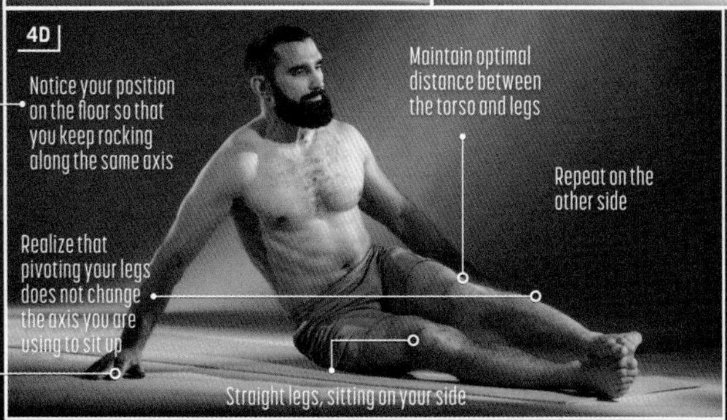

4D
Notice your position on the floor so that you keep rocking along the same axis
Maintain optimal distance between the torso and legs
Repeat on the other side
Realize that pivoting your legs does not change the axis you are using to sit up
Straight legs, sitting on your side

In the same way that we dissociated the legs from one axis, we will now combine a hip pivot with the dissociation of the legs through a distance that depends on how fast you perform the exercise. As in the previous exercise, keep the rocking motion along the same axis (do not move off the floor mat); your hips are pivoting while your torso lifts up in the same line. Press your back into the floor, control the distance between the torso and the legs, and alternate between fast and slow versions of this exercise.

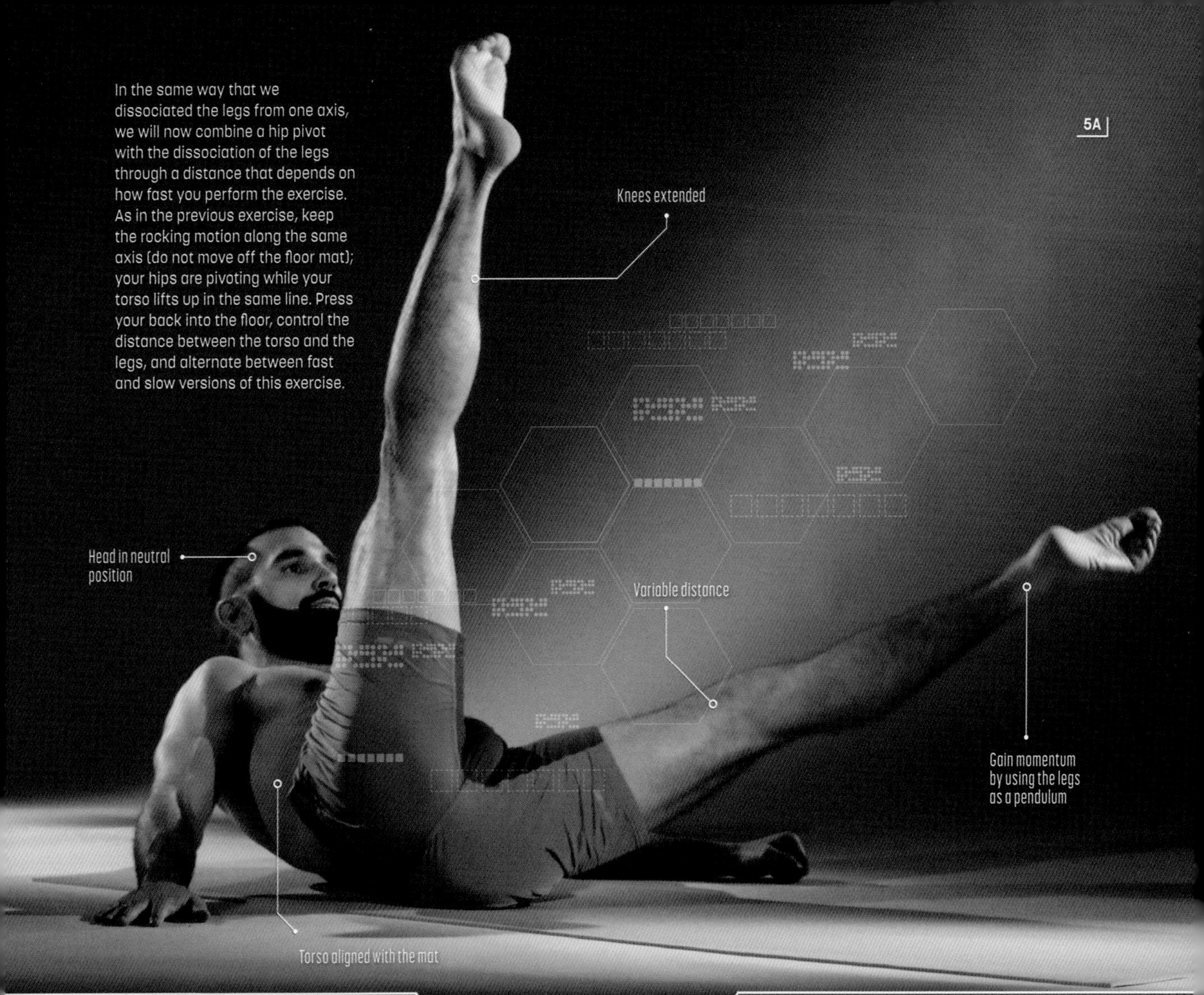
5A
Knees extended
Head in neutral position
Variable distance
Gain momentum by using the legs as a pendulum
Torso aligned with the mat

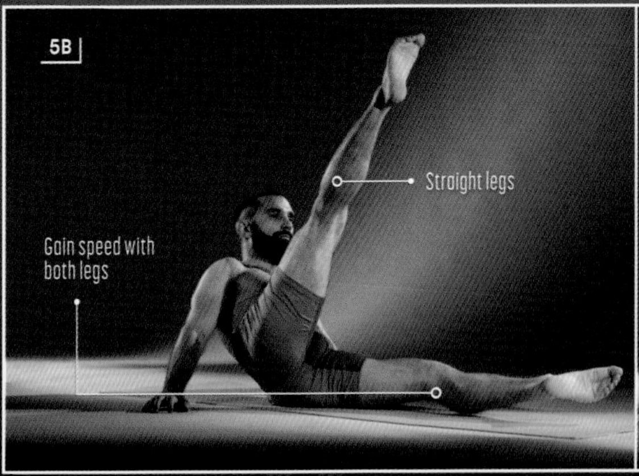
5B
Straight legs
Gain speed with both legs

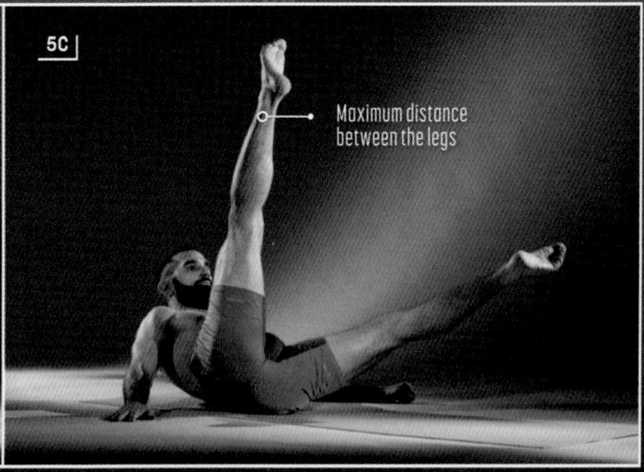
5C
Maximum distance between the legs

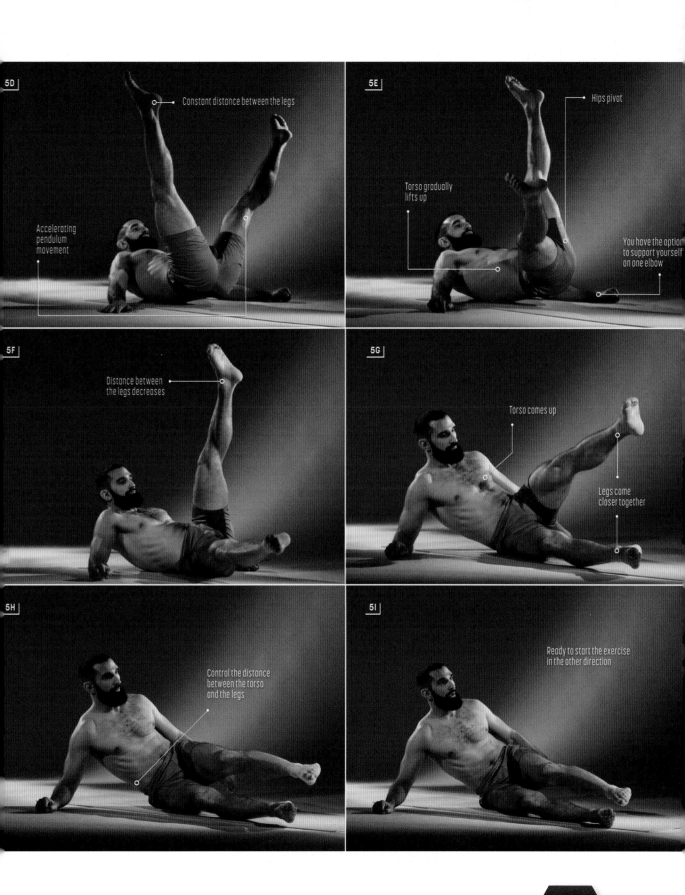

5D
Constant distance between the legs
Accelerating pendulum movement

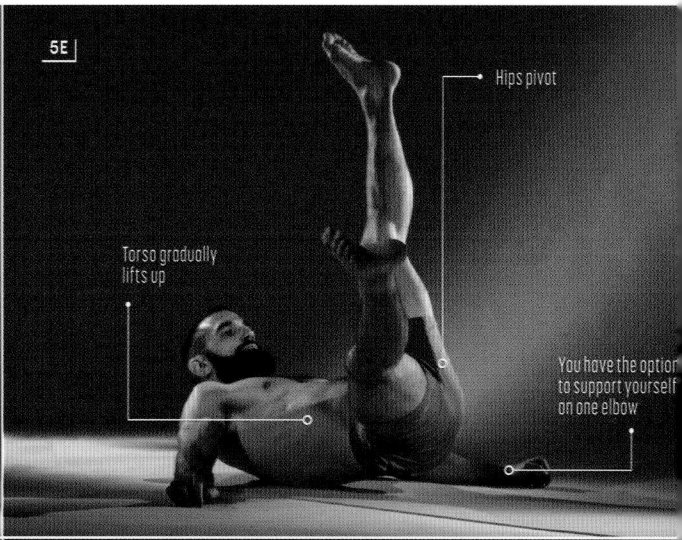
5E
Hips pivot
Torso gradually lifts up
You have the option to support yourself on one elbow

5F
Distance between the legs decreases

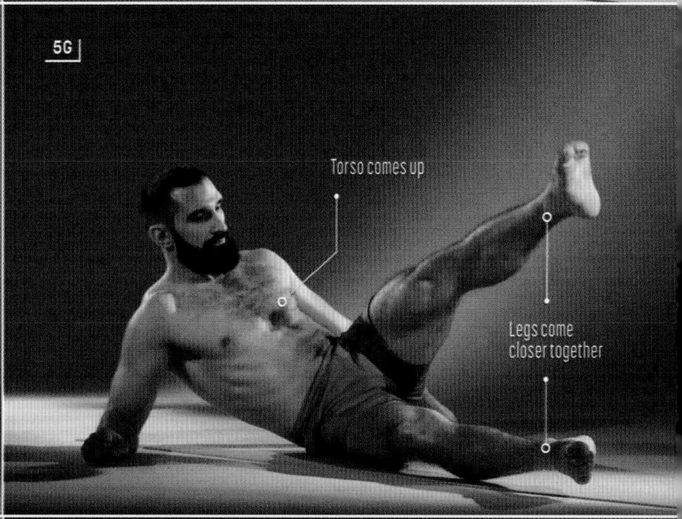
5G
Torso comes up
Legs come closer together

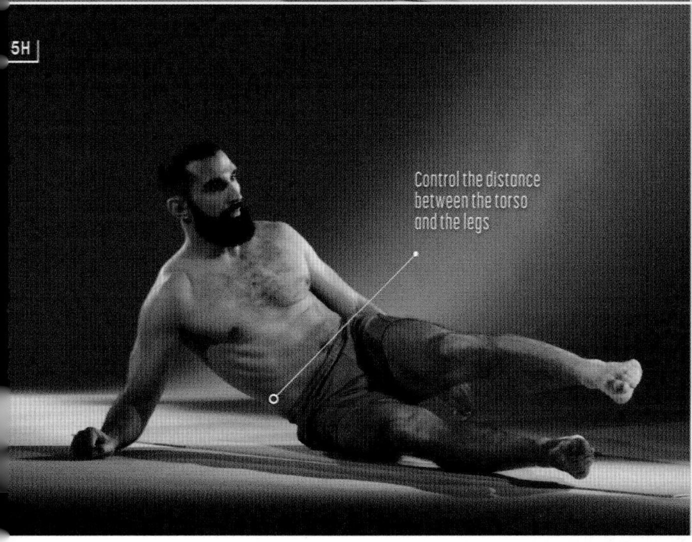
5H
Control the distance between the torso and the legs

5I
Ready to start the exercise in the other direction

The ultimate exercise version of this series ends with both hips rotated (one rotated internally and the other rotated externally). This is a similar movement as the previous exercise, but the pendulum becomes so efficient that you can start the movement from a stretched position and continue it through to the same stretched position on the other side. You simply need to sit up and move your legs as you did before but with enough speed so you can swing the legs, sit up, and reverse the position of your legs. Pause for a moment in the fully stretched position (step 6J) before reaching the basic SMS position (step 7) with one knee on the floor and one knee lifted.

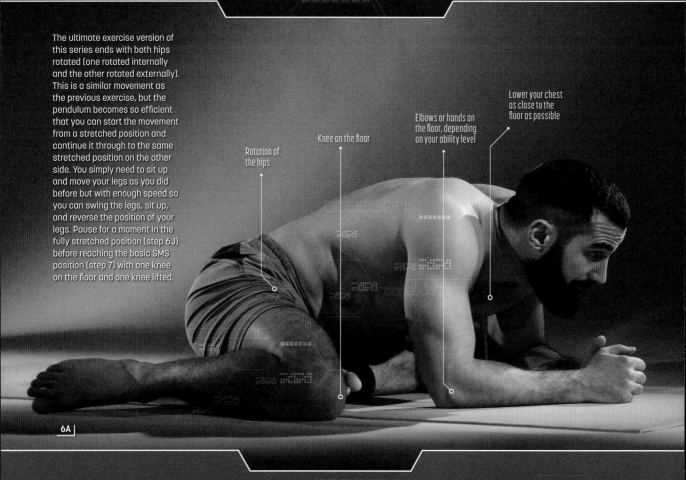

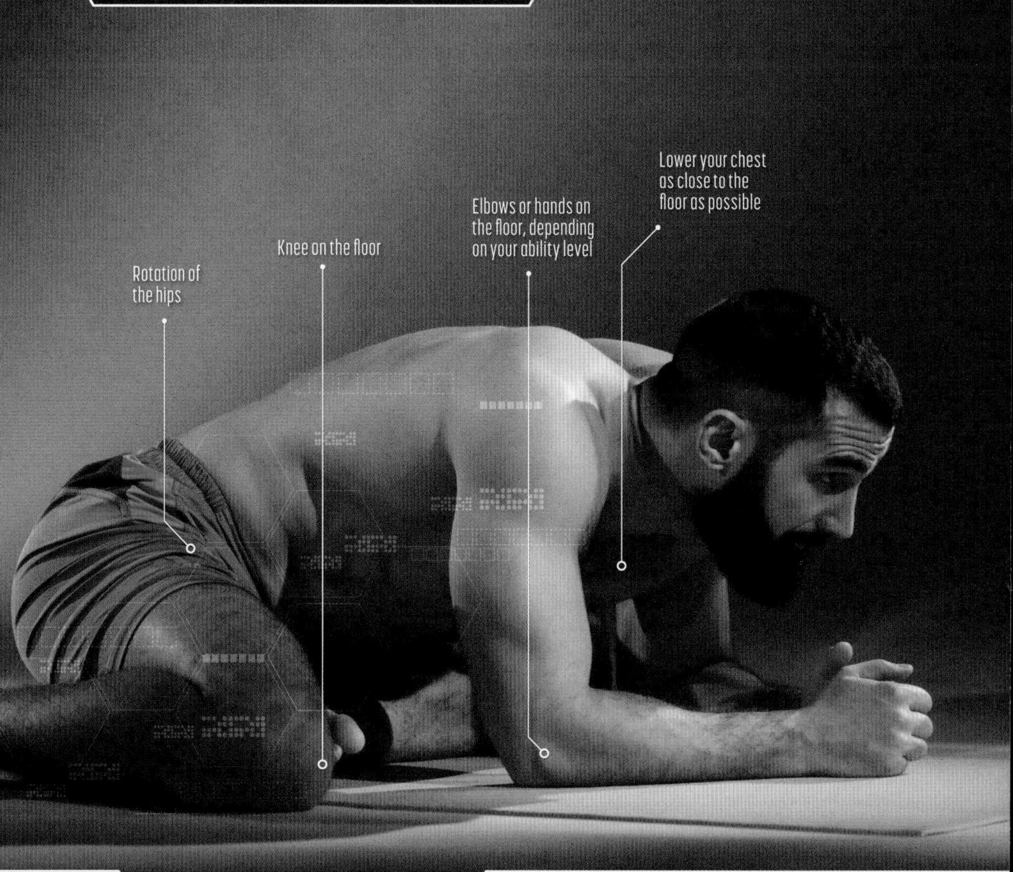

Rotation of the hips
Knee on the floor
Elbows or hands on the floor, depending on your ability level
Lower your chest as close to the floor as possible
6A

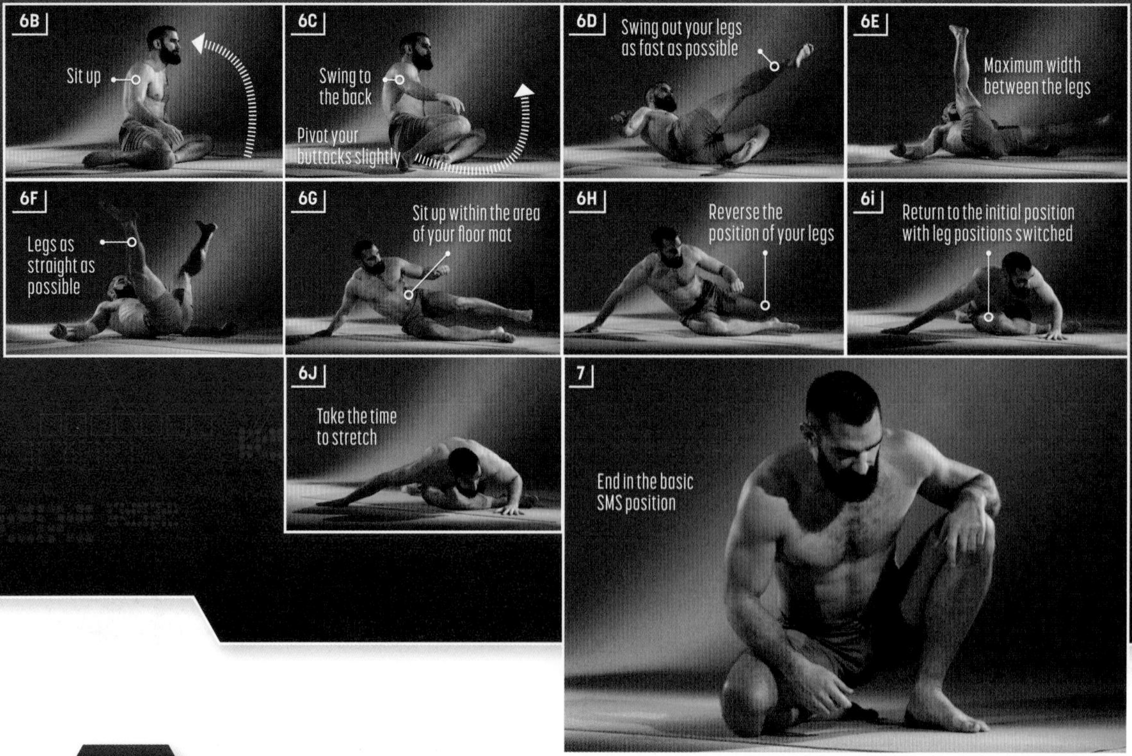

6B
Sit up
6C
Swing to the back
Pivot your buttocks slightly
6D
Swing out your legs as fast as possible
6E
Maximum width between the legs
6F
Legs as straight as possible
6G
Sit up within the area of your floor mat
6H
Reverse the position of your legs
6i
Return to the initial position with leg positions switched
6J
Take the time to stretch
7
End in the basic SMS position

TURKISH GET-UP
SERIES

The Turkish get-up combines strength and mobility for all the muscle chains like very few exercises can. When done without weight, each step of this exercise is an opportunity to improve joint mobility and stability.

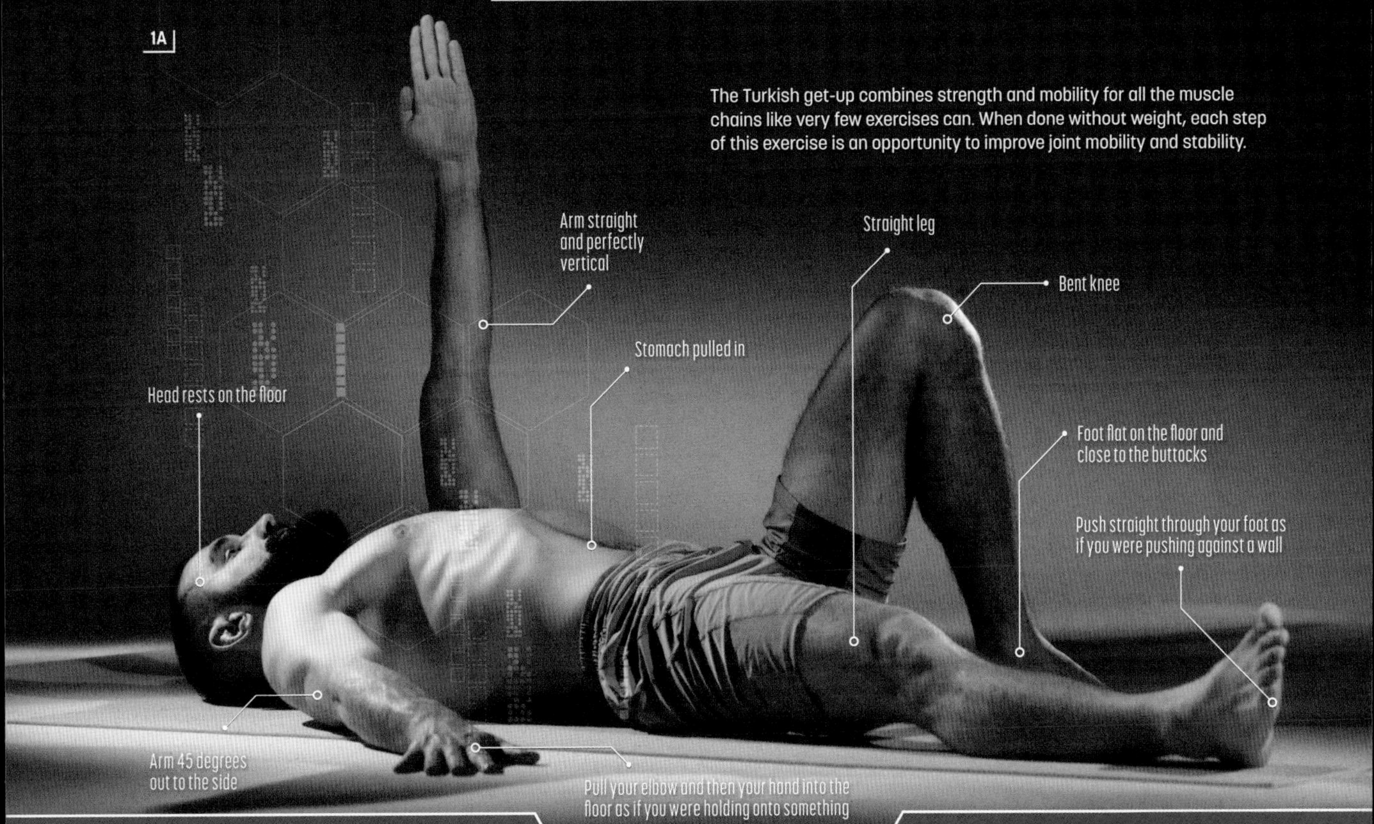

1A
Arm straight and perfectly vertical
Straight leg
Bent knee
Stomach pulled in
Head rests on the floor
Foot flat on the floor and close to the buttocks
Push straight through your foot as if you were pushing against a wall
Arm 45 degrees out to the side
Pull your elbow and then your hand into the floor as if you were holding onto something

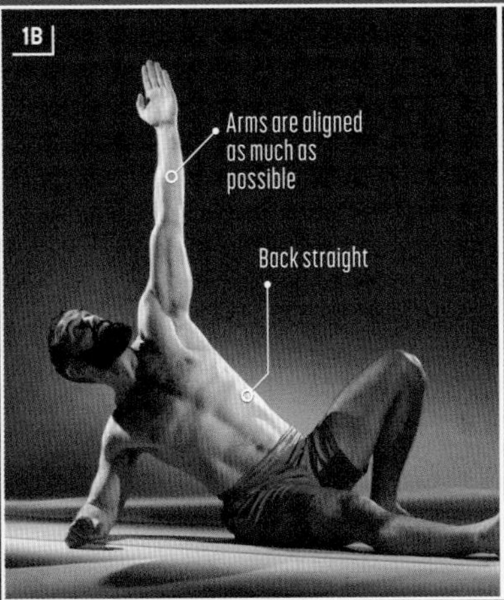

1B
Arms are aligned as much as possible
Back straight

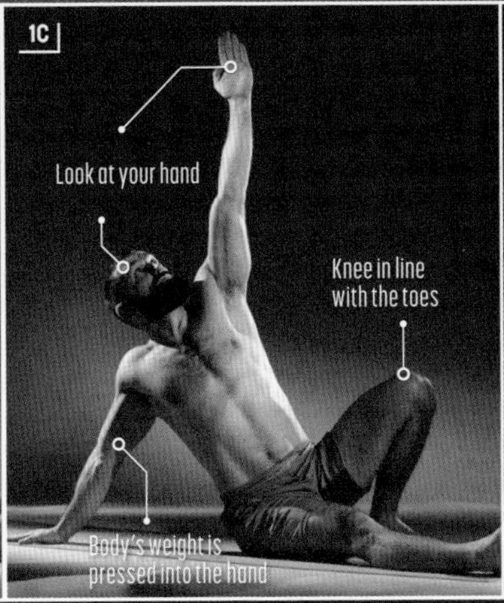

1C
Look at your hand
Knee in line with the toes
Body's weight is pressed into the hand

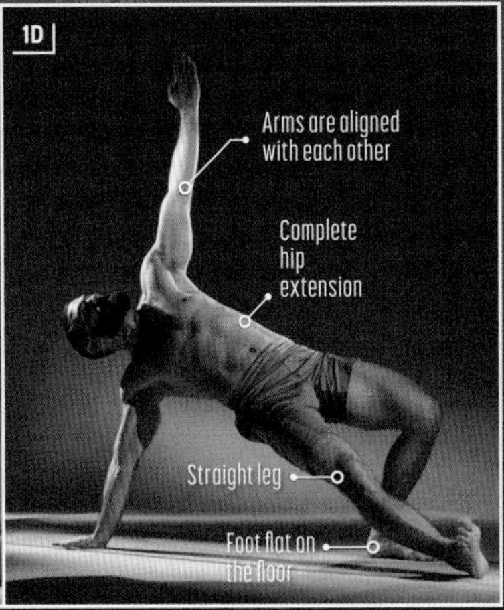

1D
Arms are aligned with each other
Complete hip extension
Straight leg
Foot flat on the floor

1E

Each step is essential, uses the principle of diagonal support introduced in the basic get-up 2 series, and requires you to carefully stabilize yourself along the way. Take note that the foot that is flat on the floor at the beginning does not move at all throughout the exercise. After reaching a standing position, go back down by doing the reverse of all the same steps. Do not rush. Take time for each step; these steps correspond to many exercises for core support, stability, and mobility. The classic mistake is to round the upper back, so be careful to open your chest and look at your hand to keep your back from rounding.

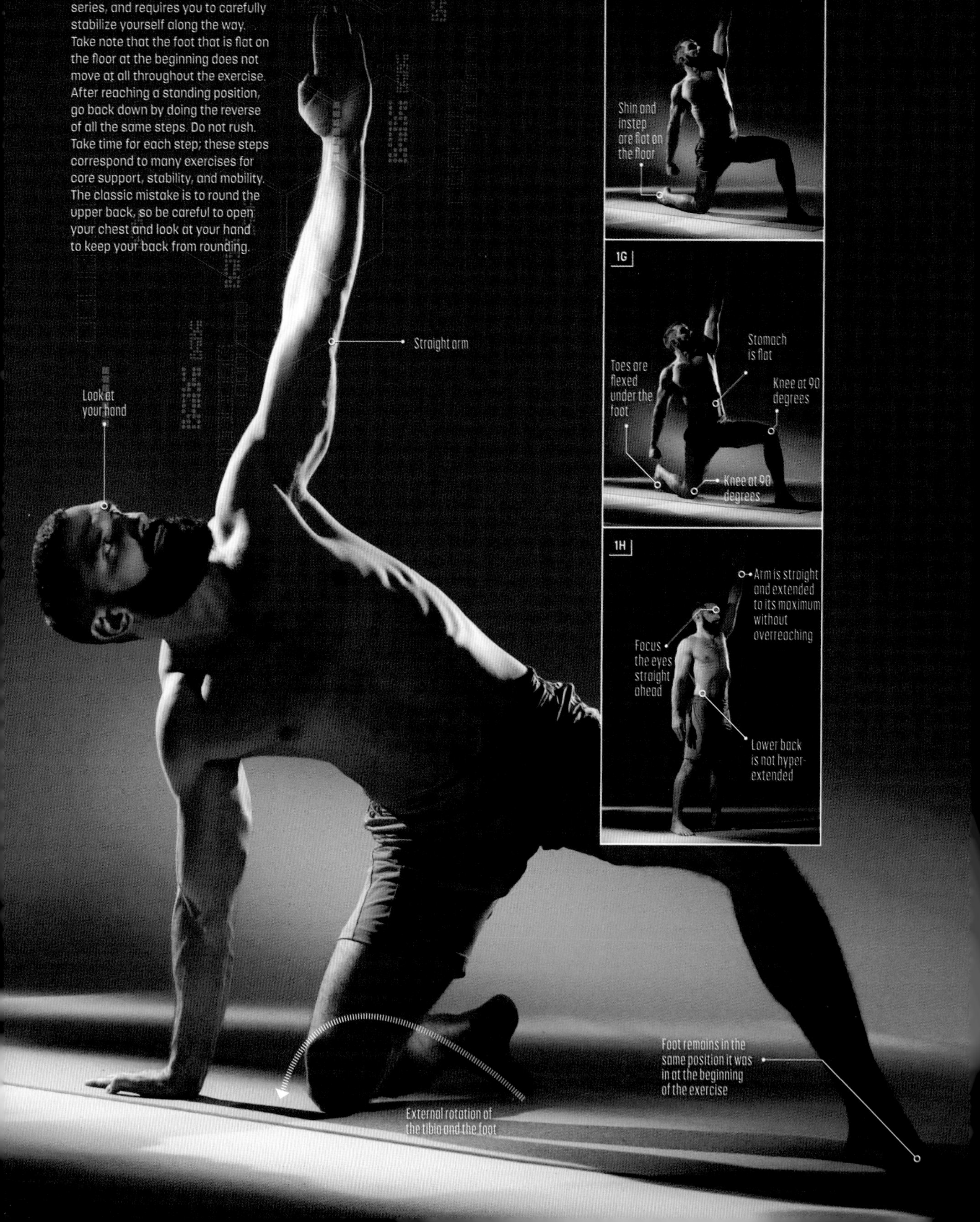

Straight arm
Look at your hand
External rotation of the tibia and the foot
Foot remains in the same position it was in at the beginning of the exercise
1F
Shin and instep are flat on the floor
1G
Stomach is flat
Toes are flexed under the foot
Knee at 90 degrees
Knee at 90 degrees
1H
Arm is straight and extended to its maximum without overreaching
Focus the eyes straight ahead
Lower back is not hyper-extended

TABLE 1
SERIES

The table is found in many disciplines that use an all-fours posture, such as Brazilian jiu-jitsu, Afro-Brazilian capoeira, and hip hop. It also involves moving the body in a diagonal trajectory with two bases of support that are diagonally opposite, which creates an interaction between the anterior and posterior chains through the functional and spiral chains. This interaction inspired us to create this series that blends stability and mobility in the pelvis and the shoulders. The first exercise is static and limits movement in the hips to a single plane in space.

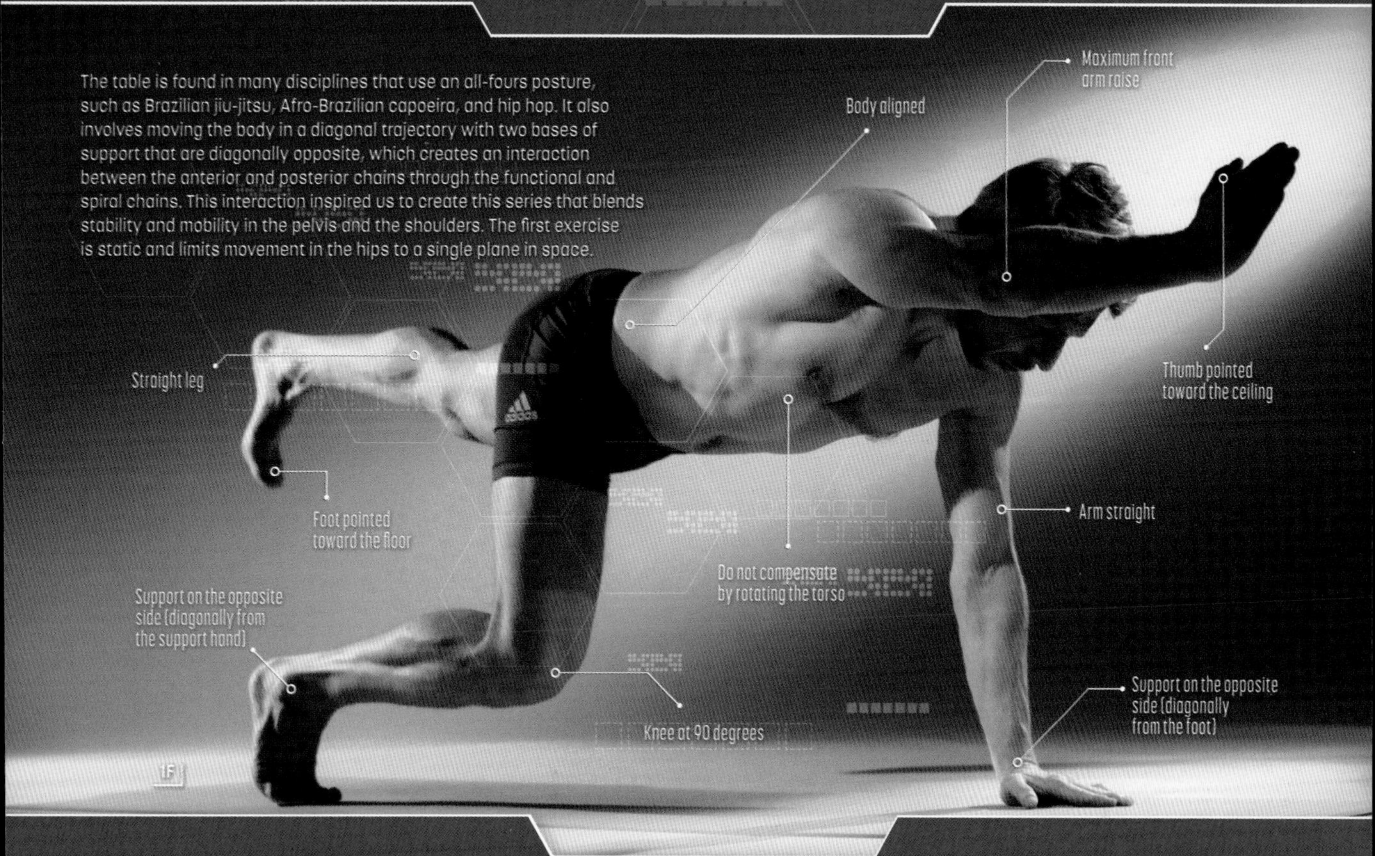

Maximum front arm raise
Body aligned
Straight leg
Thumb pointed toward the ceiling
Foot pointed toward the floor
Arm straight
Do not compensate by rotating the torso
Support on the opposite side (diagonally from the support hand)
Support on the opposite side (diagonally from the foot)
Knee at 90 degrees
1F

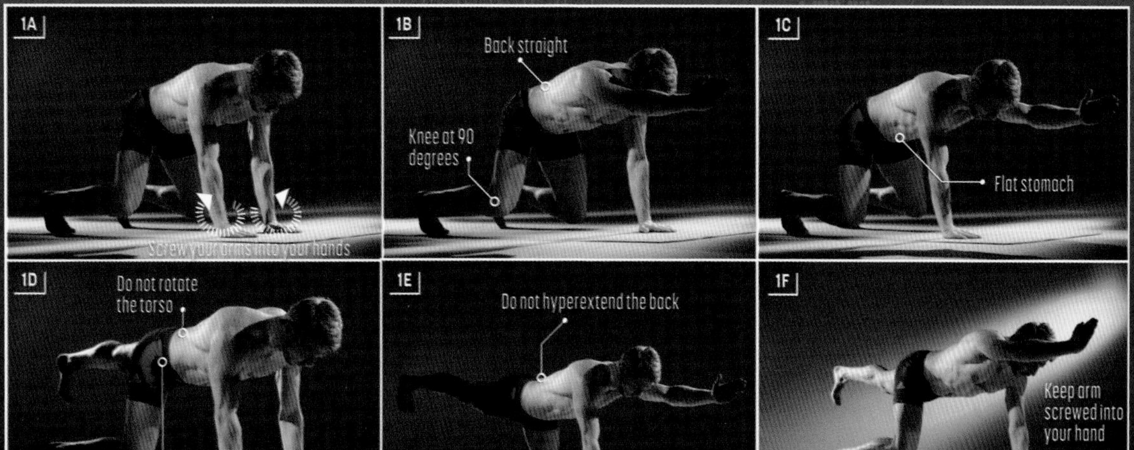

1A
Screw your arms into your hands
1B
Back straight
Knee at 90 degrees
1C
Flat stomach
1D
Do not rotate the torso
Complete hip extension
1E
Do not hyperextend the back
1F
Keep arm screwed into your hand

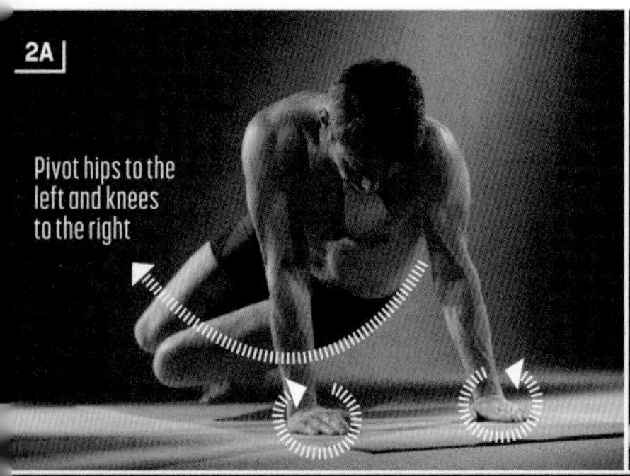
2A
Pivot hips to the left and knees to the right

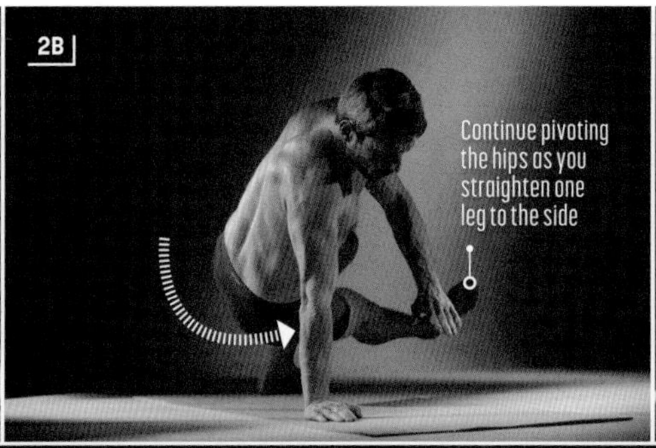
2B
Continue pivoting the hips as you straighten one leg to the side

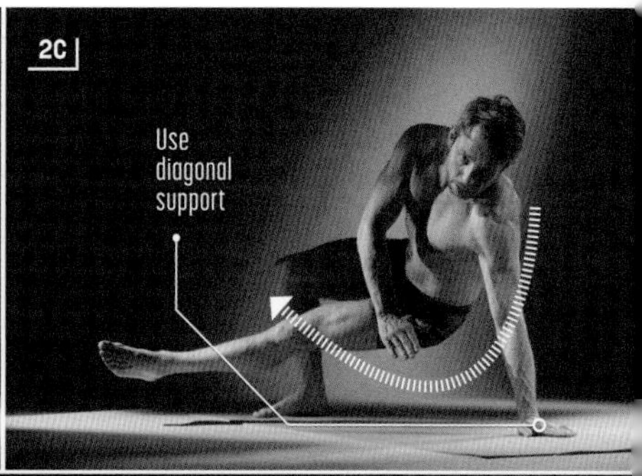
2C
Use diagonal support

For this second exercise, unleash your hips' mobility in the frontal and horizontal planes. More than ever, it is essential to use diagonal support. Always work at two different speeds: first by using maximum control as you extend your legs and arms as the movement slows down and second by taking plenty of time to rotate your hips. Additionally, strive for maximum fluidity, range of motion, and relaxation to get the most out of the exercise.

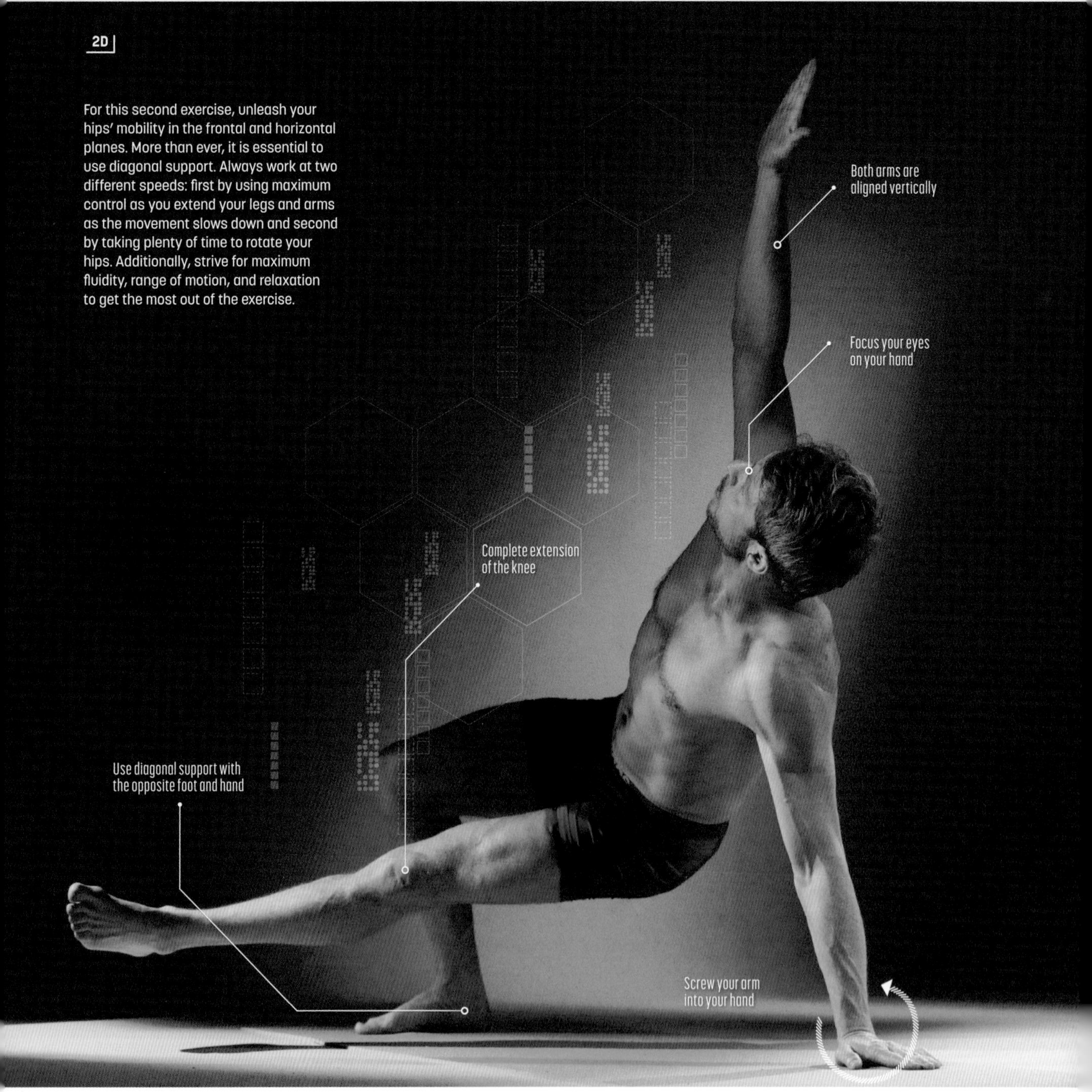
2D
Both arms are aligned vertically
Focus your eyes on your hand
Complete extension of the knee
Use diagonal support with the opposite foot and hand
Screw your arm into your hand

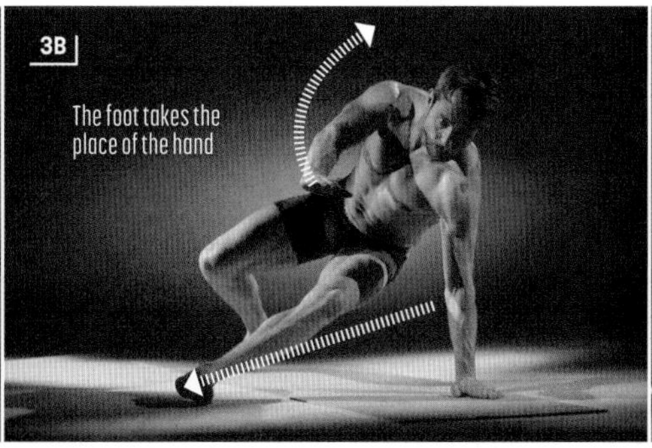

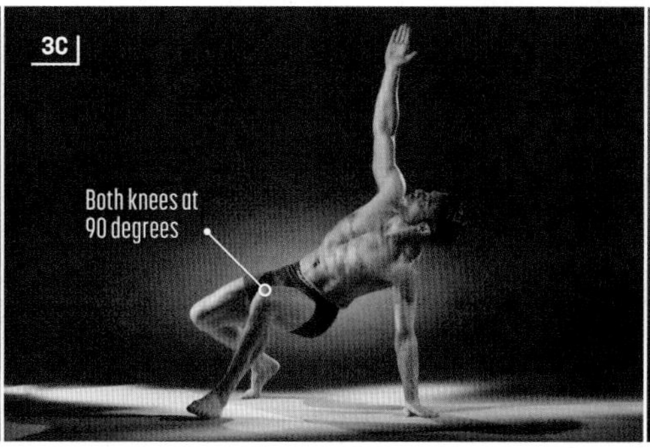

It is possible to extend the hips to different degrees
The hand switches places with the foot

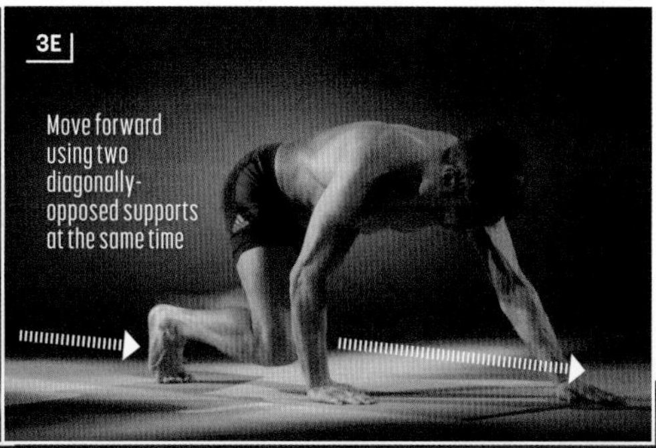

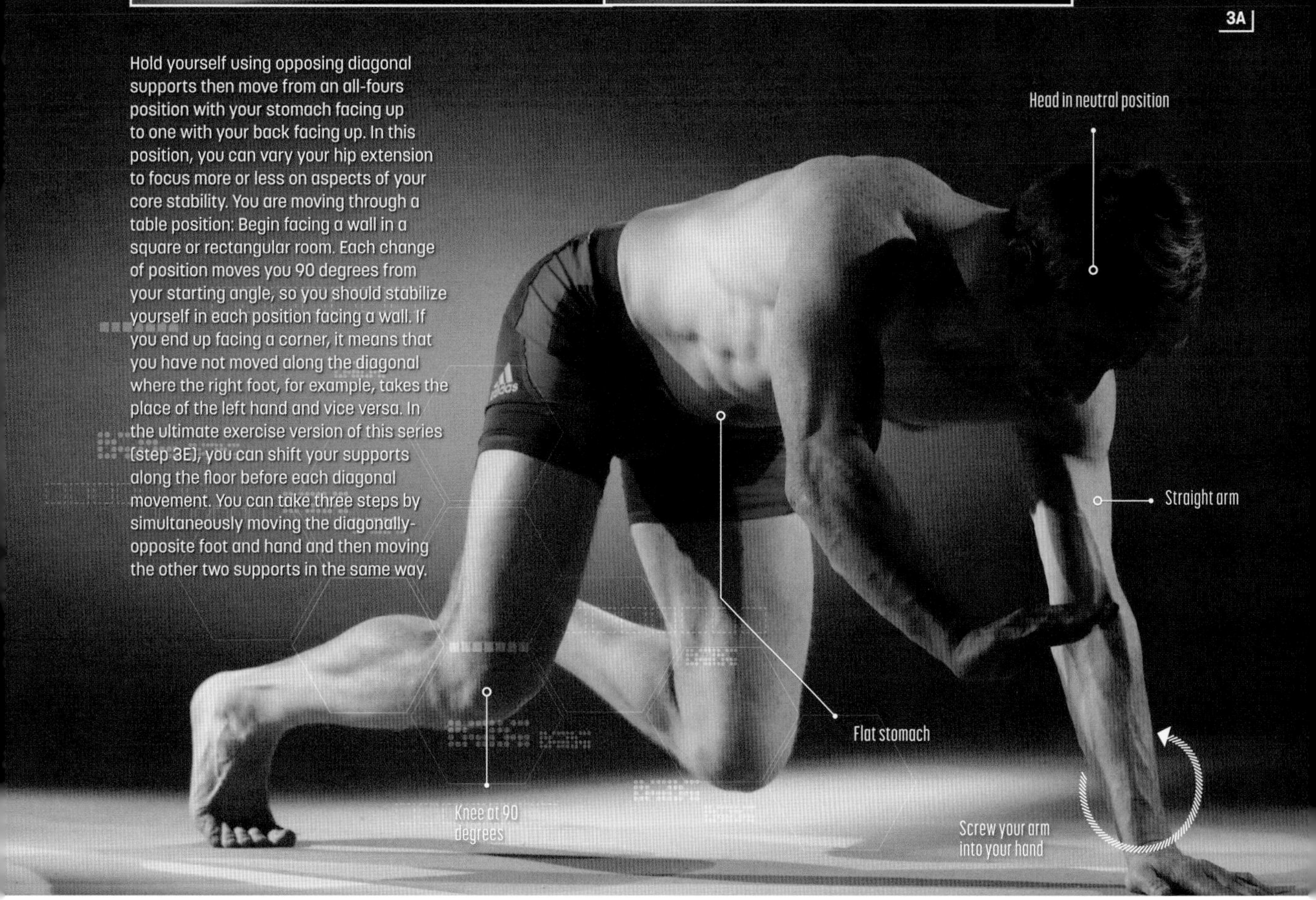

Move forward using two diagonally-opposed supports at the same time

Hold yourself using opposing diagonal supports then move from an all-fours position with your stomach facing up to one with your back facing up. In this position, you can vary your hip extension to focus more or less on aspects of your core stability. You are moving through a table position: Begin facing a wall in a square or rectangular room. Each change of position moves you 90 degrees from your starting angle, so you should stabilize yourself in each position facing a wall. If you end up facing a corner, it means that you have not moved along the diagonal where the right foot, for example, takes the place of the left hand and vice versa. In the ultimate exercise version of this series (step 3E), you can shift your supports along the floor before each diagonal movement. You can take three steps by simultaneously moving the diagonally-opposite foot and hand and then moving the other two supports in the same way.

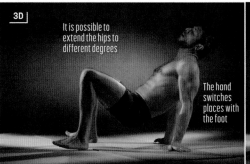

ARABESQUE SERIES

The *arabesque* is a body position in which a person stands on one leg with the other leg extended behind the body, with both legs held straight. It was included in exercises that train the superficial posterior chain, and it is an excellent mobility exercise when it is combined with diagonal rotation.

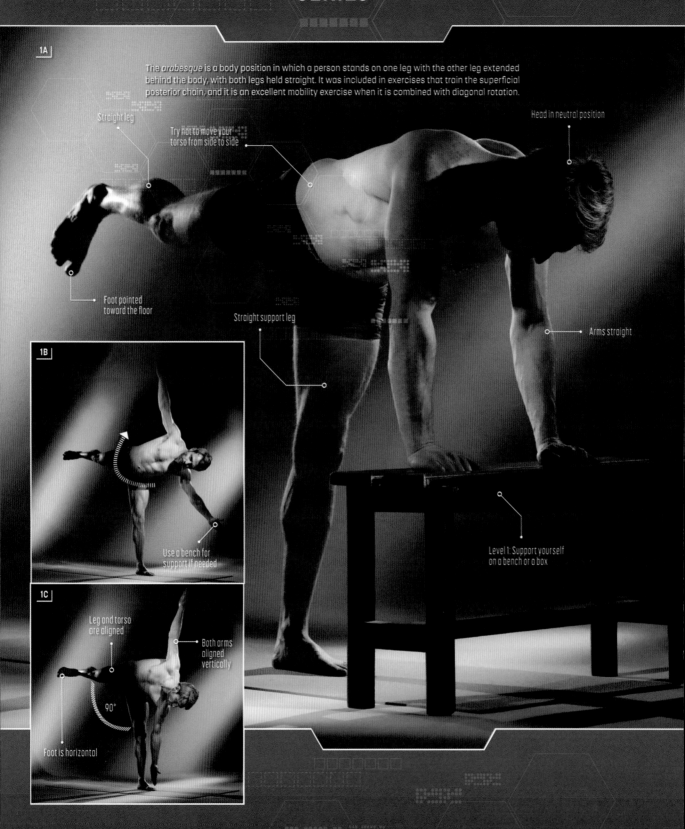

This second version alternates between an arabesque and a knee raise in the sagittal or frontal plane. Maintain your posture, especially your torso, and avoid compensating using the foot that is on the floor or by flexing the knee or the elbow.

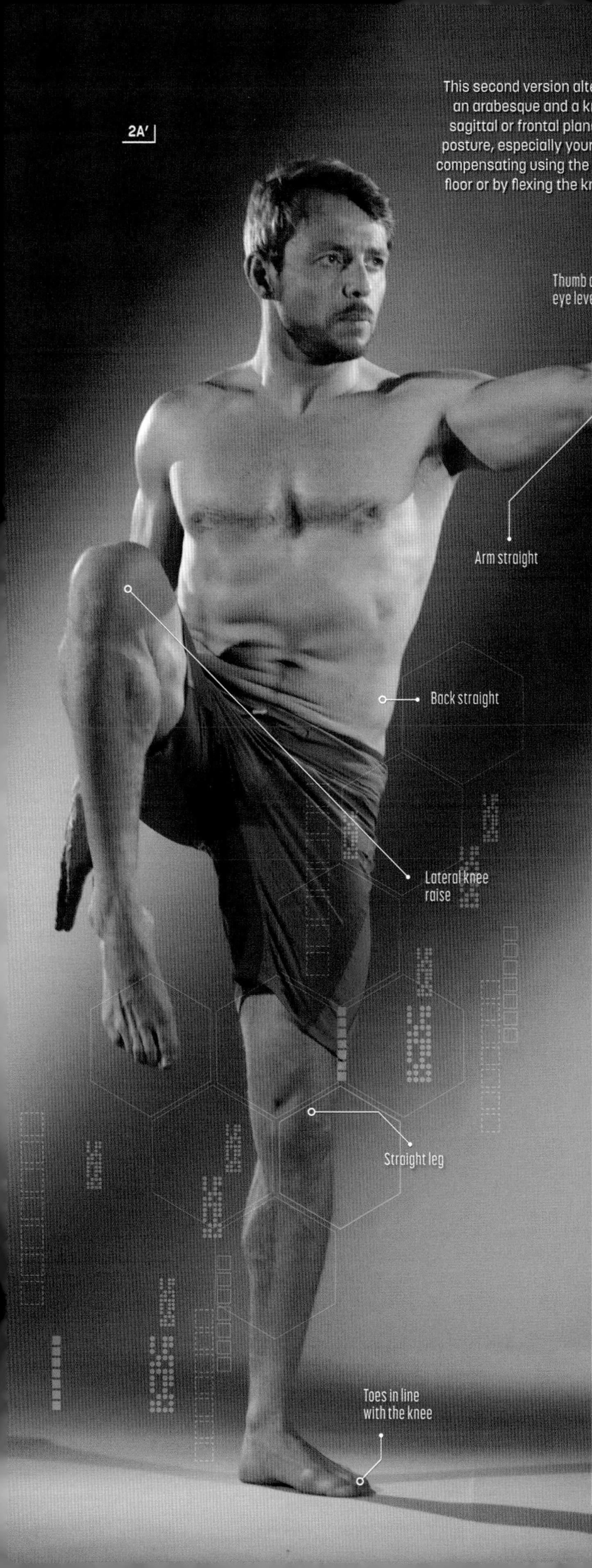
2A′
Thumb at eye level
Arm straight
Back straight
Lateral knee raise
Straight leg
Toes in line with the knee

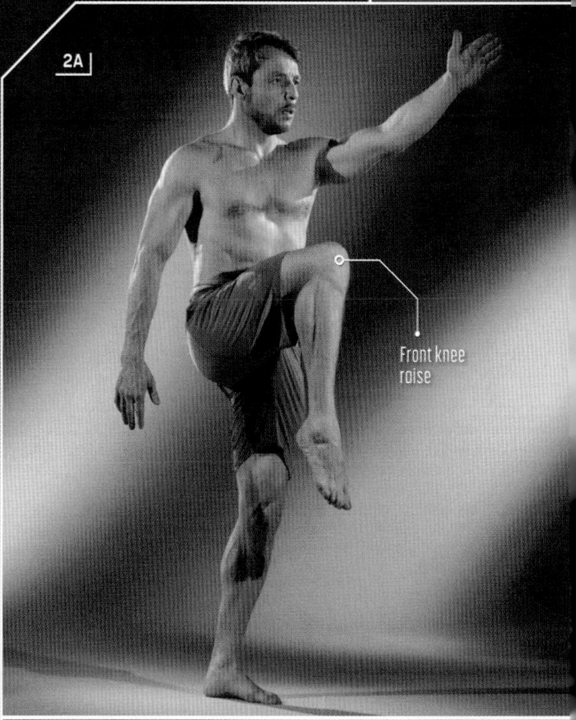
2A
Front knee raise

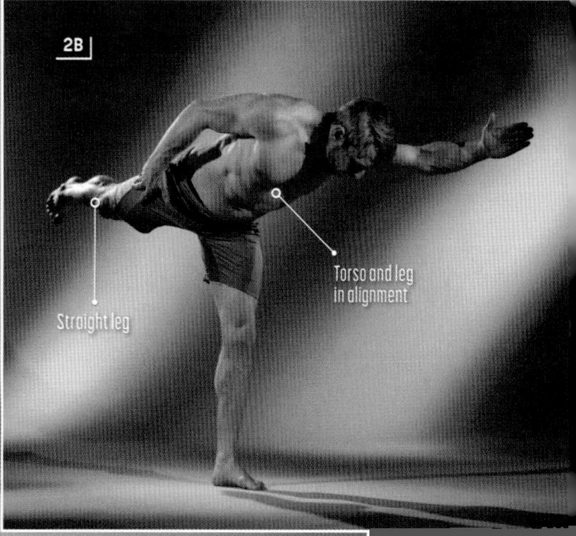
2B
Straight leg
Torso and leg in alignment

LUNGE AND TRIPOD SERIES

Inspired by yoga moves, tripod poses are excellent warm-up and mobility exercises. They are so complete in their involvement of muscle chains that they apply to nearly all sports and activities. Unlike the exercises up to now, this series involves holding each pose for a specified amount of time that can be adjusted by 20 seconds.

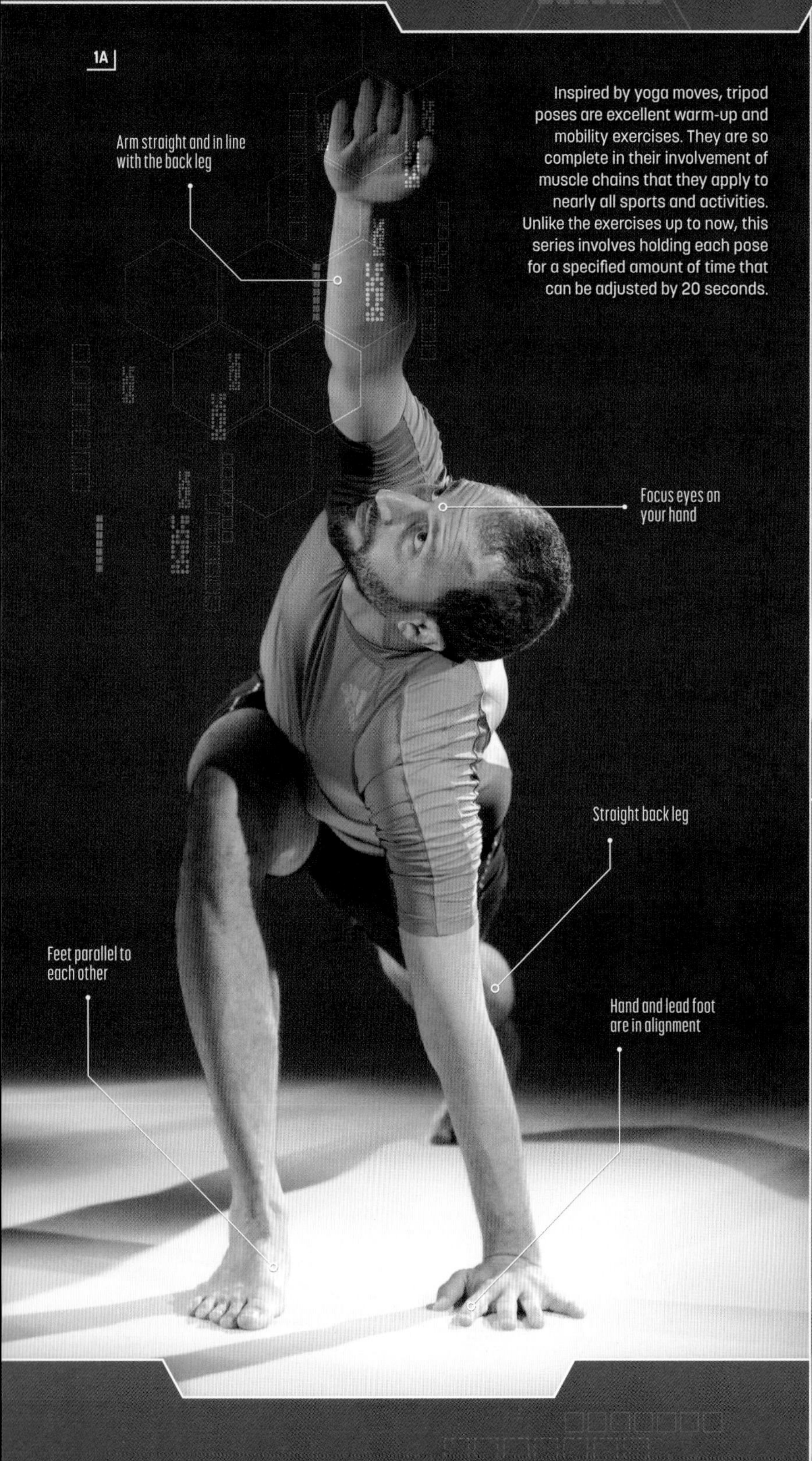

1A
Arm straight and in line with the back leg
Focus eyes on your hand
Straight back leg
Feet parallel to each other
Hand and lead foot are in alignment

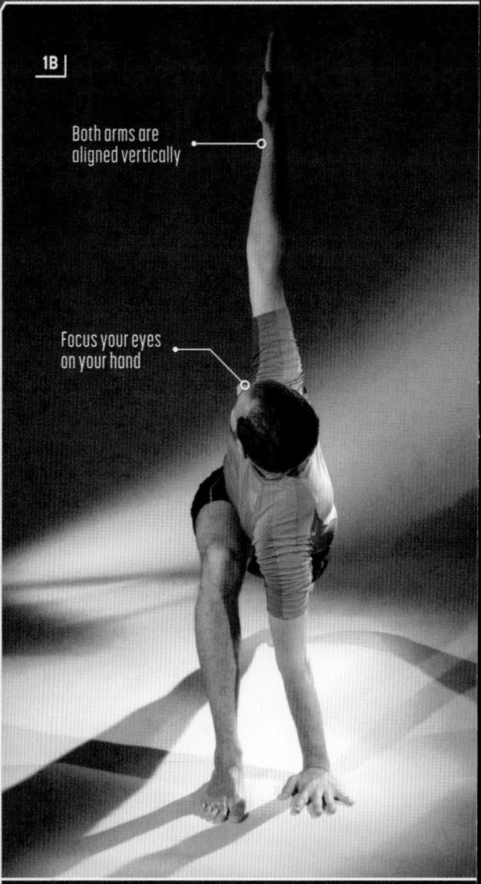

1B
Both arms are aligned vertically
Focus your eyes on your hand

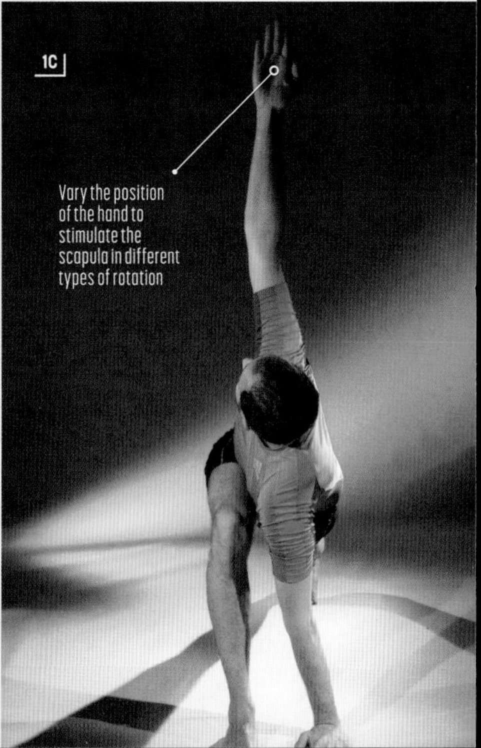

1C
Vary the position of the hand to stimulate the scapula in different types of rotation

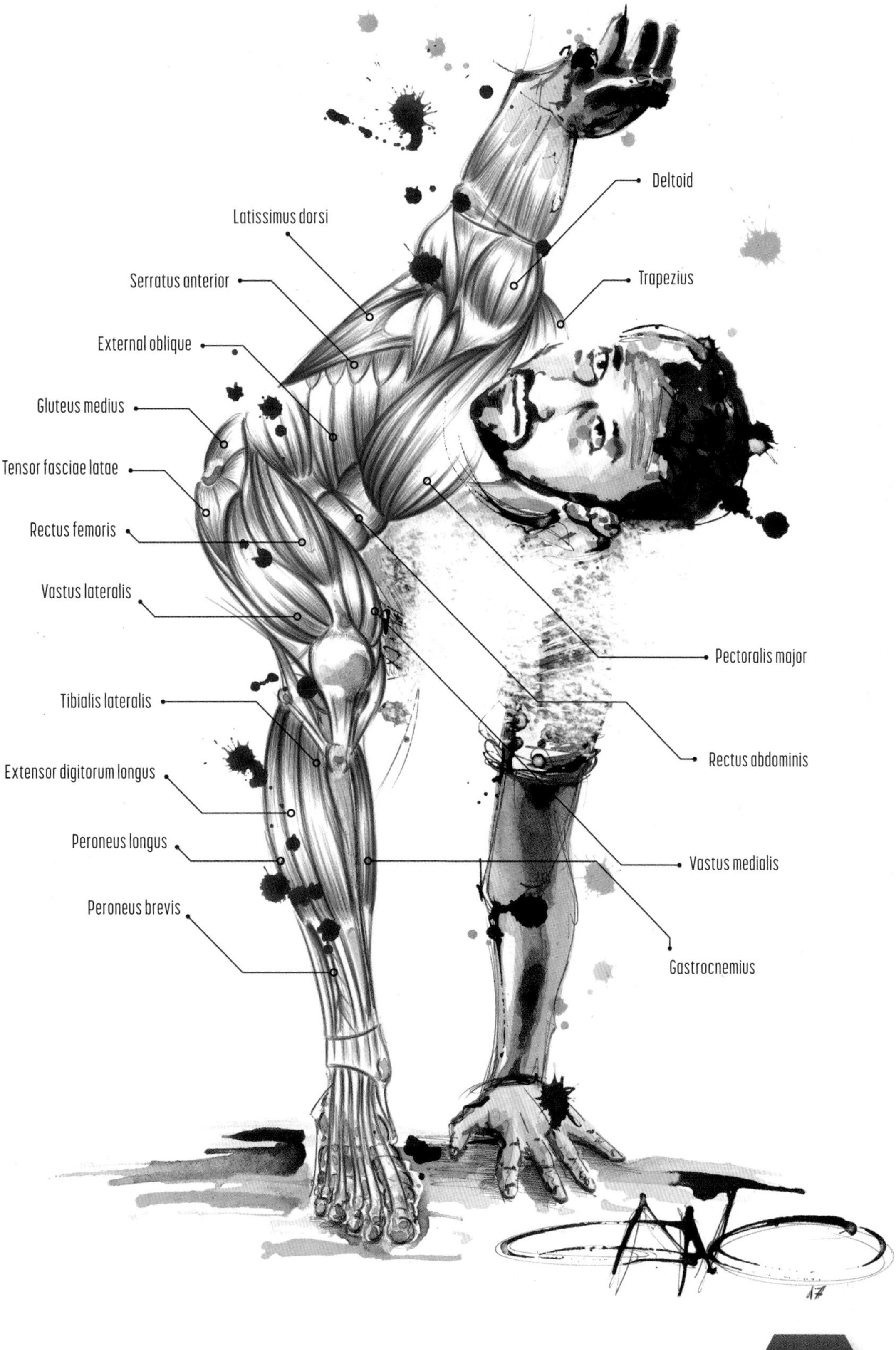
Deltoid
Latissimus dorsi
Serratus anterior
Trapezius
External oblique
Gluteus medius
Tensor fasciae latae
Rectus femoris
Vastus lateralis
Pectoralis major
Tibialis lateralis
Rectus abdominis
Extensor digitorum longus
Peroneus longus
Vastus medialis
Peroneus brevis
Gastrocnemius

This lunge series provides a complete extension of the posterior chain. Take the time to hold each pose and gradually increase your range of motion. Combine this series with your breathing (see page 78).

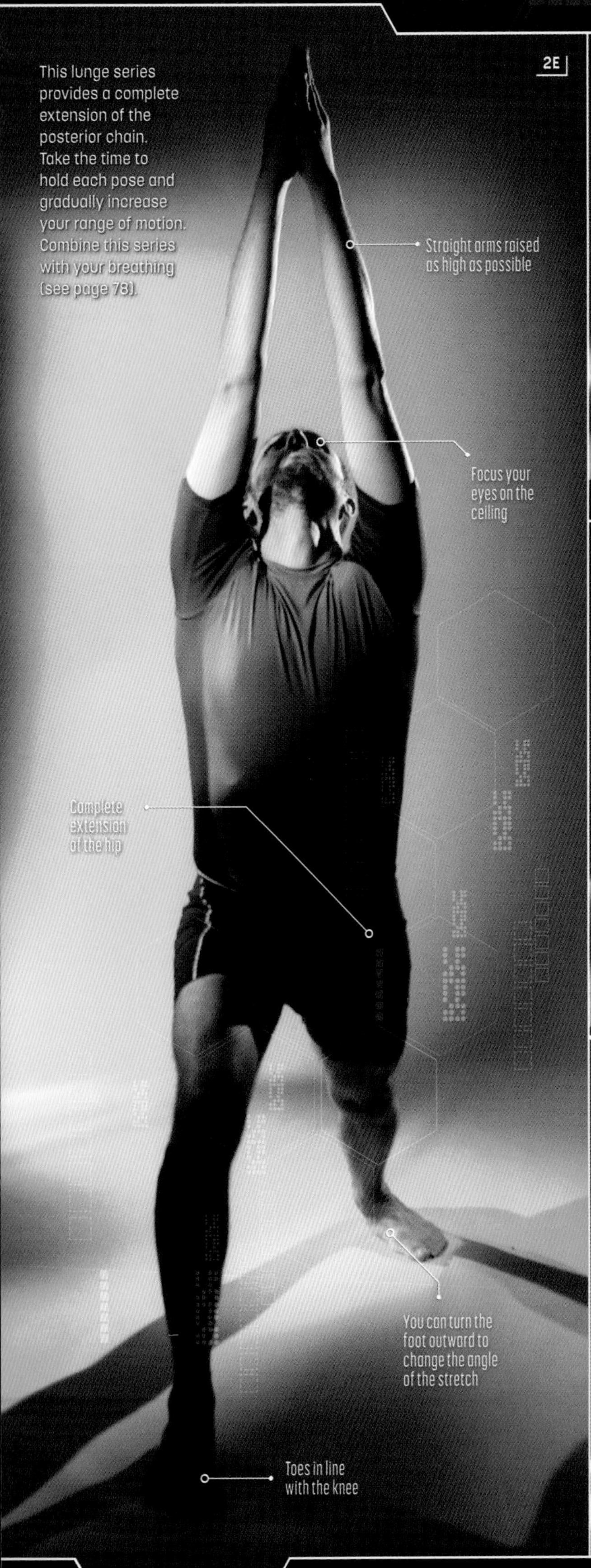
2E
Straight arms raised as high as possible
Focus your eyes on the ceiling
Complete extension of the hip
You can turn the foot outward to change the angle of the stretch
Toes in line with the knee

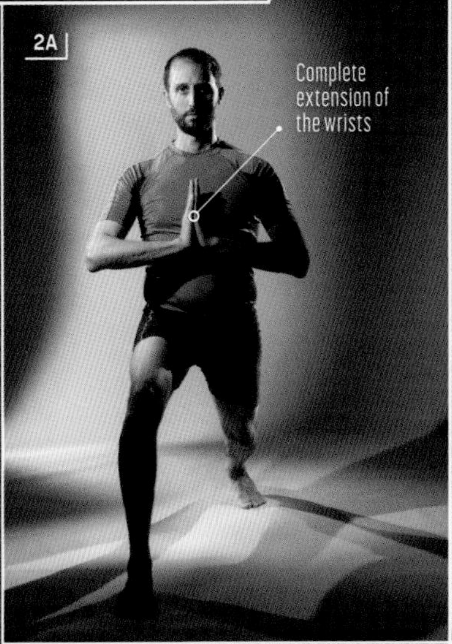
2A
Complete extension of the wrists

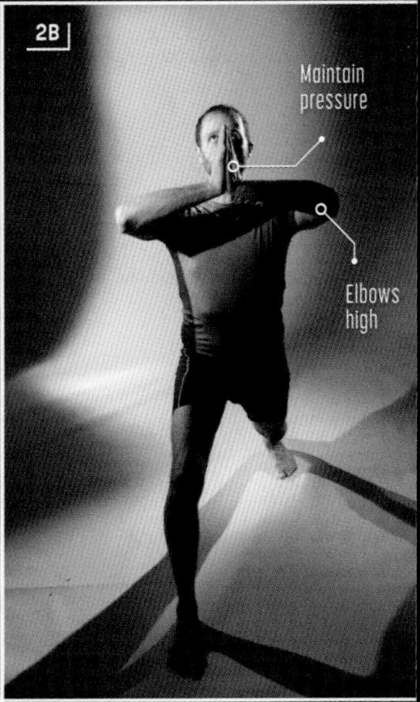
2B
Maintain pressure
Elbows high

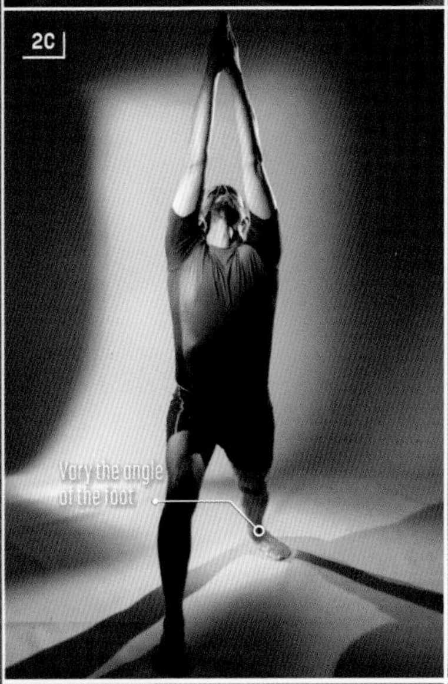
2C
Vary the angle of the foot

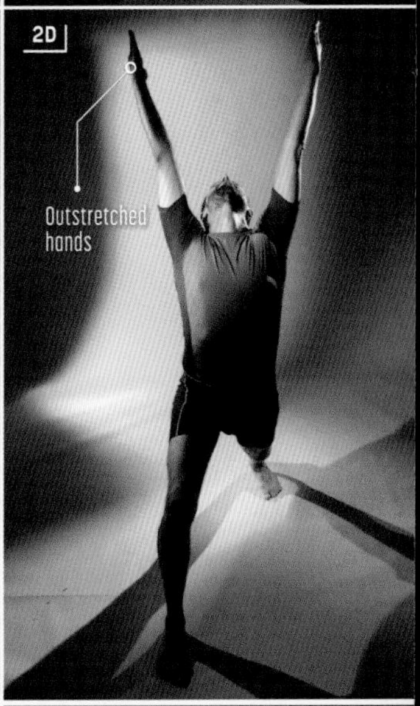
2D
Outstretched hands

SIDE VIEW

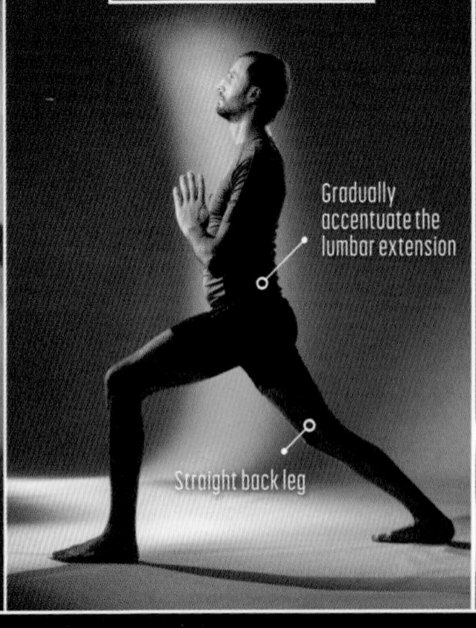
Gradually accentuate the lumbar extension
Straight back leg

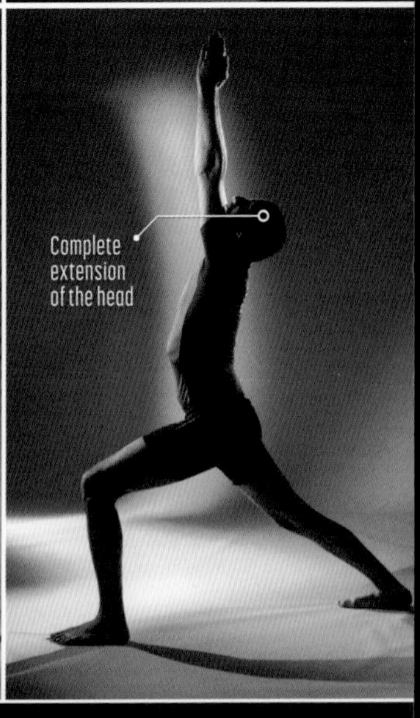
Complete extension of the head

The second version includes torso rotation and flexing so you can train different combinations of muscle chains. As always, avoid compensating, work on your breathing, and hold each position. There are three final positions; alternate between them during the same set.

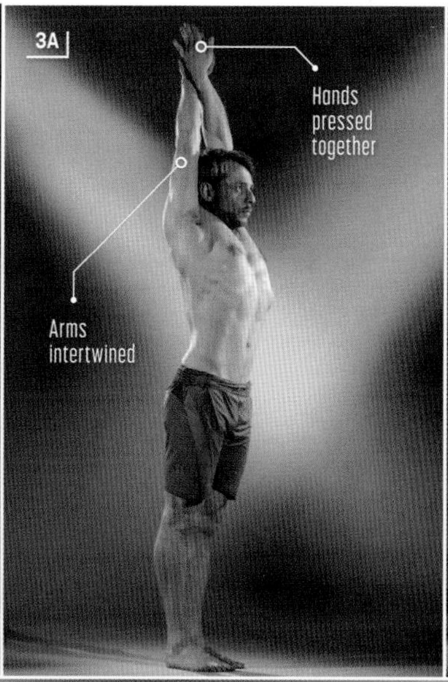

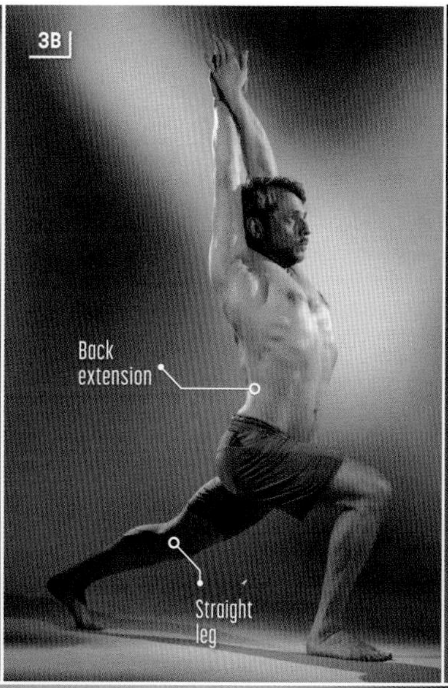

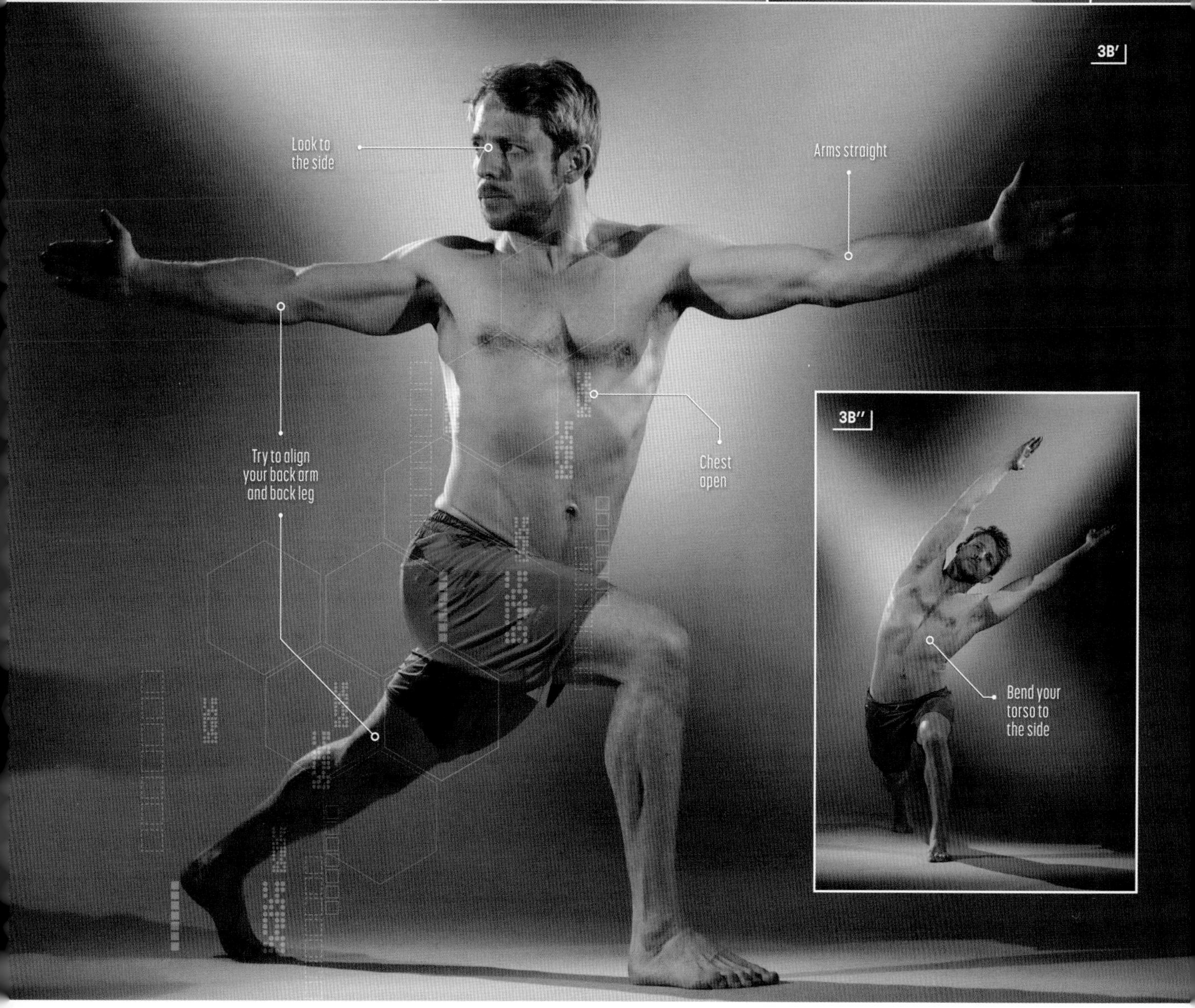

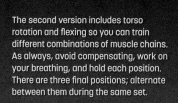

In the most advanced versions, the tripod lunge multiplies the support options to train mobility and stability even more intensely.

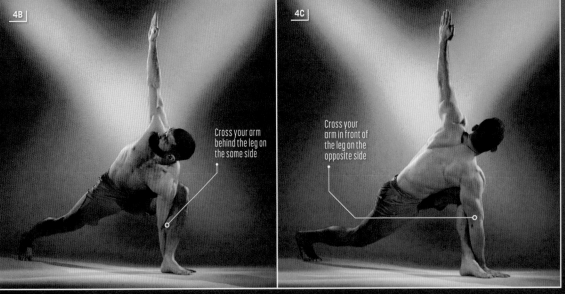

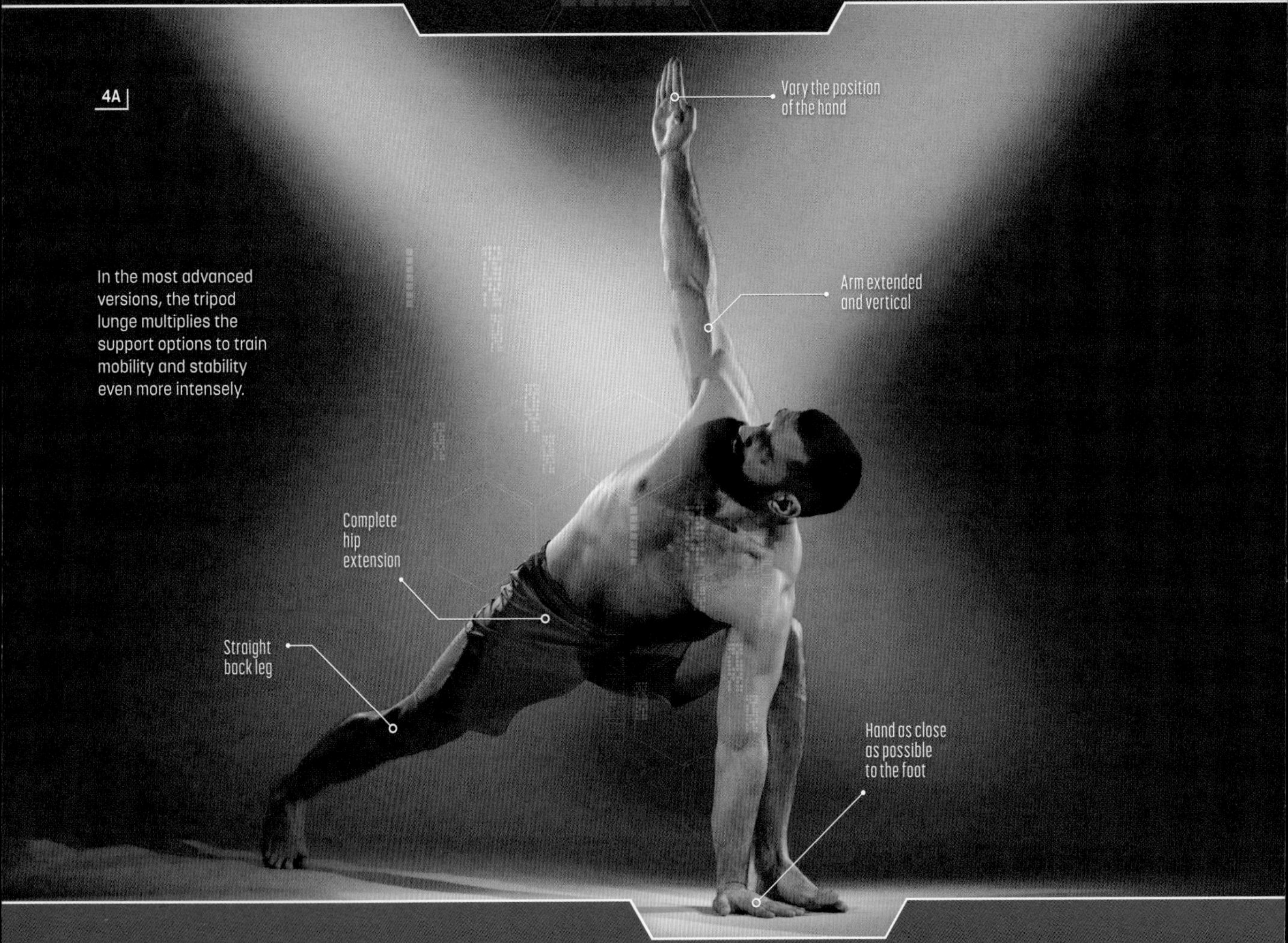
4A
Vary the position of the hand
Arm extended and vertical
Complete hip extension
Straight back leg
Hand as close as possible to the foot

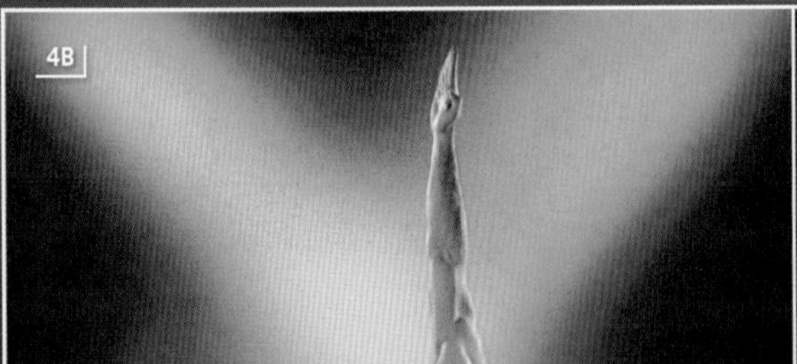
4B
Cross your arm behind the leg on the same side

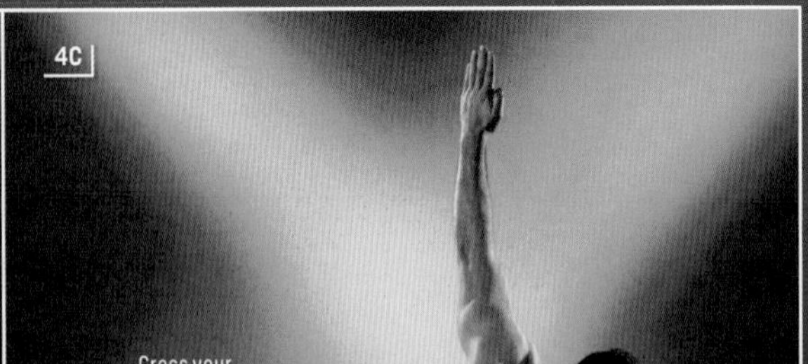
4C
Cross your arm in front of the leg on the opposite side

LUNGE
SERIES

The lunge series is found in yoga and often in martial arts. We have borrowed these lower series, with complementary support from the knee on the floor to allow you to intensify the emphasis on the hips.

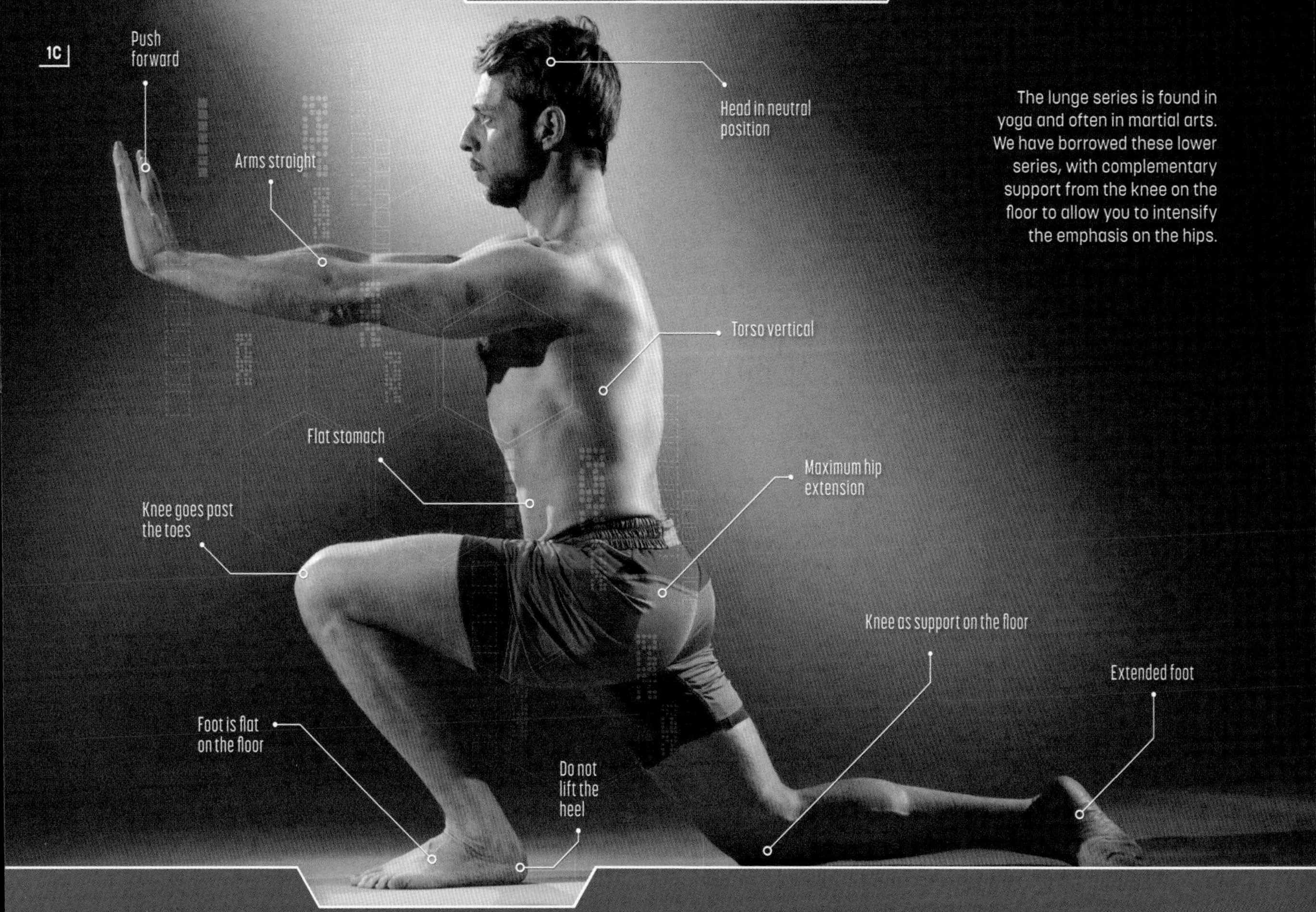

1C
Push forward
Arms straight
Head in neutral position
Torso vertical
Flat stomach
Maximum hip extension
Knee goes past the toes
Knee as support on the floor
Extended foot
Foot is flat on the floor
Do not lift the heel

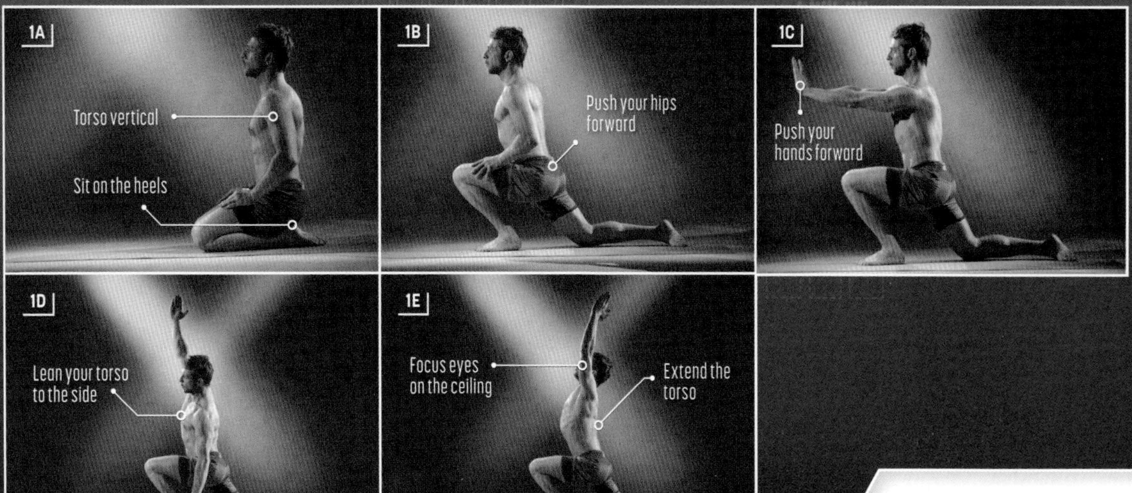

1A
Torso vertical
Sit on the heels
1B
Push your hips forward
1C
Push your hands forward
1D
Lean your torso to the side
1E
Focus eyes on the ceiling
Extend the torso

SHRIMP SERIES

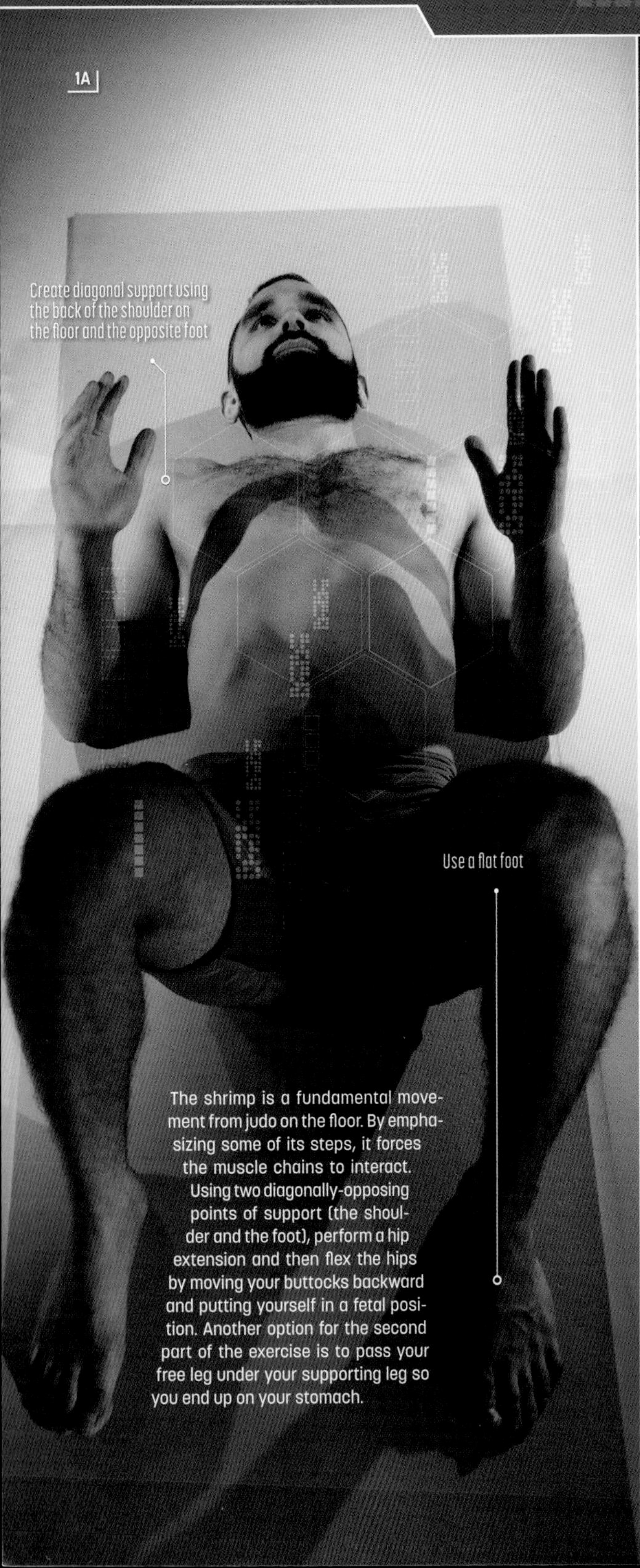
1A
Create diagonal support using the back of the shoulder on the floor and the opposite foot
Use a flat foot

The shrimp is a fundamental movement from judo on the floor. By emphasizing some of its steps, it forces the muscle chains to interact. Using two diagonally-opposing points of support (the shoulder and the foot), perform a hip extension and then flex the hips by moving your buttocks backward and putting yourself in a fetal position. Another option for the second part of the exercise is to pass your free leg under your supporting leg so you end up on your stomach.

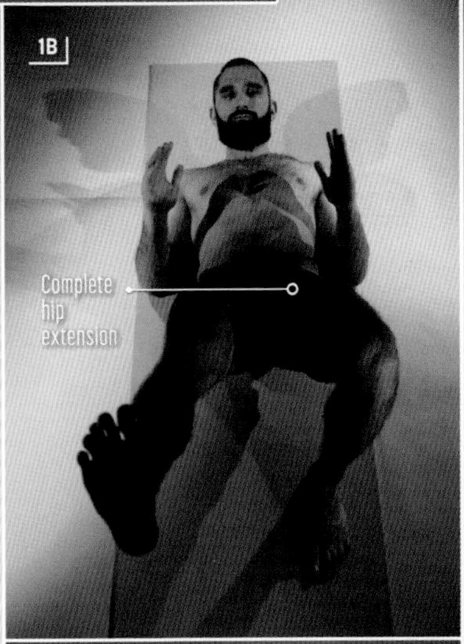
1B
Complete hip extension

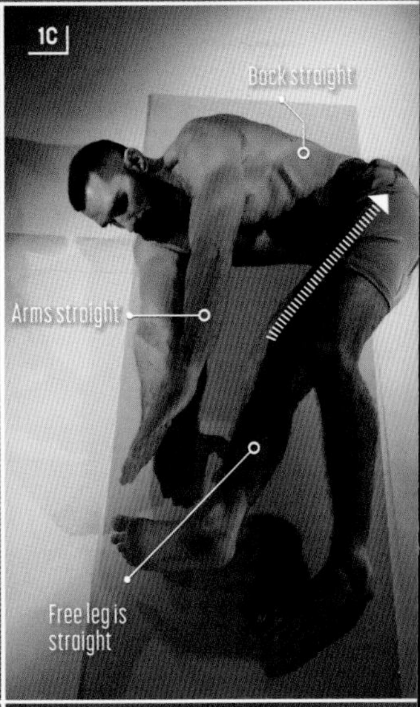
1C
Back straight
Arms straight
Free leg is straight

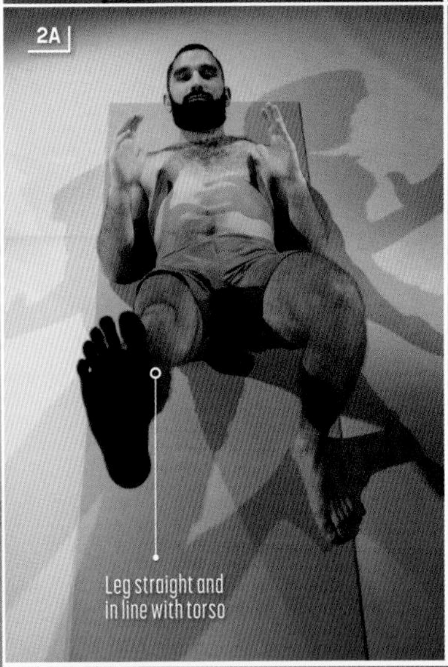
2A
Leg straight and in line with torso

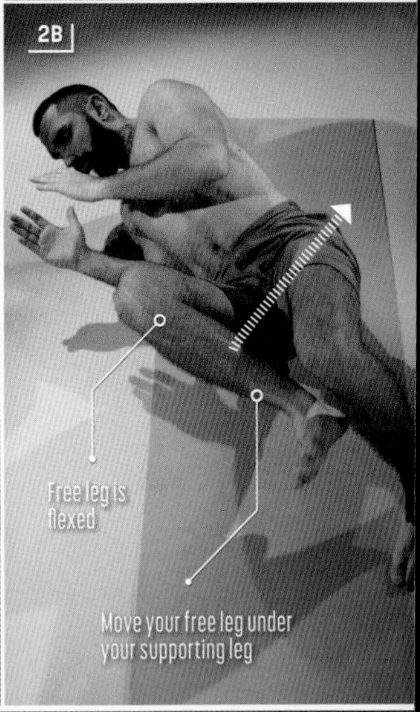
2B
Free leg is flexed
Move your free leg under your supporting leg

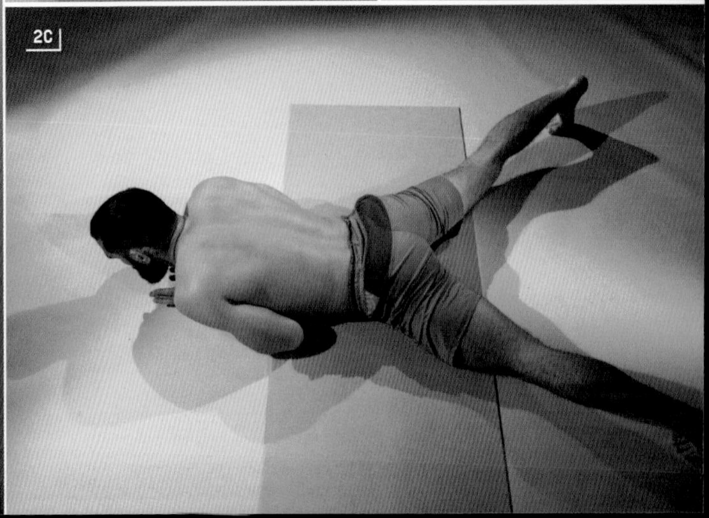
2C

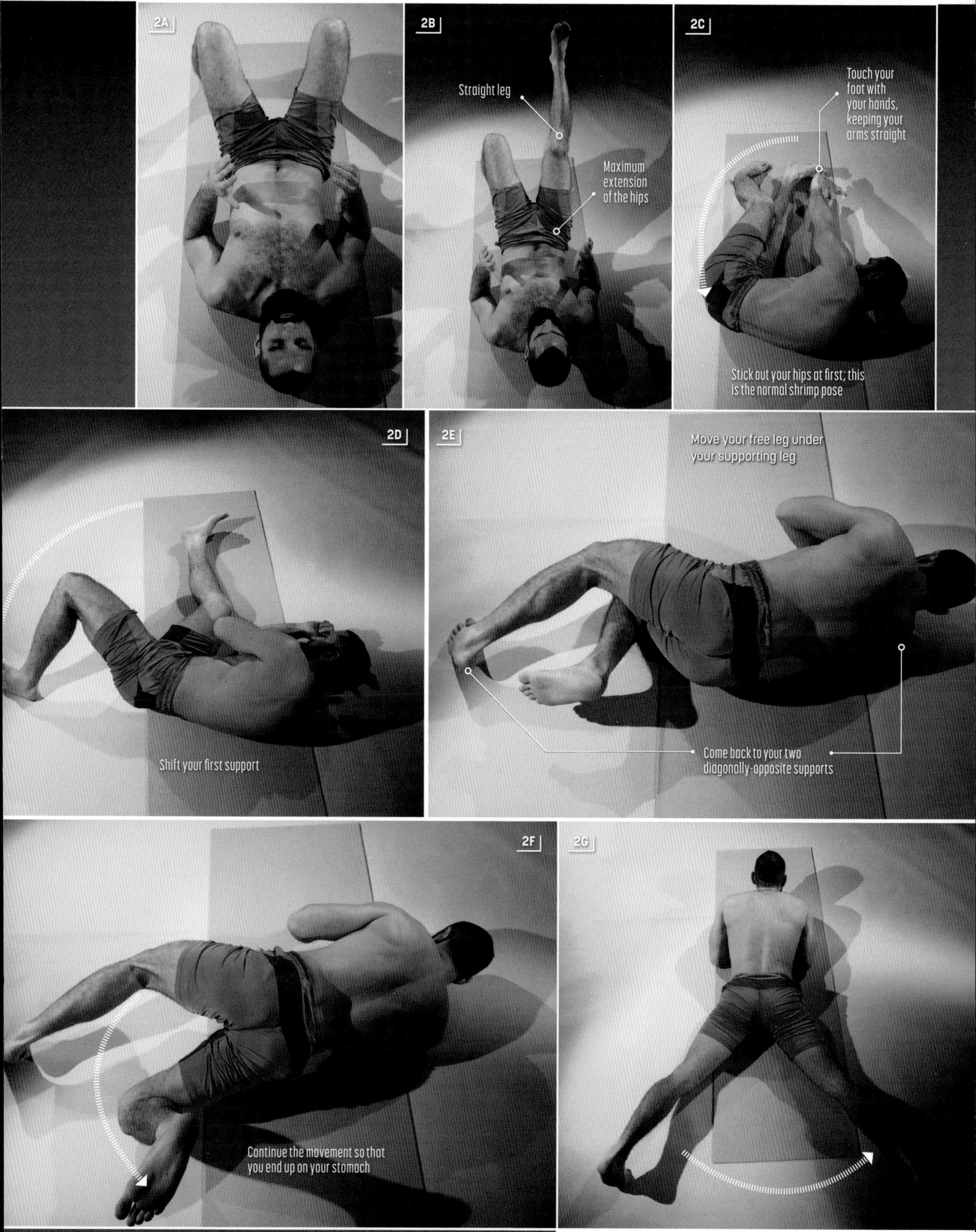
2A
2B
Straight leg
Maximum extension of the hips
2C
Touch your foot with your hands, keeping your arms straight
Stick out your hips at first; this is the normal shrimp pose
2D
Shift your first support
2E
Move your free leg under your supporting leg
Come back to your two diagonally-opposite supports
2F
Continue the movement so that you end up on your stomach
2G

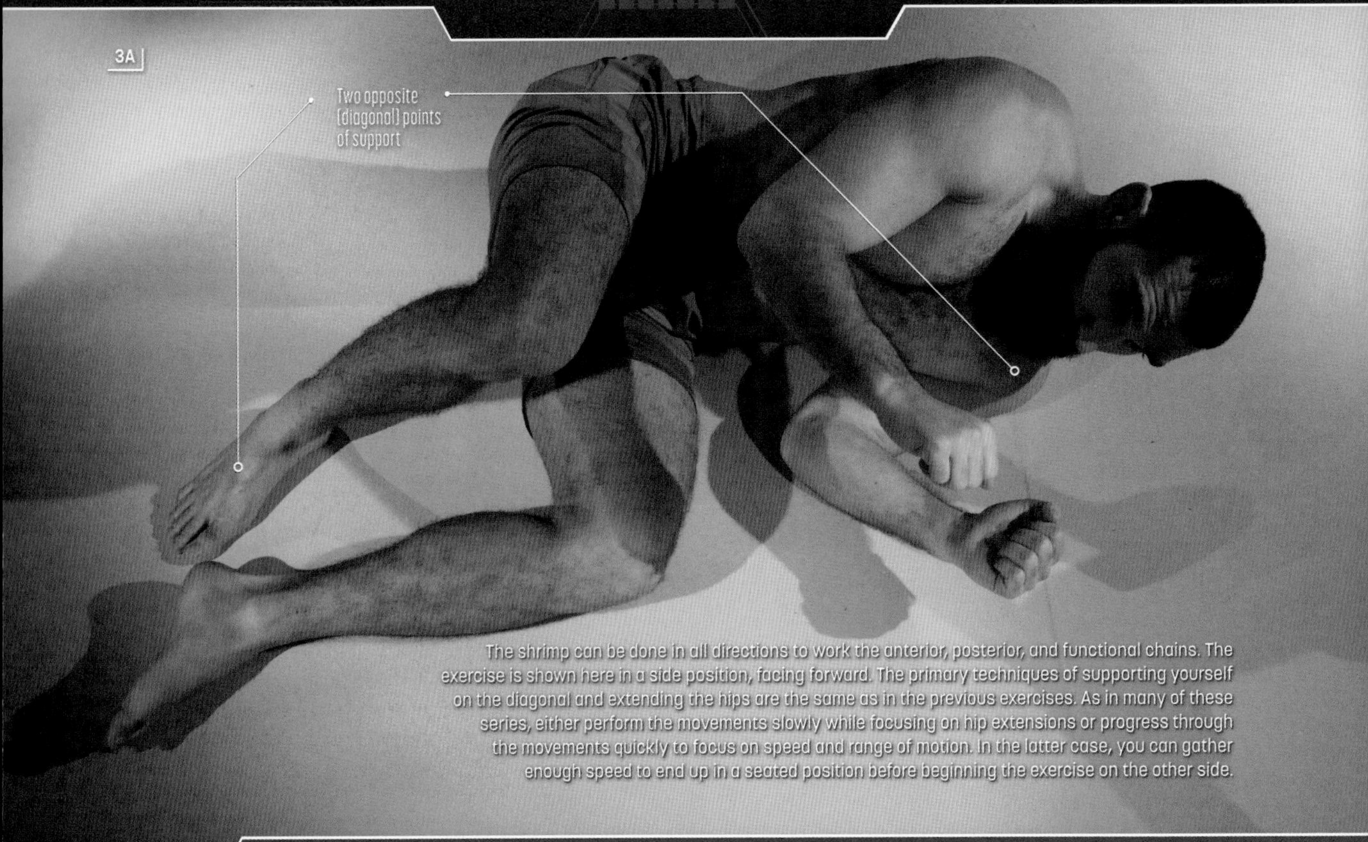
3A
Two opposite (diagonal) points of support

The shrimp can be done in all directions to work the anterior, posterior, and functional chains. The exercise is shown here in a side position, facing forward. The primary techniques of supporting yourself on the diagonal and extending the hips are the same as in the previous exercises. As in many of these series, either perform the movements slowly while focusing on hip extensions or progress through the movements quickly to focus on speed and range of motion. In the latter case, you can gather enough speed to end up in a seated position before beginning the exercise on the other side.

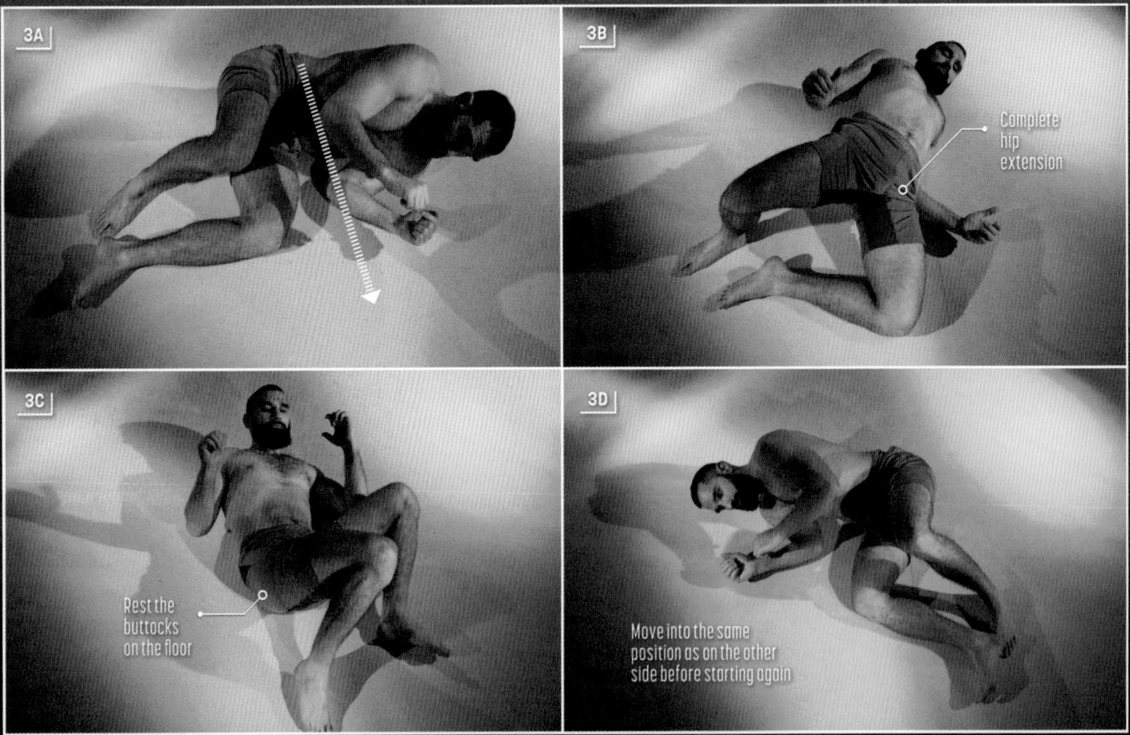
3A
3B
Complete hip extension
3C
Rest the buttocks on the floor
3D
Move into the same position as on the other side before starting again

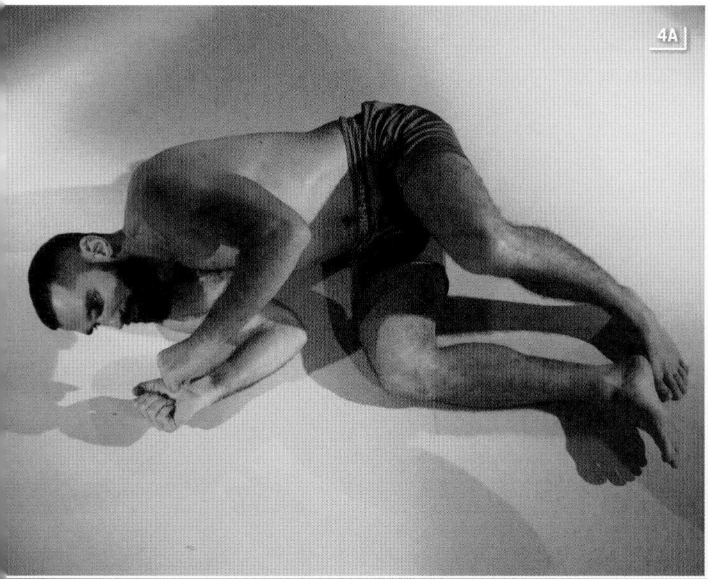
4A

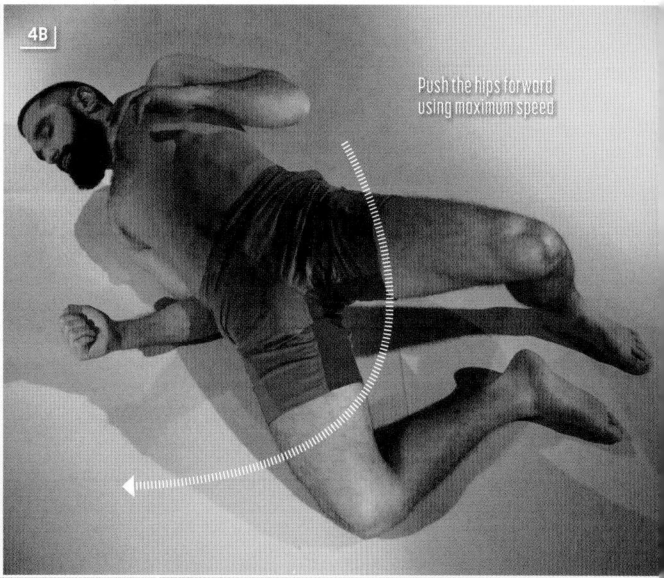
4B
Push the hips forward using maximum speed

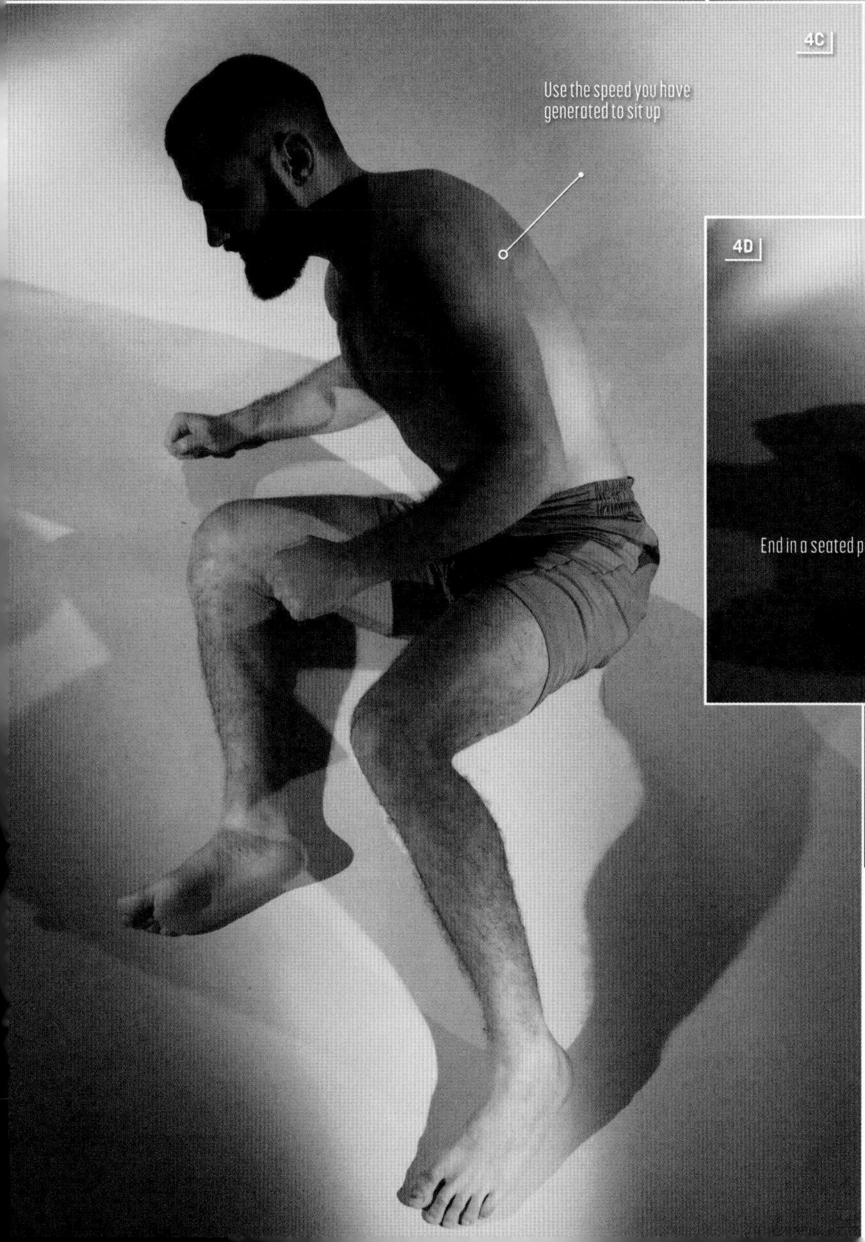
4C
Use the speed you have generated to sit up

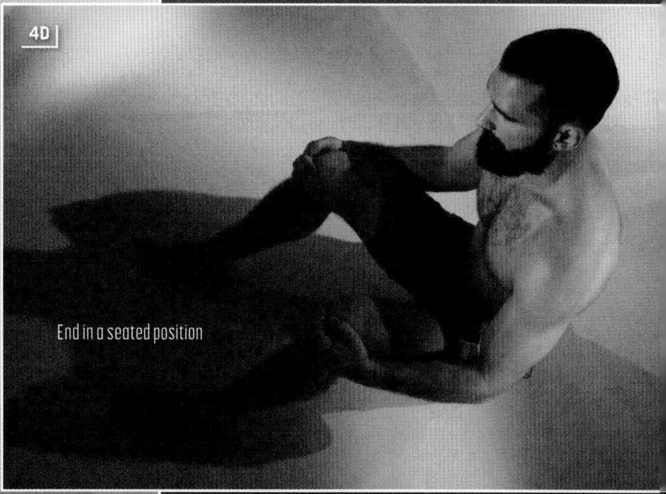
4D
End in a seated position

TABLE 2
SERIES

1A

Table movements done in a square have application to many exercises. Here is another series with a starting position that is more focused on lengthening the posterior chain (i.e., back straight and feet flat on the floor).

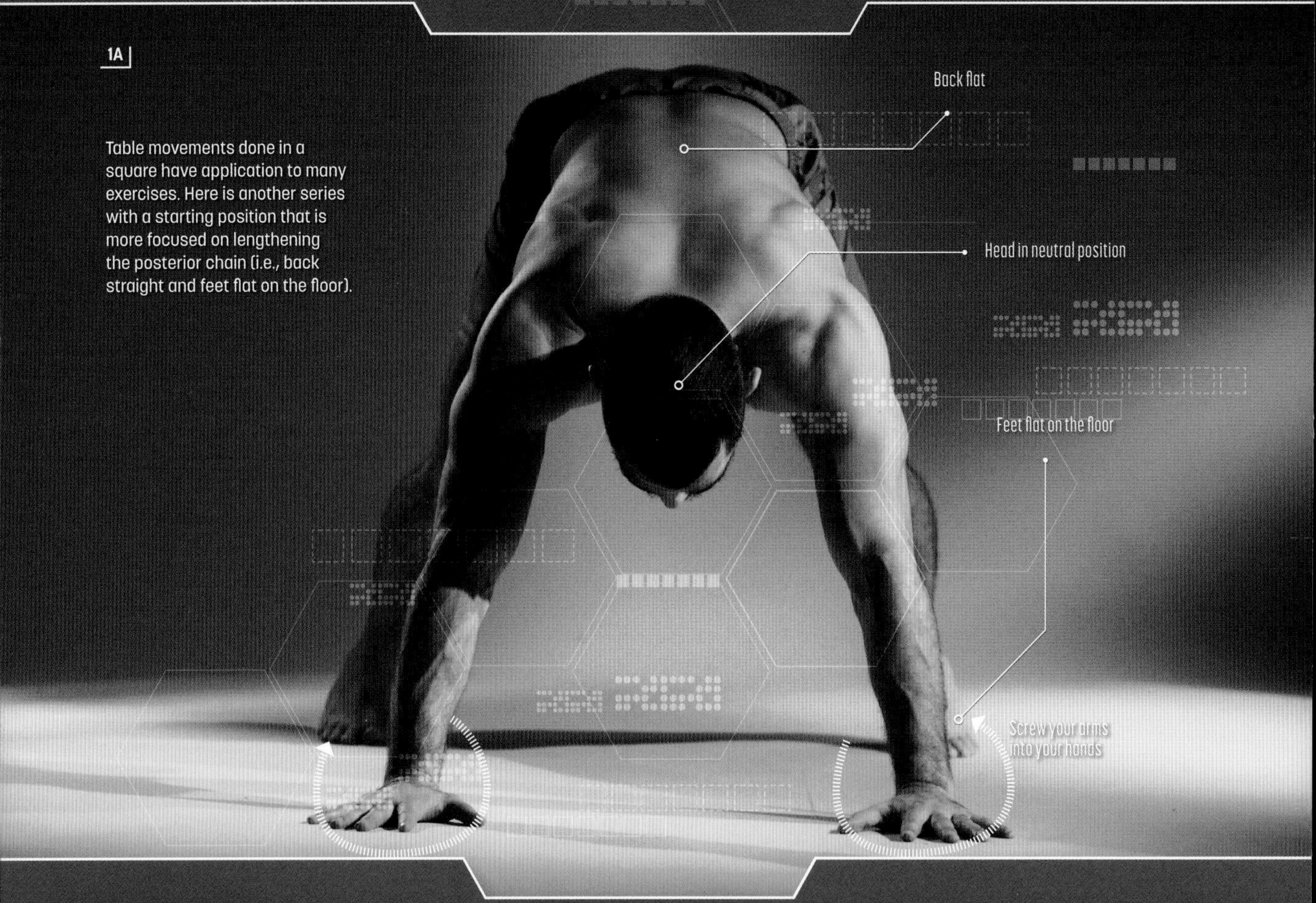

1B'

Do not change the position of your hands

1C'

The position of the foot does not change, but it does pivot upon itself to allow the torso to rotate to the side

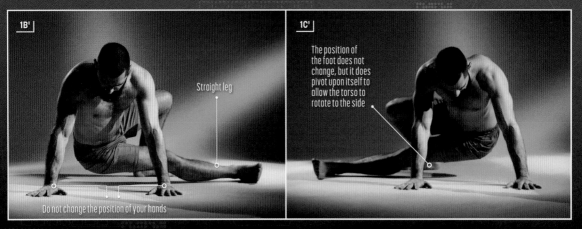

In this version, you will not end your movement in a square. You will simply divide the square movement diagonally and then move your back supports perpendicularly to the original axis so you can shift and return to the raised all-fours position.

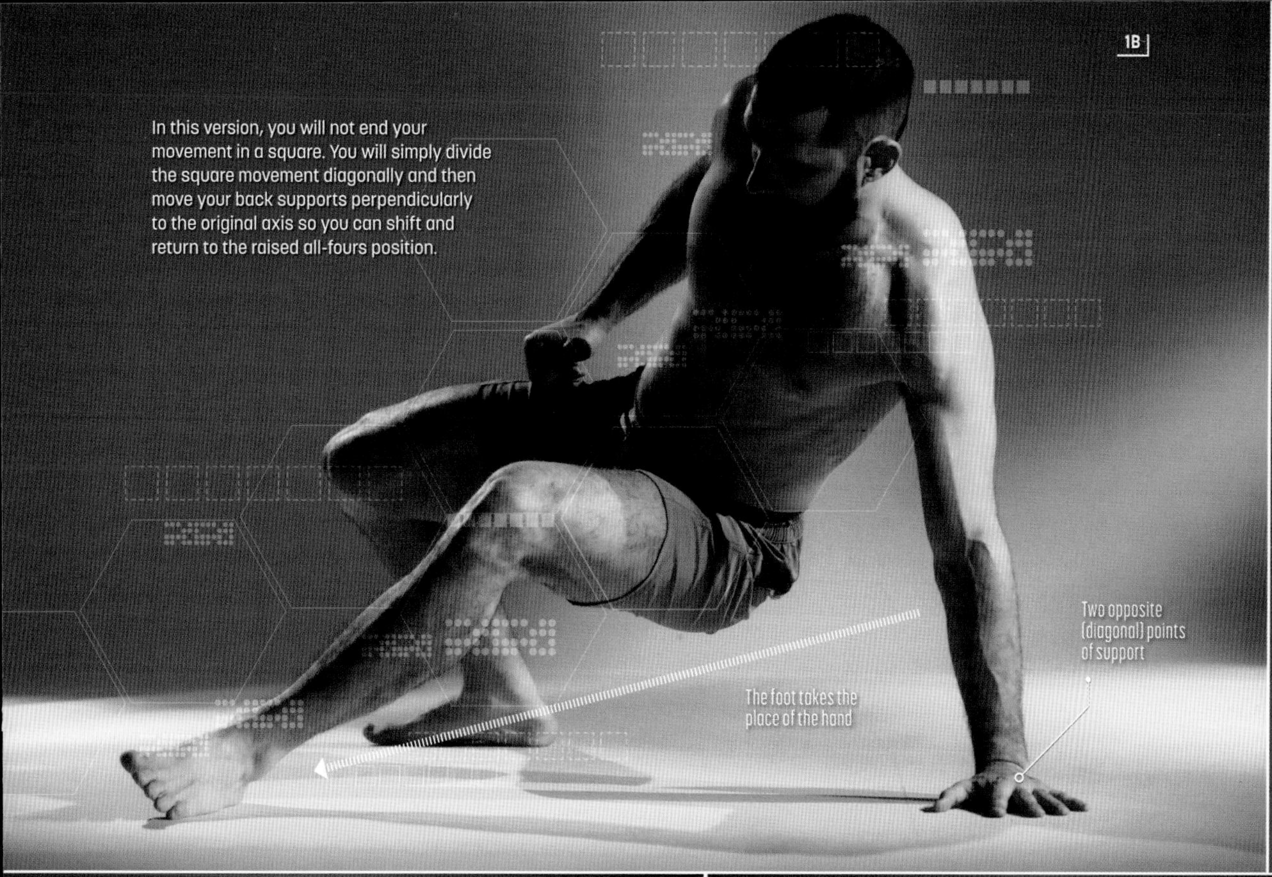

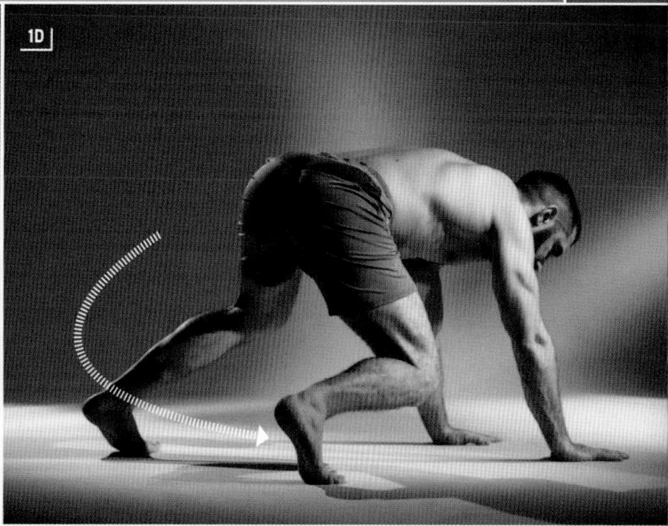

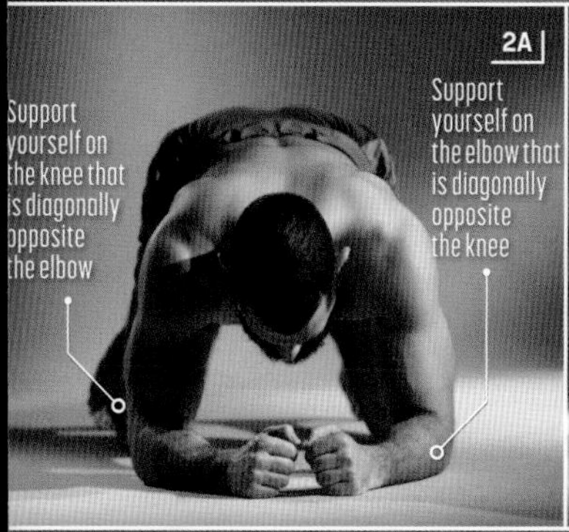

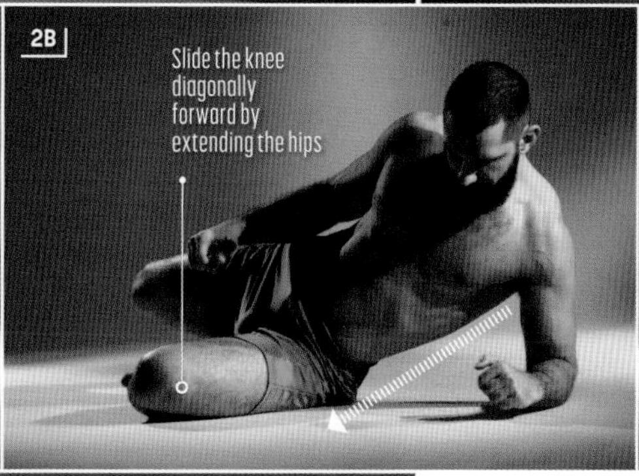

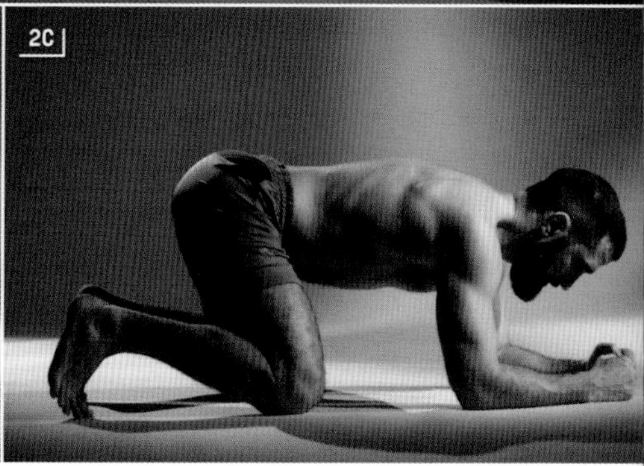

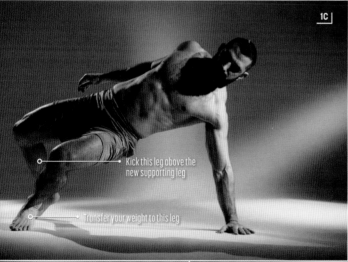

1B
Two opposite (diagonal) points of support
The foot takes the place of the hand

1C
Kick this leg above the new supporting leg
Transfer your weight to this leg

1D

2A
Support yourself on the knee that is diagonally opposite the elbow
Support yourself on the elbow that is diagonally opposite the knee

2B
Slide the knee diagonally forward by extending the hips

2C

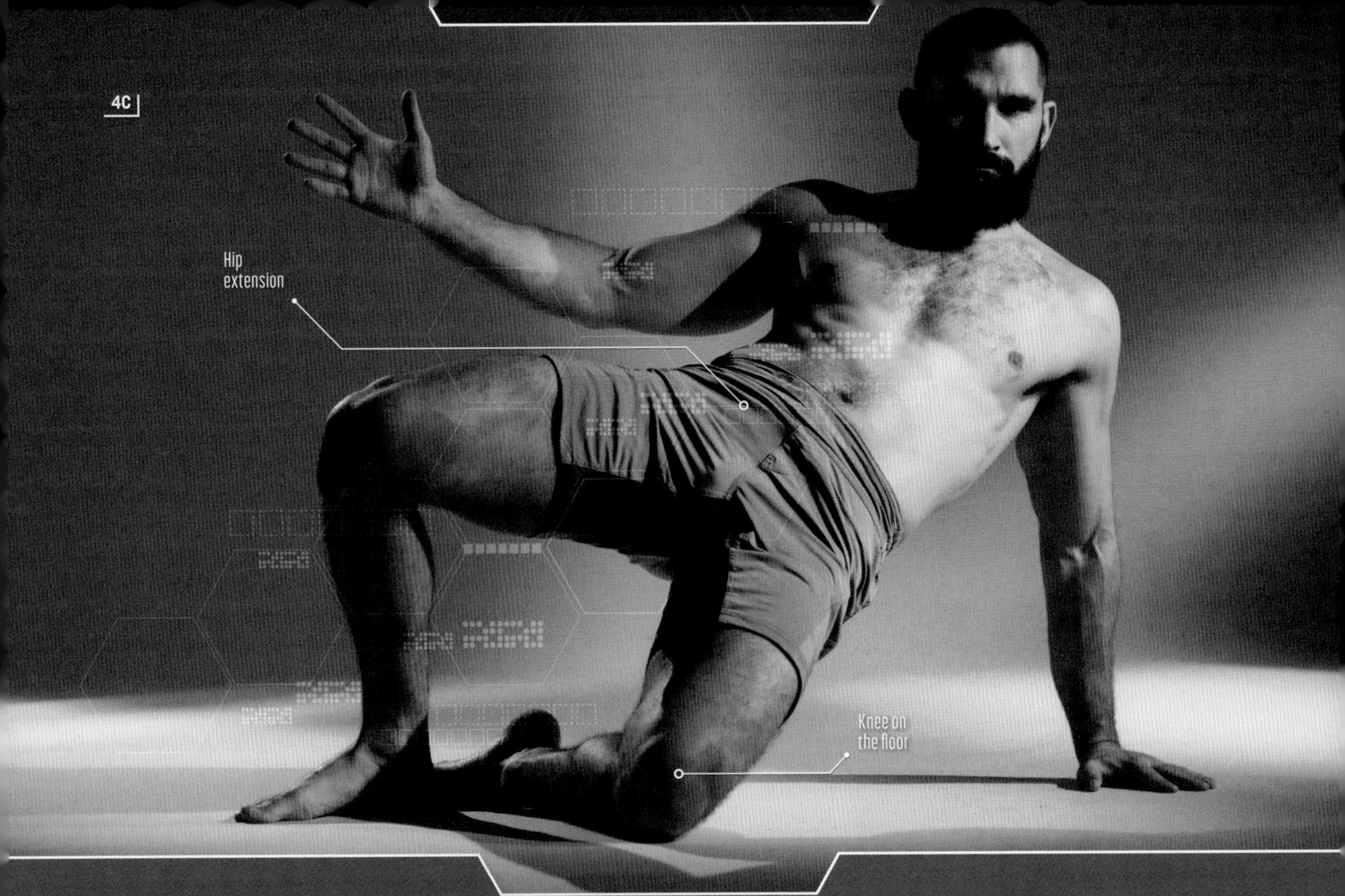
4C
Hip extension
Knee on the floor

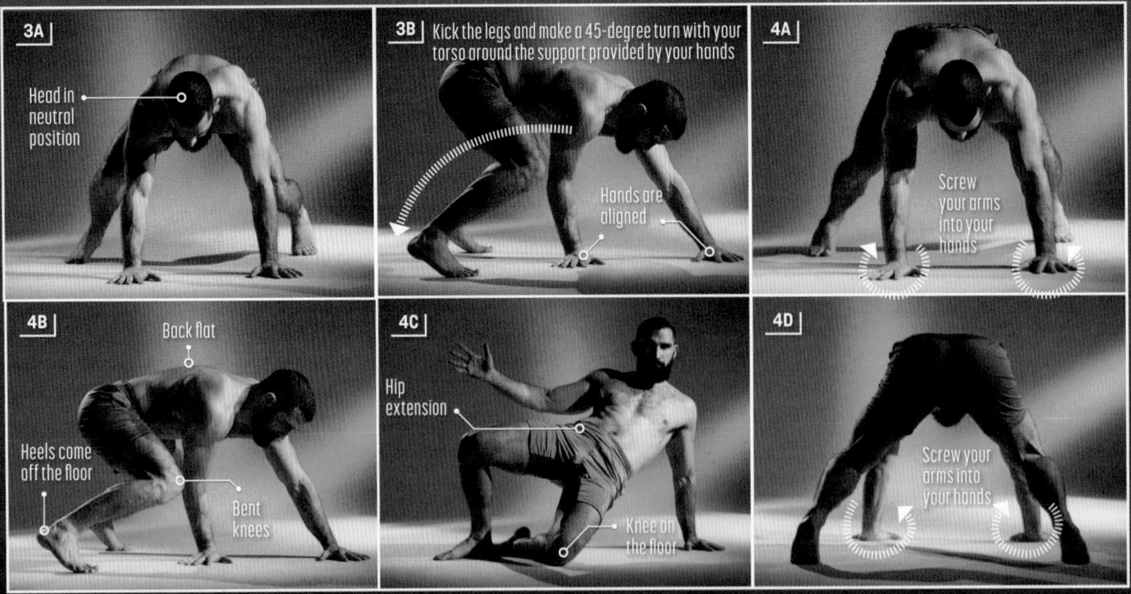
3A
Head in neutral position
3B
Kick the legs and make a 45-degree turn with your torso around the support provided by your hands
Hands are aligned
4A
Screw your arms into your hands
4B
Back flat
Heels come off the floor
Bent knees
4C
Hip extension
Knee on the floor
4D
Screw your arms into your hands

BUTTERFLY AND SIDE ROLL
SERIES

This exercise, which is used to teach children how to roll, is particularly useful for maintaining the health of the hips and dynamic flexibility in the posterior chain. From the initial butterfly position, get ready to roll in all directions.

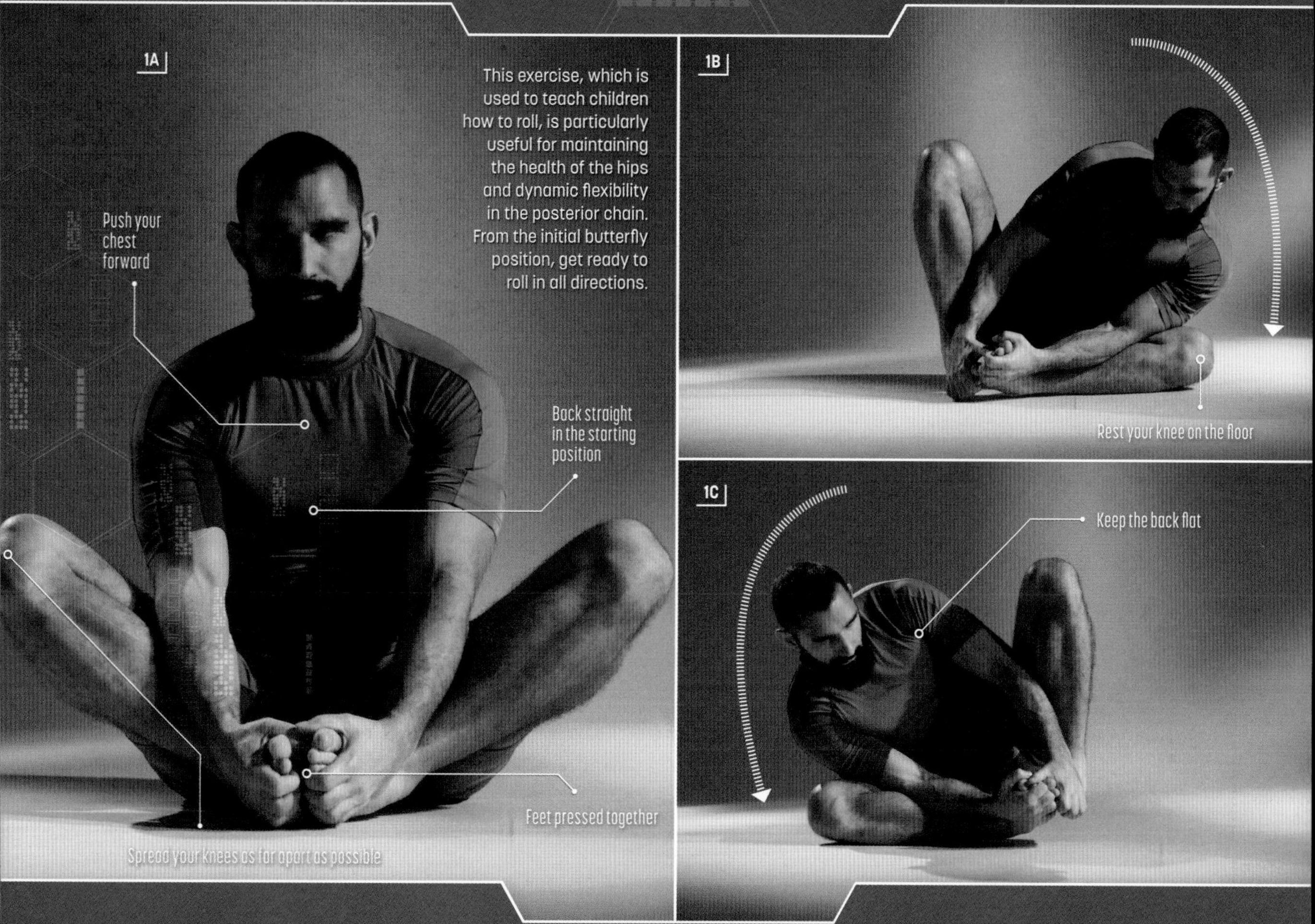
1A
Push your chest forward
Back straight in the starting position
Feet pressed together
Spread your knees as far apart as possible
1B
Rest your knee on the floor
1C
Keep the back flat

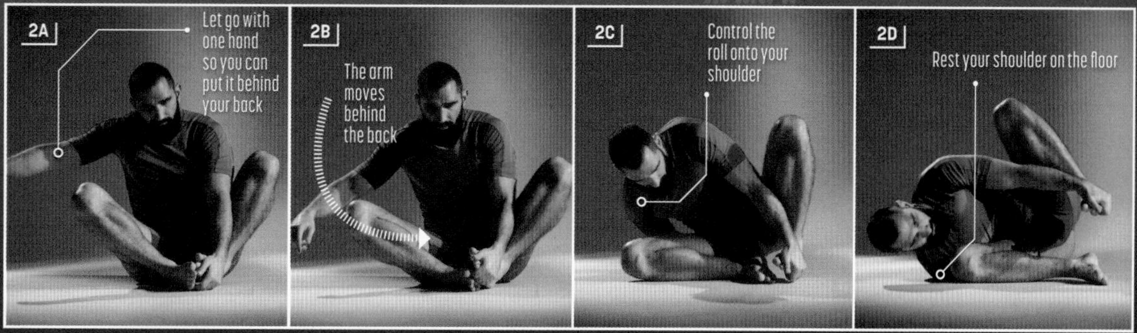
2A
Let go with one hand so you can put it behind your back
2B
The arm moves behind the back
2C
Control the roll onto your shoulder
2D
Rest your shoulder on the floor

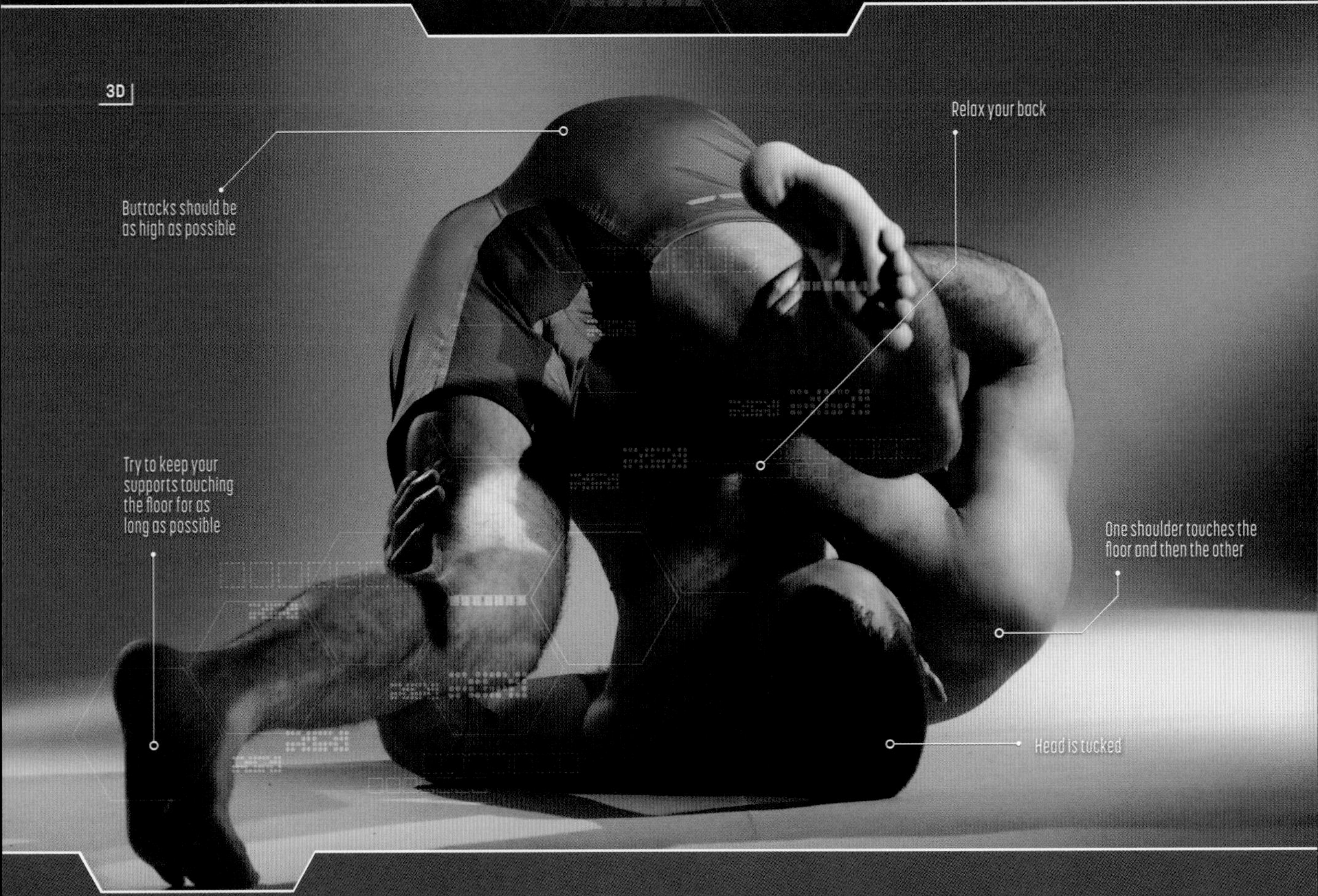
3D
Buttocks should be as high as possible
Relax your back
Try to keep your supports touching the floor for as long as possible
One shoulder touches the floor and then the other
Head is tucked

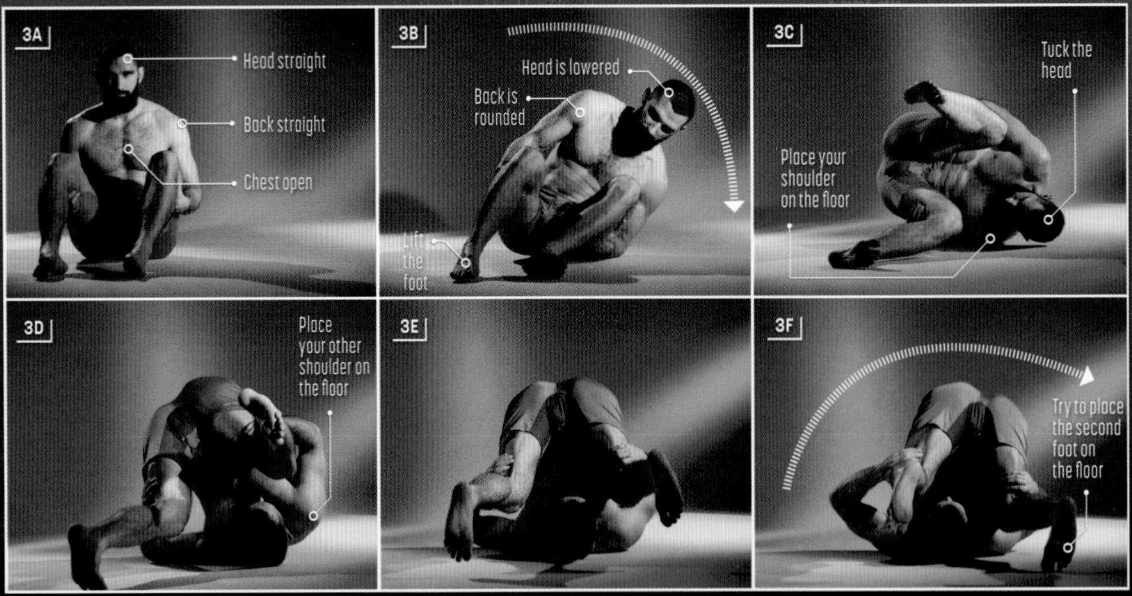
3A
Head straight
Back straight
Chest open
3B
Head is lowered
Back is rounded
Lift the foot
3C
Tuck the head
Place your shoulder on the floor
3D
Place your other shoulder on the floor
3E
3F
Try to place the second foot on the floor

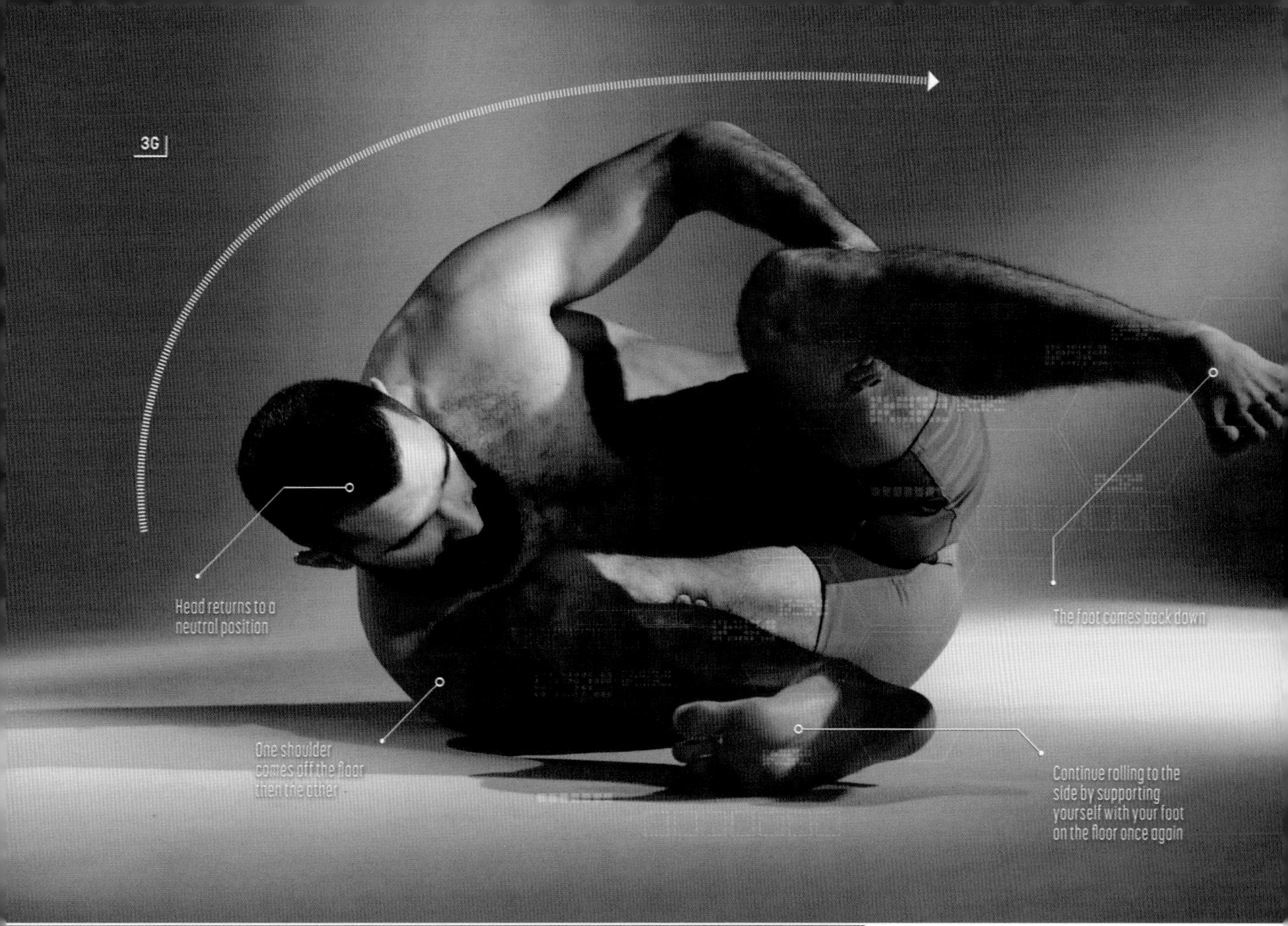
3G
Head returns to a neutral position
The foot comes back down
One shoulder comes off the floor then the other
Continue rolling to the side by supporting yourself with your foot on the floor once again

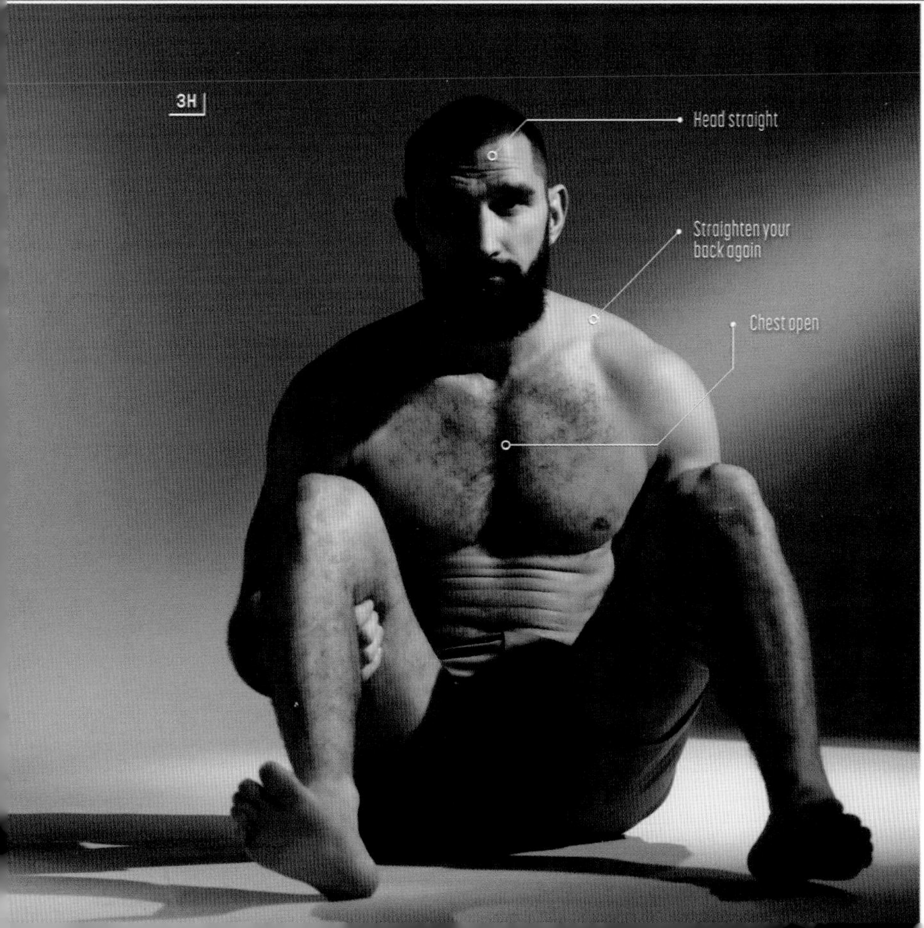
3H
Head straight
Straighten your back again
Chest open

4A

From this seated position, you can achieve a profound and dynamic flexion of the torso and neck as you do a complete rotation on your neck. From the opposite side to which you will be turning, place one point of support on the floor (try not to remove this base of support at all during the exercise). Gently rest your shoulder on the floor, tuck your head, and roll on your neck around the anchor point of your supporting foot.

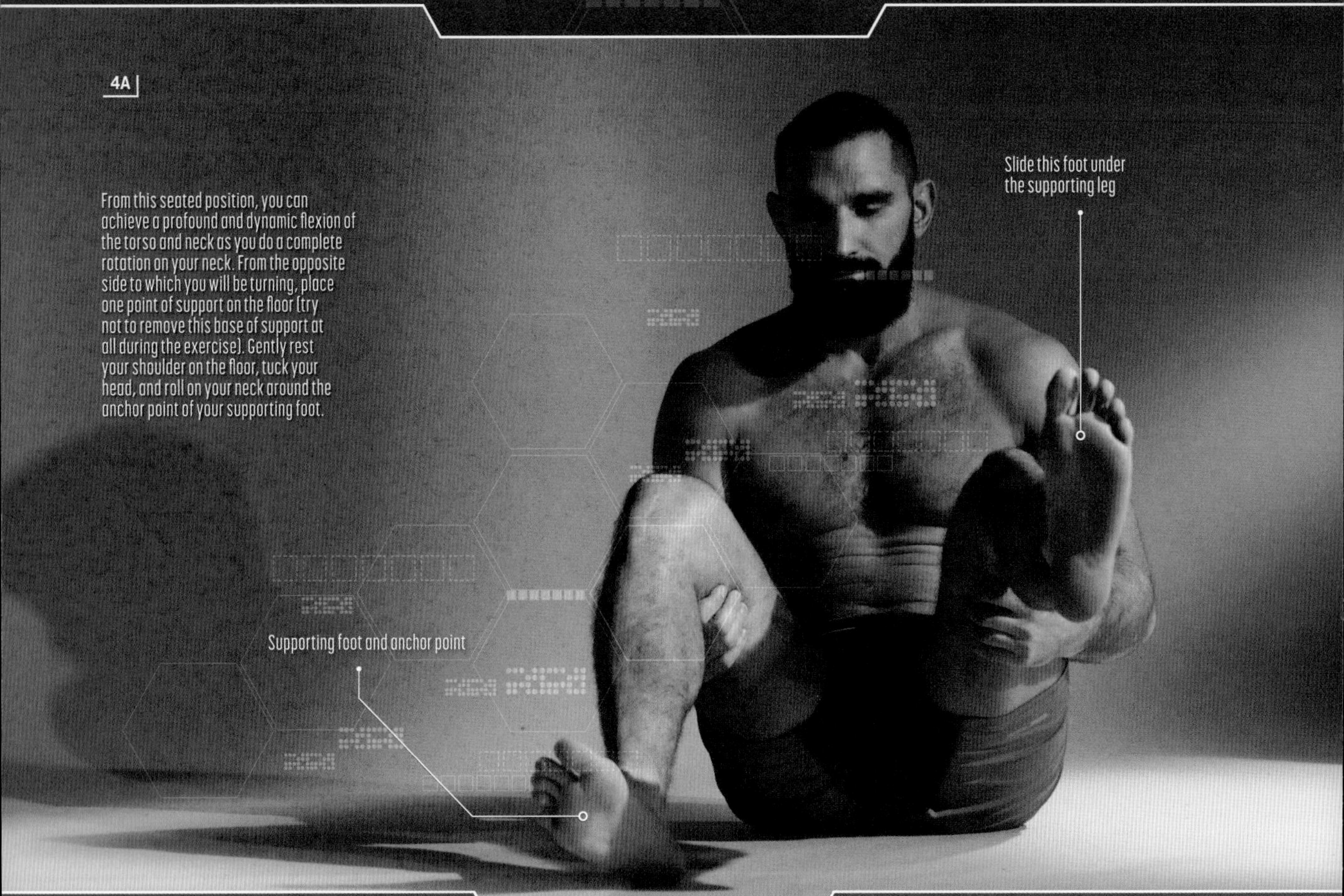

Slide this foot under the supporting leg
Supporting foot and anchor point

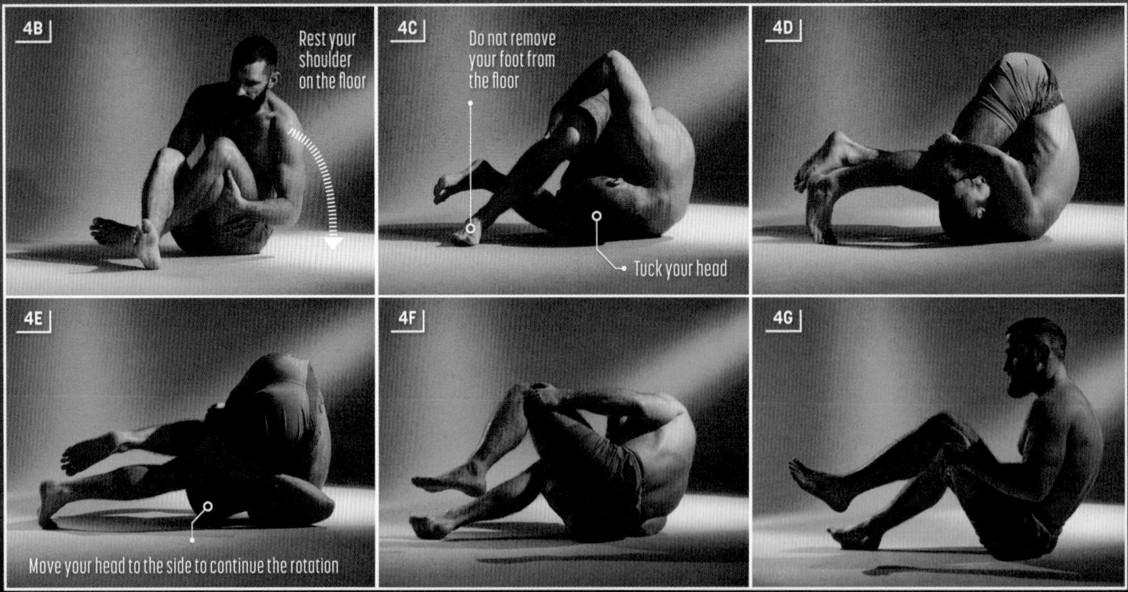

4B
Rest your shoulder on the floor
4C
Do not remove your foot from the floor
Tuck your head
4D
4E
Move your head to the side to continue the rotation
4F
4G

5B

Once you have learned the previous side roll sequence, you can use variations of the starting position. You can do the side roll from the starting position of this series in the butterfly position, but you can also try to roll forward and backward, systematically returning to the butterfly position, which is effective for maintaining the health of the hips.

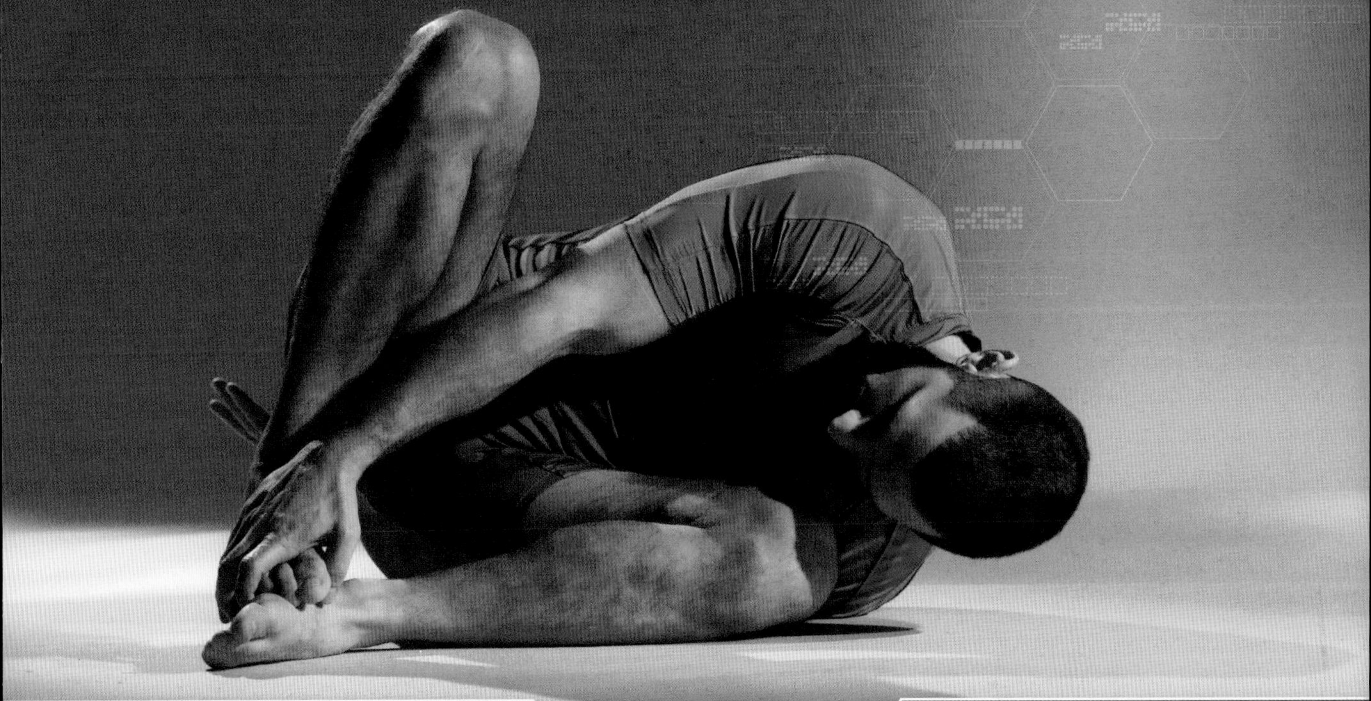

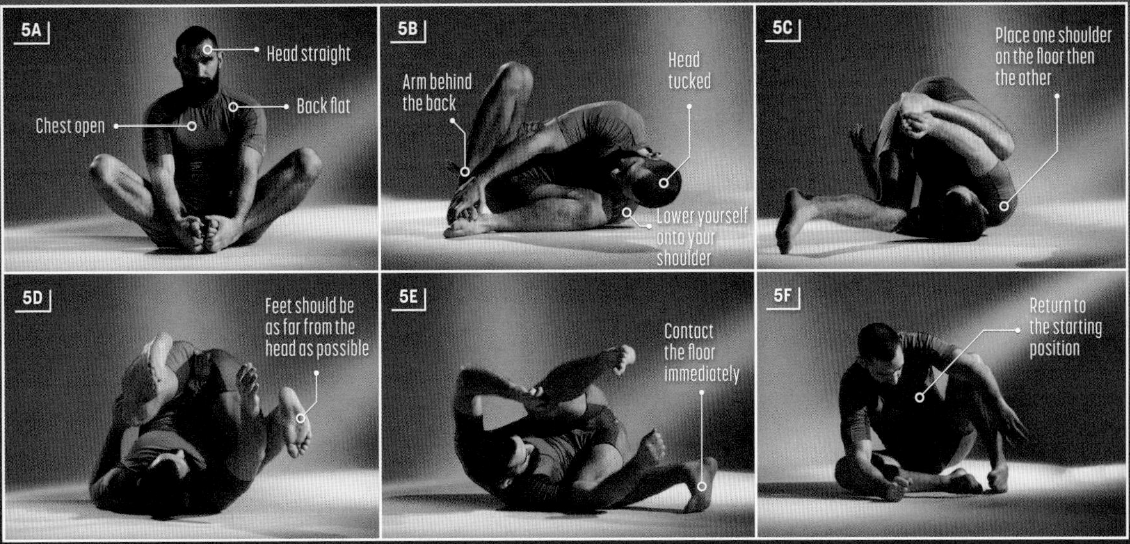

5A
Head straight
Back flat
Chest open
5B
Arm behind the back
Head tucked
Lower yourself onto your shoulder
5C
Place one shoulder on the floor then the other
5D
Feet should be as far from the head as possible
5E
Contact the floor immediately
5F
Return to the starting position

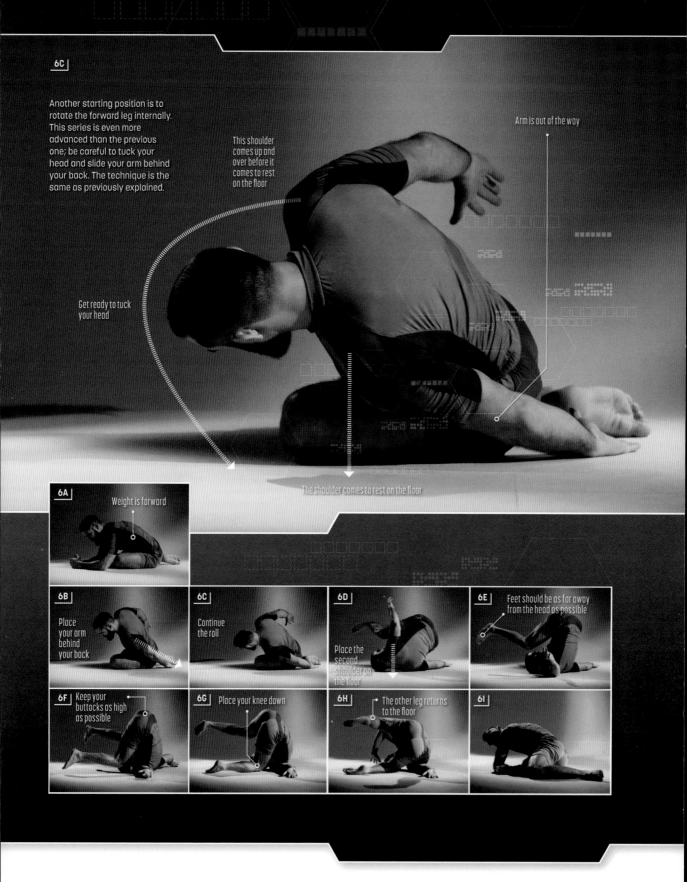

6C

Another starting position is to rotate the forward leg internally. This series is even more advanced than the previous one; be careful to tuck your head and slide your arm behind your back. The technique is the same as previously explained.

This shoulder comes up and over before it comes to rest on the floor
Arm is out of the way
Get ready to tuck your head
The shoulder comes to rest on the floor

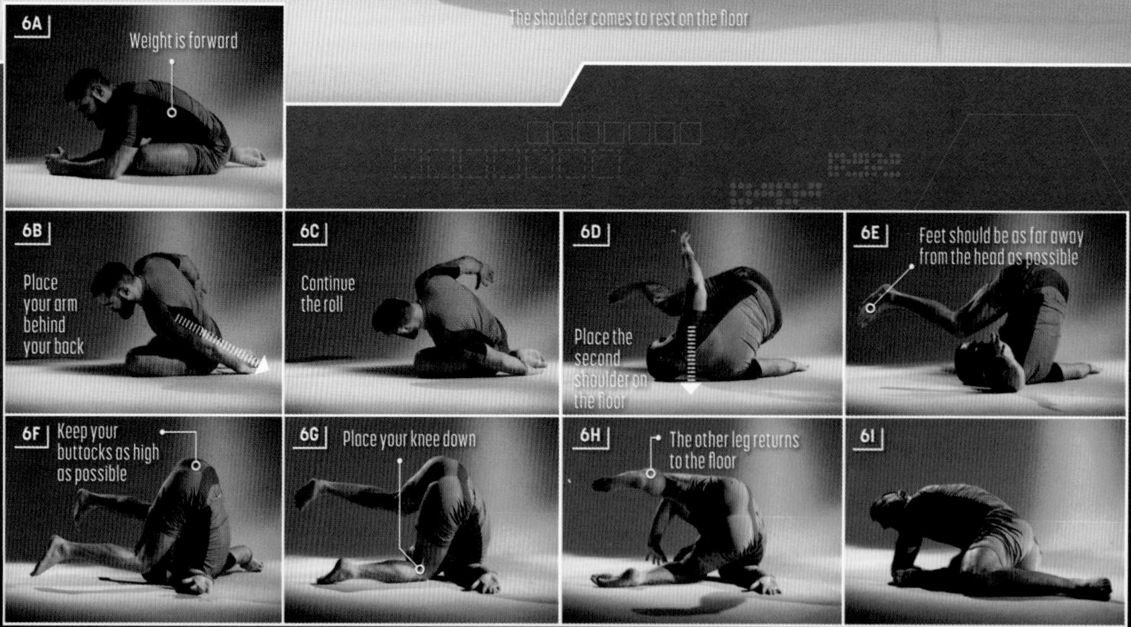

6A
Weight is forward
6B
Place your arm behind your back
6C
Continue the roll
6D
Place the second shoulder on the floor
6E
Feet should be as far away from the head as possible
6F
Keep your buttocks as high as possible
6G
Place your knee down
6H
The other leg returns to the floor
6I

The most complex level of this series begins with you on your back. It uses the shrimp position to promote mobility in the neck. More than ever, you will rely on diagonal support to perform this exercise and maintain your initial support using your foot as a permanent anchor point.

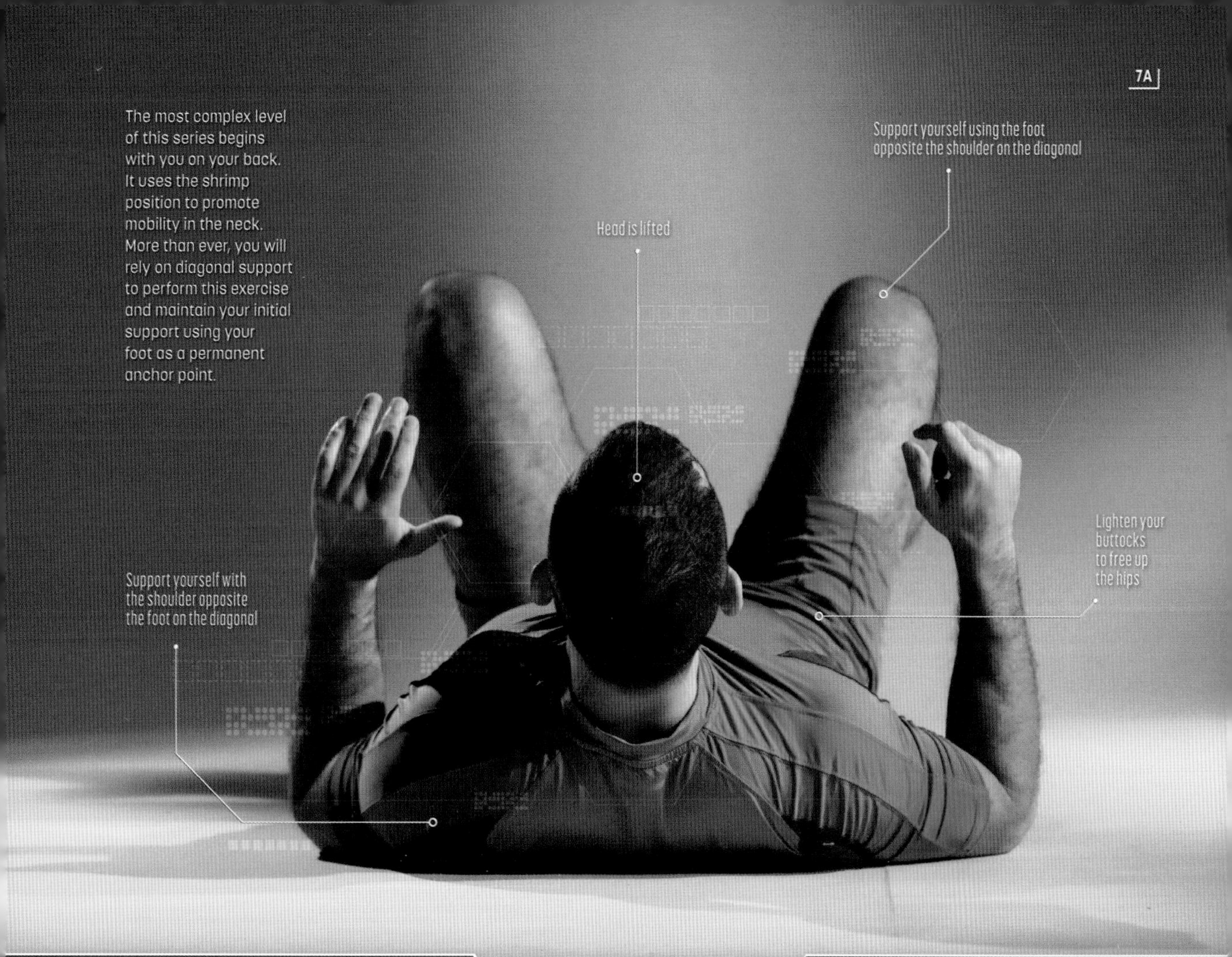

7A
Support yourself using the foot opposite the shoulder on the diagonal
Head is lifted
Lighten your buttocks to free up the hips
Support yourself with the shoulder opposite the foot on the diagonal

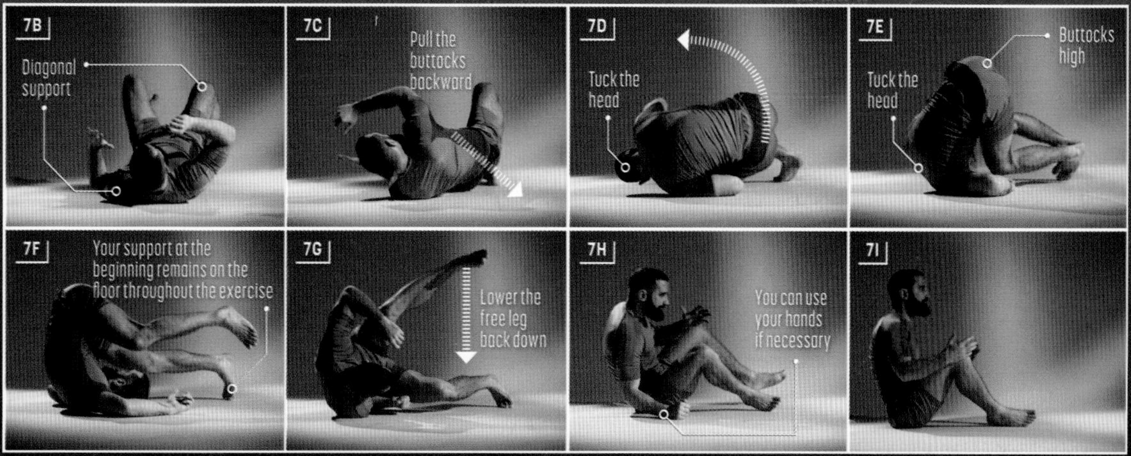

7B
Diagonal support
7C
Pull the buttocks backward
7D
Tuck the head
7E
Buttocks high
Tuck the head
7F
Your support at the beginning remains on the floor throughout the exercise
7G
Lower the free leg back down
7H
You can use your hands if necessary
7I

SQUAT LEVEL 1
SERIES

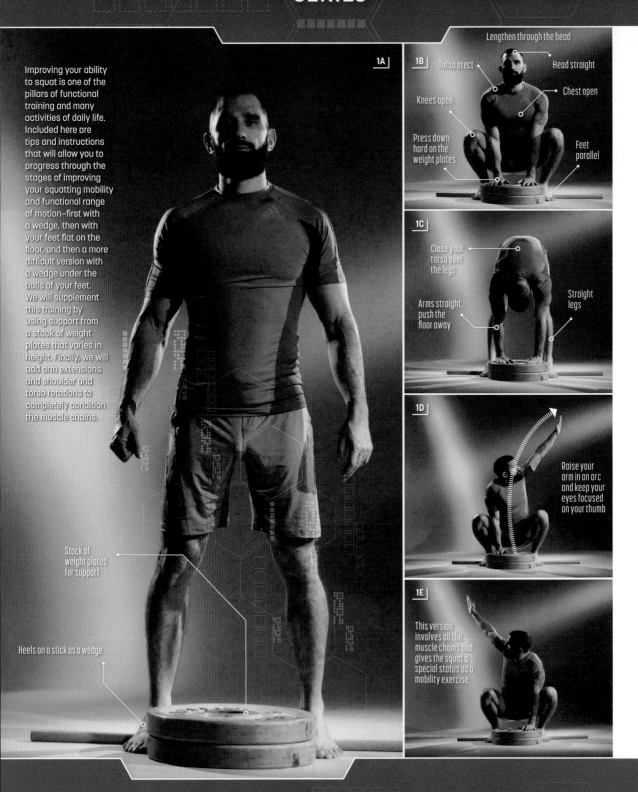

Improving your ability to squat is one of the pillars of functional training and many activities of daily life. Included here are tips and instructions that will allow you to progress through the stages of improving your squatting mobility and functional range of motion—first with a wedge, then with your feet flat on the floor, and then a more difficult version with a wedge under the balls of your feet. We will supplement this training by using support from a stack of weight plates that varies in height. Finally, we will add arm extensions and shoulder and torso rotations to completely condition the muscle chains.

1A
Stack of weight plates for support
Heels on a stick as a wedge

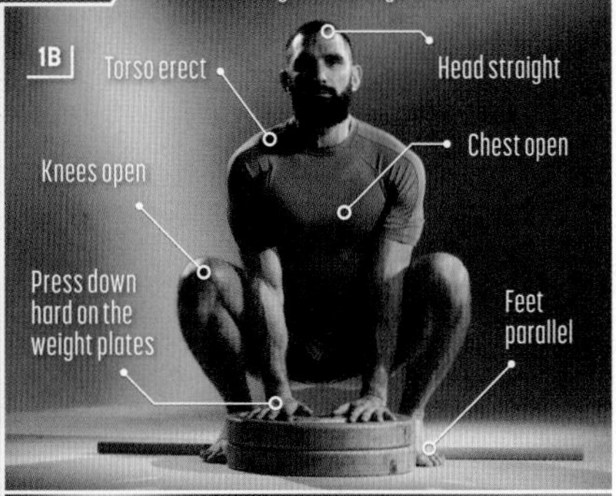

1B
Lengthen through the head
Torso erect
Head straight
Chest open
Knees open
Press down hard on the weight plates
Feet parallel

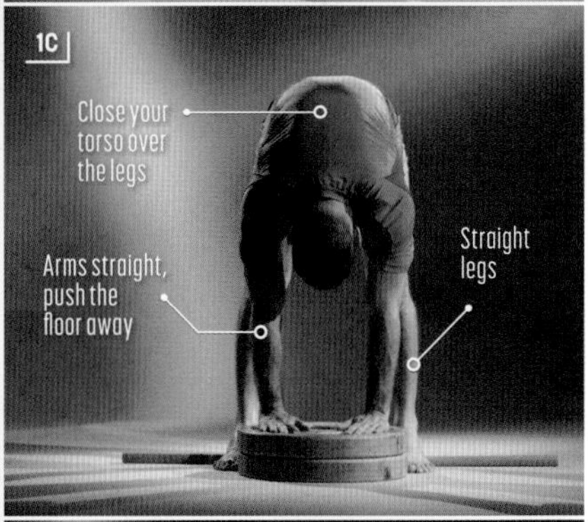

1C
Close your torso over the legs
Straight legs
Arms straight, push the floor away

1D
Raise your arm in an arc and keep your eyes focused on your thumb

1E
This version involves all the muscle chains and gives the squat a special status as a mobility exercise.

Version 2 is the same exercise but done with feet flat on the floor

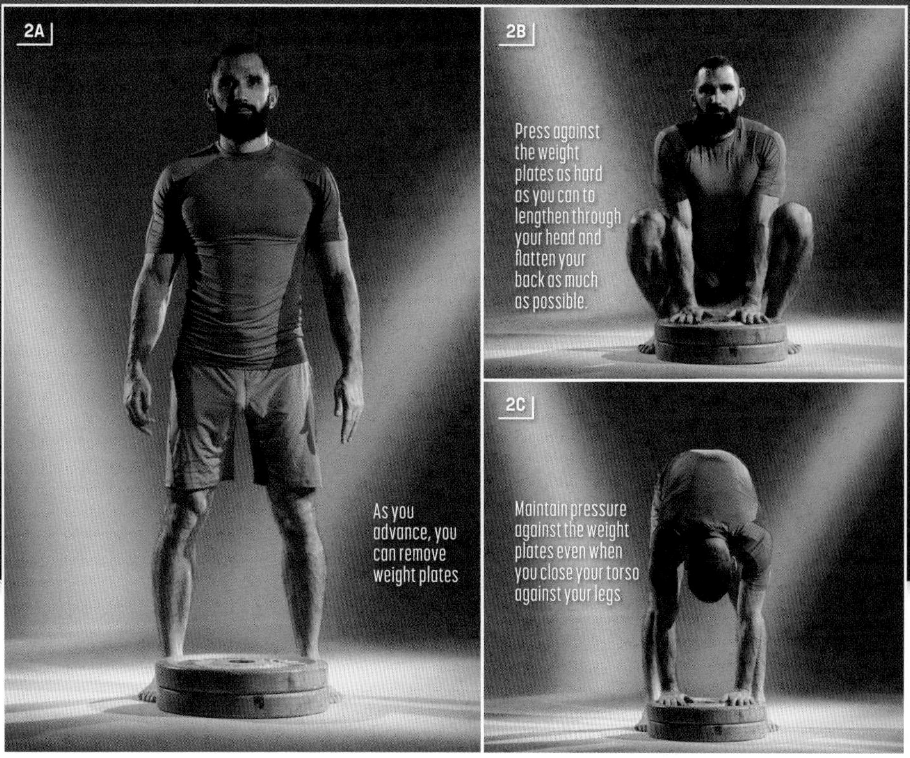

2A
As you advance, you can remove weight plates
2B
Press against the weight plates as hard as you can to lengthen through your head and flatten your back as much as possible.
2C
Maintain pressure against the weight plates even when you close your torso against your legs

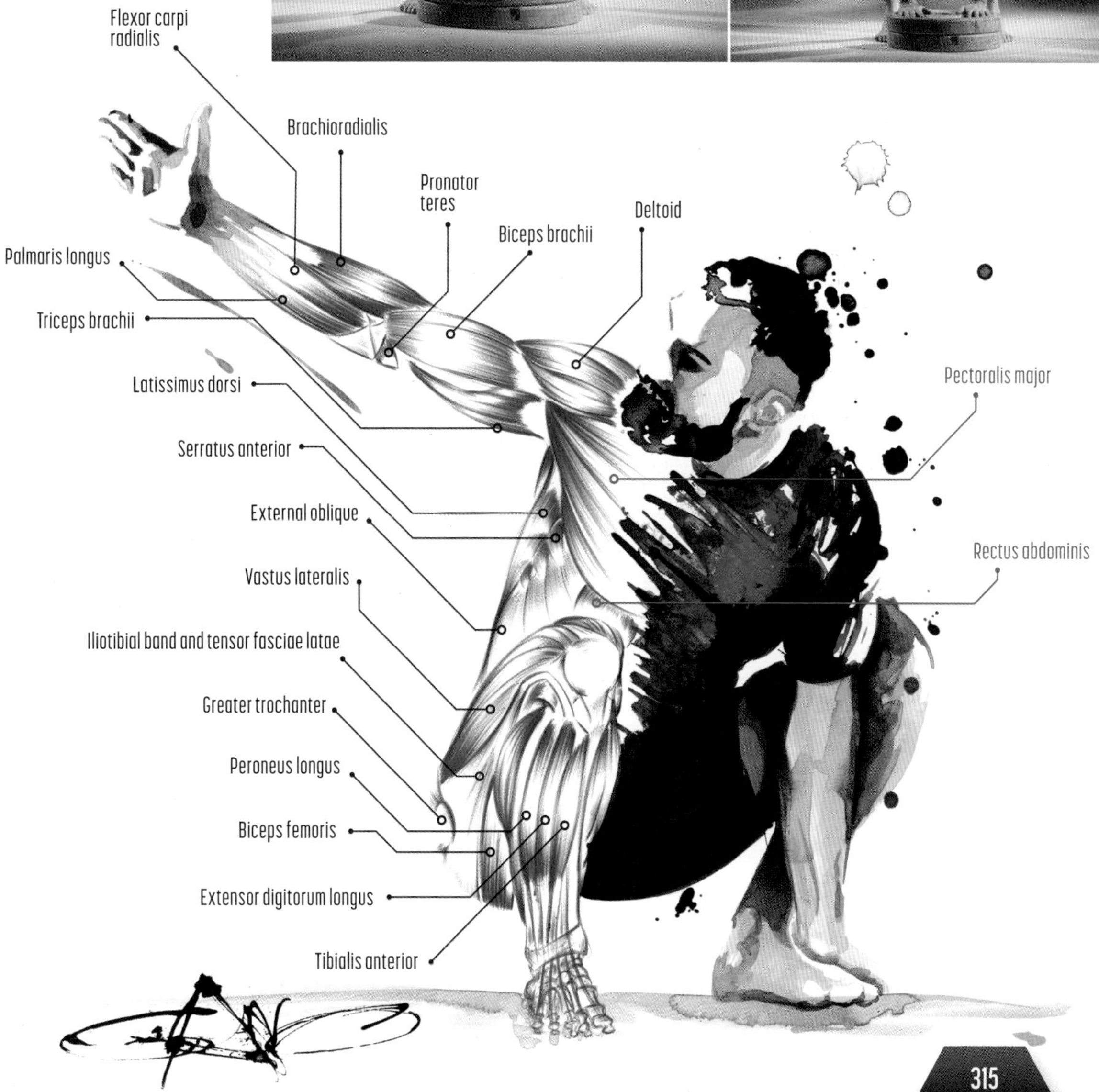

Varying the position of the wedge can make the exercise easier or harder.

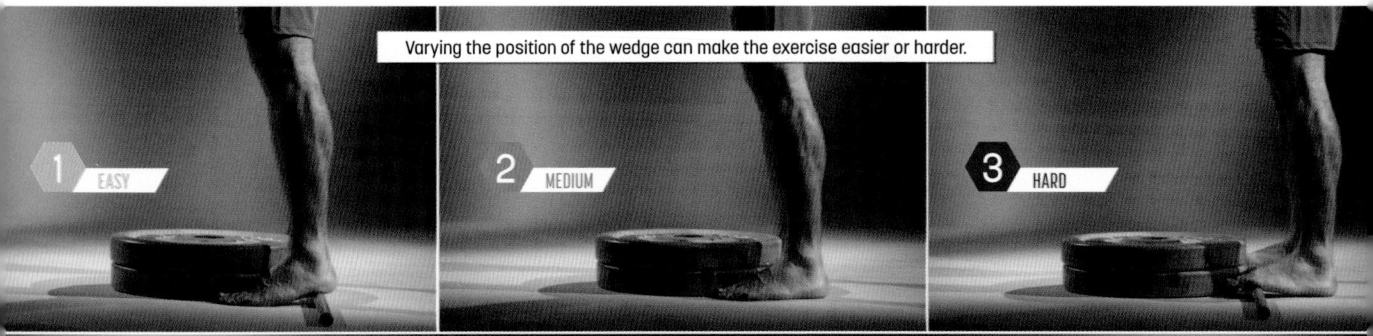
1 EASY
2 MEDIUM
3 HARD

3A

Once you are very comfortable in the bottom squatting position, you can add arm extensions to the movement. It is important to start off as compact as possible; keep your arms tightly pressed into your torso. When you are ready, extend them upward as far as you can without shifting your torso to compensate.

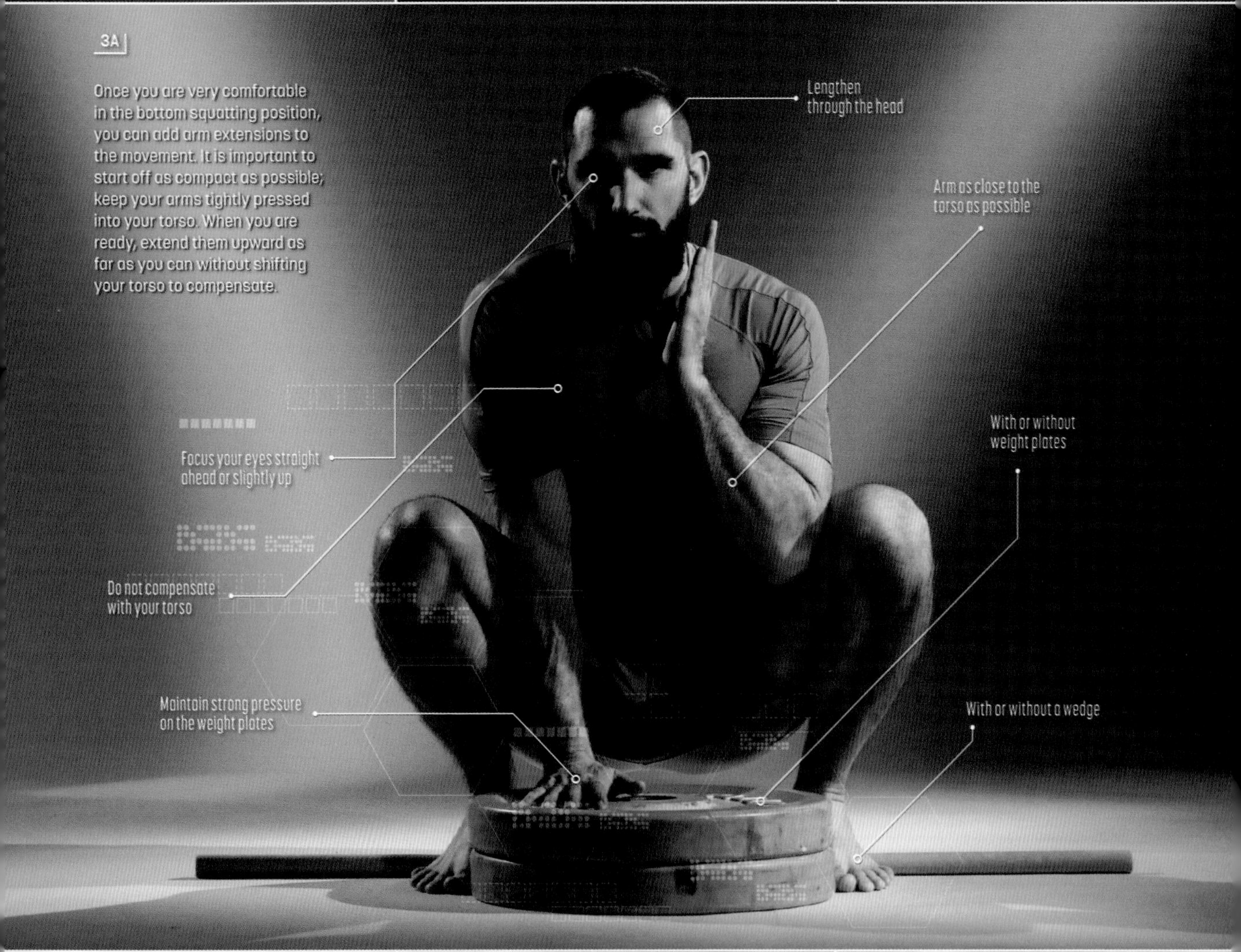
Lengthen through the head
Arm as close to the torso as possible
Focus your eyes straight ahead or slightly up
With or without weight plates
Do not compensate with your torso
Maintain strong pressure on the weight plates
With or without a wedge

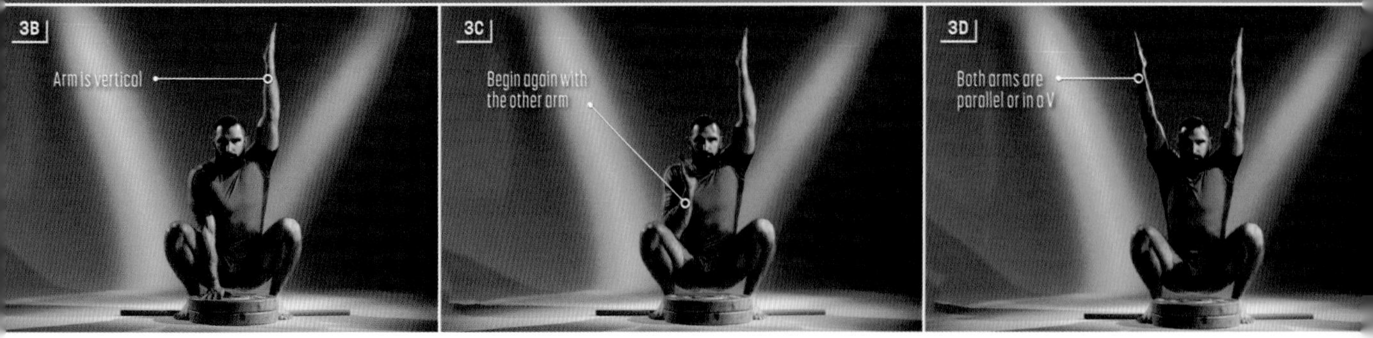
3B
Arm is vertical
3C
Begin again with the other arm
3D
Both arms are parallel or in a V

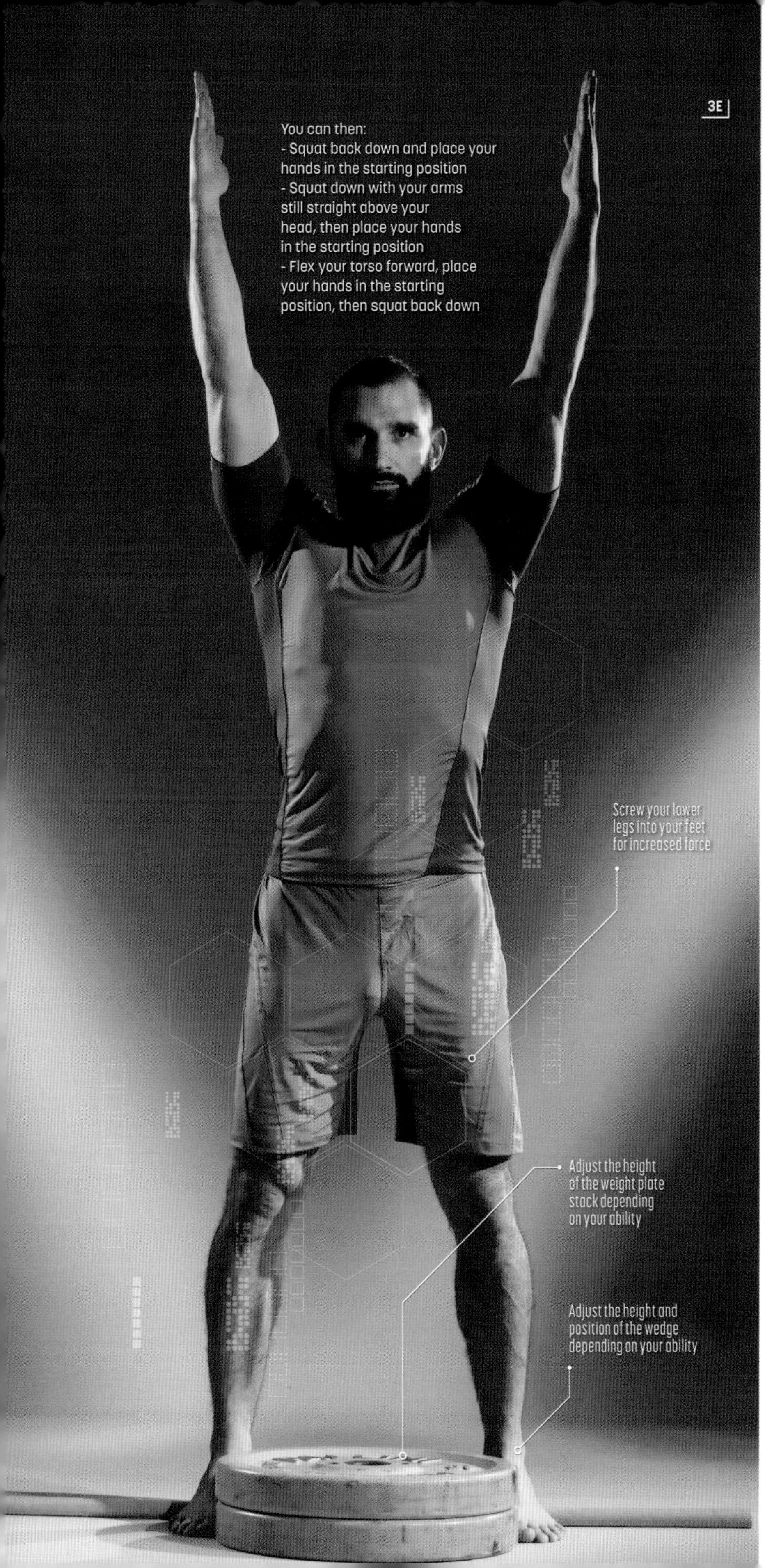
3E
Screw your lower legs into your feet for increased force
Adjust the height of the weight plate stack depending on your ability
Adjust the height and position of the wedge depending on your ability

You can then:
- Squat back down and place your hands in the starting position
- Squat down with your arms still straight above your head, then place your hands in the starting position
- Flex your torso forward, place your hands in the starting position, then squat back down

SQUAT LEVEL 2
SERIES

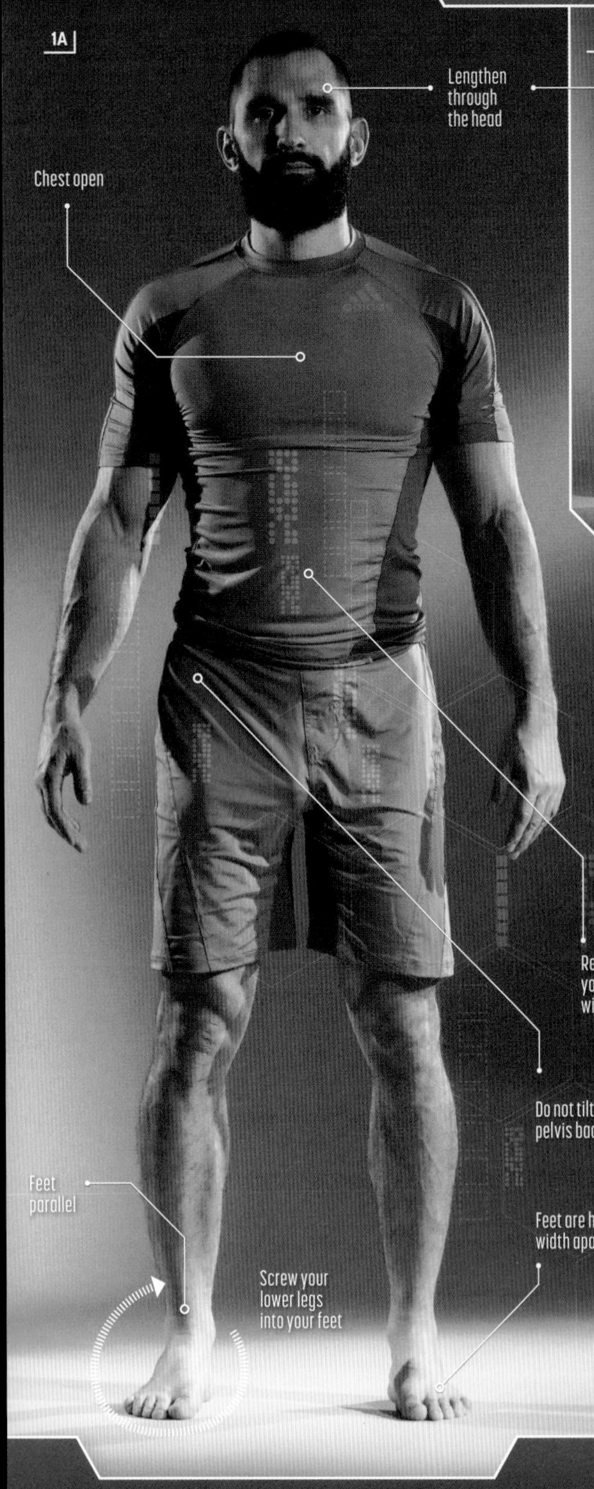
1A
Lengthen through the head
Chest open
Relax your stomach; you must breathe with your diaphragm
Do not tilt your pelvis backward
Feet parallel
Feet are hip-width apart
Screw your lower legs into your feet

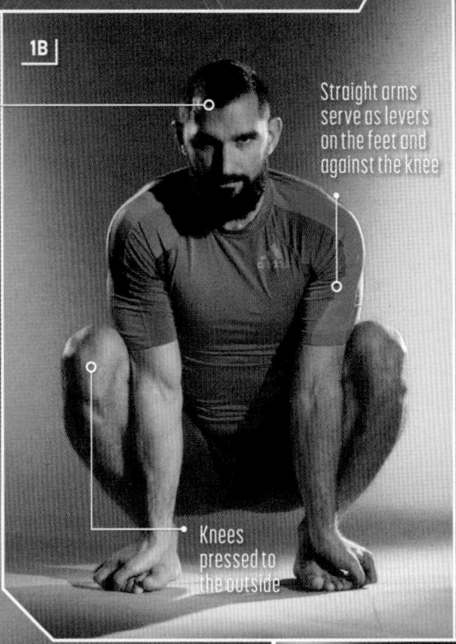
1B
Straight arms serve as levers on the feet and against the knee
Knees pressed to the outside

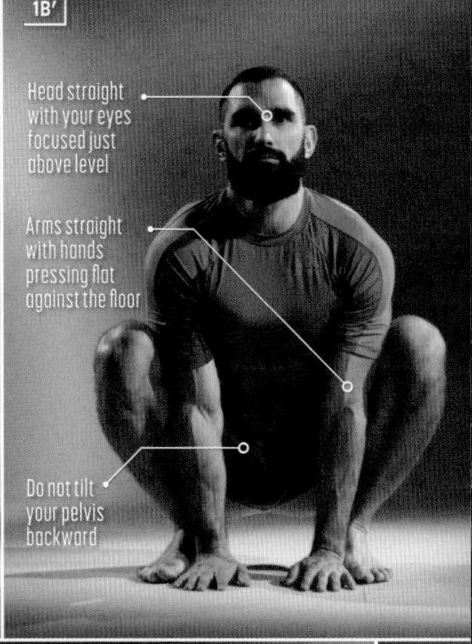
1B′
Head straight with your eyes focused just above level
Arms straight with hands pressing flat against the floor
Do not tilt your pelvis backward

If you are extremely comfortable with the first squat series progression, move to the next level. This is the advanced level with your feet firmly flat on the floor with no weight plate stack or wedge under the heels.

1C
Strong support on the floor
Avoid compensating with the legs

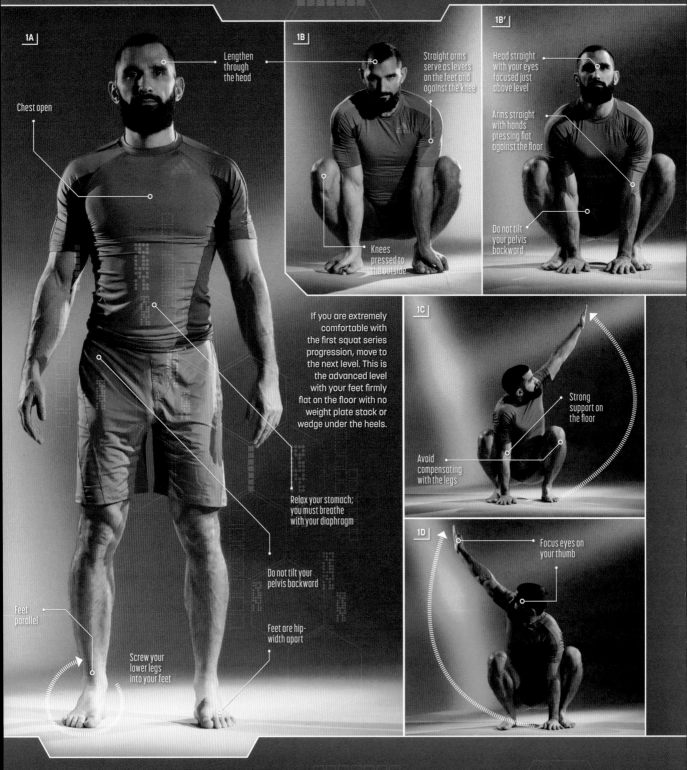

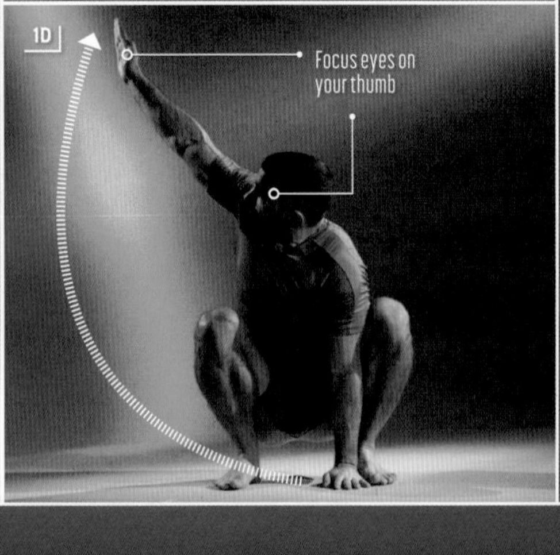
1D
Focus eyes on your thumb

This progression of the squat with the arms extended overhead is more difficult; you will use your arms as much as you can to push your knees toward the outside and support yourself on your arms to stretch your back to its maximum and to lengthen through your head. As in the other squat exercises, begin with parallel feet that are hip-width apart. Screw your lower legs into your feet and keep your back straight. Do not let your pelvis tilt backward.

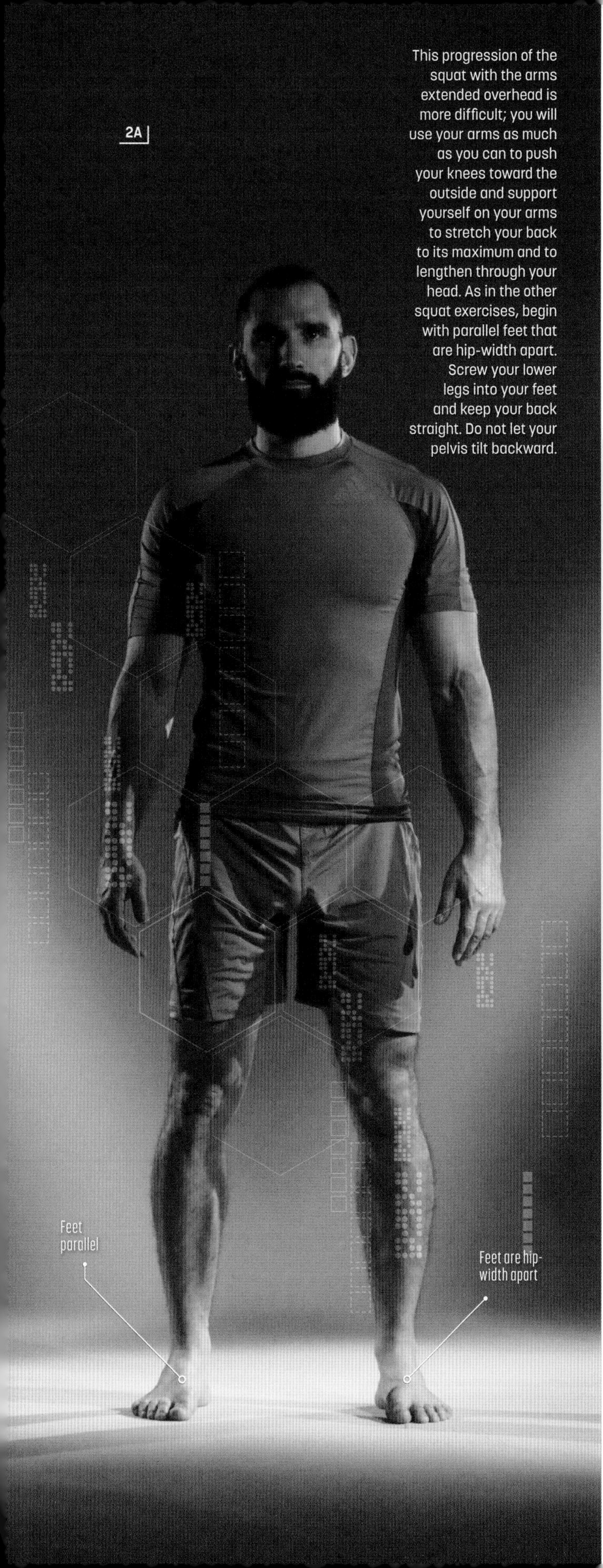
2A
Feet parallel
Feet are hip-width apart

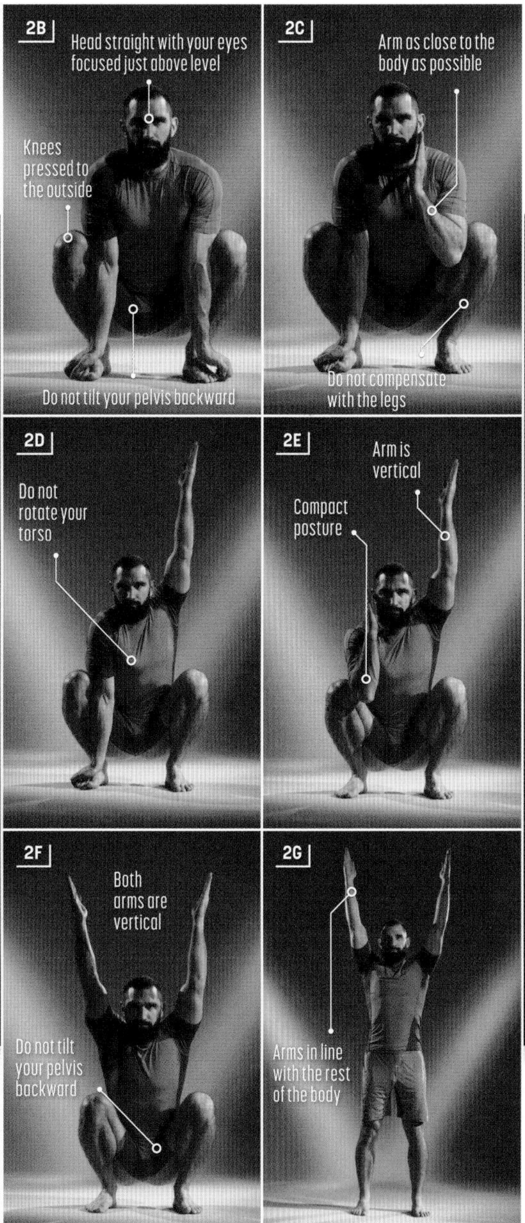
2B
Head straight with your eyes focused just above level
Knees pressed to the outside
Do not tilt your pelvis backward
2C
Arm as close to the body as possible
Do not compensate with the legs
2D
Do not rotate your torso
2E
Arm is vertical
Compact posture
2F
Both arms are vertical
Do not tilt your pelvis backward
2G
Arms in line with the rest of the body

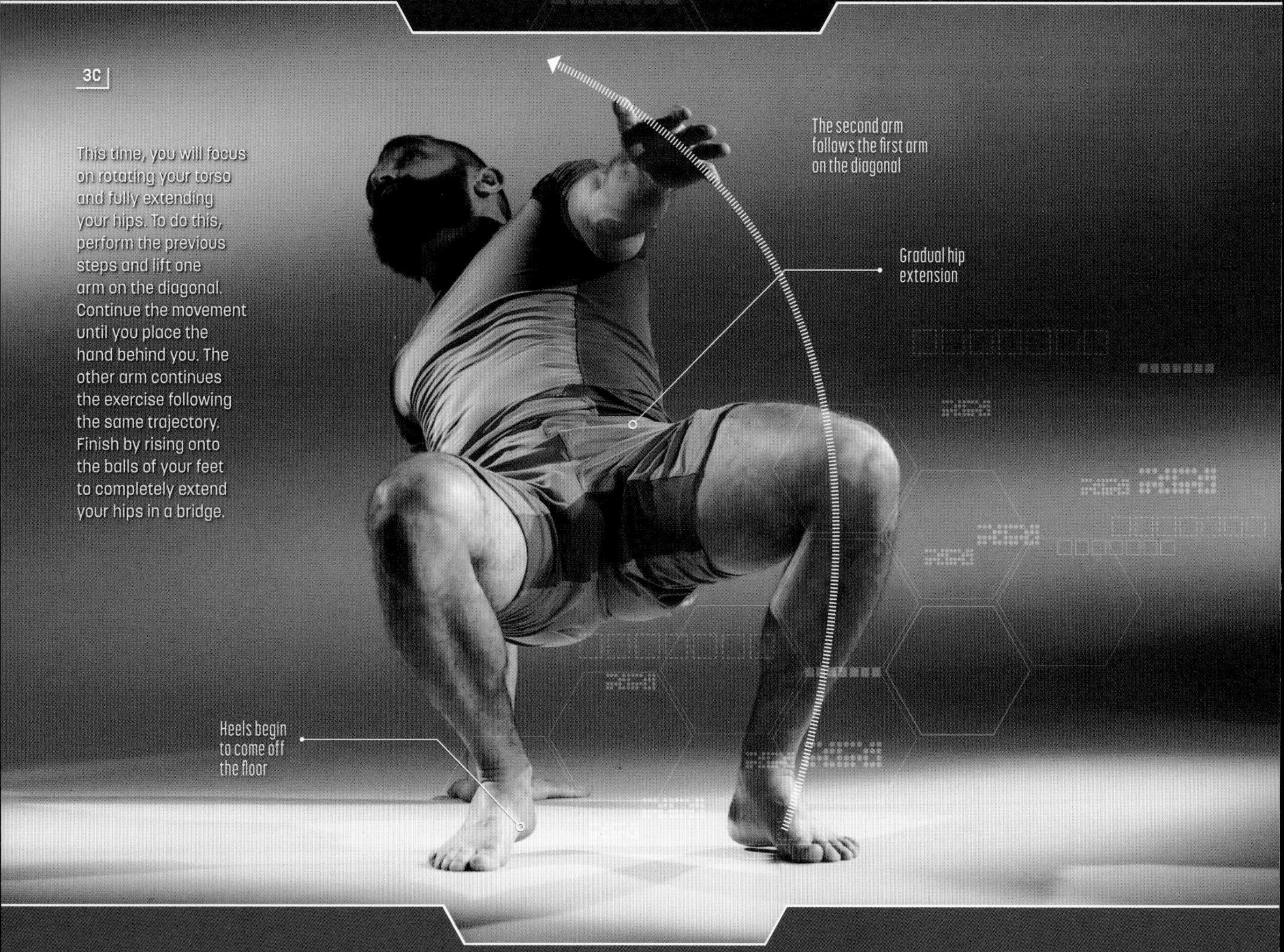
3C
The second arm follows the first arm on the diagonal
Gradual hip extension
Heels begin to come off the floor

This time, you will focus on rotating your torso and fully extending your hips. To do this, perform the previous steps and lift one arm on the diagonal. Continue the movement until you place the hand behind you. The other arm continues the exercise following the same trajectory. Finish by rising onto the balls of your feet to completely extend your hips in a bridge.

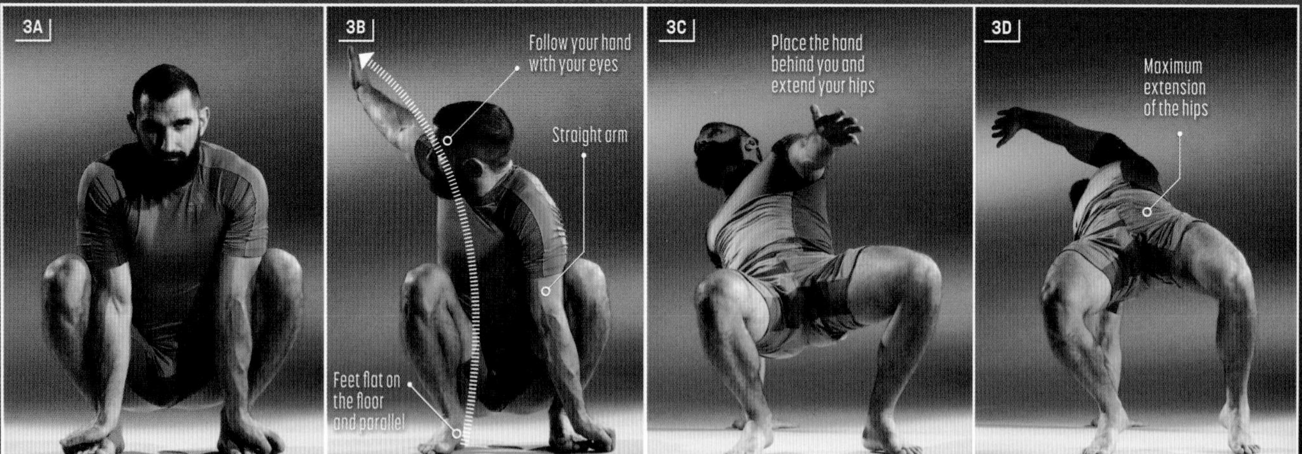
3A
3B
Follow your hand with your eyes
Straight arm
Feet flat on the floor and parallel
3C
Place the hand behind you and extend your hips
3D
Maximum extension of the hips

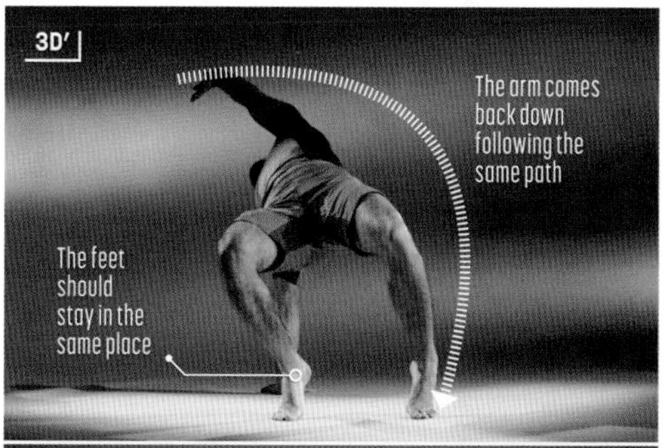

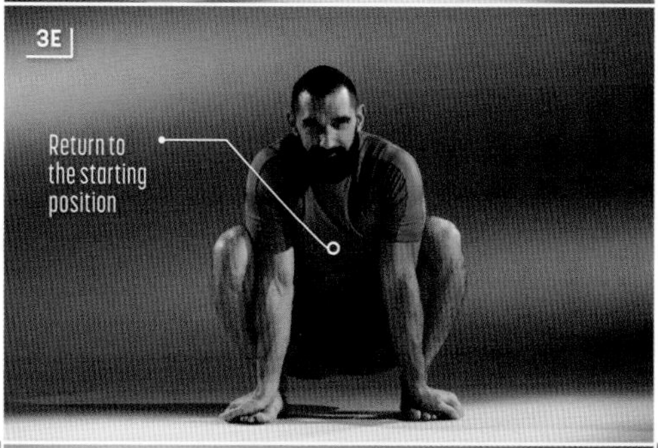

The arm comes back down following the same path
The feet should stay in the same place

3E
Return to the starting position

3F
Move to an elevated all-fours position

This combination can be easily repeated from step 3A to step 3D, or you can continue to step 3G. You will go through a squat before progressing to the all-fours position. From that point, you can work on diagonal movements from the table square position (see the Table 1 series on page 289).

Chest open
Support yourself on the foot that is diagonally opposite your supporting hand
Support yourself with the hand that is diagonally opposite the supporting foot
Slide the knee diagonally

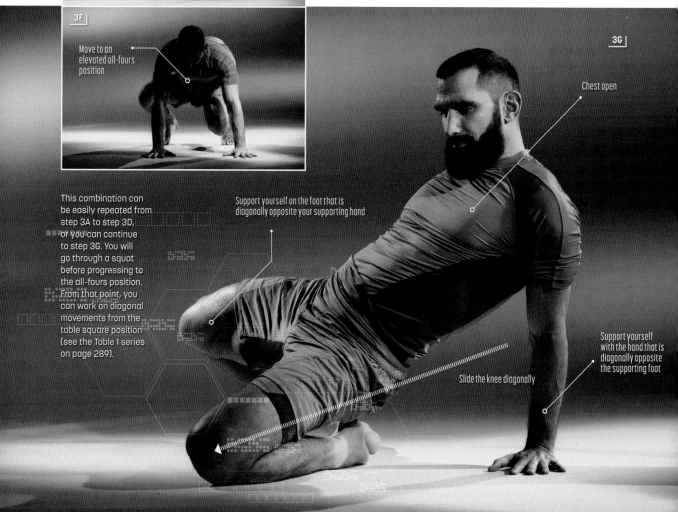

STAR SERIES

Star exercises are a reliable way to develop core strength and balance. They are also powerful activators of the lateral and spiral chains. When doing these, be sure to align your body segments for maximum effectiveness (see the recommended alignments for each individual exercise).

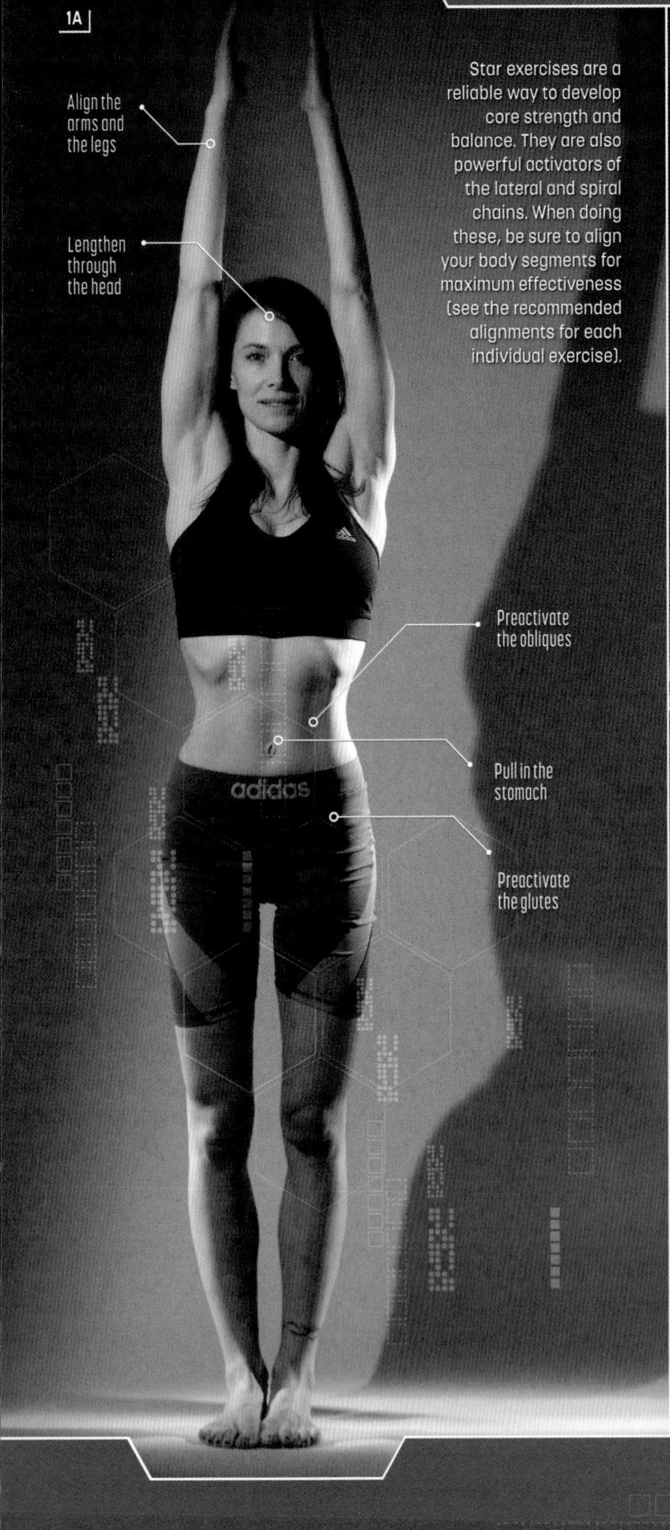
1A
Align the arms and the legs
Lengthen through the head
Preactivate the obliques
Pull in the stomach
Preactivate the glutes

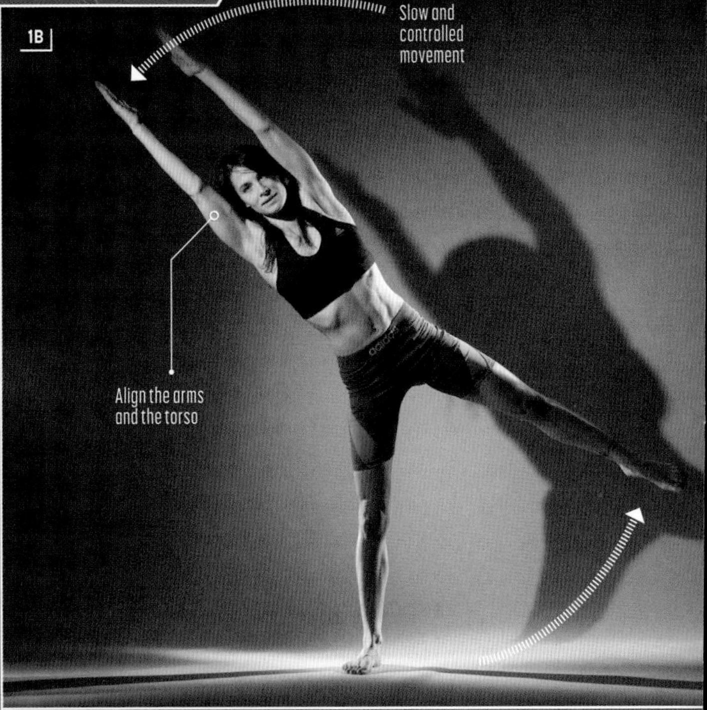
1B
Slow and controlled movement
Align the arms and the torso

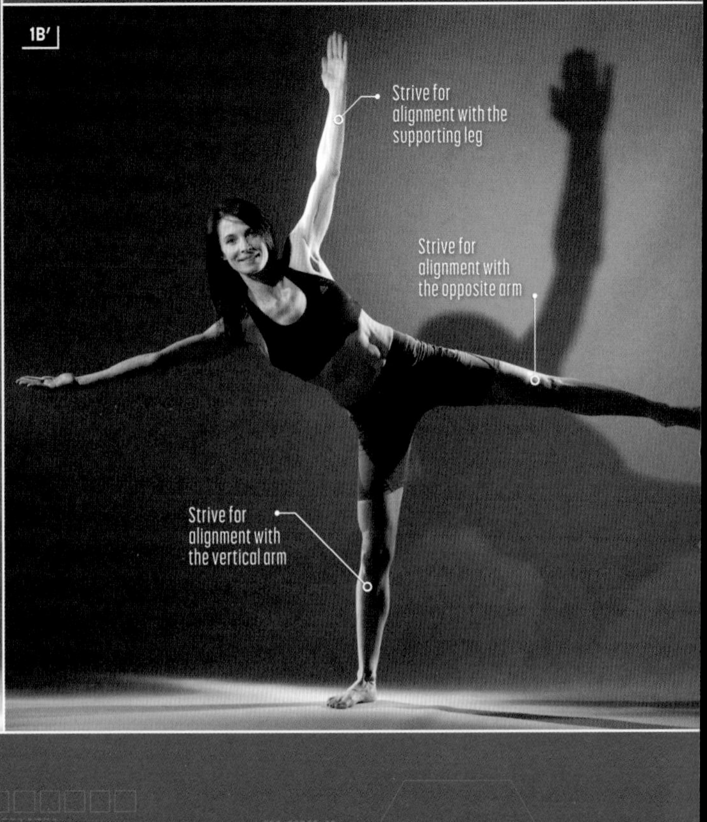
1B′
Strive for alignment with the supporting leg
Strive for alignment with the opposite arm
Strive for alignment with the vertical arm

This series was inspired by the athletic movements of hurdle jumpers to extend the leg out in front of the body. Because we rarely move in only one plane; this combination involves the sagittal plane as well as the frontal plane. Be sure to not allow your posture to be compromised at any point in the movement (i.e., do not lean your torso forward or backward).

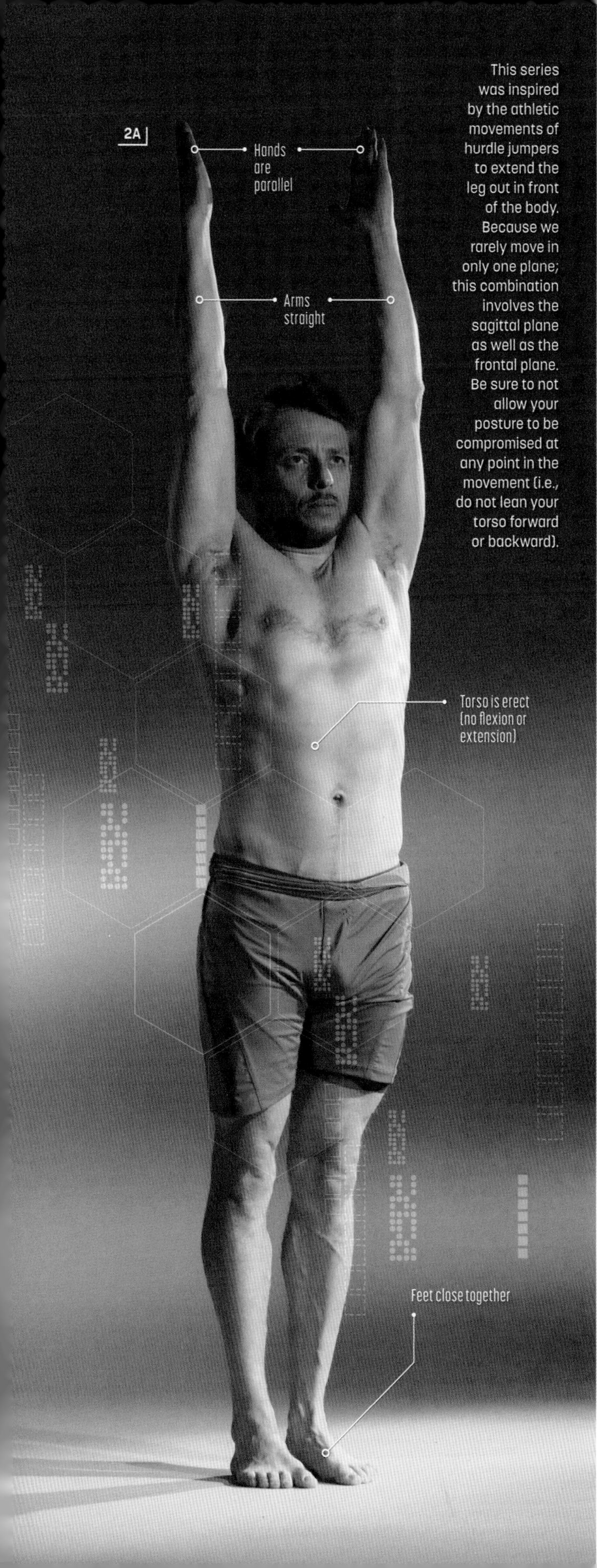
2A
Hands are parallel
Arms straight
Torso is erect (no flexion or extension)
Feet close together

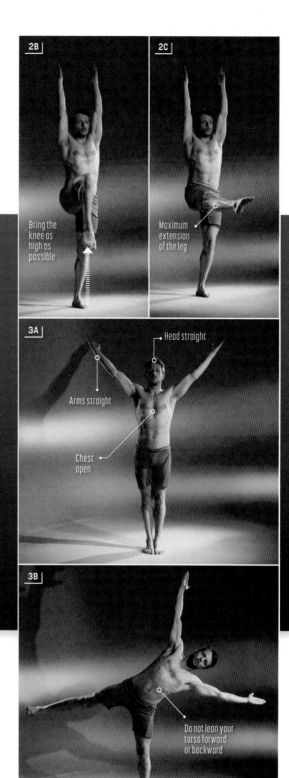

2B
Bring the knee as high as possible

2C
Maximum extension of the leg

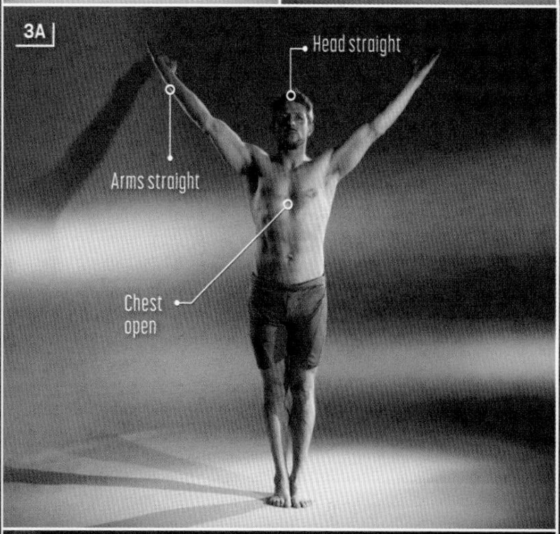
3A
Head straight
Arms straight
Chest open

3B
Do not lean your torso forward or backward

4A

The cartwheel is one of the best applications of the dynamics of the star series. Due to the squat series, you are now especially comfortable in the squat position and can begin a cartwheel right from that position.

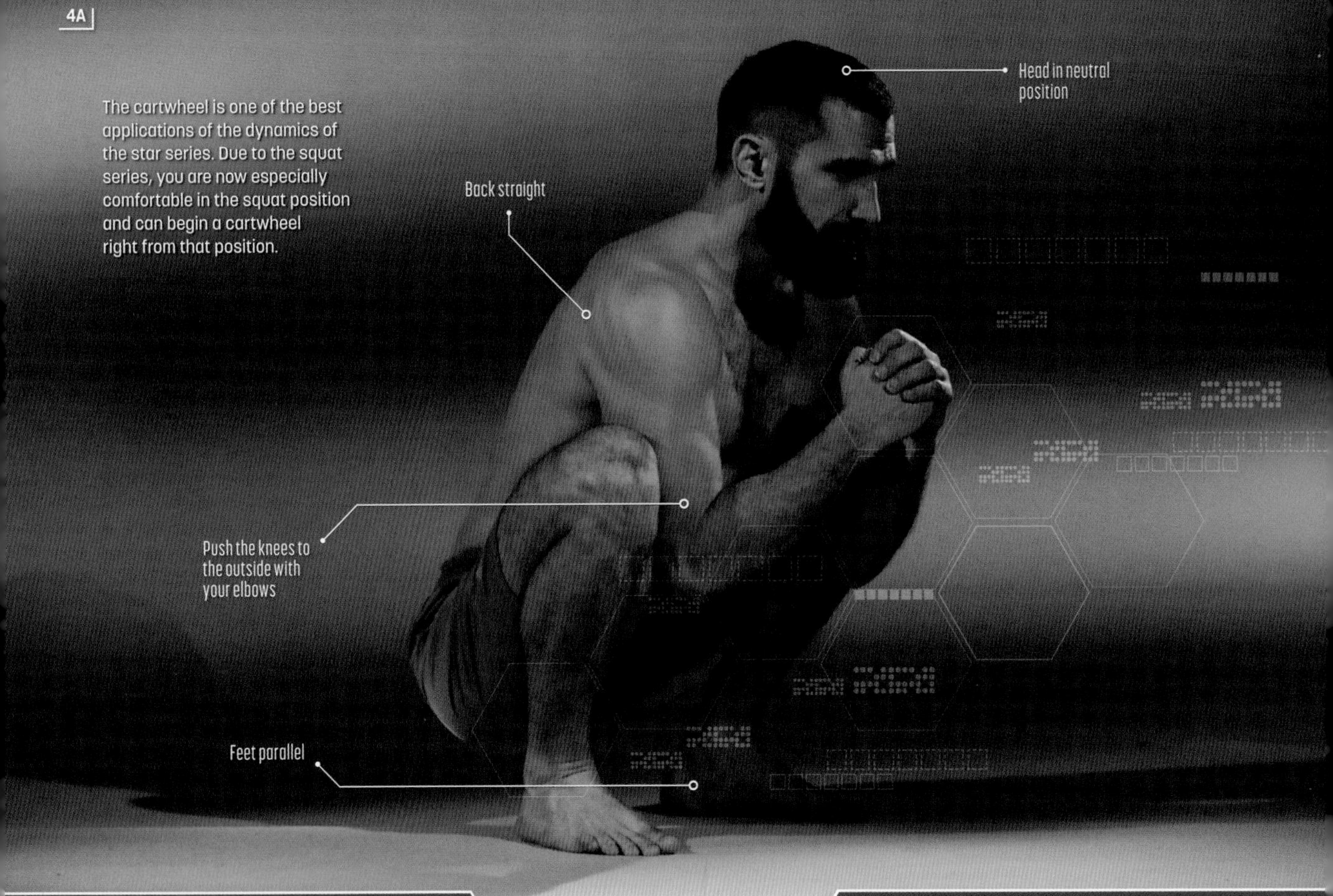

Head in neutral position
Back straight
Push the knees to the outside with your elbows
Feet parallel

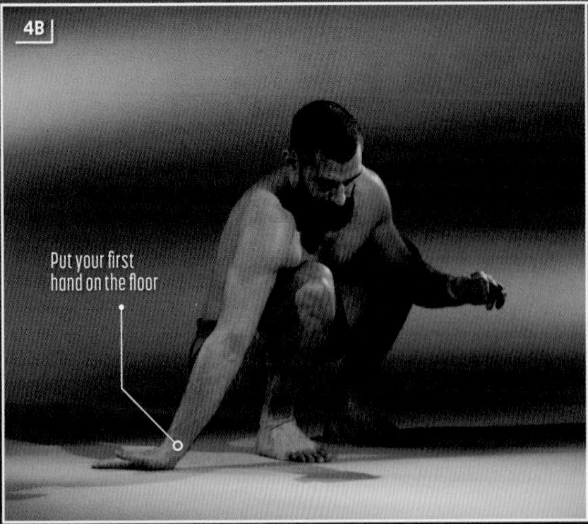

4B
Put your first hand on the floor

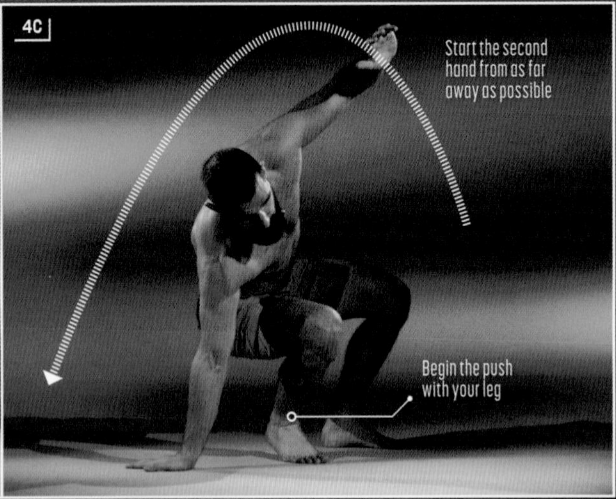

4C
Start the second hand from as far away as possible
Begin the push with your leg

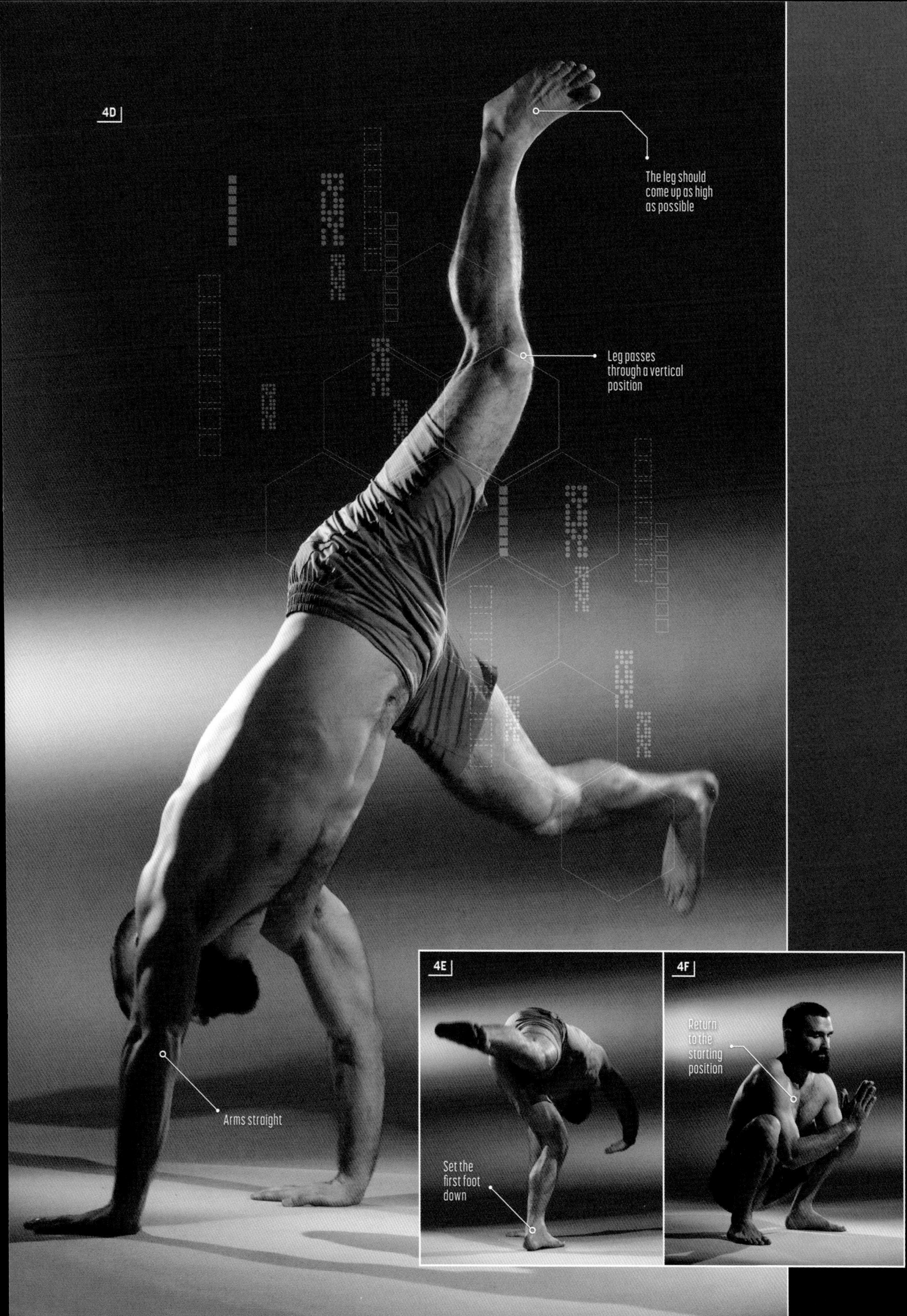
4D
The leg should come up as high as possible
Leg passes through a vertical position
Arms straight
4E
Set the first foot down
4F
Return to the starting position

JUDO SALUTE
SERIES

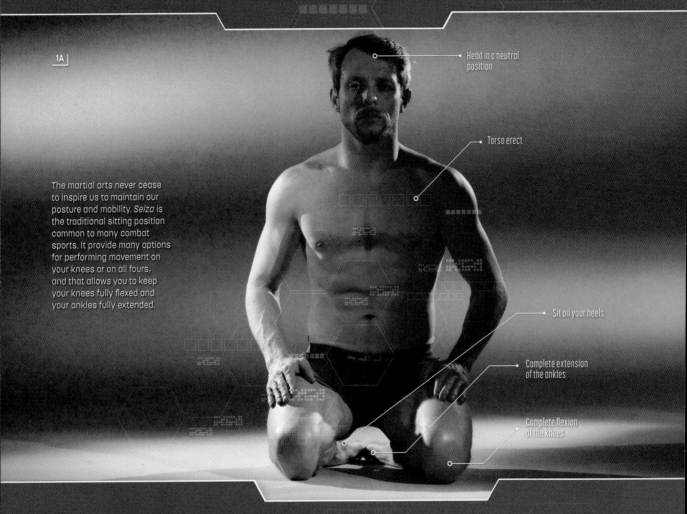

The martial arts never cease to inspire us to maintain our posture and mobility. *Seiza* is the traditional sitting position common to many combat sports. It provide many options for performing movement on your knees or on all fours, and that allows you to keep your knees fully flexed and your ankles fully extended.

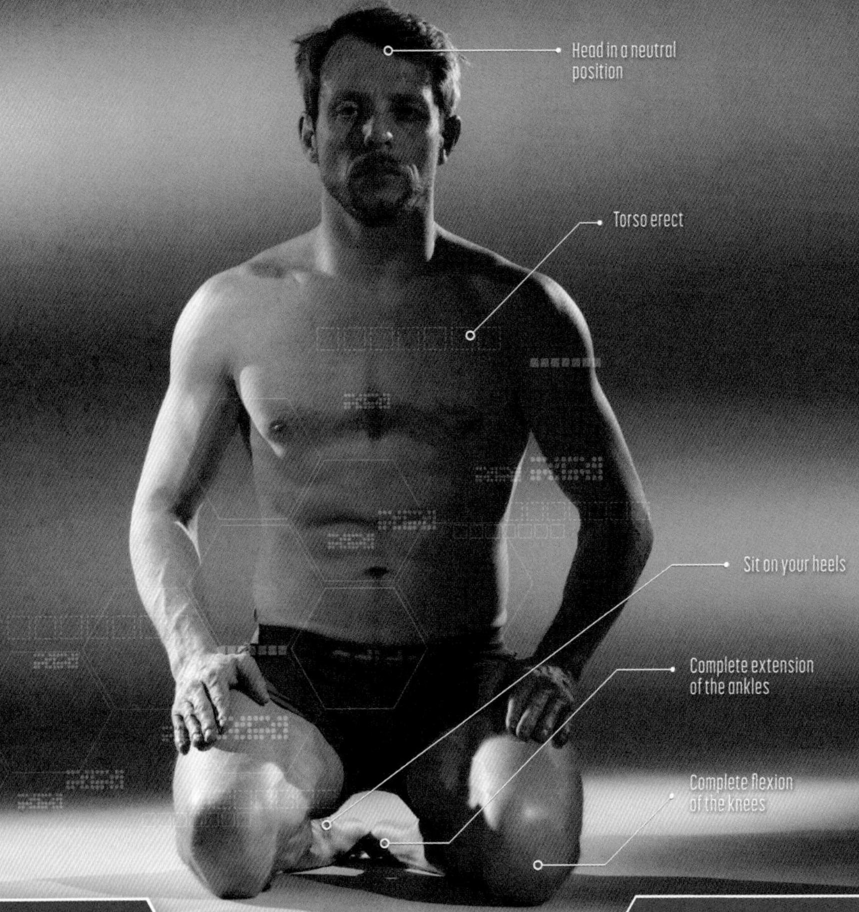

1A
Head in a neutral position
Torso erect
Sit on your heels
Complete extension of the ankles
Complete flexion of the knees

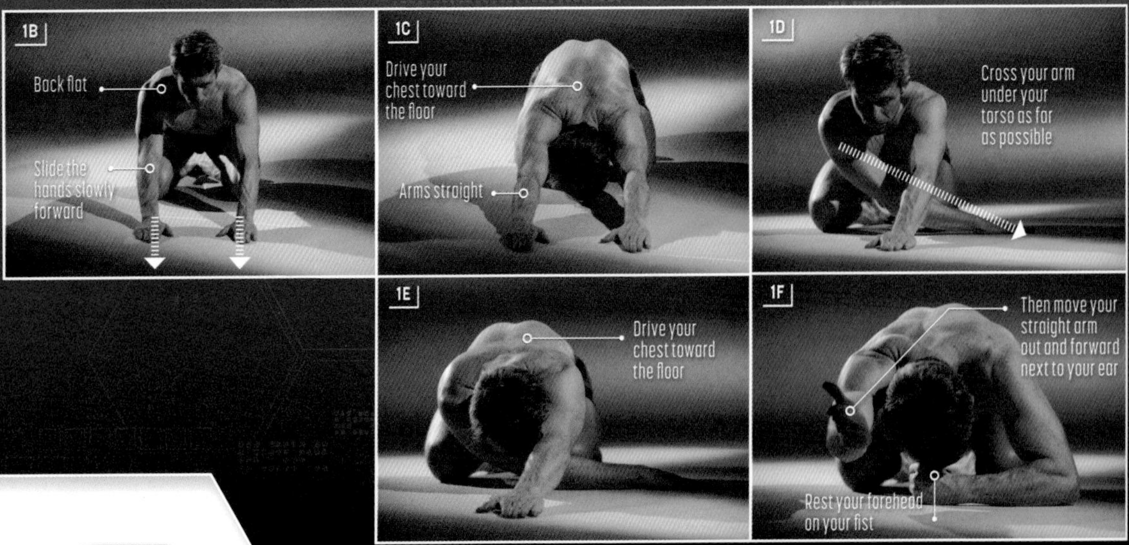

1B
Back flat
Slide the hands slowly forward
1C
Drive your chest toward the floor
Arms straight
1D
Cross your arm under your torso as far as possible
1E
Drive your chest toward the floor
1F
Then move your straight arm out and forward next to your ear
Rest your forehead on your fist

2A

An evolution of the classic salute from martial arts involves adding a stick as you perform the exercise, which helps you learn where to place your back and helps improve shoulder mobility. The more points of contact you achieve with the stick, the more mobile you are becoming.

2B

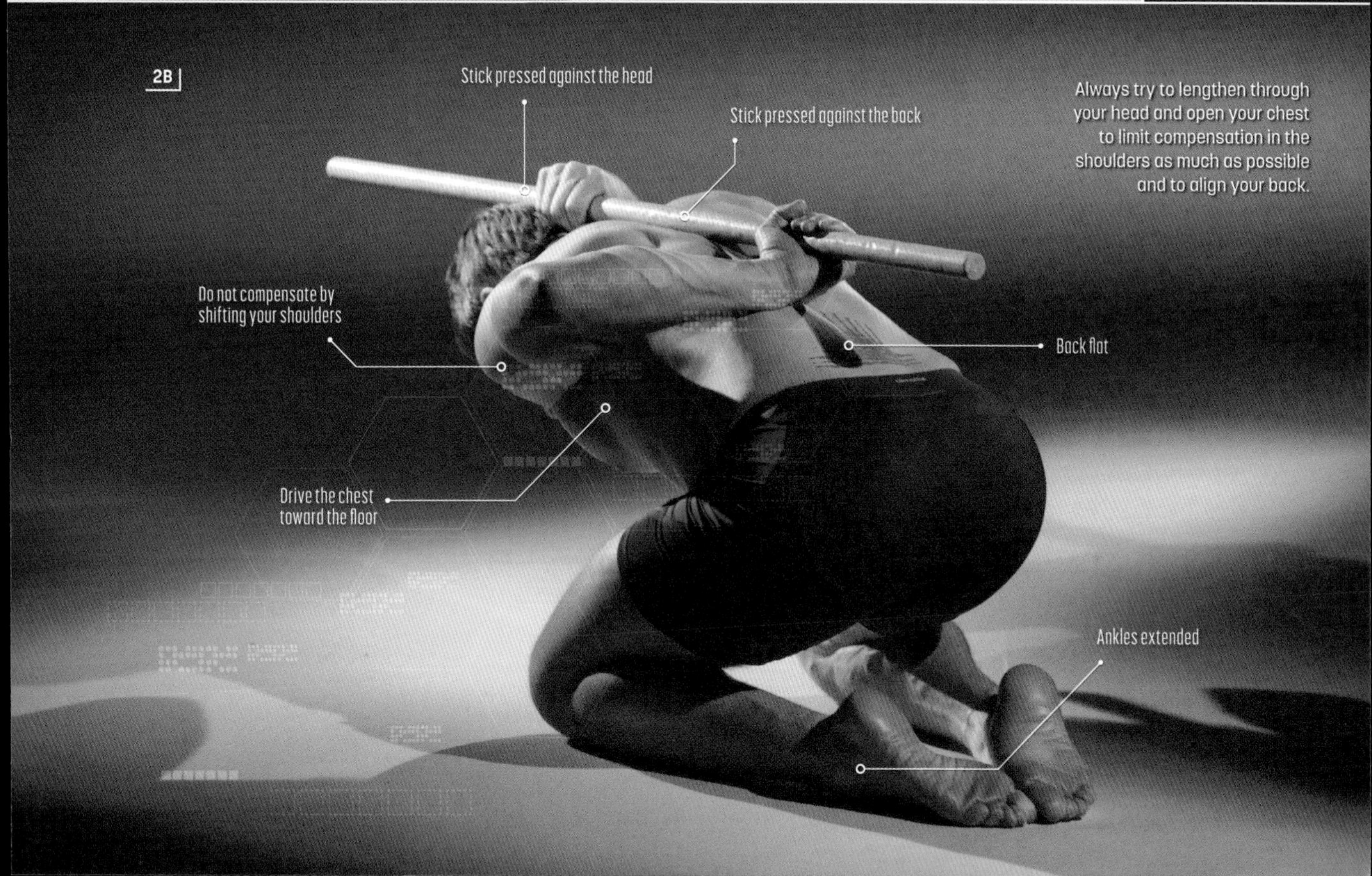

Always try to lengthen through your head and open your chest to limit compensation in the shoulders as much as possible and to align your back.

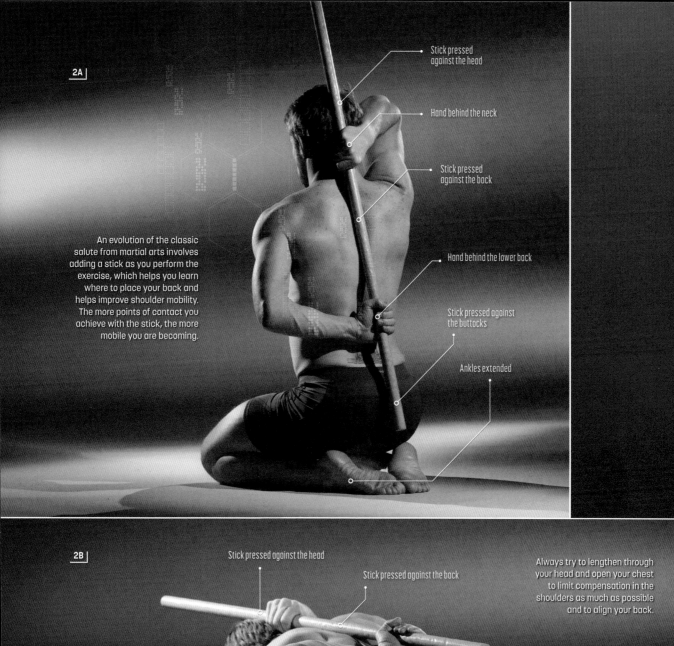

The bowl of rice exercise is also borrowed from ancient oriental practices. It combines mobility and strengthening of the spine and the shoulders. You will slide a small weight (mimicking a bowl of rice) out in front of you, first along the floor and then close to the floor.

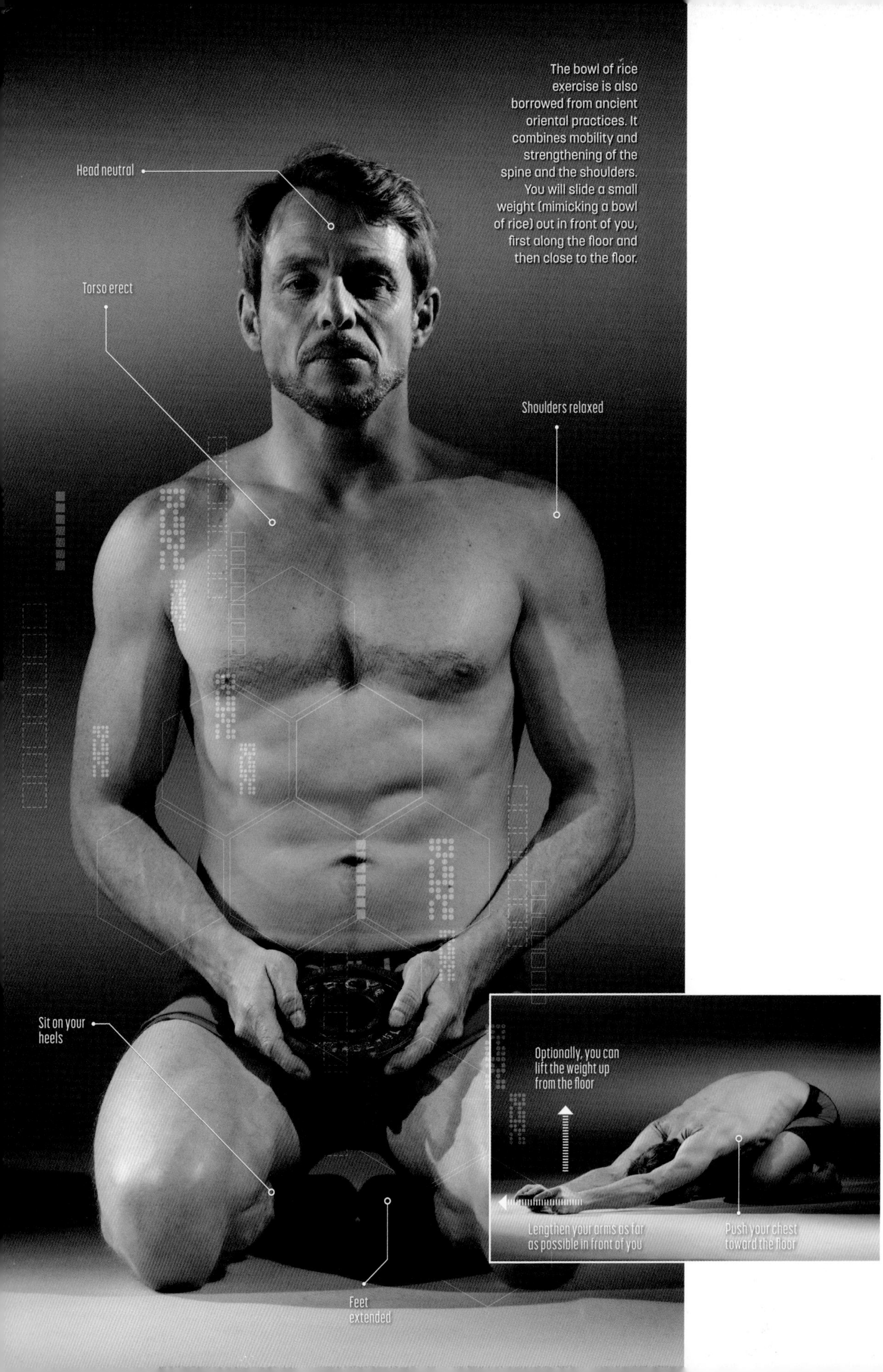

Head neutral
Torso erect
Shoulders relaxed
Sit on your heels
Feet extended
Optionally, you can lift the weight up from the floor
Lengthen your arms as far as possible in front of you
Push your chest toward the floor

SHOULDER MOBILITY ON AN EXERCISE BALL 1
SERIES

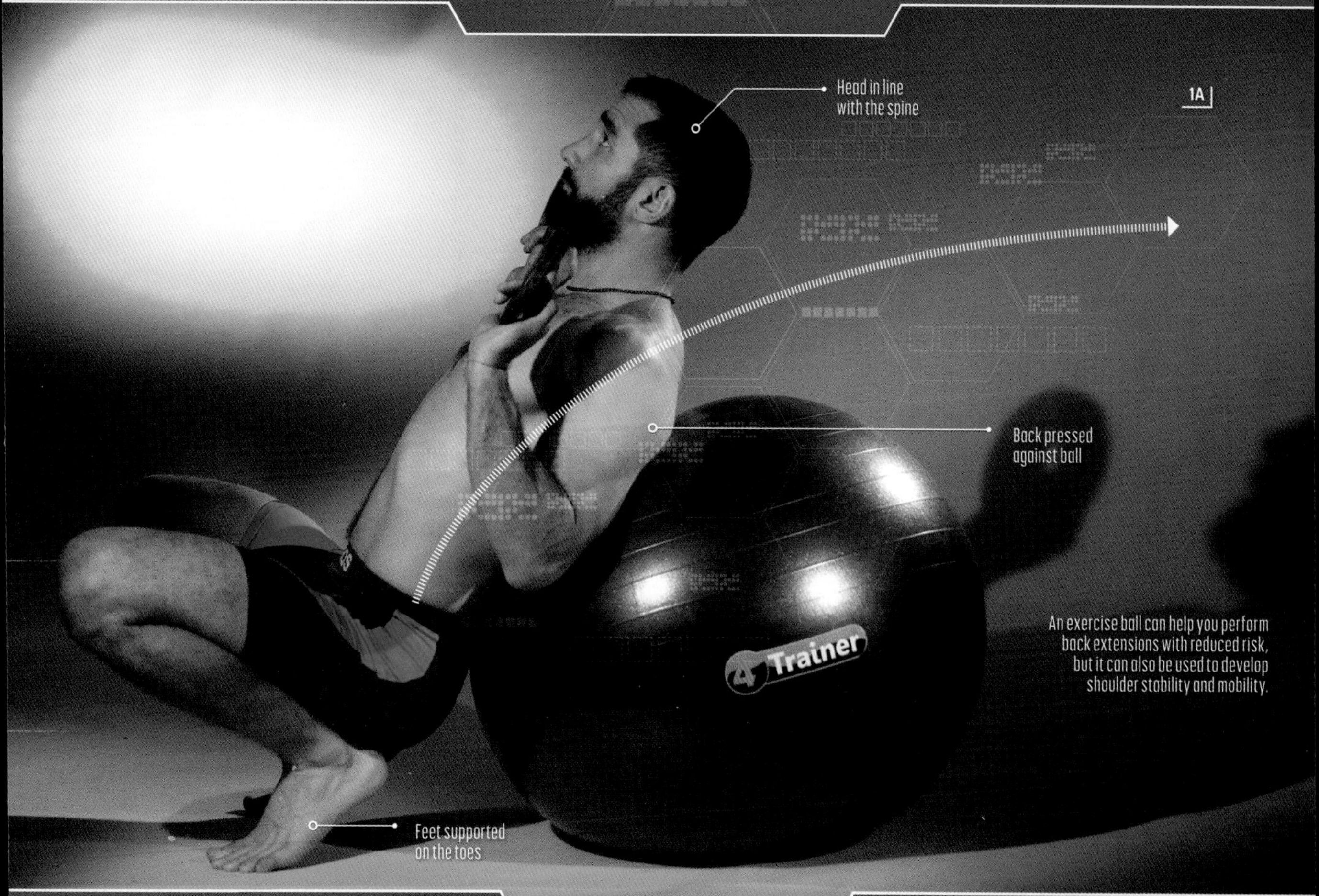

An exercise ball can help you perform back extensions with reduced risk, but it can also be used to develop shoulder stability and mobility.

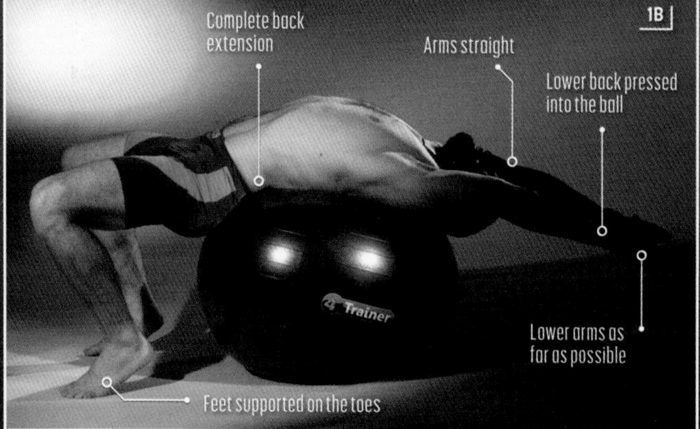

2A

This exercise improves shoulder stability and mobility in all planes of movement. After performing step 1A, move one arm straight out to be parallel to the floor and perpendicular to your torso. The other arm should be extended above your head. Then move that overhead arm down in a semicircle to your hip and then reverse the position of the hand by rotating the shoulder internally and flexing your elbow. Wrap your arm over your torso to return to the starting position. Strive for fluidity, not fatigue. Little by little, as you improve, you can perform the movements faster.

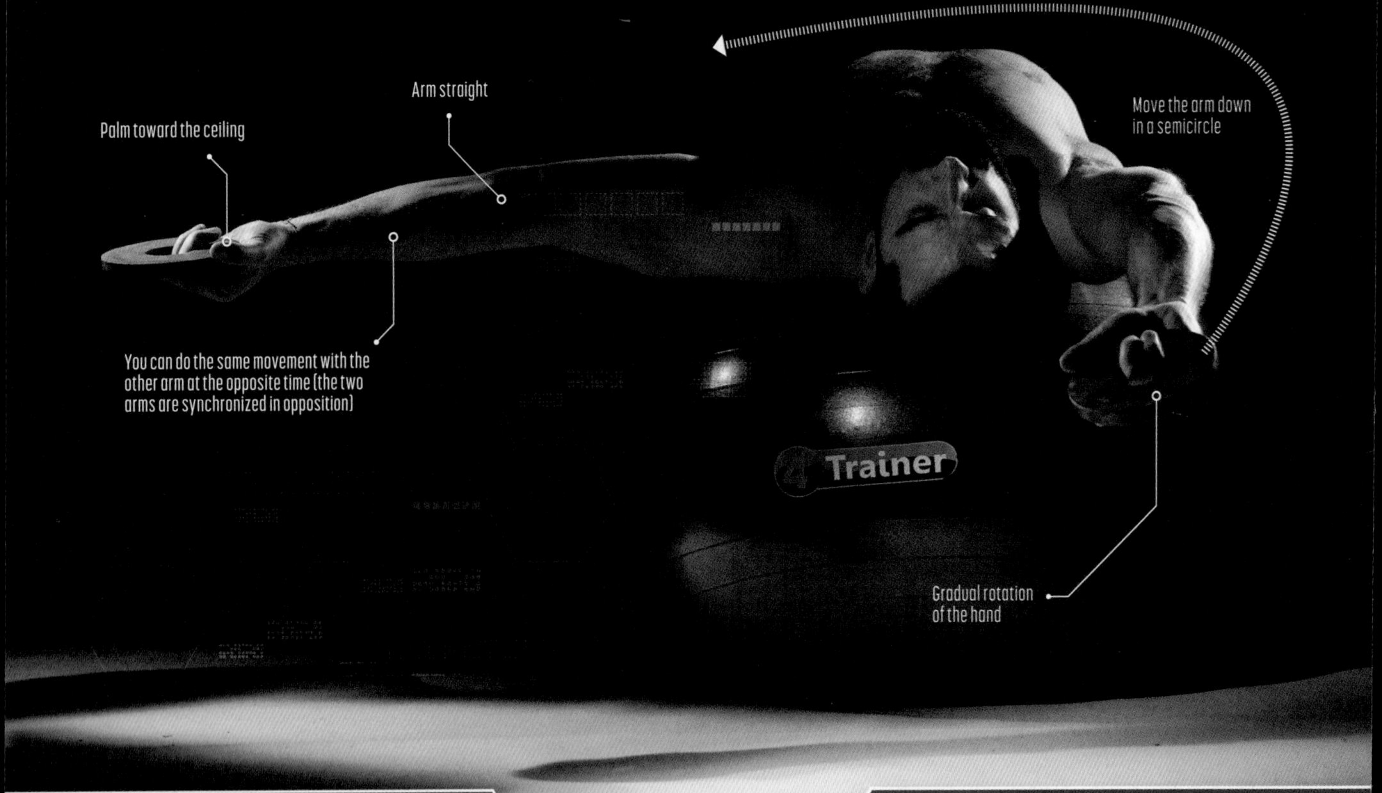
Arm straight
Palm toward the ceiling
Move the arm down in a semicircle
You can do the same movement with the other arm at the opposite time (the two arms are synchronized in opposition)
Trainer
Gradual rotation of the hand

2B

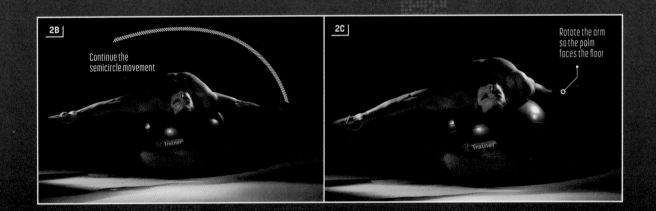

Continue the semicircle movement
Trainer

2C

Rotate the arm so the palm faces the floor
Trainer

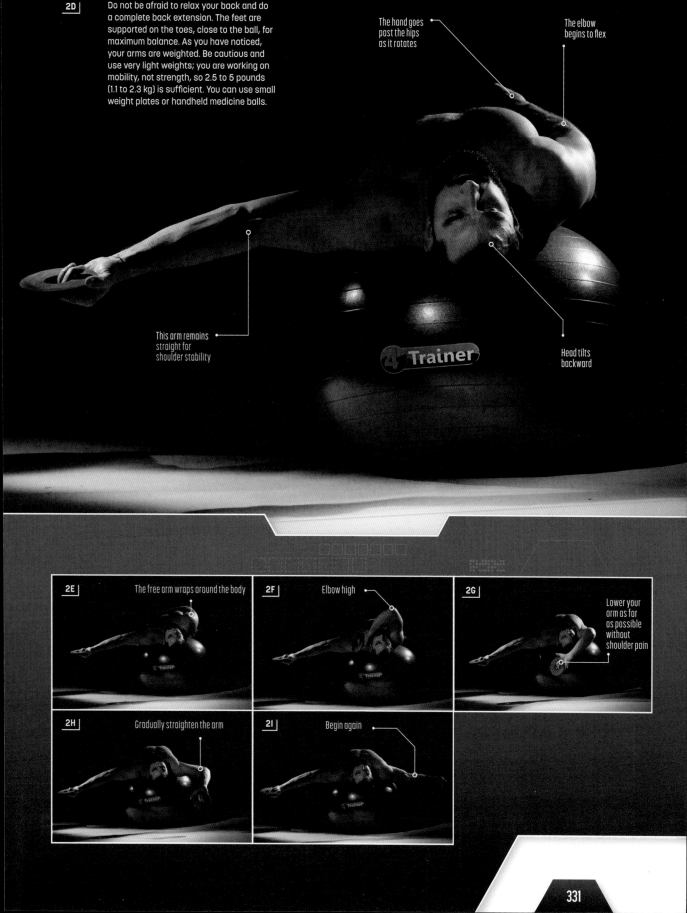

2D

Do not be afraid to relax your back and do a complete back extension. The feet are supported on the toes, close to the ball, for maximum balance. As you have noticed, your arms are weighted. Be cautious and use very light weights; you are working on mobility, not strength, so 2.5 to 5 pounds (1.1 to 2.3 kg) is sufficient. You can use small weight plates or handheld medicine balls.

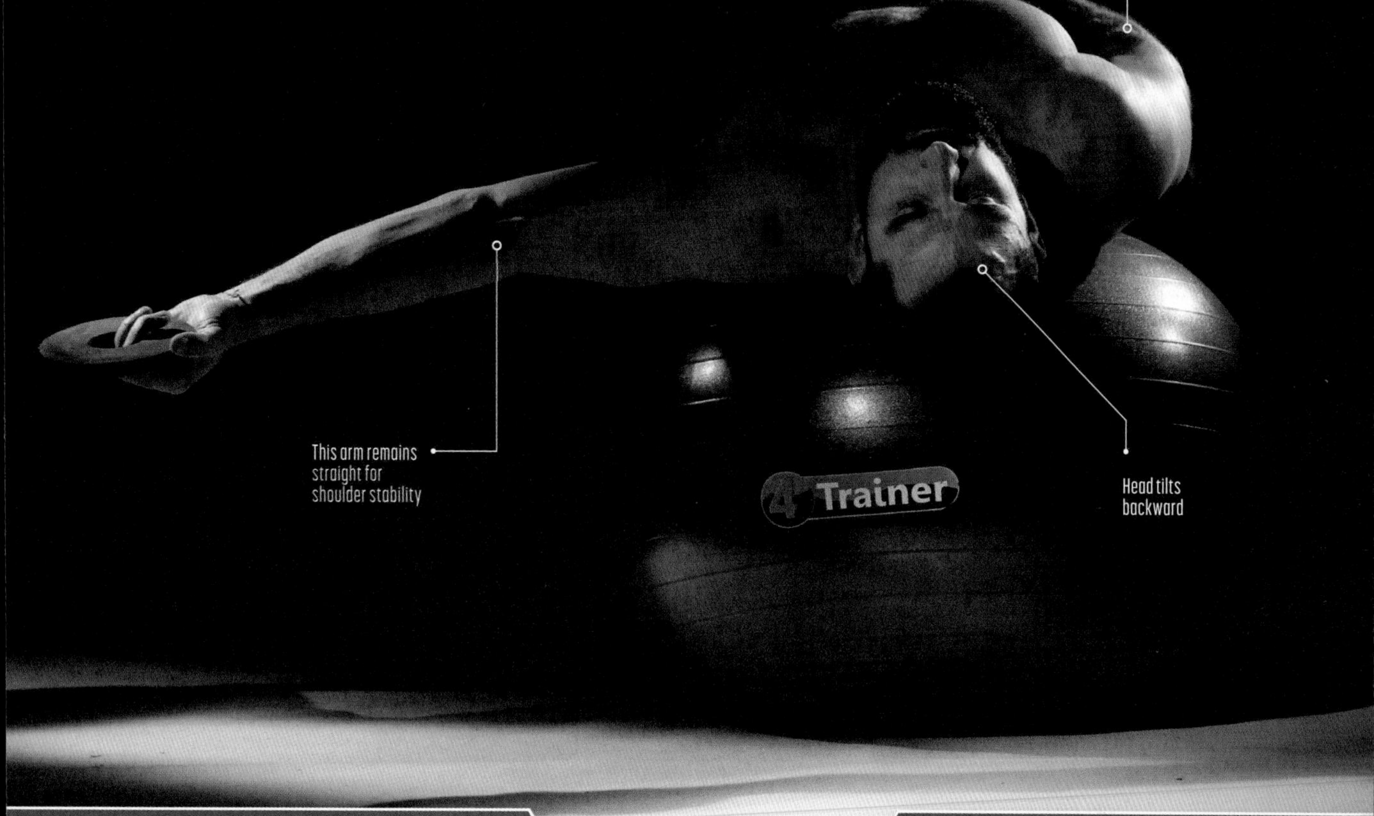

The hand goes past the hips as it rotates
The elbow begins to flex
This arm remains straight for shoulder stability
Head tilts backward
Trainer

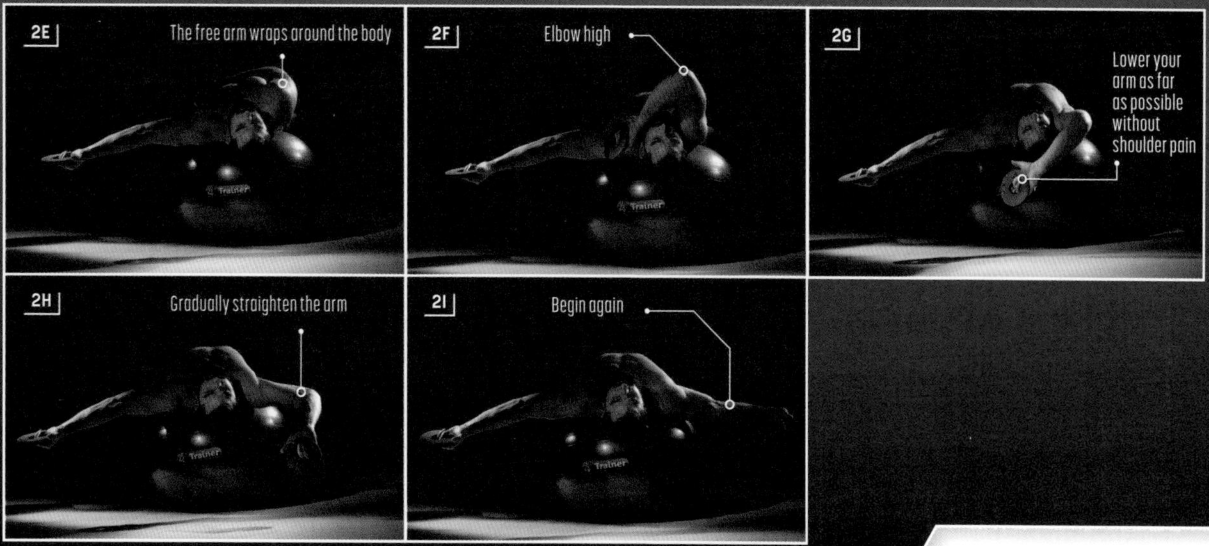

2E
The free arm wraps around the body
2F
Elbow high
2G
Lower your arm as far as possible without shoulder pain
2H
Gradually straighten the arm
2I
Begin again

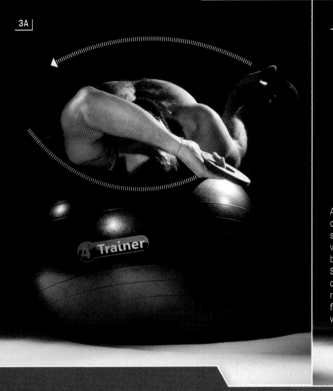

3A

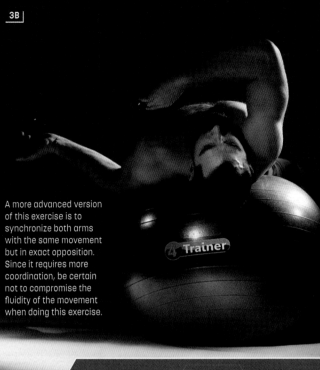

3B

A more advanced version of this exercise is to synchronize both arms with the same movement but in exact opposition. Since it requires more coordination, be certain not to compromise the fluidity of the movement when doing this exercise.

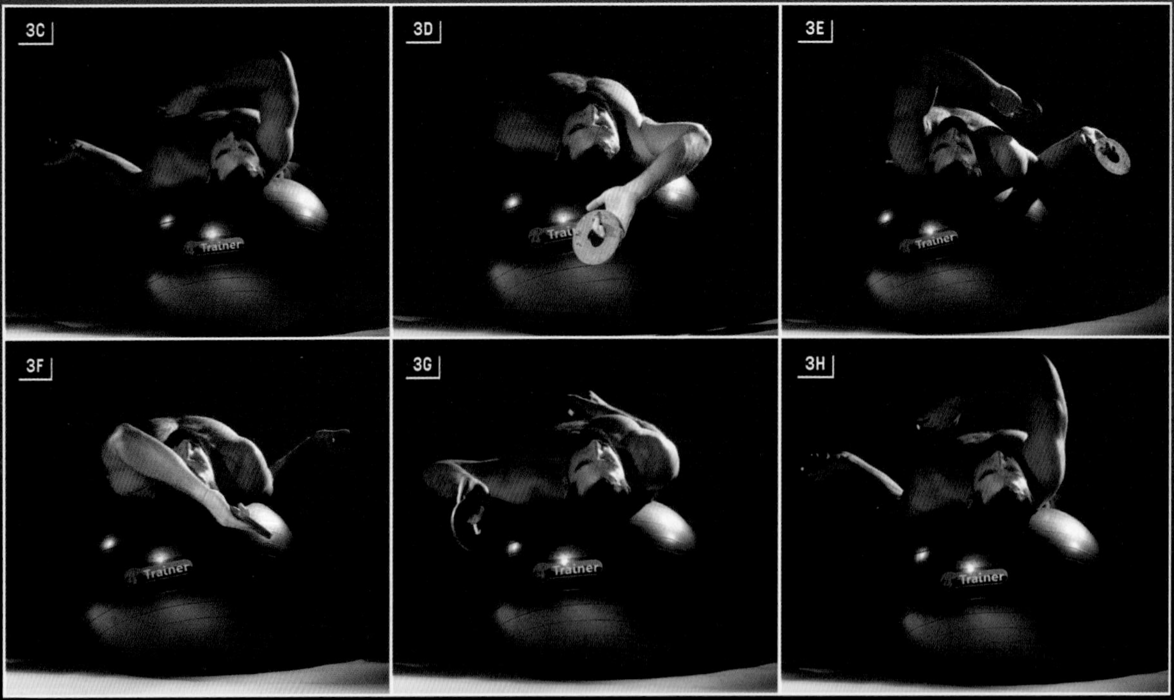

SHOULDER MOBILITY ON AN EXERCISE BALL 2
SERIES

The exercise ball is a remarkable tool for shoulder mobility. The first exercise in this series is to alternate a relaxed opening of the arms (with or without bouncing) and a crossing of the arms (with or without bouncing) using weights. The feet are always supported on the toes, and the back is completely extended. There are always two methods to perform these exercises: slow and controlled or dynamic and relaxed, taking time to extend your straight arms and rebound your crossed arms on the ball.

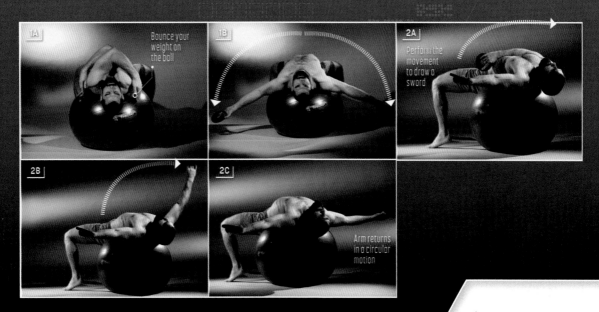

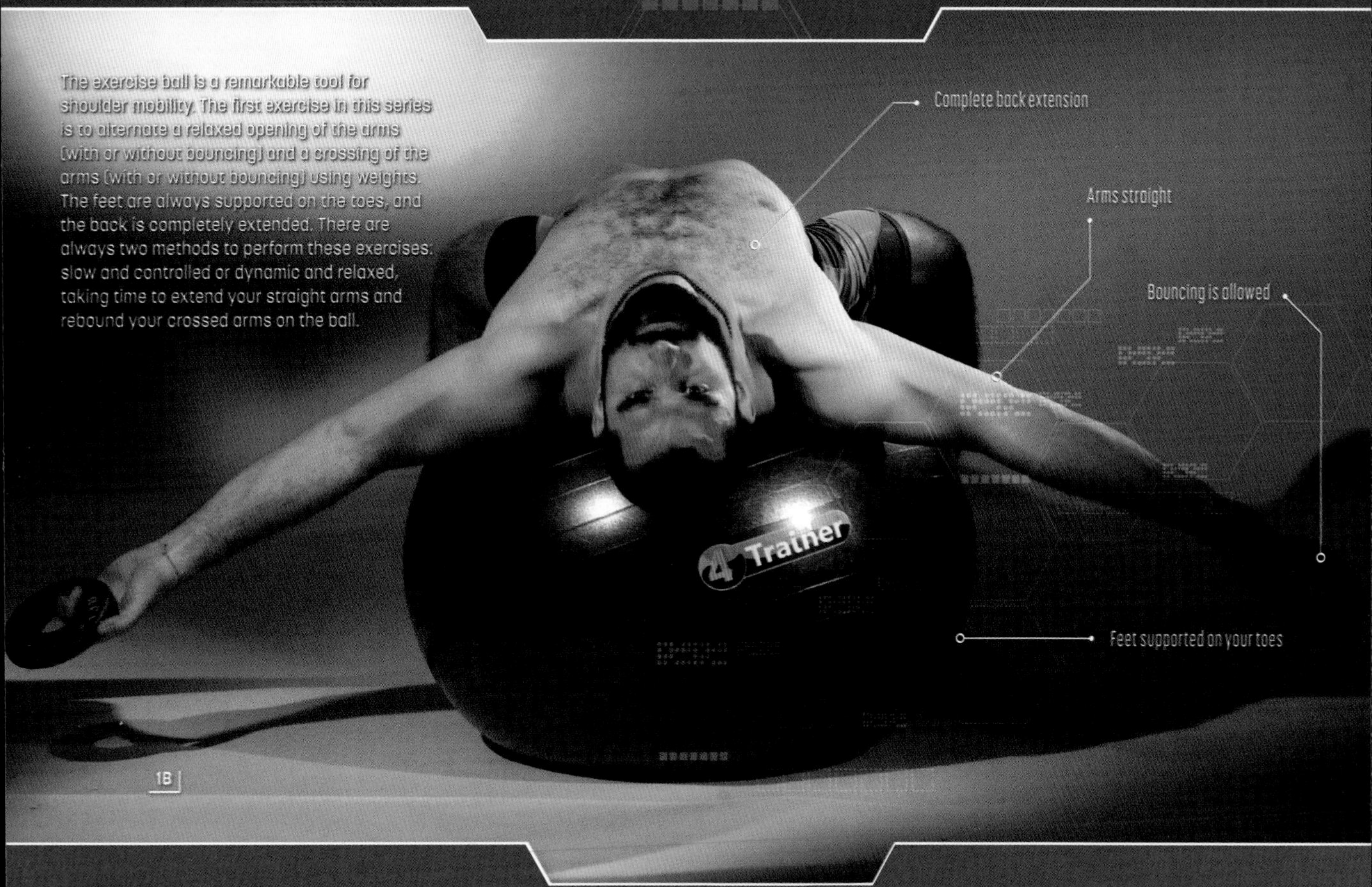

Complete back extension
Arms straight
Bouncing is allowed
Feet supported on your toes
1B

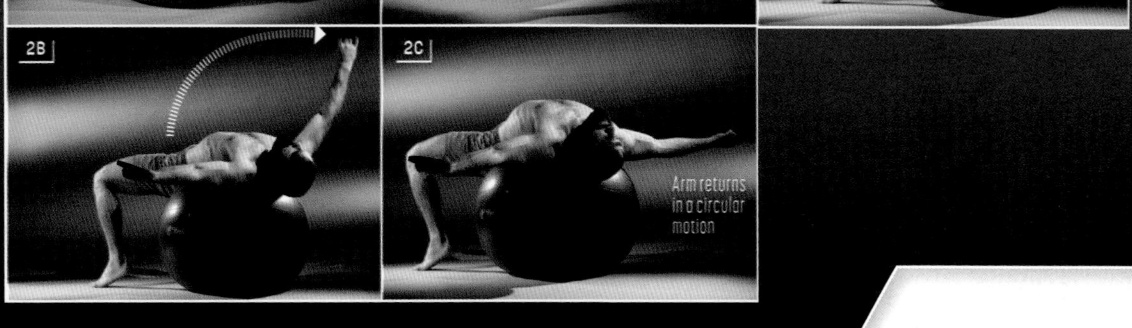

1A
Bounce your weight on the ball
1B
2A
Perform the movement to draw a sword
2B
2C
Arm returns in a circular motion

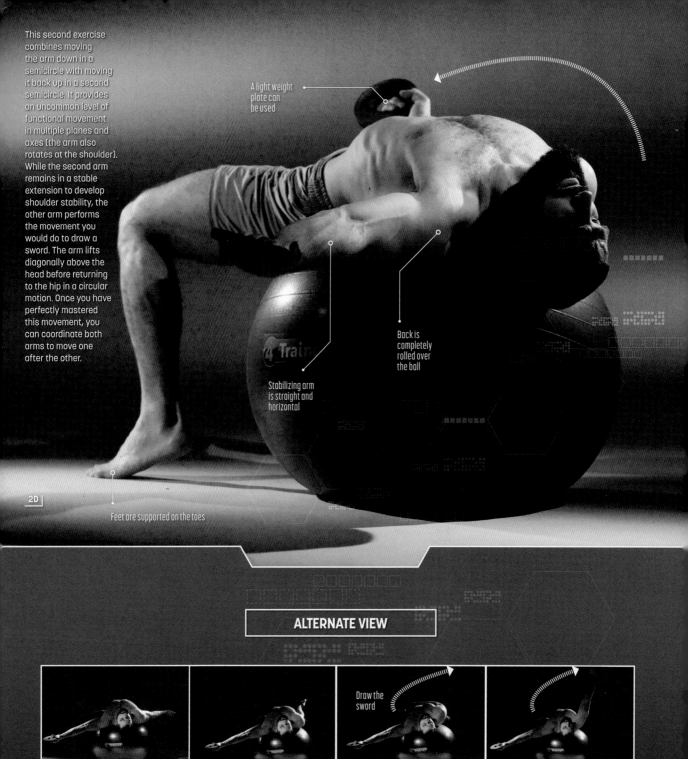

This second exercise combines moving the arm down in a semicircle with moving it back up in a second semicircle. It provides an uncommon level of functional movement in multiple planes and axes (the arm also rotates at the shoulder). While the second arm remains in a stable extension to develop shoulder stability, the other arm performs the movement you would do to draw a sword. The arm lifts diagonally above the head before returning to the hip in a circular motion. Once you have perfectly mastered this movement, you can coordinate both arms to move one after the other.

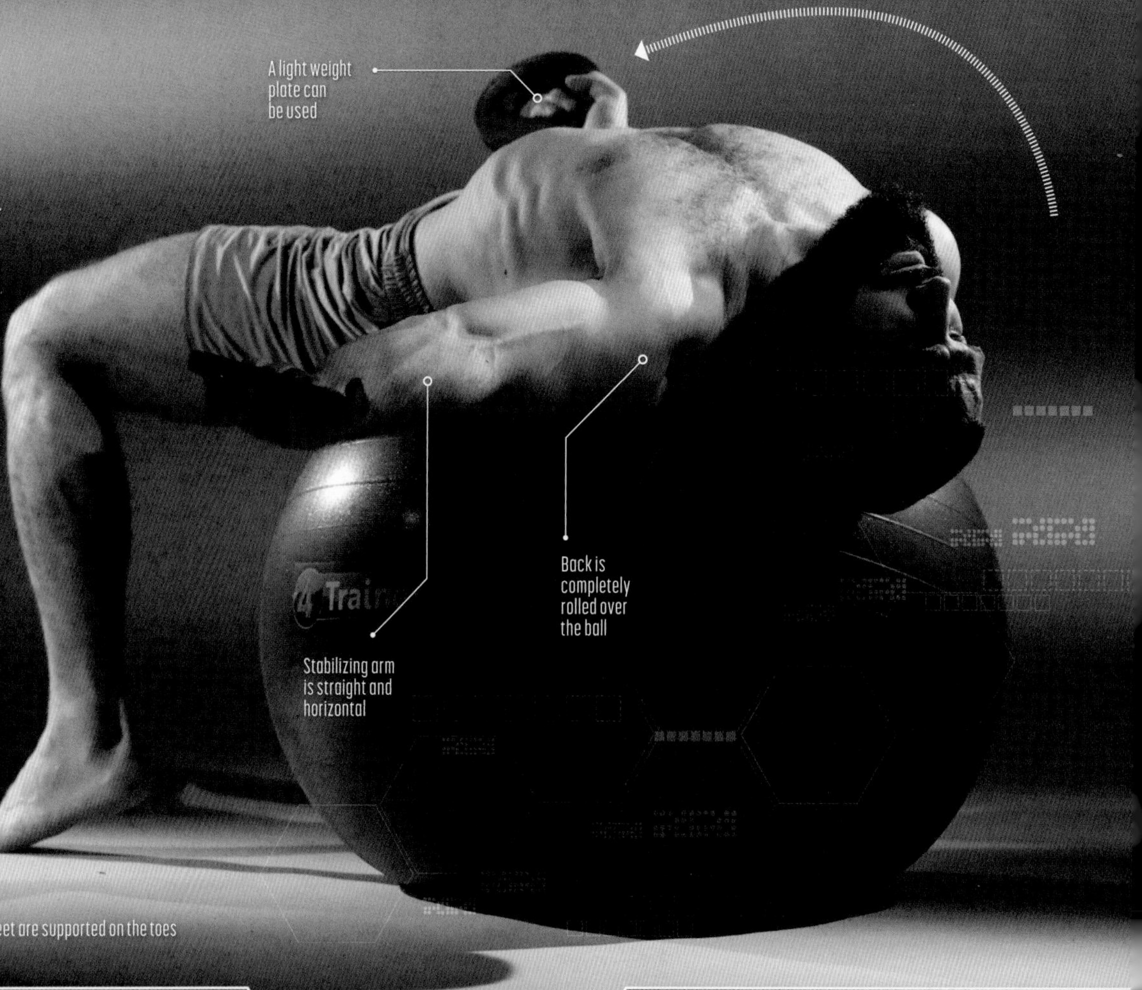

A light weight plate can be used
Back is completely rolled over the ball
Stabilizing arm is straight and horizontal
2D
Feet are supported on the toes

ALTERNATE VIEW

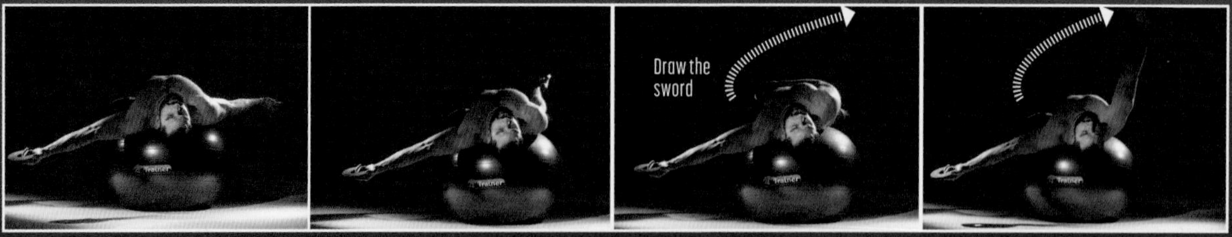

Draw the sword

PELVIS/SHOULDER DISSOCIATION ON AN EXERCISE BALL SERIES

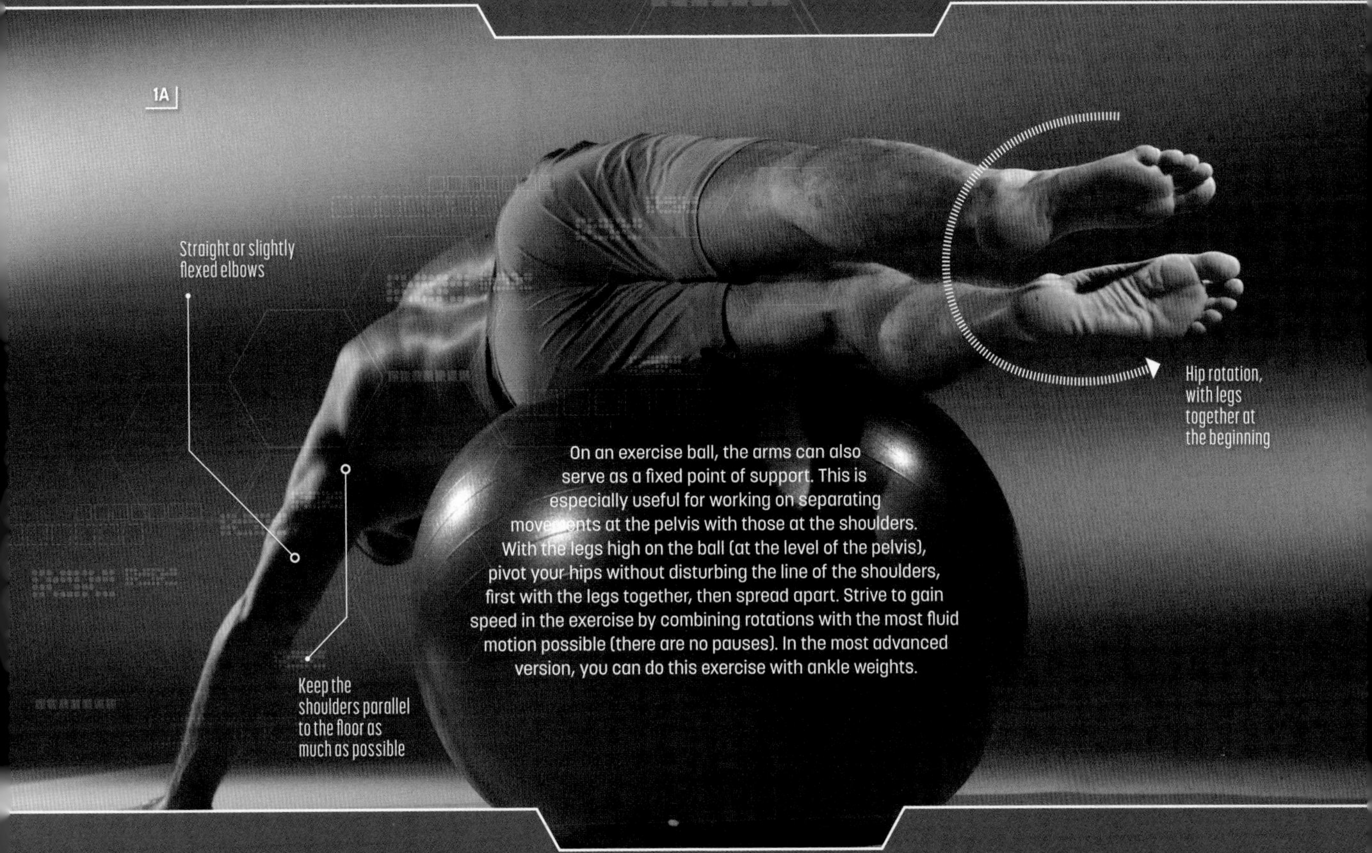
1A
Straight or slightly flexed elbows
Keep the shoulders parallel to the floor as much as possible
Hip rotation, with legs together at the beginning

On an exercise ball, the arms can also serve as a fixed point of support. This is especially useful for working on separating movements at the pelvis with those at the shoulders. With the legs high on the ball (at the level of the pelvis), pivot your hips without disturbing the line of the shoulders, first with the legs together, then spread apart. Strive to gain speed in the exercise by combining rotations with the most fluid motion possible (there are no pauses). In the most advanced version, you can do this exercise with ankle weights.

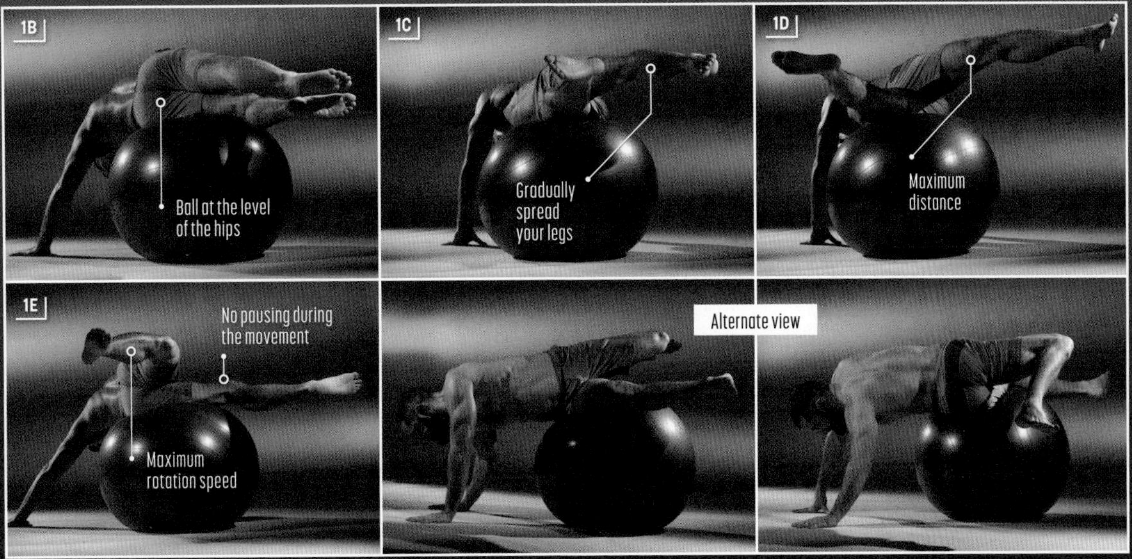
1B
Ball at the level of the hips
1C
Gradually spread your legs
1D
Maximum distance
1E
No pausing during the movement
Maximum rotation speed
Alternate view

TSUGI ASHI
SERIES

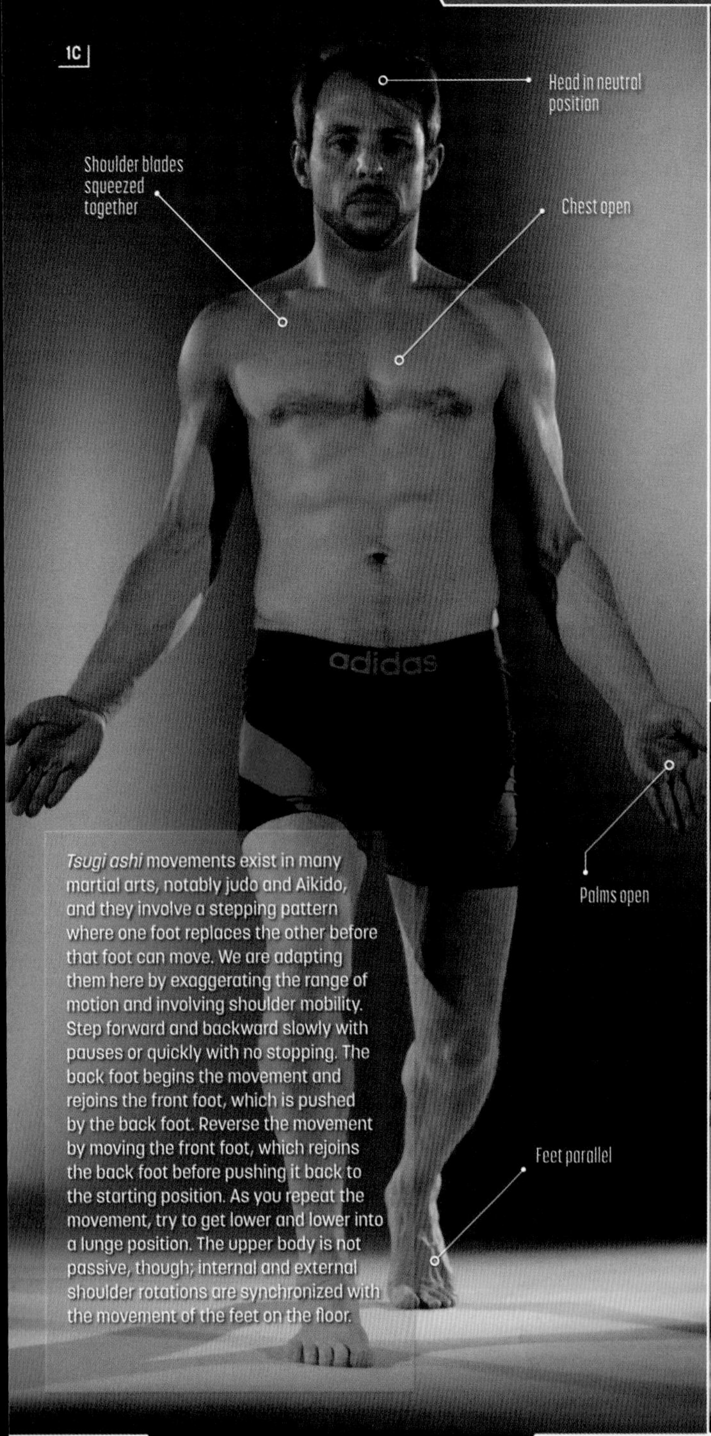

1C
Head in neutral position
Shoulder blades squeezed together
Chest open
Palms open
Feet parallel

Tsugi ashi movements exist in many martial arts, notably judo and Aikido, and they involve a stepping pattern where one foot replaces the other before that foot can move. We are adapting them here by exaggerating the range of motion and involving shoulder mobility. Step forward and backward slowly with pauses or quickly with no stopping. The back foot begins the movement and rejoins the front foot, which is pushed by the back foot. Reverse the movement by moving the front foot, which rejoins the back foot before pushing it back to the starting position. As you repeat the movement, try to get lower and lower into a lunge position. The upper body is not passive, though; internal and external shoulder rotations are synchronized with the movement of the feet on the floor.

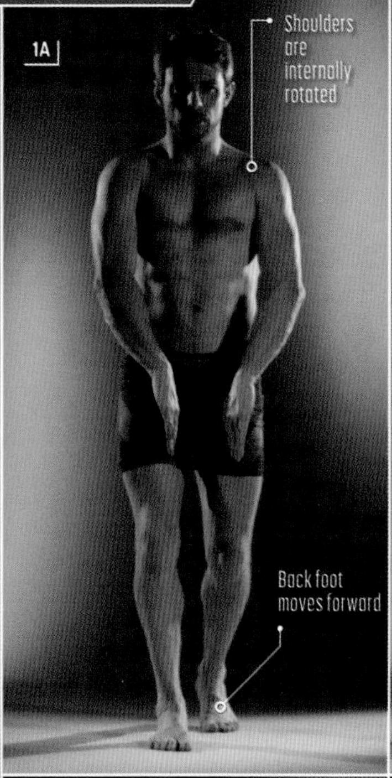

1A
Shoulders are internally rotated
Back foot moves forward

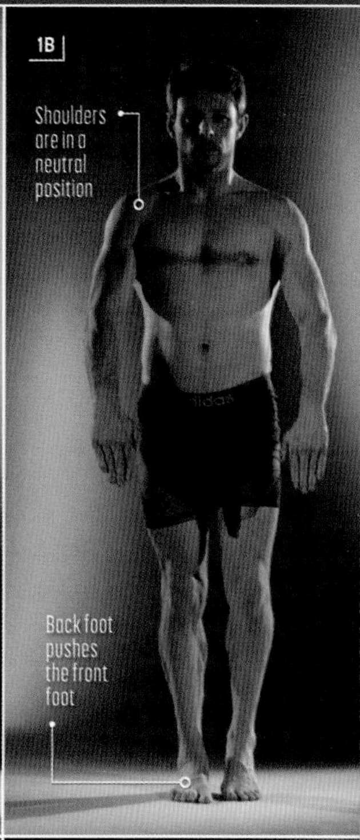

1B
Shoulders are in a neutral position
Back foot pushes the front foot

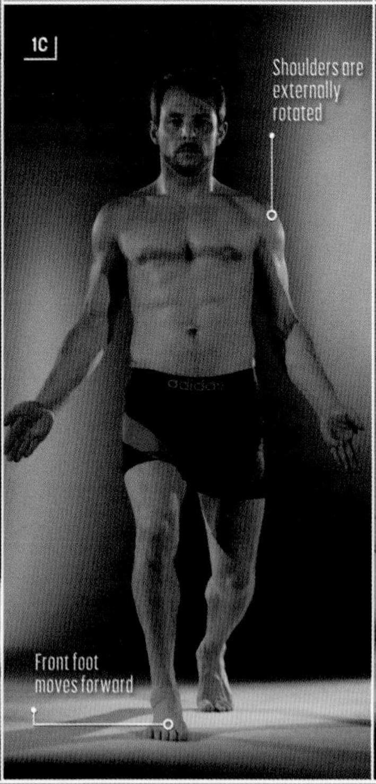

1C
Shoulders are externally rotated
Front foot moves forward

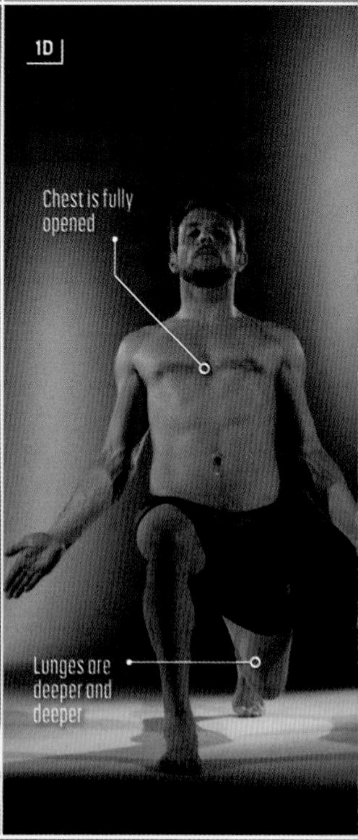

1D
Chest is fully opened
Lunges are deeper and deeper

2A | These same stepping movements can be done to the side. Just as before, the right foot moves first and rejoins then pushes the left foot, allowing for movement to the side. You can vary the depth of the squatted position or add arm flexions and extensions behind the head in a low or high position. We are inspired by the snatch exercise of Olympic weightlifting, so a stick was used to mimic an Olympic bar. You can do all these variations at full speed or with pauses.

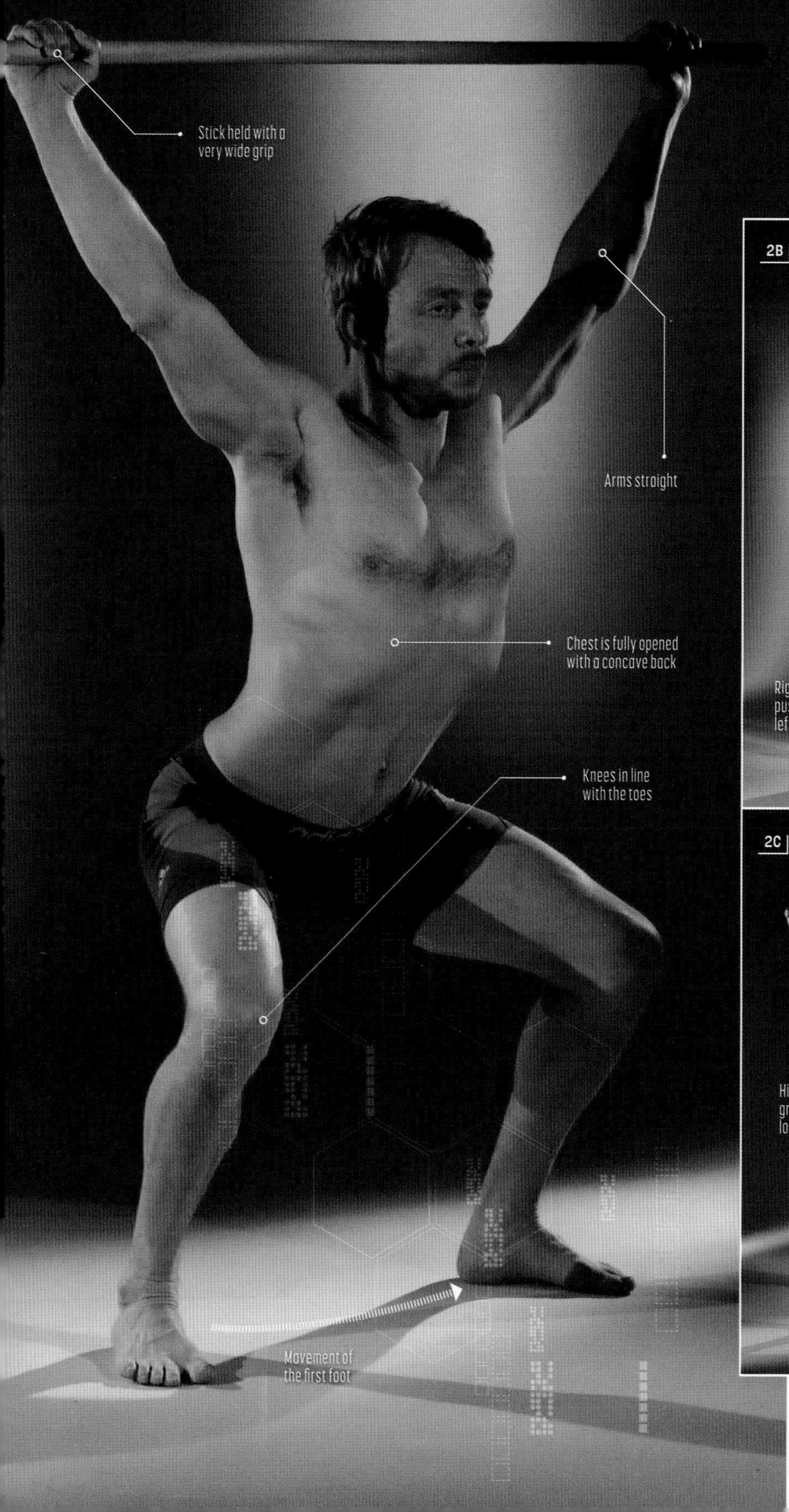
Stick held with a very wide grip
Arms straight
Chest is fully opened with a concave back
Knees in line with the toes
Movement of the first foot

2B |

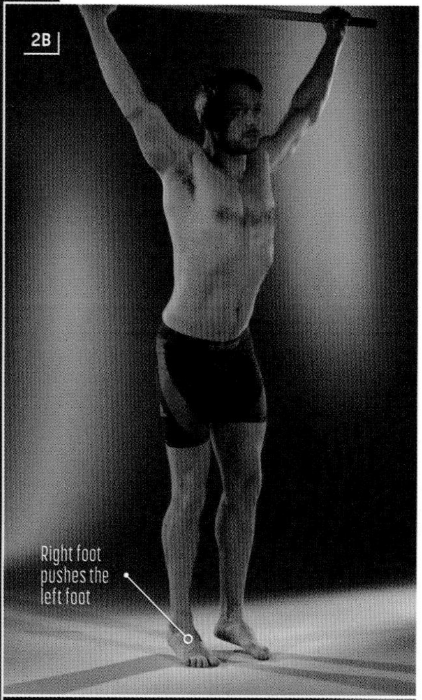
Right foot pushes the left foot

2C |

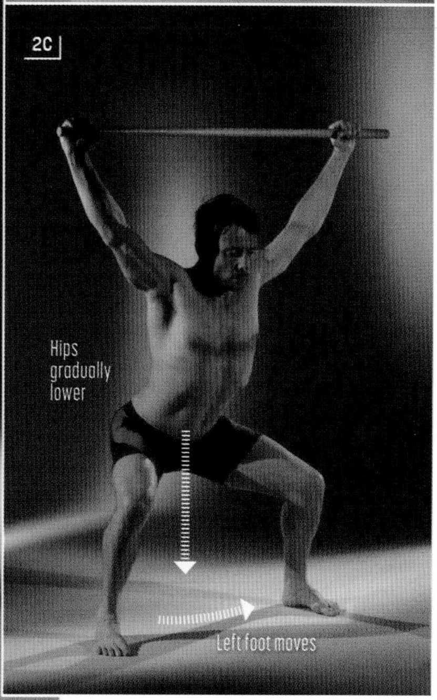
Hips gradually lower
Left foot moves

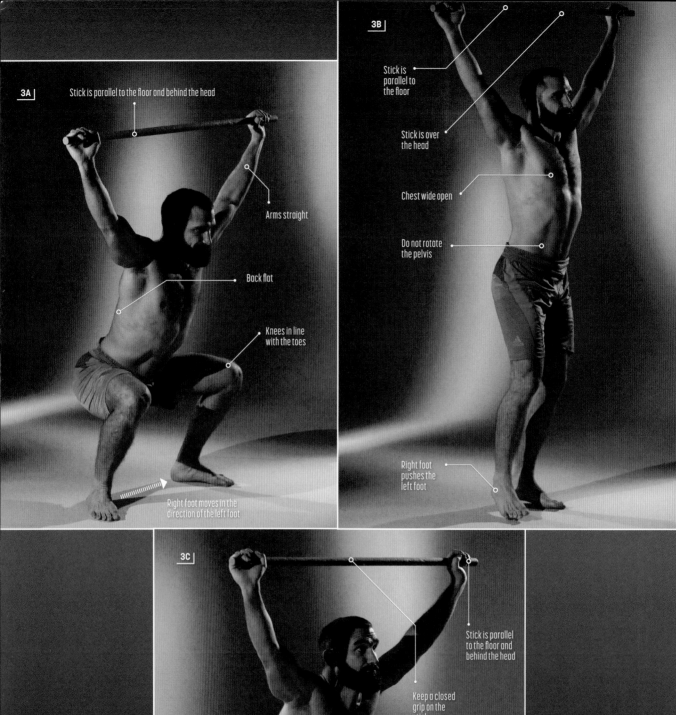

3A
Stick is parallel to the floor and behind the head
Arms straight
Back flat
Knees in line with the toes
Right foot moves in the direction of the left foot

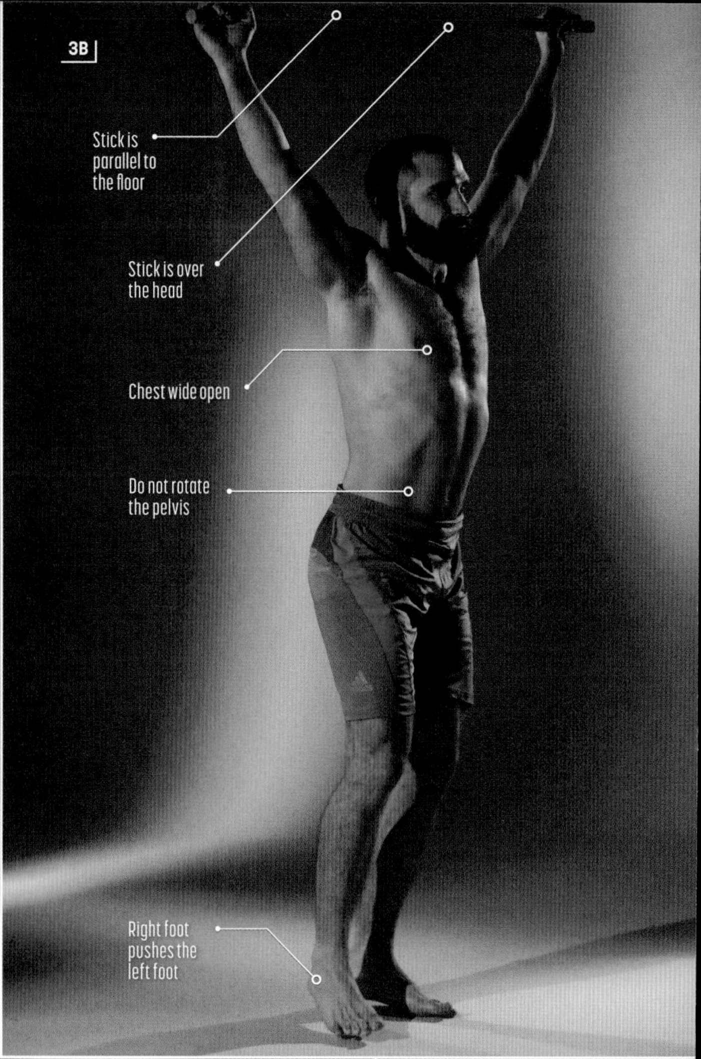
3B
Stick is parallel to the floor
Stick is over the head
Chest wide open
Do not rotate the pelvis
Right foot pushes the left foot

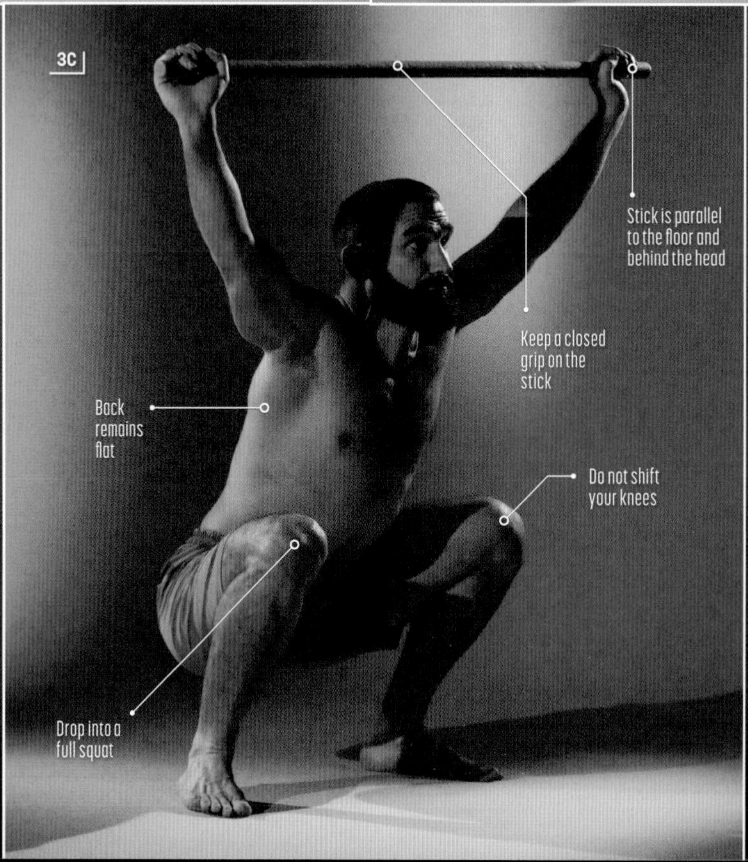
3C
Stick is parallel to the floor and behind the head
Keep a closed grip on the stick
Back remains flat
Do not shift your knees
Drop into a full squat

TAI SABAKI
SERIES

Tai sabaki is another exercise inspired by martial arts that involves a twisting movement in a half circle that promotes body awareness and ankle stability. The first foot advances on the diagonal, and the second comes to rest nearby with the knee somewhat flexed. The legs are then crossed; by uncrossing them, you make a half turn.

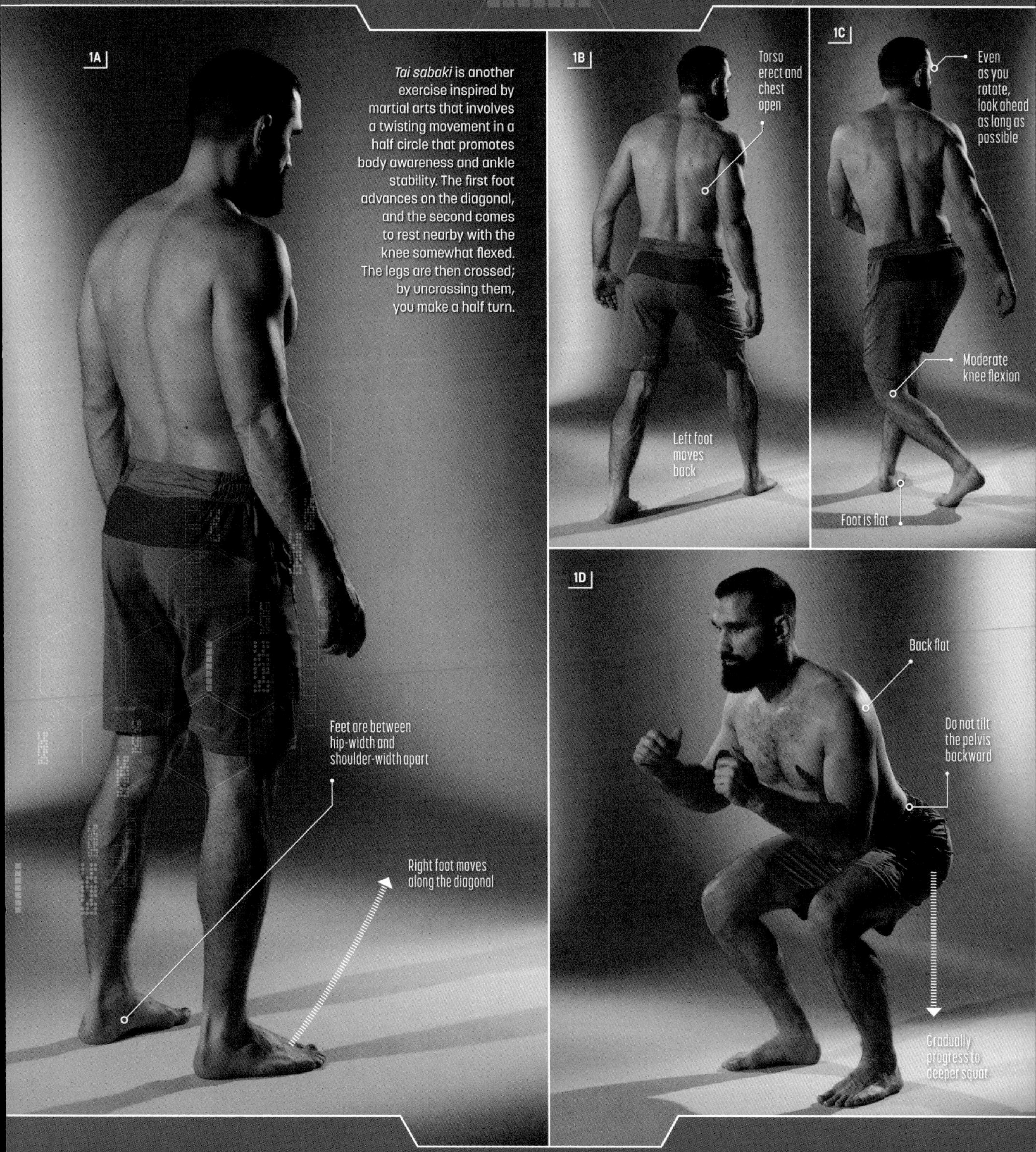

1A
Feet are between hip-width and shoulder-width apart
Right foot moves along the diagonal
1B
Torso erect and chest open
Left foot moves back
1C
Even as you rotate, look ahead as long as possible
Moderate knee flexion
Foot is flat
1D
Back flat
Do not tilt the pelvis backward
Gradually progress to deeper squat

It is always beneficial to train the entire muscle chain. By keeping a resistance band taut as the exercise is performed, the upper body chains will be kept activated throughout the movement.

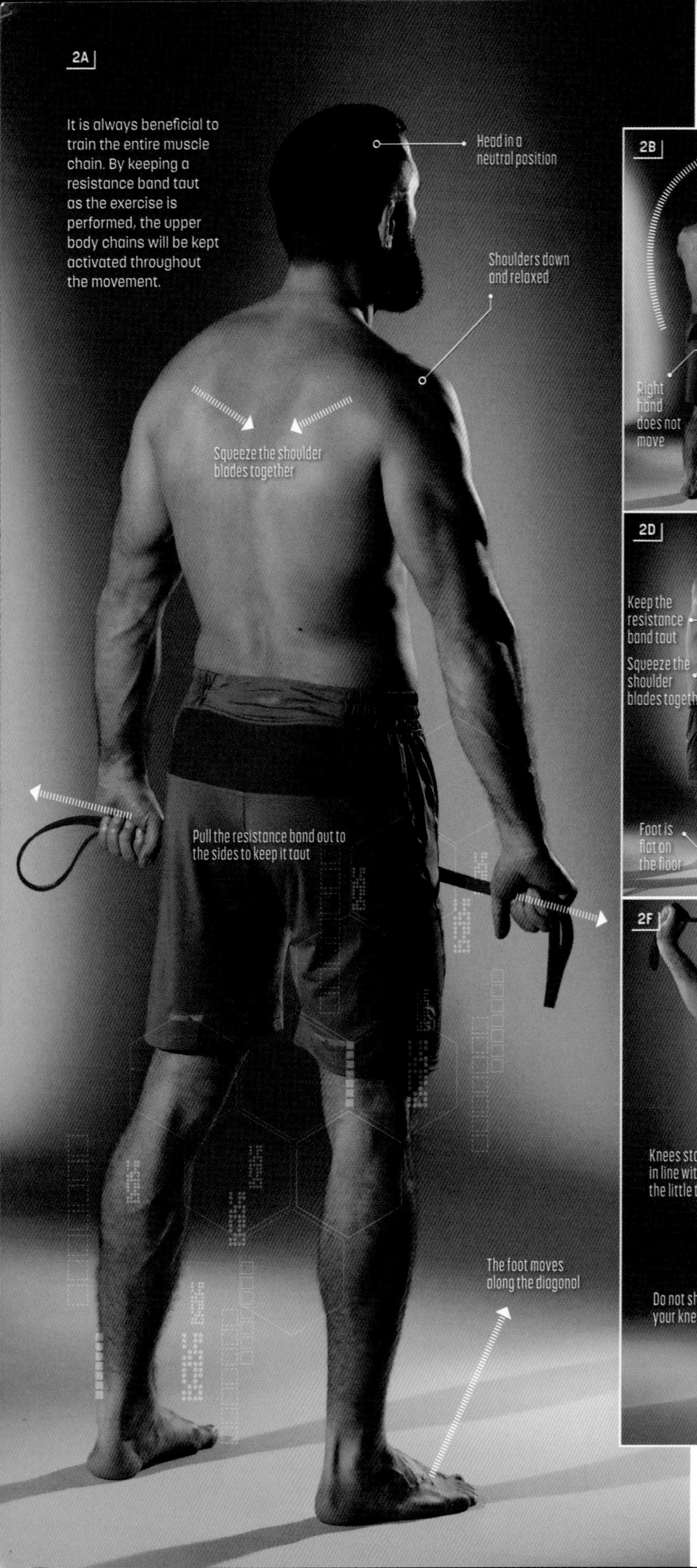
2A
Head in a neutral position
Shoulders down and relaxed
Squeeze the shoulder blades together
Pull the resistance band out to the sides to keep it taut
The foot moves along the diagonal

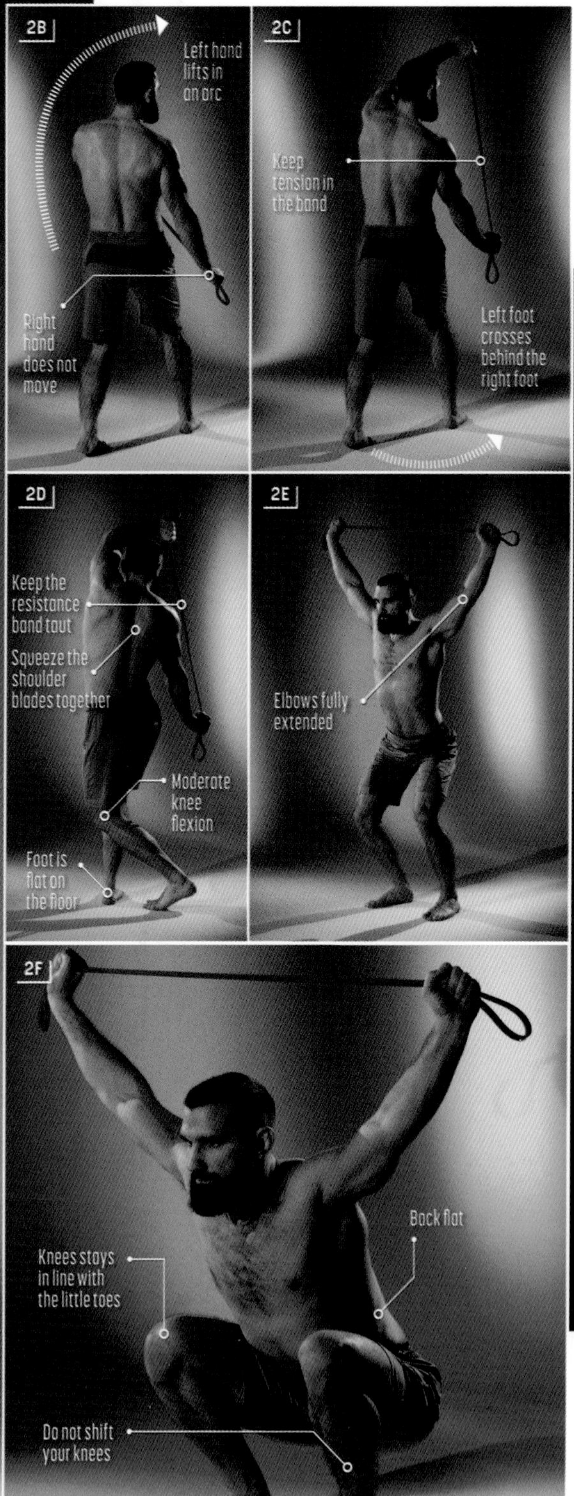
2B
Left hand lifts in an arc
Right hand does not move
2C
Keep tension in the band
Left foot crosses behind the right foot
2D
Keep the resistance band taut
Squeeze the shoulder blades together
Moderate knee flexion
Foot is flat on the floor
2E
Elbows fully extended
2F
Back flat
Knees stays in line with the little toes
Do not shift your knees

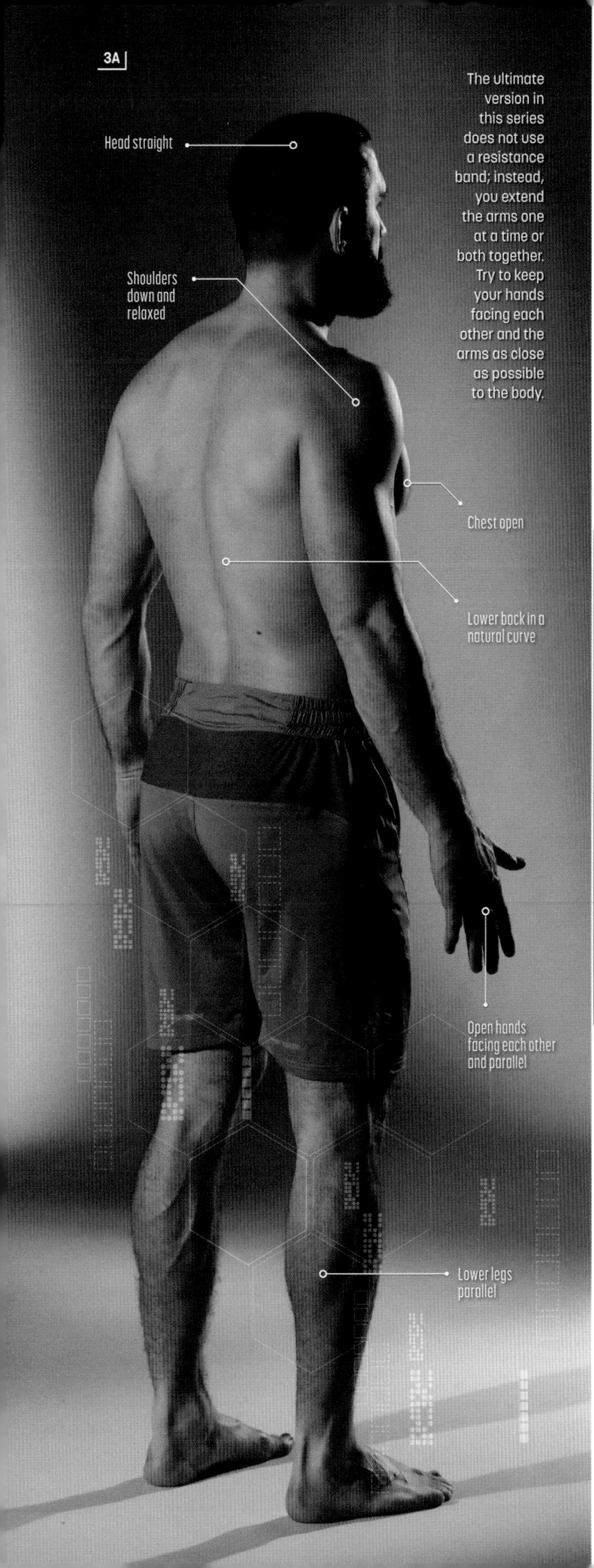

The ultimate version in this series does not use a resistance band; instead, you extend the arms one at a time or both together. Try to keep your hands facing each other and the arms as close as possible to the body.

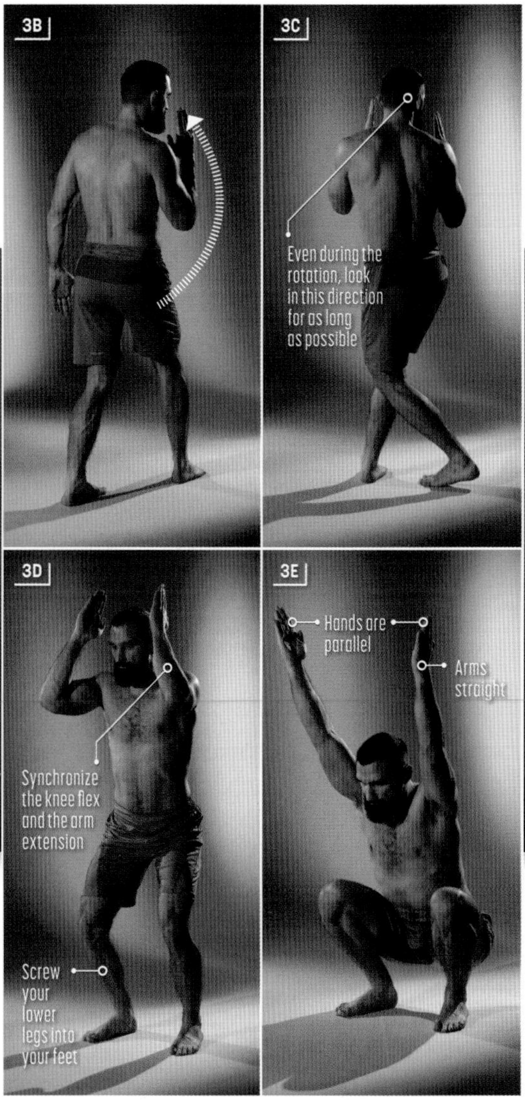

STANDING UP SQUAT
SERIES

2G

We are always squatting, but we were made to stand just as we were made to squat. Once again, beginning in the Seiza position works marvels.

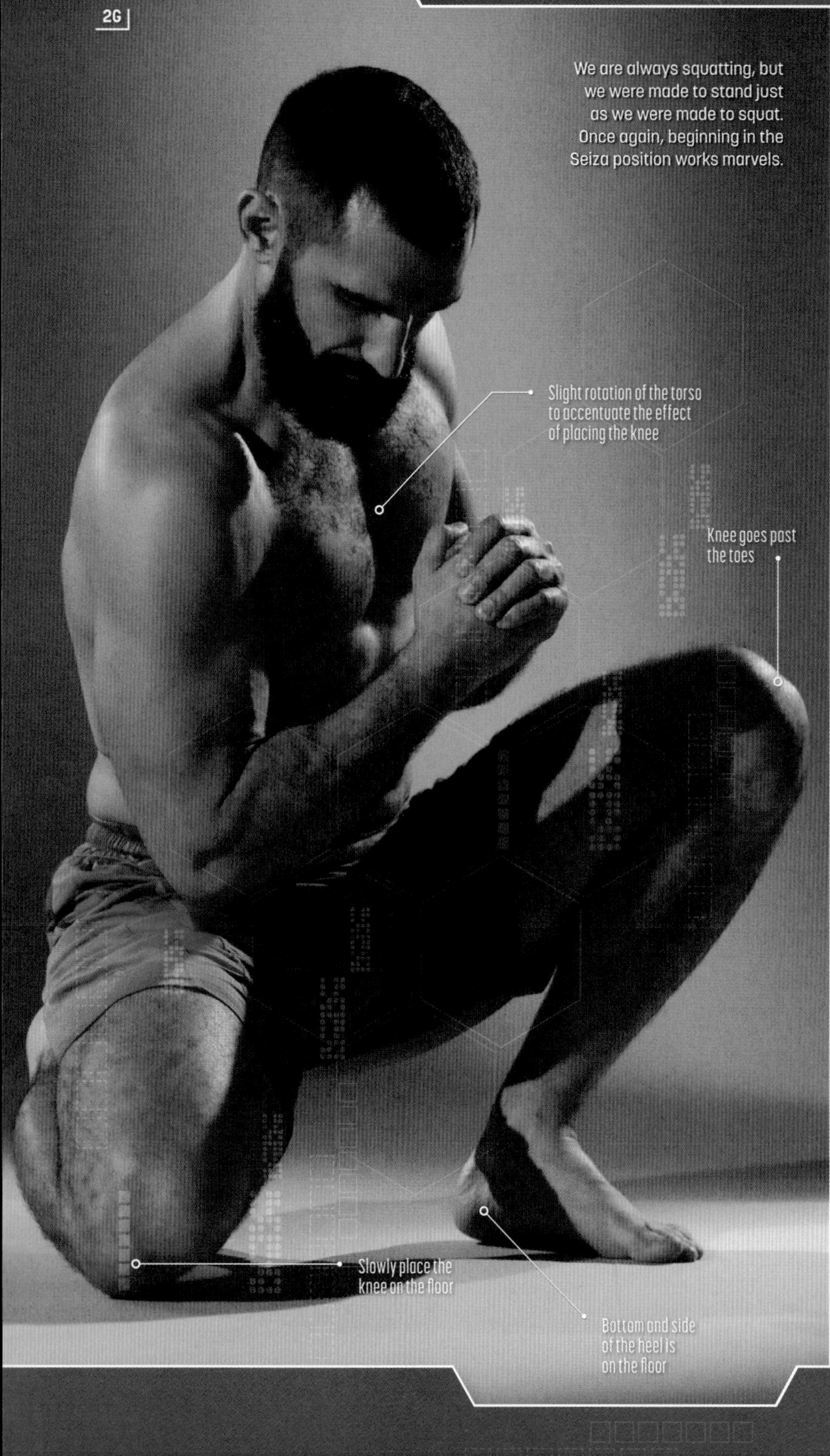
Slight rotation of the torso to accentuate the effect of placing the knee
Knee goes past the toes
Slowly place the knee on the floor
Bottom and side of the heel is on the floor

1A

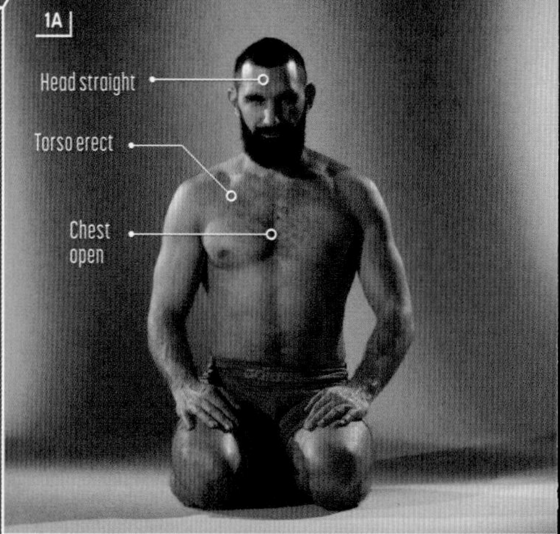
Head straight
Torso erect
Chest open

1B

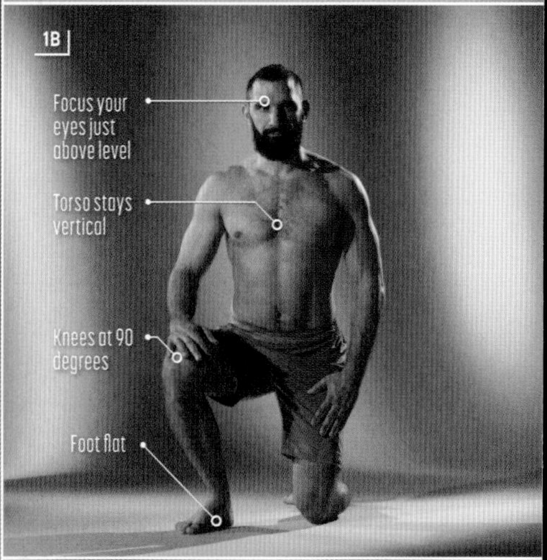
Focus your eyes just above level
Torso stays vertical
Knees at 90 degrees
Foot flat

1C

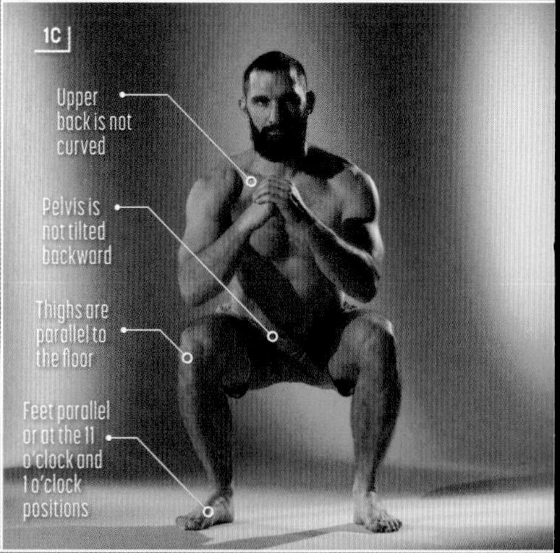
Upper back is not curved
Pelvis is not tilted backward
Thighs are parallel to the floor
Feet parallel or at the 11 o'clock and 1 o'clock positions

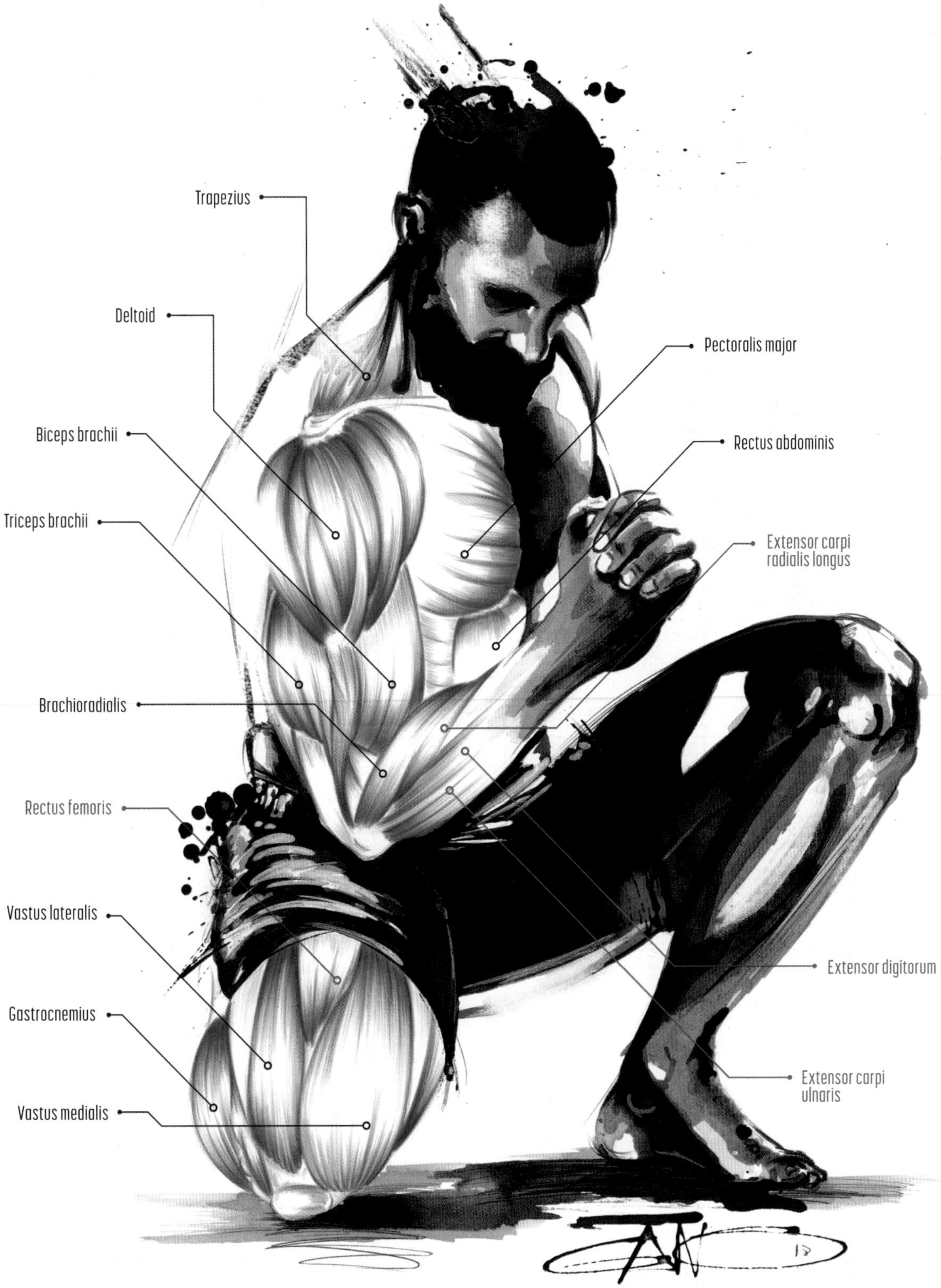
Trapezius
Deltoid
Biceps brachii
Triceps brachii
Brachioradialis
Rectus femoris
Vastus lateralis
Gastrocnemius
Vastus medialis
Pectoralis major
Rectus abdominis
Extensor carpi radialis longus
Extensor digitorum
Extensor carpi ulnaris

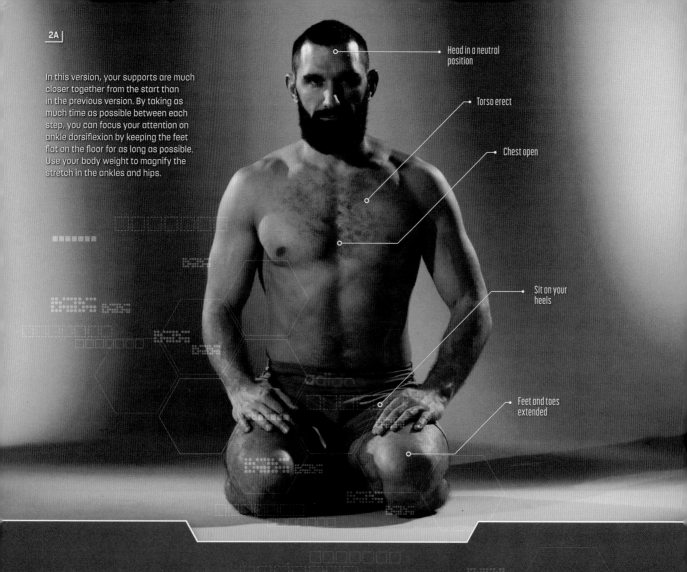

2A

In this version, your supports are much closer together from the start than in the previous version. By taking as much time as possible between each step, you can focus your attention on ankle dorsiflexion by keeping the feet flat on the floor for as long as possible. Use your body weight to magnify the stretch in the ankles and hips.

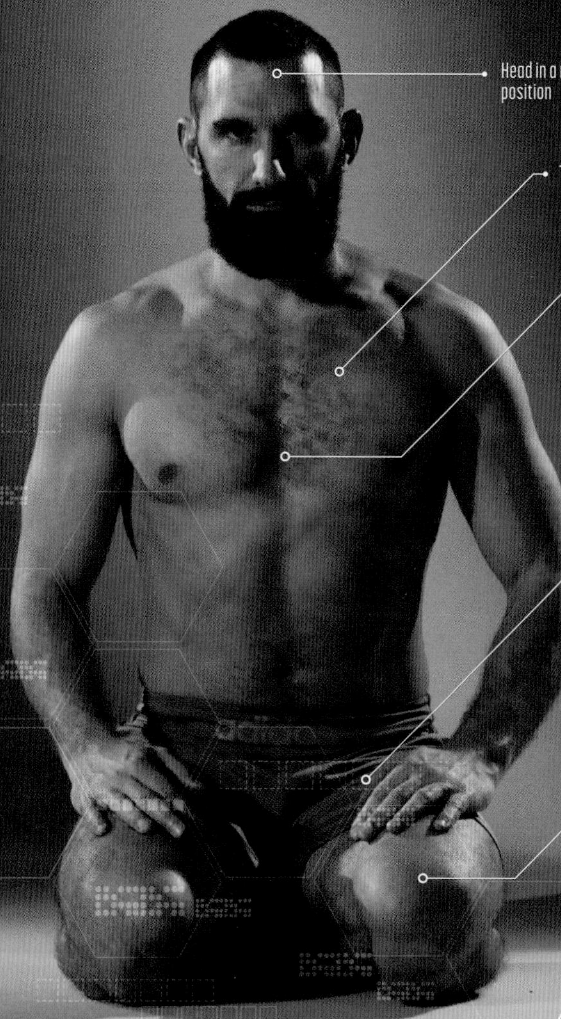

Head in a neutral position
Torso erect
Chest open
Sit on your heels
Feet and toes extended

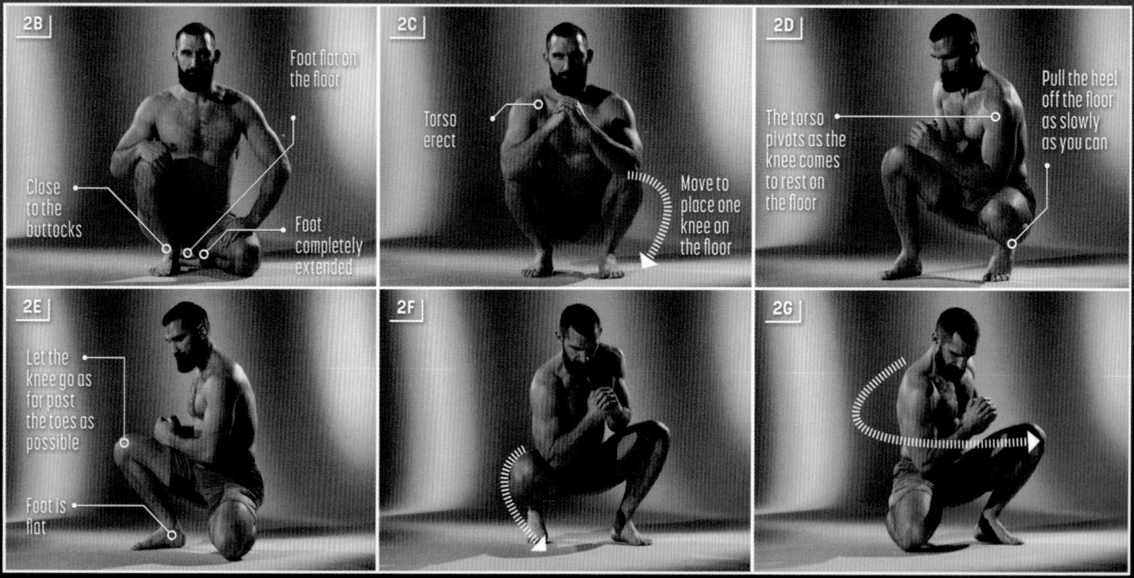

2B
Foot flat on the floor
Close to the buttocks
Foot completely extended
2C
Torso erect
Move to place one knee on the floor
2D
The torso pivots as the knee comes to rest on the floor
Pull the heel off the floor as slowly as you can
2E
Let the knee go as far past the toes as possible
Foot is flat
2F
2G

3A

The previous steps in the series were done slowly, with perfect control for a good stretch. The following steps should be done at full speed to work on explosiveness and stability. The first variation involves moving from your knees to a half-squat in one move. Depending on your physical ability, you may need to practice this before you can do it correctly. You can use your arms to help generate power, but remember that if you are not moving at full speed, you will not be able to get up off your knees.

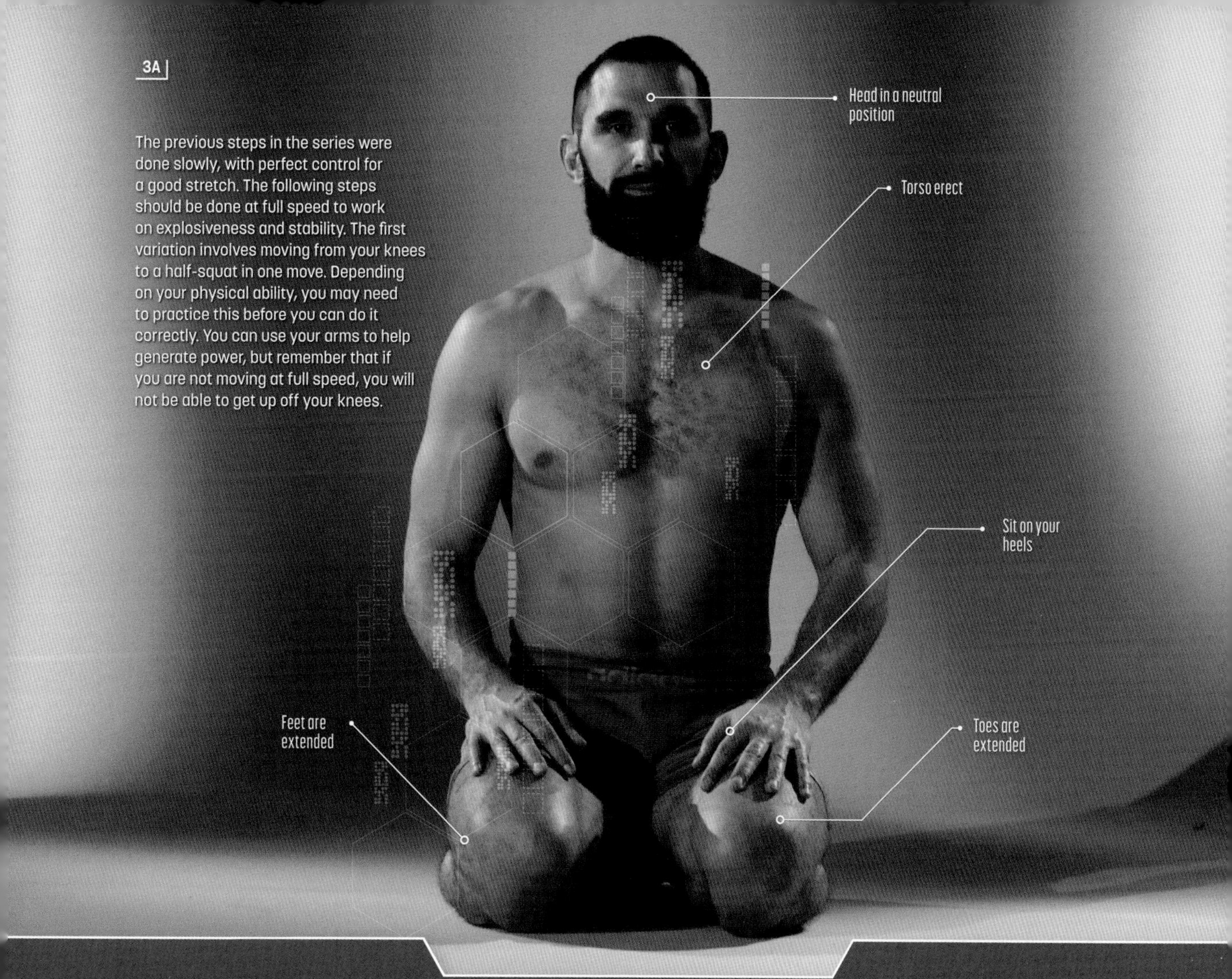
Head in a neutral position
Torso erect
Sit on your heels
Feet are extended
Toes are extended

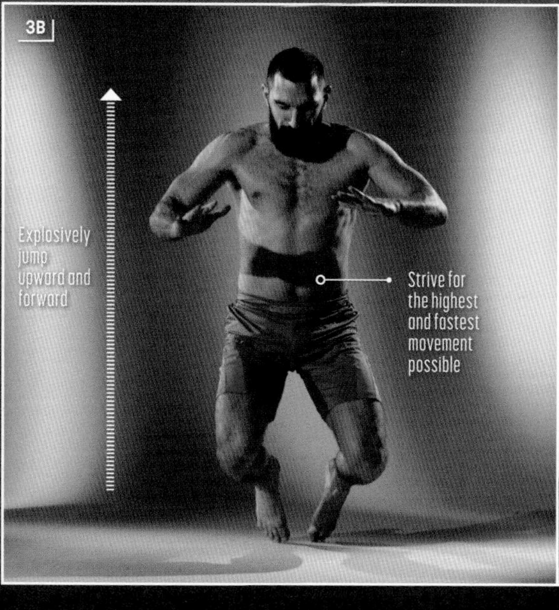
3B
Explosively jump upward and forward
Strive for the highest and fastest movement possible

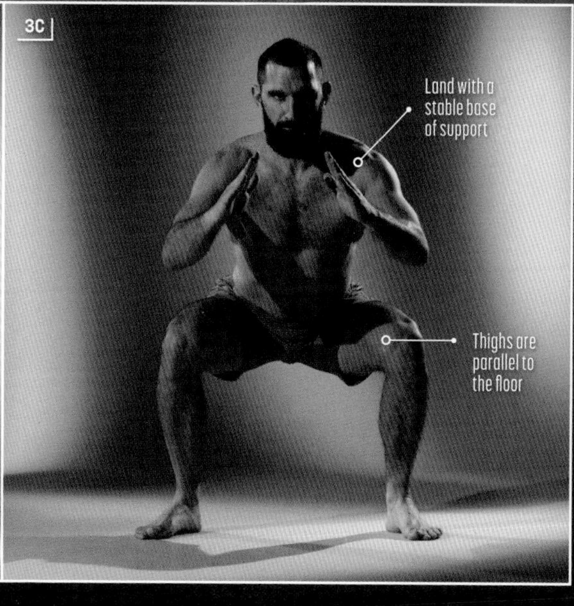
3C
Land with a stable base of support
Thighs are parallel to the floor

4A

After you've mastered the previous version and have improved your mobility to perform a deep squat, you can land directly in the deep squat position. It is critical to use perfect form, however. Do not compromise the position of your back (by leaning forward) or the full support of your feet (by keeping your heels lifted). Move with enough power and speed to get up off your knees.

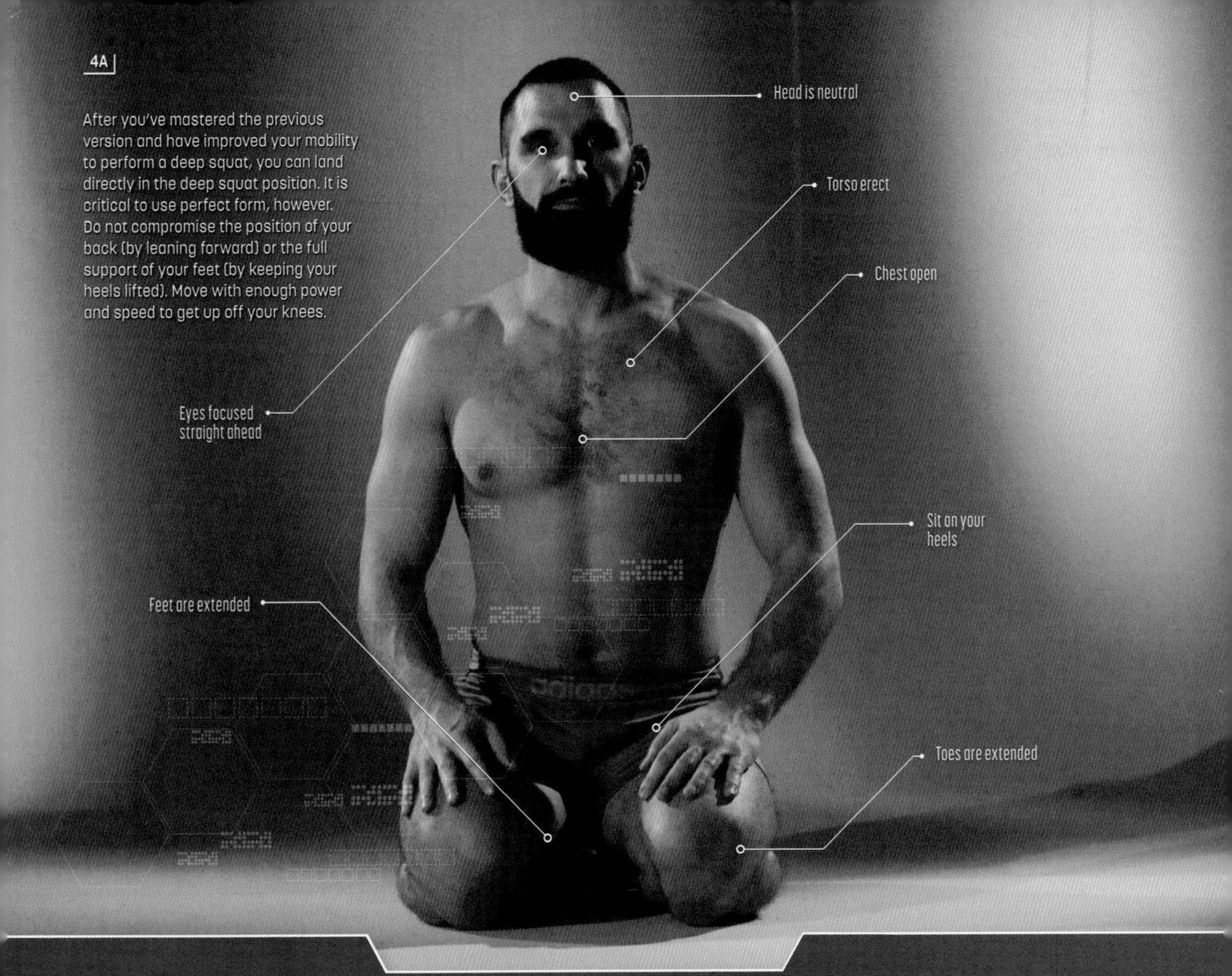
Head is neutral
Torso erect
Chest open
Eyes focused straight ahead
Sit on your heels
Feet are extended
Toes are extended

4B

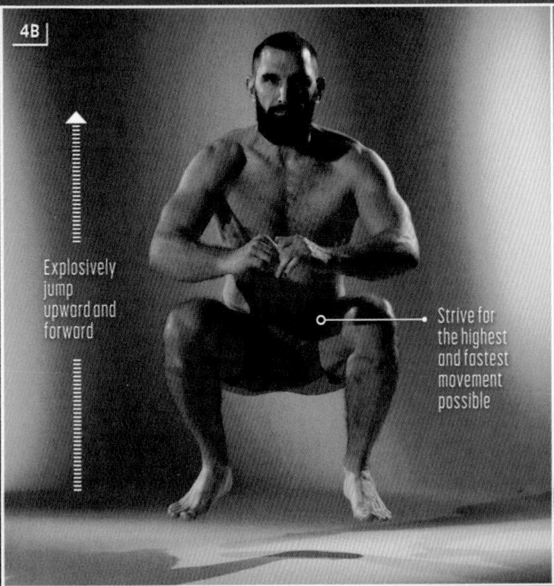
Explosively jump upward and forward
Strive for the highest and fastest movement possible

4C

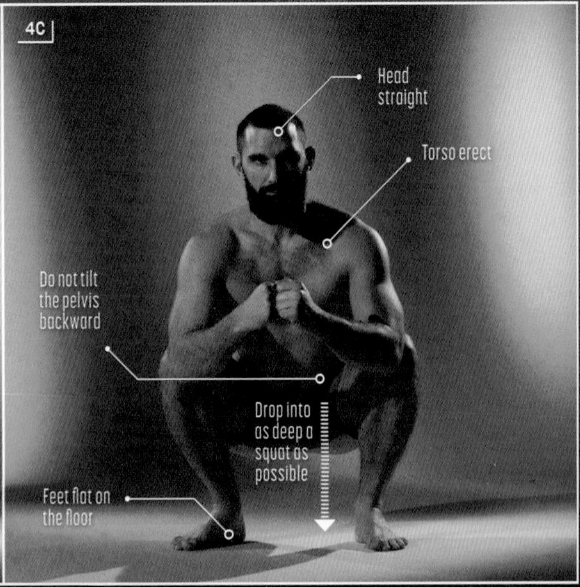
Head straight
Torso erect
Do not tilt the pelvis backward
Drop into as deep a squat as possible
Feet flat on the floor

CORCOVADO
SERIES

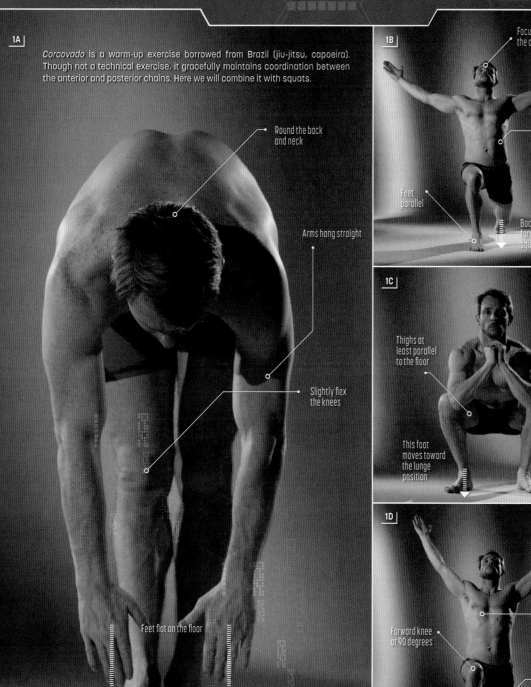

1A

Corcovado is a warm-up exercise borrowed from Brazil (jiu-jitsu, capoeira). Though not a technical exercise, it gracefully maintains coordination between the anterior and posterior chains. Here we will combine it with squats.

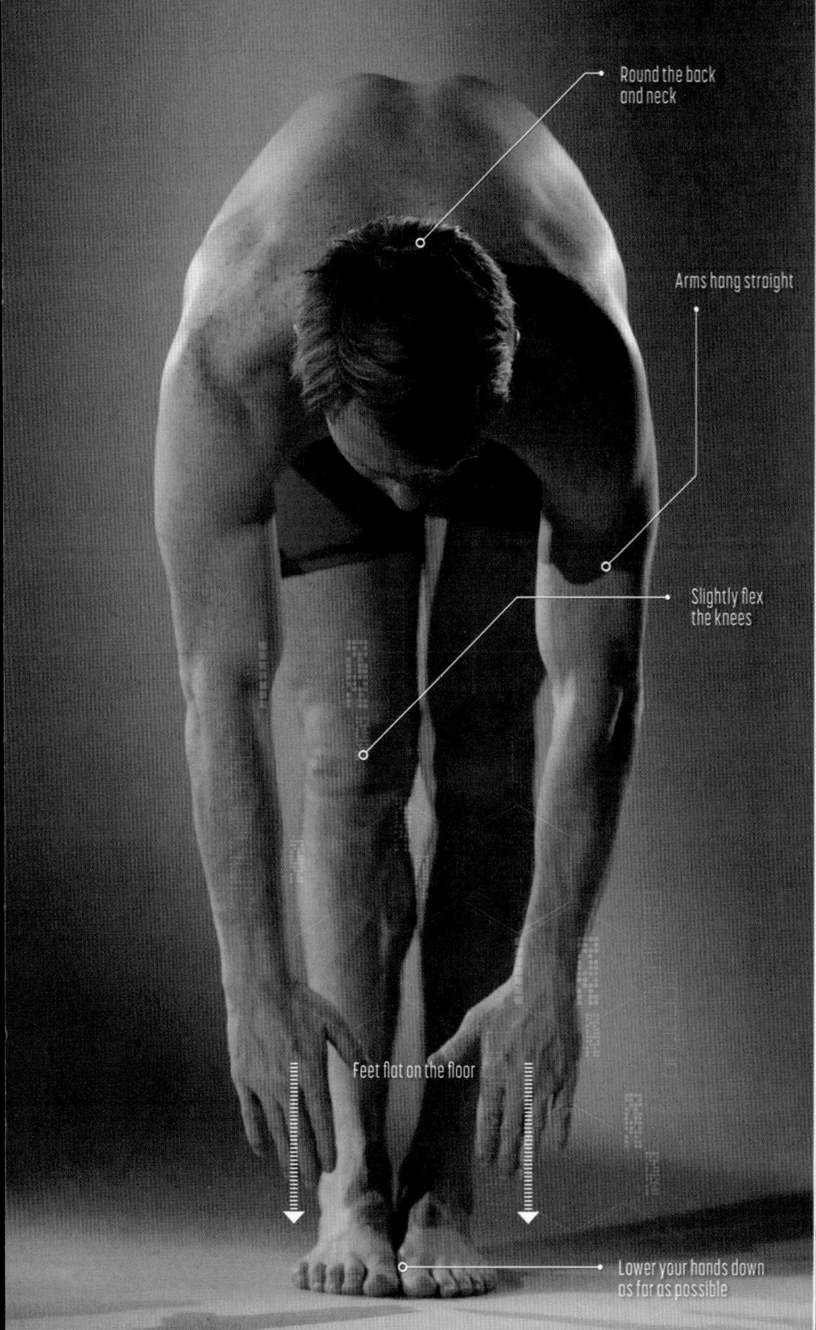

Round the back and neck
Arms hang straight
Slightly flex the knees
Feet flat on the floor
Lower your hands down as far as possible

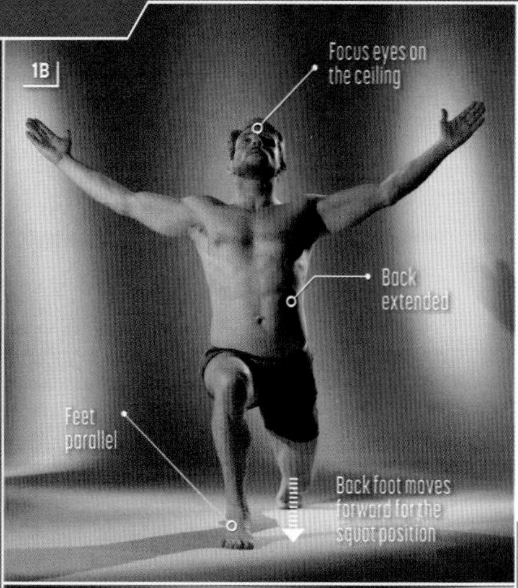

1B
Focus eyes on the ceiling
Back extended
Feet parallel
Back foot moves forward for the squat position

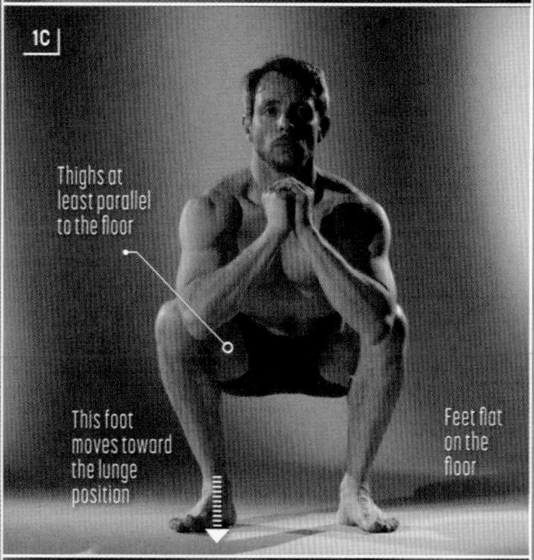

1C
Thighs at least parallel to the floor
This foot moves toward the lunge position
Feet flat on the floor

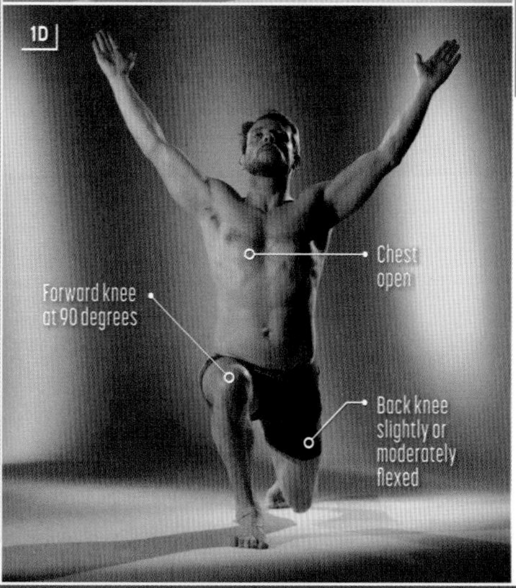

1D
Chest open
Forward knee at 90 degrees
Back knee slightly or moderately flexed

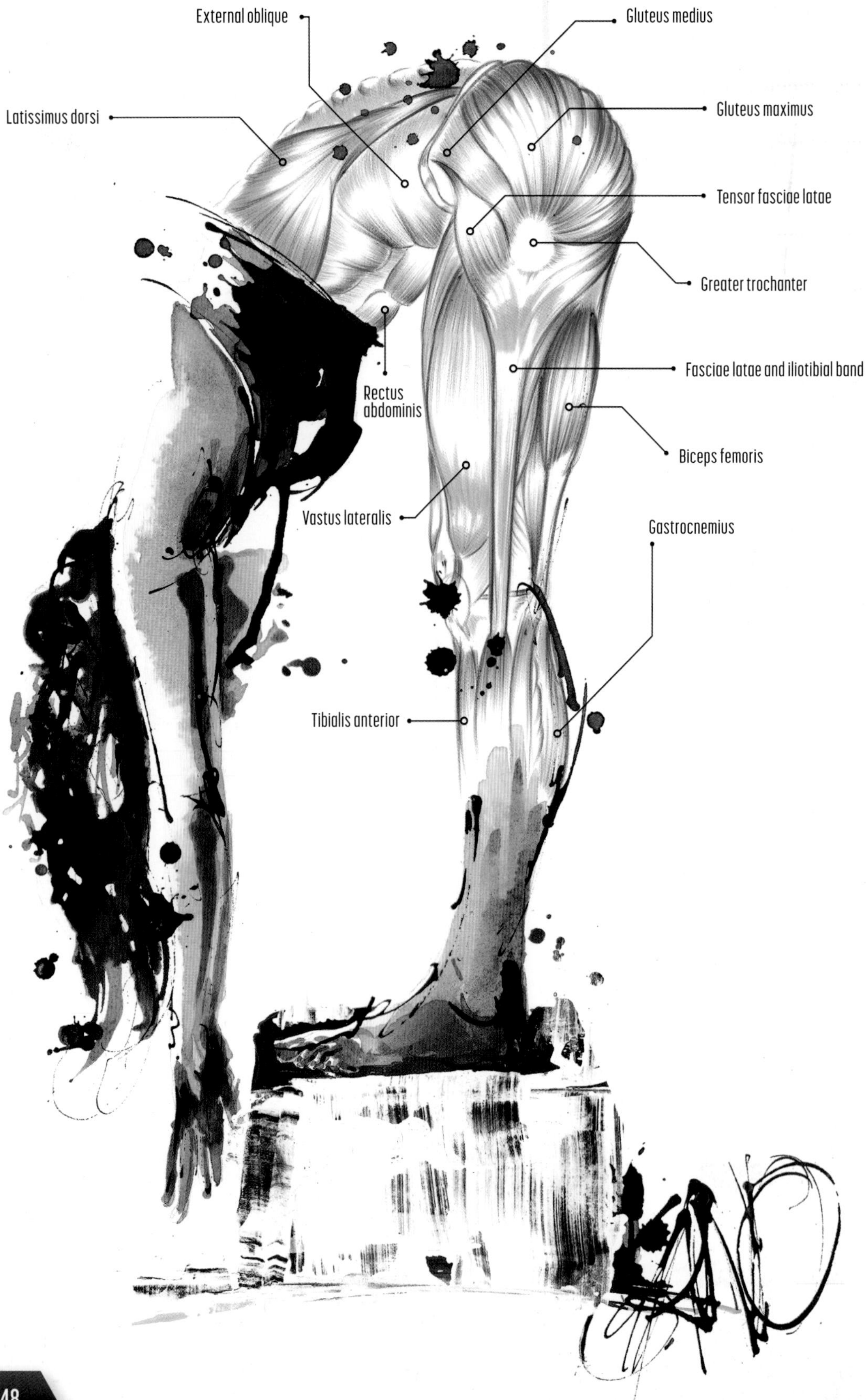
External oblique
Gluteus medius
Latissimus dorsi
Gluteus maximus
Tensor fasciae latae
Greater trochanter
Fasciae latae and iliotibial band
Rectus abdominis
Biceps femoris
Vastus lateralis
Gastrocnemius
Tibialis anterior

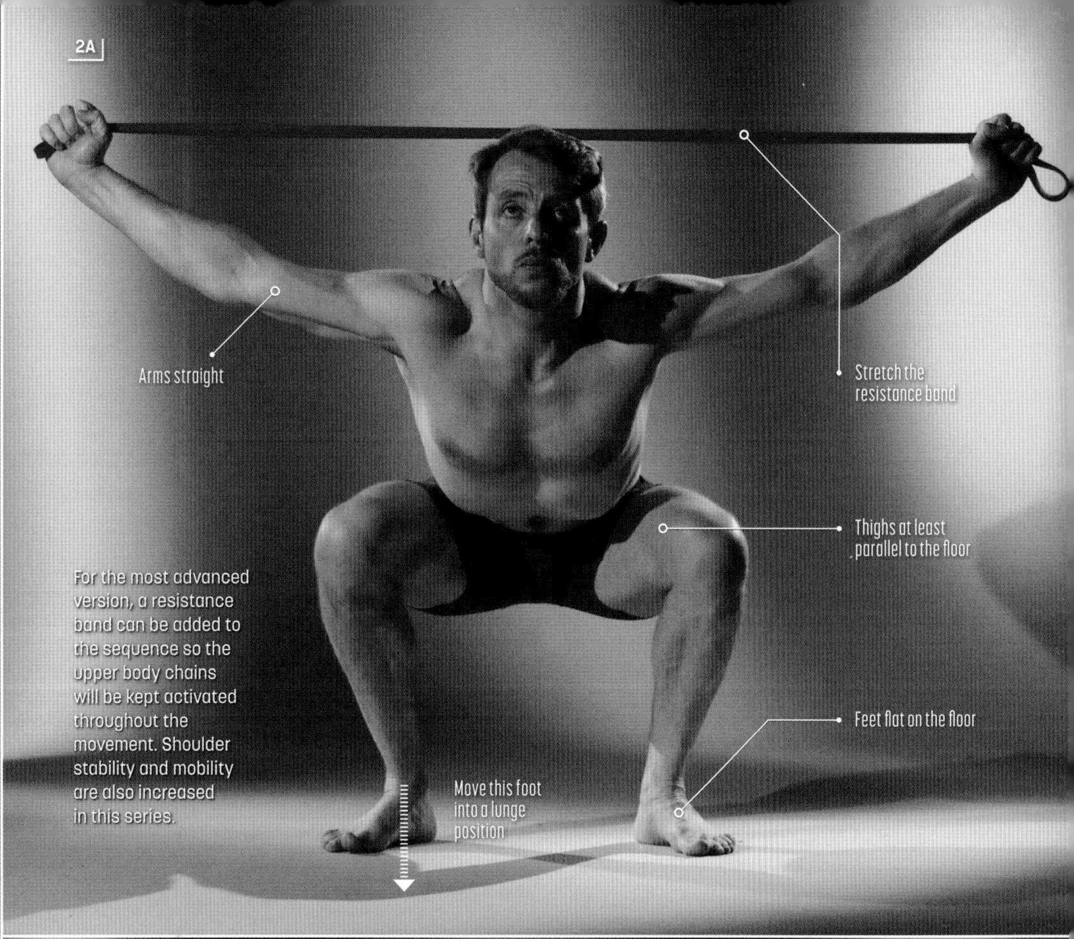
2A
Arms straight
Stretch the resistance band
Thighs at least parallel to the floor
Feet flat on the floor
Move this foot into a lunge position

For the most advanced version, a resistance band can be added to the sequence so the upper body chains will be kept activated throughout the movement. Shoulder stability and mobility are also increased in this series.

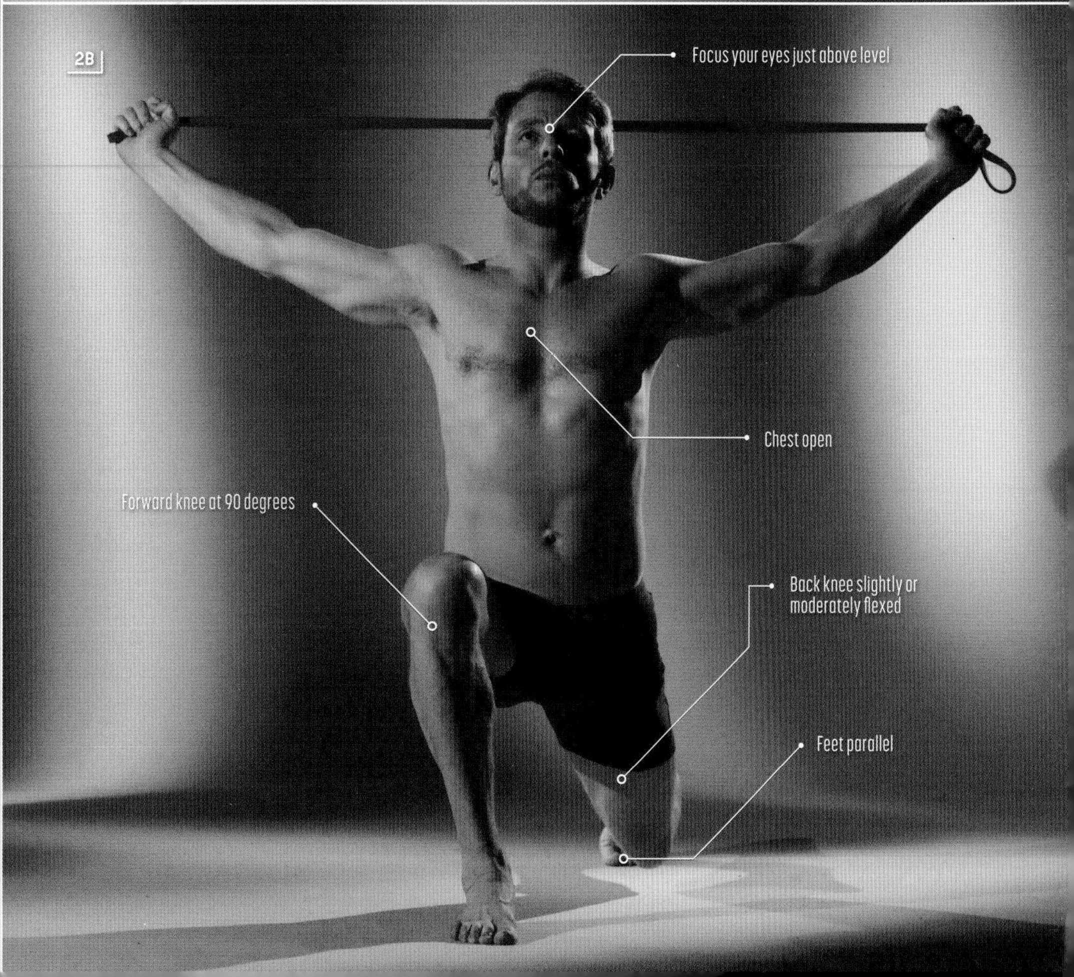
2B
Focus your eyes just above level
Chest open
Forward knee at 90 degrees
Back knee slightly or moderately flexed
Feet parallel

BIBLIOGRAPHY

Arend M, Kivastik J, Mäestu J. Maximal inspiratory pressure is influenced by intensity of the warm-up protocol. *Respir Physiol Neurobiol*. 2016;230:11-15.

Behm DG. The effects and potential mechanisms of foam rolling on athletic performance. *ECSS Congress*; 2017.

Bordoni B, Marelli F, Bordoni G. A review of analgesic and emotive breathing: A multidisciplinary approach. *J Multidiscip Health*. 2016;9:97-102.

Bouisset S, Duchêne JL. Is body balance more perturbed by respiration in seating than in standing posture? *Neuroreport*. 1994;5:957-960.

Bushell JE, Dawson SM, Webster MM. Clinical relevance of foam rolling on hip extension angle in a functional lunge position. *J Strength Cond Res*. 2015;29(9):2397-2403.

Butler J, Plisky PJ, Kiesel KB. Interrater reliability of videotaped performance on the functional movement screen using the 100-point scoring scale. *Athletic Training & Sports Health Care*. 2012;4(3):103-109.

Carrio C. *Sport Sans Blessure*. CTS Editions; 2017.

Carrio C. *Savoir s'*étirer. Ed Thierry Soucard; 2010.

Cavanaugh MT, Aboodarda SJ, Hodgson DD, Behm DG. Foam rolling of quadriceps decreases biceps femoris activation. *J Strength Cond Res*. 2017;31(8):2238-2245.

Chatrenet, Y. Chaîne cinétique ouverte versus chaîne cinétique fermée: etat des lieux en 2013. *Kinesither Scient*. 2013;547:29-34.

Cheatham SW, Kolber MJ, Cain M, Lee M. The effects of self-myofascial release using a foam roll or roller massager on joint range of motion, muscle recovery, and performance: A systematic review. *Int J Sports Phys Ther*. 2015;10(6):827-838.

Comerford MJ, Mottram SL. Functional stability retraining: Principles and strategies for managing mechanical dysfunction. *Manual Therapy*. 2001;6:3-14.

Comerford MJ, Mottram SL. *Kinetic Control*. Ed Churchill Livingstone; 2012.

Dankaerts W, O'Sullivan P, Burnett A, Straker L. Altered patterns of superficial trunk muscle activation during sitting in nonspecific chronic low back pain patients: importance of subclassification. *Spine (Phila Pa 1976)*. 2006;31(17):2017-2023.

Davies C, Davies A. *Soulagez Vos Douleurs Par Les Trigger Points*. Ed Soucard; 2014.

Falla D, Bilenkij G, Jull G. Patients with chronic neck pain demonstrate altered patterns of muscle activation during performance of a functional upper limb task. *Spine (Phila Pa 1976)*. 2004;29(13):1436-1440.

Falla DL, Jull GA, Hodges PW. Patients with neck pain demonstrate reduced electromyographic activity of the deep cervical flexor muscles during performance of the craniocervical flexion test. *Spine (Phila Pa 1976)*. 2004;29(19):2108-2114.

Gabbe BJ, Bennell KL, Finch CF. Why are older Australian football players at greater risk of hamstring injury? *Journal of Science and Medicine in Sport*. 2006;9:327-333.

Gabbe BJ, Bennell KL, Wajswelner H, Finch CF. Reliability of common lower extremity musculoskeletal screening tests. *Physical Therapy in Sport*. 2004;5(2):90-97.

Grieve R, Goodwin F, Alfaki M, et al. The immediate effect of bilateral self-myofascial release on the plantar surface of the feet on hamstring and lumbar spine flexibility: A pilot randomised controlled trial. *J Bodyw Mov Ther*. 2014;19(3):544-552.

Halperin I, Aboodarda SJ, Button DC, Andersen LL, Behm D. Roller massager improves range of motion of plantar flexor muscles without subsequent decreases in force parameters. *Int J Sports Phys Ther*. 2014;9(1):92-102.

Hamaoui A, Gonneau E, Le Bozec S. Respiratory disturbance to posture varies according to the respiratory mode. *Neurosci Lett*. 2010;475:141-144.

Hamaoui A, Do M, Poupard L, Bouisset S. Does respiration perturb body balance more in chronic low back pain subjects than in healthy subjects? *Clin Biomech (Bristol, Avon)*. 2002;17:548-550.

Hart N, Sylvester K, Ward S, Cramer D, Moxham J, Polkey MI. Valuation of an inspiratory muscle trainer in healthy humans. *Respir Med*. 2001;95(6):526-531.

Hellyer N, Andreas NM, Bernstetter AS, et al. Comparison of diaphragm thickness measurements among postures via ultrasound imaging. *PMR*. 2017;9(1):21-25.

Hodges PW, Moseley GL, Gabrielsson A, Gandevia SC. Experimental muscle pain changes feedforward postural responses of the trunk muscles. *Exp Brain Res*. 2003;151(2):262-271.

Hodges PW, Moseley GL. Pain and motor control of the lumbopelvic region: Effect and possible mechanisms. *J Electromyogr Kinesiol*. 2003;13(4):361-370.

Hudson AL, Joulia F, Butler AA, Fitzpatrick RC, Gandevia SC, Butler JE. Activation of human inspiratory muscles in an upside-down posture. *Respir Physiol Neurobiol*. 2015;226:152-159.

Jacobs JV, Henry SM, Nagle KJ. People with chronic low back pain exhibit decreased variability in the timing of their anticipatory postural adjustments. *Behav Neurosci*. 2009;123(2):455-458.

Jay K, Sundstrup E, Søndergaard SD, Behm D, Saervoll CA, Jakobsen MD, Andersen LL. Specific and cross over effects of massage for muscle soreness: randomized controlled trial. *Int J Sports Phys Ther*. 2014;9(1):82-91.

Jull GA, Richardson CA. Motor control problems in patients with spinal pain: A new direction for therapeutic exercise. *J Manipulative Physiol Ther*. 2000;23(2):115-117.

Kellens I, Cannizzaro F, Gouilly P, Crielaard JM. Inspiratory muscles strength training in recreational athletes. *Rev Mal Respir*. 2011;28(5):602-8.

Kelly S, Beardsley C. Specific and cross-over effects of foam rolling on ankle dorsiflexion range of motion. *Int J Sports Phys Ther*. 2016;11(4):544-551.

Klyne DM, Schmid AB, Moseley GL, Sterling M, Hodges PW. Effect of types and anatomic arrangement of painful stimuli on conditioned pain modulation. *J Pain*. 2015;16(2):176-185.

Sundstrup JK, Sondergaard SD. Specific and cross over effects of massage for muscle soreness: Randomized controlled trial. *Int J Sports Phys Ther*. 2014;9(1):82-91.

Lee, D. *The Pelvic Girdle: An Integration of Clinical Expertise and Research*. 4th ed. Edinburgh: Churchill Livingstone; 2011.

Macdonald D, Moseley GL, Hodges PW. People with recurrent low back pain respond differently to trunk loading despite remission from symptoms. *Spine (Phila Pa 1976)*. 2010;35(7):818-824.

Macdonald D, Moseley GL, Hodges PW. Why do some patients keep hurting their back? Evidence of ongoing back muscle dysfunction during remission from recurrent back pain. *Pain*. 2009;142(3):183-188.

Macdonald GZ, Button DC, Drinkwater EJ. Foam rolling as a recovery tool after an intense bout of physical activity. *Med Sci Sports Exerc*. 2014;46(1):131-142.

MacDonald GZ, Penney MD, Mullaley ME. An acute bout of self-myofascial release increases range of motion without a subsequent decrease in muscle activation or force. *J Strength Cond Res*. 2013;27(3):812-821.

Mikkelsen C, Werner S, Eriksson E. Closed kinetic chain alone compared to combined open and closed kinetic chain exercises for quadriceps strengthening after anterior cruciate ligament reconstruction with respect to return to sports: A prospective matched follow-up study. *Knee Surg Sports Traumatol Arthrosc*. 2000;8(6):337-342.

Minahan C, Sheehan B, Doutreband R, Kirkwood T, Reeves D, Cross T. Repeated-sprint cycling does not induce respiratory muscle fatigue in active adults: Measurements from the Powerbreathe® inspiratory muscle trainer. *J Sports Sci Med*. 2015;14(1):233-238.

Minick KI, Kiesel KB, Burton L, Taylor A, Plisky P, Butler RJ. Interrater reliability of the functional movement screen. *J Strength Cond Res*. 2010;24(2):479-486.

Monteiro ER, Cavanaugh MT, Frost DM, Novaes JD. Is self-massage an effective joint range-of-motion strategy? A pilot study. *J Bodyw Mov Ther*. 2017;21(1):223-226.

Moseley GL, Brhyn L, Ilowiecki M, Solstad K, Hodges PW. The threat of predictable and unpredictable pain: Differential effects on central nervous system processing? *Aust J Physiother*. 2003;49(4):263-267.

Moseley GL, Nicholas MK, Hodges PW. Pain differs from non-painful attention-demanding or stressful tasks in its effect on postural control patterns of trunk muscles. *Exp Brain Res*. 2004;156(1):64-71.

Myers TW. *Anatomy Trains: Myofascial Meridians for Manual and Movement Therapists*. Edinburgh: Churchill Livingstone; 2013.

O'Leary S, Falla D, Jull G. The relationship between superficial muscle activity during the cranio-cervical flexion test and clinical features in patients with chronic neck pain. *Man Ther*. 2011;16(5):452-455.

O'Sullivan K, O'Sullivan P. The ineffectiveness of paracetamol for spinal pain provides opportunities to better manage low back pain. *Br J Sports Med*. 2016;50(4):197-198.

Pearcey GEP, Bradbury-Squires DJ, Kawamoto JE, Drinkwater EJ, Behm DG, Button DC. Foam tolling for delayed-onset muscle soreness and recovery of dynamic performance measures. *J Athl Train*. 2015;50(1):5-13.

Richardson C, Jull G, Hodges P, Hides J. *Therapeutic Exercise for Spinal Segmental Stabilization in Low Back Pain*. Edinburgh: Churchill Livingstone;1998:12.

Richardson C, Hodges P, Hides J. *Therapeutic Exercise for Lumbopelvic Stabilization*. 2nd ed. Edinburgh: Churchill Livingstone; 2004.

Sahrmann, SA. *Diagnosis and Treatment of Move–ment Impairments Syndromes*. Mosby: St. Louis; 2002.

Sahrmann, SA. Does postural assessment contribute to patient care? *J Orthop Sports Phys Ther*. 2002;32(8):376-379.

Schleip R, Klingler W, Lehmann-Horn F. Active fascial contractility: Fascia may be able to contract in a smooth muscle-like manner and thereby influence musculoskeletal dynamics. *Med Hypotheses*. 2005;65(2):273-277.

Smith MD, Russell A, Hodges PW. Do incontinence, breathing difficulties, and gastrointestinal symptoms increase the risk of future back pain? *J Pain*. 2009;10(8):876-886.

Shirley D, Hodges PW, Eriksson AEM, Gandevia SC. Spinal stiffness changes throughout the respiratory cycle. *J Appl Physiol*. 2003;95:1467-1475.

Spracklin K, Button DC, Halperin I. Looped band placed around thighs increases EMG of gluteal muscles without hindering performance during squatting. *Journal of Performance Health Research*; 2017;1(1):60-71.

Starrett K, Cordoza G. *Becoming a Supple Leopard*. Victory Belt Publishing; 2015.

Starrett K, Cordoza G. *Deskbound*. Victory Belt Publishing; 2016.

Travell JG, Simons DG. *Myofascial Pain and Dysfunction: The Trigger Point Manual: The Lower Extremities*, Vol 2. Lippincott Williams and Wilkins; 1992.

Travell JG, Simons DG. *Myofascial Pain and Dysfunction: The Trigger Point Manual: Upper Half of Body*, Vol. 1. Lippincott Williams and Wilkins; 1998.

Willard FH, Vleeming A, Schuenke MD, Danneels L, Schleip R. The thoracolumbar fascial anatomy, function and clinical considerations. *J Anat*. 2012;221(6):507-536.

About the Authors

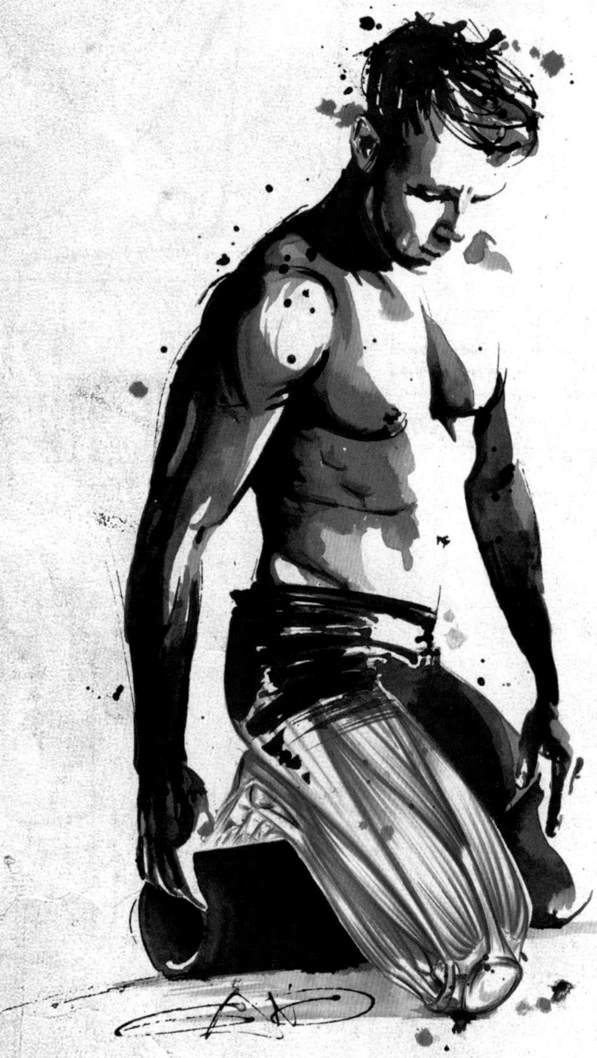

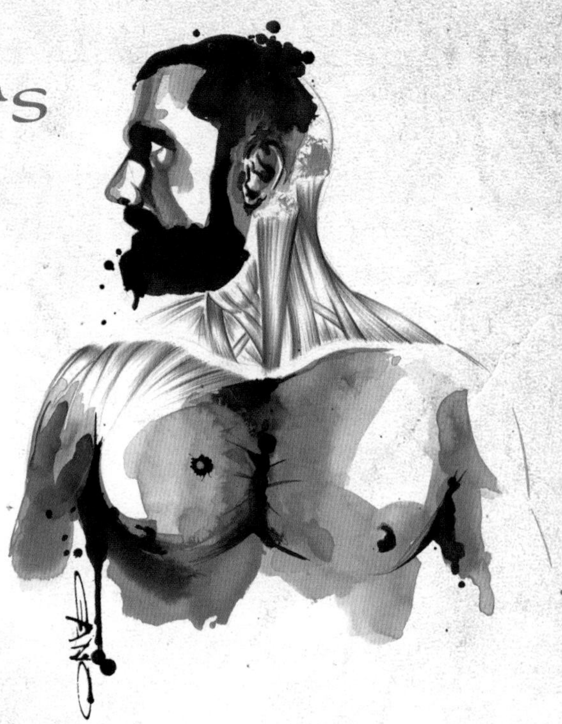

Aurélien Broussal-Derval holds master's degrees in strength and conditioning, sport and rehabilitation, and performance engineering. He also has a degree in sport sciences from the National Institute of Sport and Physical Education (INSEP) in Paris, France. He is the author of *The Modern Art of High Intensity Training* and French best sellers *Modern Physique Training, Judo Physique Training, Proprioception,* and *Field Tests: Protocols for Measuring Sport Performance.* Highlights of Broussal-Derval's career as a strength and conditioning coach include his training of Olympic medalists, professional athletes, the French Olympic weightlifting team, the French boxing teams, and the British and Russian judo teams. He led research for France Volleyball for years and is the technical director to one of the world's premier martial arts studios, the prestigious Cercle Tissier in Vincennes. Today he is head of French Weightlifting Coaches Development. Broussal-Derval lives in Paris.

Stéphane Ganneau is a professional illustrator and graphic designer. After training in applied arts in Nantes, France, he launched his career in advertising and product design. After 15 years, Ganneau's independent spirit, need for creativity, and desire for challenge drew him away from industry work. He now merges his love for illustration with his passion for resistance training. His strong graphics, expressive lines, and vibrant colors result in a distinctive style that pairs perfectly with *The Modern Art of High Intensity Training* and now *The Modern Art and Science of Mobility.*